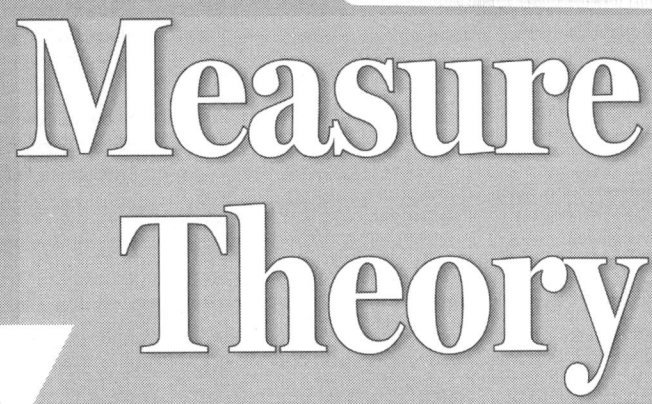

Measure Theory

Useful for

Post Graduate Students of All Indian Universities
and Various Competitive Examination

Dr. SUDHIR KUMAR PUNDIR

M.Sc., M.Phil, NET (C.S.I.R.), Ph.D.
HEAD,
Department of Mathematics
S.D. (P.G.) College,
Muzaffarnagar (U.P.)

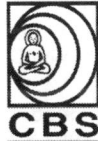

CBS

CBS Publishers & Distributors Pvt Ltd

New Delhi • Bengaluru • Chennai • Kochi • Kolkata • Mumbai
Hyderabad • Nagpur • Patna • Pune • Jharkhand • Uttarakhand

Measure Theory

ISBN: 978-93-88527-67-5

First Edition: 2019

Copyright © Author

Published by **Satish Kumar Jain** and produced by **Varun Jain** for
CBS Publishers & Distributors Pvt. Ltd.,
4819/XI Prahlad Street, 24 Ansari Road, Daryaganj, New Delhi - 110002
delhi@cbspd.com, cbspubs@airtelmail.in • www.cbspd.com
Ph.: 23289259, 23266861, 23266867 • Fax: 011-23243014
Corporate Office: 204 FIE, Industrial Area, Patparganj, Delhi - 110 092
Ph: 49344934 • Fax: 011-49344935
E-mail: publishing@cbspd.com • publicity@cbspd.com
Branches:
• *Bengaluru:* 2975, 17th Cross, K.R. Road, Bansankari 2nd Stage,
  Bengaluru   70 • Ph: +91-80-26771678/79 • Fax: +91-80-26771680
  E-mail: cbsbng@gmail.com, bangalore@cbspd.com
• *Chennai:* No. 7, Subbaraya Street, Shenoy Nagar, Chennai - 600030
  Ph: +91-44-26681266, 26680620 • Fax: +91-44-42032115
  E-mail: chennai@cbspd.com
• *Kochi:* Ashana House, 39/1904, A.M. Thomas Road, Valanjambalam,
  Ernakulum, Kochi • Ph: +91-484-4059061-65
  Fax: +91-484-4059065 • E-mail: cochin@cbspd.com
• *Kolkata:* 6-B, Ground Floor, Rameshwar Shaw Road, Kolkata - 700014
  Ph: +91-33-22891126/7/8 • E-mail: kolkata@cbspd.com
• *Mumbai:* 83-C, Dr. E. Moses Road, Worli, Mumbai - 400018
  Ph: +91-9833017933, 022-24902340/41 • E-mail: mumbai@cbspd.com
Representatives:
• Hyderabad: 0-9885175004   • Nagpur: 0-9021734563
• Patna: 0-9334159340   • Pune: 0-9623451994
• Jharkhand: 0-9811541605   • Uttarakhand: 0-9716462459

Printed at:
India Binding House, Noida, UP (India)

Preface

The present book entitled "MEASURE THEORY" is meant for PG students of all Indian universities. Besides, it will be very useful for those students preparing for various competitive examinations.

This book provide theoretical background of the subject with will graded set of detailed solved examples. It is a collection and compilation work from vanrus sources and has been endeavored to include as much as information could be possible. There is a plenty of slope in the form of exercise for the reader to try and solve the problem on his own.

I express my gratitude to the authors and publishers of various books I consulted.

I wish to sincerely thank Sh S.K. Jain and Sh Varun Jain Managing Director, CBS Publishers and Distributors, New Delhi for his encouragement and help in bringing out this publication in a present nice form.

My special thanks to Sh. B.M. Singh, Sh. Sunil Dutt, Sh. Puneet Verma and entire team of CBS Publishers and Distributors, New Delhi whose encouragement and unstinted support enabled me to complete my book. Mr. Peeyush Goel, M/s Dreamshapers also deserve special mention for nice type setting.

I must also record my appreciation due to my wife Dr. Rimple, daughter Rijuta and son Shrish for their understanding and love during the long period that I have taken to complete this book.

Above all I am thankful to The Almighty God, without whose grace nothing is possible for any one.

Readers are welcomed to point out errors, if any and send their valuable suggestions for improving the quality of the book.

Dr. SUDHIR KUMAR PUNDIR
email : skpundir05@yahoo.co.in

Preface

CONTENTS

Ch 13.   More Theorems on Convergence and Integrations   349-362

Ch 14.   Fourier Series   363-382

Chapter

1 Introduction

1.1 INTRODUCTION

In previous classes, we have studied about the concept of sets and their types and properties. We are also familiar about the Venn diagrams and its uses. In this chapter we shall discuss about the relation and functions, concept of topological spaces and review of bounded set which are widely used in the further study.

1.2 RELATION

Let us take two sets of natural numbers N_1 and N_2. We define R as a relation between them such that N_1 is a square of N_2. Then we can write $1R1$, $2R4$, $3R9$, ...

In terms of ordered pair, we can write
$$R = \{(1, 1), (2, 4), (3, 9), (4, 16), ...\} = \{(x, y : x, y \in N \text{ and } y = x^2\}$$
The relation from set N to N is a subset of $N \times N$ such that $y = x^2$.

Definition. *Let A and B be two sets. Then a relation R from A to B is a subset of A×B.*

Symbolically: R is a relation from A to $B \Leftrightarrow R \subseteq A \times B$.

☞ REMARKS
- If R is a relation from A to B, then A is called the domain and B the range of R.
- If R is a relation from a non-empty set A to a non-empty set B and if $(a, b) \in R$, then we write aRb, read as "a is related to b by the relation R." On the other hand, if $(a, b) \notin R$, we write $a\mathcal{R}b$ and say that 'a is not related to b by the relation R'.
- In particular, any subset $A \times A$ defined a relation in A, known as Binary relation.

Illustrations

♦ If $a, b \in N$ and R is defined as "a is divisor of b" then R is relation on N.

The subset $N \times N$, which corresponds to the relation R is $S = \{(n, r): n \in N, r \in N\}$
Here, it is clear that $(1, 3)$, $(2, 4)$, $(3, 9)$ $(4, 8)$, $(4, 4)$, are in S, whereas $(2, 3)$, $(4, 5)$, $(5, 6)$ are not in S.

♦ If R is a relation from set $A = \{1,2,3\}$ to the set $B = \{-1, -2\}$ defined by $x + y = 0$, then $R = \{(1, -1), (2, -2)\}$
Here, domain of R is $\{1, 2\}$ and Range = $\{-1, -2\}$.

♦ If $A = \{a, b, c, d, e\}$ and $B = \{f, g, h, i\}$ and let $R = \{(a, g), (a, i), (d, h), (e, f)\}$ by a relation from A to B then
Domain of $R = \{a, d, e\}$ and
Range of $R = \{g, i, h, f\}$

♦ If $a, b \in R$, the set of real numbers and R is "$|a - b|$ is a rational number" then R is a relation on R. The subset S of $R \times R$ which corresponds to the relation is
$S = \{(a, b + a): a \in R, b \in Q\}$

It is observed that $\left(1, 2\frac{1}{2}\right), \left(\pi, \pi - \frac{1}{2}\right)$

belongs to S, while $(\sqrt{2}, \pi + \sqrt{2}) \notin S$.

◆ If $A = \{2, 3, 4\}$ and $B = \{a, b, c\}$, then $R = \{(2, b), (3, c), (2, a), (4, a)\}$ being a subset of $A \times B$, is a relation from $A \times B$. Here $(2, b)$, $(3, c), (2, a), (4, a) \in R$, so we may write $2Rb$, $3Rc, 2Ra, 4Ra$. But $(3, b) \notin R$ therefore, $3 \not R b$.

◆ If $a, b \in N$ and R is defined by "$a - b$ is divisible by a number $n \in N$", then R is a relation on N. The subset S of $N \times N$ corresponding to the relation by
$S = \{n, n + rm : n \in N, r \in N\}$
Here, $m = 3$, $(2, 8)$, $(5, 11) \in S$
[∵ $2 - 8 = 6$, which is divisible by 3]
While $(3, 8) \notin S$
[∵ $3 - 8 = 5$, which is not divisible by 3]

1.2.1 TOTAL NUMBER OF RELATIONS

Let A and B be two non-empty finite sets consisting p and q elements respectively, then $A \times B$ consists of $p\,q$ ordered pairs. Therefore, total number of subset of $A \times B$ is 2^{pq}.

☛ REMARKS
- For a non-empty set A, $\phi \in A \times A$, therefore it is a relation on A, called void or empty relation on A.
- The void relation ϕ and the universal relation $A \times B$ are called trivial relations from A to B.
- The void and universal relation on set A respectively the smallest and the largest relation on A.

1.2.2 IDENTITY RELATION

Let A be a set. The identity relation on A is the relation $I_A = \{(x, x) : x \in A\}$ on A.

For example : If $A = \{a, b, c\}$ then the relation $I_A = \{(a, a), (b, b), (c, c)\}$ is the identity relation. $R = \{(a, a), (b, b)\}$ is not an identity relation as $(c, c) \notin R$.

1.2.3 INVERSE OF A RELATION

Let A, B be two non-empty sets and R be a relation from a set A to B and let (x,y), number of the subset D of $A \times B$ corresponding to the relation R from A to B.

To the relation R from the set A to the set B, there corresponds a relation from the set B to the set A called the inverse of the relation, denoted by R^{-1} such that the subset $B \times A$ corresponding to the relation R^{-1} is $= \{(y, x): (x, y) \in D\}$.

i.e., $$yR^{-1}x \Leftrightarrow xRy$$

Illustrations

◆ Let $A = \{a, b, c\}$ and $B = \{1,2,3\}$ be two sets and let $R = \{(a, 1), (a, 2), (b, 1), (b, 2)\}$ be a relation from A to B then $R-1 = \{(1, a), (2, a), (1, b), (2, b)\}$

◆ If $A = \{1, 2, 3\}$, $B = \{5, 6, 7\}$ and let $R = \{(1, 5), (2, 5), (2, 7)\}$ be a relation from A to B.

Then $R^{-1} = \{(5, 1), (5, 2), (7, 2)\}$ which is a relation from B to A.
Also, Domain $(R) = \{1, 2\} =$ Range (R^{-1})
And, Range $(R) = \{5, 7\} =$ Domain (R^{-1})

◆ The inverse of the relation "is less than" in R "is greater than".

☛ REMARK
- Sometimes, the inverse of a relation coincides with the relation itself.
For example, the inverse of the relation "perpendicular to" in the set of straight lines coincides with itself.

1.3 CLASSIFICATION OF RELATIONS

(a) **Reflexive Relation:** Let R be a relation on a set A.
"A relation R is said to be reflexive if $(x, x) \in R \; \forall \; x \in A$", i.e., $x R x \; \forall \; x \in A$

Illustrations

♦ In a set of integers, a relation R defined by $x \, R \, y$ iff $x - y$ is divisible by 4, then R is a reflexive relation because $x - x = 0$ which is divisible by 4.

♦ The universal relation on a non-empty set A is reflexive.

♦ The relation "is less than," *i.e.*, '<' in the set of rational number is not reflexive, because no member have the relation is less than to itself.

♦ The relation "is a factor of" in the set of rational number is reflexive, since every rational number is a factor of itself.

♦ The relation "is less than or equal to." *i.e.*, ≤ in the set of natural number is reflexive.

$$n \leq n \; \forall \, n \in N$$

(b) Symmetric Relation. *A relation R on a set A is said to be symmetric if*

$$(y, x) \in R \text{ whenever } (x, y) \in R \; \forall \, x, y \in R$$

i.e., $\qquad x \, R \, y \Leftrightarrow y \, R \, x \; \forall \, x, y \in R$

 Illustrations

♦ Let l_1, l_2 be two lines such that l_1 is perpendicular to l_2,

i.e., $l_1 \perp l_2$. Then $l_1 \perp l_2 \Rightarrow l_2 \perp l_1$. Therefore the relation $\perp$ is symmetric.

♦ The identity and the universal relation on a non-empty set are symmetric relations.

♦ Consider the set N of natural numbers and the relation 'is less than'. This relation is not symmetric. Since if $2 < 3$ then $3 \not< 2$.

Let $A = \{1, 2, 3\}$ and relations R_1 and R_2 defined by $R_1 = \{(1, 2), (1, 3), (3, 1), (2, 1)\}$ and $R_2 = \{(1, 2), (2, 3), (3, 1)\}$

Then R_1 is a symmetric relation, but R_2 is not symmetric.

(c) Transitive Relation: *A relation R on a set A is said to be transitive iff $(x, y) \in R$ and $(y, z) \in R \Rightarrow (x, z) \in R \; \forall \, x, y, z \in A$, i.e., $x \, R \, y, \, y \, R \, z \Rightarrow xRz$.*

 Illustrations

♦ Let a, b, c be three numbers such that a is a factor of b and b is a factor of c, then obviously a is a factor of c. Therefore, 'is a factor of' is a transitive relation.

♦ If l_1, l_2, l_3 are three lines such that $l_1 \perp l_2$ and $l_2 \perp l_3$ then it is obvious that l_1 is parallel to l_3. Therefore the relation "$\perp$" is not transitive.

♦ The identity and universal relation on a non-empty set are transitive.

♦ Let l_1, l_2, l_3 be three straight lines, such that l_1 is parallel to l_2 and l_2 is parallel to l_3 then it is clear that l_1 is parallel to l_3. Therefore, 'is parallel to' is a transitive relation.

(d) Anti-symmetric Relation. *A relation R on a non-empty set A is said to be an anti-symmetric relation iff $(x, y) \in R$ and $(y, x) \in R \Rightarrow x = y \; \forall \, x, y \in R$*

☞ REMARKS

• The identity relation R on a set A is an anti – symmetric relation.

• If $(x, y) \in R$ and $(y, x) \notin R$, then it may be noted that $x = y$.

• The universal relation on a set A containing at least two elements is not anti – symmetric.

1.3.1 EQUIVALENCE RELATIONS

A relation R on a set E is said to be equivalence if it is

    (i) Reflexive,   (ii) Symmetric and   (iii) Tansitive

Illustrations

+ In a set of integers, a relation R is defined by $x\,R\,y$ if and only if $x - y$ is divisible by 4. Then R is an equivalence relation. Since

(a) For $x\,R\,x$, $x - x = 0$ is divisible by 4. Therefore, it is reflexive.

(b) For $x\,R\,y$. Let $x - y = 4m$ so $y - x = 4m$, which is also divisible by 4. Therefore, it is symmetric.

(c) For $x\,R\,y$, let $x - y = 4m$; for $y\,R\,z$, let $y - z = 4n$. By adding these two equations, we get $x - z = -4(m + n)$, which is divisible by 4. Therefore it is transitive.

+ Let R be a relation on the set of all lines in a plane L defined by $(l_1, l_2) \in R$ if and only if line l_1 is parallel to l_2, then R is an equivalence relation because

(a) For each line $l \in L$, we have l is parallel to l $\Rightarrow lRl \Rightarrow R$ is reflexive.

(b) Let $l_1, l_2 \in L$ such that $(l_1, l_2) \in R$, then $\Rightarrow (l_1, l_2) \in R \Rightarrow l_1$ is parallel to $l_2 \Rightarrow l$ is symmetric.

(c) Let $l_1, l_2, l_3 \in L$ such that (l_1, l_2) and $(l_2, l_3) \in R$, then obviously $(l_1, l_3) \in R$ because if l_1 is parallel to l_2 and l_2 is parallel to l_3, then l_3 should be parallel to l_1.

1.3.2 Congruence Modulo 'm'

Let m be an arbitrary but fixed integer. If $x - y$ is divisible by m, then two integers x and y are said to be congruence modulo m of one another.

Symbolically : $x \equiv y \pmod{m}$ if $x - y$ divisible by m.

For example : $32 \equiv 2 \pmod 3$, as $32 - 2 = 30$ which is divisible by 3.

1.3.3 Composition of Relations

Let R_1 and R_2 be two relations from set A to B and B to C respectively, then we can define a relation $R_1 \cup R_2$ from A to C, such that $(x, z) \in R_1 \cup R_2$ if and only if there exist $y \in Y$ such that $(x, y) \in R_1$ and $(y, z) \in R_2$.

This relation is called composition of R_1 and R_2.

☞ Remarks

• $R_1 o R_2 \neq R_2 o R_1$

• $(R_2 o R_1)^{-1} = R_1^{-1} o R_2^{-1}$

• The intersection of two equivalence relations on a set is an equivalence relation.

• The union of two equivalence relations on a set is not necessarily an equivalence relation.

• If R is an equivalence relation, then R^{-1} is also an equivalence relation.

1.3.4 Ordered Set

(i) **Partially Ordered Set:** A relation $\leq$ defined on any set A is said to be partially ordered if it is

(I) **Reflexive:** i.e., $x \leq x$

(II) **Anti symmetric:** i.e., $x \leq y, y \leq x \Rightarrow y = x$

(III) **Transitive:** i.e., $x \leq y, y \leq z \Rightarrow x \leq z$, for all $x, y, z \in A$

Here, the set A is called partially ordered set and is denoted by $(A, \leq)$.

(ii) **Natural Order Relation:** The relation in N, the set of natural numbers defined by $x < y$ is a partial ordered relation. This order is called Natural Ordered or Usual Order.

(iii) **Comparable or Uncomparable Elements:** Any two elements x, y in a partially ordered set $(A, \leq)$ are said to be comparable if either $x \leq y$ or $y \leq x$. On the other hand, x, y are said to be incomparable if $x \leq y$ and $y \leq x$ both are not true.

(iv) **Totally Ordered Set:** If every pair of elements of a partially ordered set is comparable, then the set A is called a totally ordered or linearly ordered set. It is also called 'chain'.

(v) **Ordered Complete Set:** An ordered set $(X, \leq)$ is called order complete if sup(A) exists for each subset A of X.

(vi) **Well Ordered Set:** A linearly ordered set $(A, <)$ is called well ordered if every subset of A has a first element.

(vii) **Ordinal Number:** The order type of a well ordered set is called an ordinal number.

Illustrations

✦ The set N, of natural numbers with usual order is well ordered.

✦ The empty set ϕ, is regarded as well ordered.

✦ A singleton set is regarded as well ordered set.

✦ Q, R, Z with usual order are not well ordered.

✦ A finite linearly ordered set is well ordered.

✦ Z, with ordering $0, -1, +1, -2, +2, \ldots$ is well ordered.

☞ **REMARKS**
- Every subset of a well ordered set is well ordered.
- A well ordered set can not be similar to one of its initial segment.
- Every set of ordinal numbers is a well ordered set.
- Any set consisting of only one element is assumed to be linearly ordered.

Solved Examples

EXAMPLE 1. *Let Z be the set of integers. Define a relation R on Z such that $x\,R\,y$ holds if and only if $x - y$ is divisible by 5, $x \in Z$, $y \in Z$. Show that it is an equivalence relation.*

SOLUTION.   (i) For each $x \in Z$, $x - x$ i.e., 0 is divisible by 5.
Therefore, for all $x \in Z$, $x\,R\,x \Rightarrow x$ is reflexive.

(ii) Let $x\,R\,y \Rightarrow x - y$ is divisible by 5.
$\Rightarrow y - x$ is divisible by 5.
Thus $xRy = yRx$
Therefore R is symmetric.

(iii) Let us suppose xRy and yRz, then $(x - y)$ and $(y - z)$ both are divisible by 5.
Hence, 5 is also a divisor of $(x - y) + (y - z)$.
$\Rightarrow$ 5 is a divisor of $(x - z)$.
Therefore, xRy, $yRz \Rightarrow xRz \Rightarrow R$ is transitive.
From (i), (ii) and (iii), we conclude that R is an equivalence relation.

EXAMPLE 2. *Let $N \times N$ be the set of ordered pairs of natural numbers. Also, let R be the relation in $N \times N$, defined by $(a, b)\,R\,(c, d)$ if and only if $a + d = b + c$. Show that R is an equivalence relation.*

SOLUTION.   (i) For all $(a, b) \in N \times N$, we have $a + b = b + a$, i.e., $(a, b)\,R\,(b, a)$.
Therefore, R is reflexive.

(ii) Let $(a, b)\,R\,(c, d)$, then, by definition of R
$$(a + d) = (b + c) \text{ or } (c + b) = (d + a)$$
$$(c, d)\,R\,(a, b) \Rightarrow R \text{ is symmetric.}$$

(iii) Let us suppose $(a, b) R (c, d)$ and $(c, d) R (e, f)$, then

$$a + d = b+c \text{ and } c+f = d+e$$
$$\Rightarrow \quad (a + d) + (c + f) = (b + c) + (d + e) \quad \Rightarrow \quad a + f = b + e$$
$$\Rightarrow \quad (a, b)R(e, f)$$

Therefore, R is transitive.

Hence, from (i), (ii) and (iii), we conclude that R is an equivalence relation.

EXAMPLE 3. *If R is the relation for natural number defined by x+4y = 20. Find the domain and range of the relation R.*

SOLUTION. Let $x + 4y = 20 \quad \Rightarrow \quad y = \dfrac{20 - x}{4}$

For $x = 4$, $y = 4$ and for $x = 8$, $y = 3$.

For $x = 16$, $y = 1$ and for $x = 12$, $y = 2$

Therefore, Domain $= \{4, 8, 12, 16\}$ and range $= \{4, 3, 2, 1\}$

EXAMPLE 4. *A relation R defined on the set of integers Z, as follows*

$$(x, y) \in R \Rightarrow x^2 + y^2 = 25$$

Express R and R^{-1} as the sets of ordered pairs and hence find their respective domains.

SOLUTION. Since $(x, y) \in R \Leftrightarrow x^2 + y^2 = 25 \quad \Rightarrow \quad y = \pm\sqrt{25 - x^2}$

If $\quad x = 0 \quad \Rightarrow \quad y = 5$.

Therefore, $(0, 5) \in R$ and $(0, - 5) \in R$

Now, $x = 3 \quad \Rightarrow \quad y = \sqrt{25 - 9} = \pm 4$

$(3, 4) \in R$, $(-3, 4) \in R$, $(3, -4) \in R$ and $(-3, -4) \in R$

$x = \pm 4 \quad \Rightarrow \quad y = \pm 3$

Therefore, $(4, 3) \in R$, $(-4, 3) \in R$, $(4, -3) \in R$ and $(-4, -3) \in R$

$x = \pm 5 \quad \Rightarrow \quad y = \sqrt{25 - 25} = 0 \quad \therefore \quad (5, 0) \in R$ and $(-5, 0) \in R$

Here, it is clear that for any other integral value of x, y is not an integer. Therefore,

$R = \{(0, 5), (0, -5), (3, 4), (-3, 4), (3, -4), (-3, - 4), (4, 3), (-4, 3), (4, -3),$
$(- 4, -3), (5, 0), (-5, 0)\}$

and $R^{-1} = \{(5, 0), (-5, 0), (4, 3), (4, -3), (- 4, 3), (- 4, -3), (3, 4), (3, -4),$
$(-3, 4), (-3, - 4), (0, 5), (0, -5)\}$

Also, domain $(R) = \{0, 3, -3, 4, - 4, 5, -5\} =$ domain of (R^{-1}).

1.3.5 RELATIONS OTHER THAT EQUIVALENCE

Let R be a given relation on the set X. Then R is

(1) non-reflexive if $\exists x$, such that $(x, x) \notin R$.

(2) anti-reflexive or reflexive if $i_x \cap R = \phi$ (where i_x is the identity relation on X or $\forall x \in X : (x, x) \notin R$

(3) non-symmetric if for some $(x, y) \in R$, we have $(y, x) \notin R$

(4) anti-symmetric if $R \cap R^{-1} = i$, i.e., $(x, y) \in R$ and $(y, x) \in R \Rightarrow x = y$

(5) asymmetric if $R \cap R^{-1} = \phi$, i.e., $(x, y) \in R \Rightarrow (y, x) \notin R$

(6) non-transitive if $R \circ R \not\subset R$

(7) anti-transitive if $(R \circ R) \cap R = \phi$

(8) A reflexive and symmetric, but not transitive relation is called a tolerance relation.

(9) A non-symmetric transitive relation is called an ordered relation.

(10) A reflexive, anti-symmetric and transitive relation is called partial-ordered relation.

Exercise 1.1

1. If R is the relation 'is less than' from $A = \{1, 2, 3, 4, 5\}$ to $B = \{1, 4, 5\}$, find the set of ordered pairs corresponding to R. Also find R^{-1}.

2. A relation R defined from a set $A = \{2, 3, 4, 5\}$ to a set $B = \{3, 6, 7, 10\}$ as follows :

   $(x, y) \in R \Rightarrow x$ divides y. Write R as a set of ordered pairs and determine the domain and range of R. Also find R^{-1}.

3. Find the domain and range of $A = \{1, 2, 3, 4, 5, 6\}$ when the relation are defined as

   (i) $x R_1 y$ if and only if $x - y > 0$

   (ii) $x R_2 y$ if and only if $x + y < 0$

4. Two sets A and B are given by $A = \{1, 2, 8, 9\}$ and $B = \{2, 3, 4, 6, 7\}$ and if R is the relation form A to B given by $\{(1,2), (1,3), (2,4), (2,6)\}$, then which of the following statement is true?

   (i) Domain (R) = Range (R^{-1}) and Range (R) = Domain (R^{-1})

   (ii) Domain (R) = Domain (R^{-1}) and Range (R) = Range (R^{-1})

   (iii) Domain (R) = Range (R^{-1}) and Range (R) = Domain (R^{-1})

   (iv) Domain (R) = Range (R)

5. If R is a relation on a set A, then which of the following statement is not true?

   (i) If R is reflexive then R^{-1} is reflexive.

   (ii) If R is symmetric then R^{-1} is symmetric.

   (iii) If R is transitive, then R^{-1} is transitive.

   (iv) None of these

6. Find the domain and range of the following relations:

   (i) $R = \{(x + 1, x + 5)\} : x \in \{0, 1, 2, 3, 4, 5\}$

   (ii) $R = \{(x, x^3) : x$ is a prime number, less than 10\}

   (iii) $R = \{(a, b) : a \in N, a < 5, b = 4\}$

   (iv) $R = \{(a, b) : b = |a - 1|, a \in Z,$ and $|a| \le 3\}$

7. Let R_1 be the relation defined on the set of reals R such as $(a, b) \in R_1$ if and only if $1 + ab > 0$ for all $a, b \in R$. Show that R_1 is reflexive, symmetric but not transitive.

8. Let R be relation on $N \times N$, defined by $(a, b) R (c, d)$ if and only if $ad (b + c) = bc (a + d)$. Show that R is an equivalence relation.

9. Show that the relation 'congruence modulo m' on the set of integers is an equivalence relation.

10. Let R_1 be a relation on the set of reals defined by $R_1 = \{(a, b) \in R \times R : a^2 + b^2 = 1\}$ Show that R_1 is not an equivalence relation on R.

11. In a set L of all straight lines in a plane, discuss which of the following two relations are equivalence relations on L.

    (i) $R_1 = \{(x, y): x, y \in L$ and x is parallel to $y\}$

    (ii) $R_2 = \{(x, y): x, y \in L$ and x is perpendicular to $y\}$.

12. Show that the relation $R = \{(a, b) : a - b = $ even integer $\forall\, a, b \in Z\}$, i.e., $a R b \Leftrightarrow a - b = $ even integer, is an equivalence relation.

13. Show that the relation R in N, the set of natural numbers, defined by $x R y$ if $x^2 - 4xy + 3y^2 = 0$, $(x, y \in N)$ is reflexive, not symmetric and not transitive.

14. For the given relation R on a set S, determine which are equivalence relations:

    (i) S is the set of all rational numbers, $a R b$ if and only if $a = b$

    (ii) S is the set of all real numbers iff

    (a) $|a| = |b|$ \qquad (b) $a \ge b$

    (iii) S is the set of all triangles in a plane, $a R b$ iff a is congruent to b.

    (iv) S is the set of all triangles in a plane, $a R b$ iff a and b have equal perimeters.

15. An integer m is said to be related to another integer n if m is a multiple of n. Show that this relation is reflexive and transitive but not symmetric.

16. Let R be a relation defined on the set of natural number N as $R = \{(x, y): x, y \in N, 2x + y = 41\}$. Find the domain and range of R.

17. Let O be the origin. Define a relation between two points P and Q in a plane if $PO = OQ$. Show that the relation is an equivalence relation.

18. Given the relation $R = \{(1, 2), (2, 3)\}$ on the set of natural number N, add a minimum of ordered pairs so that the enlarged relation is symmetric, transitive and reflexive.

19. Let N denote the set of all natural numbers and R be the relation on $N \times N$ defined by $(a, b) R (c, d) \Leftrightarrow ad (b + c) = bc (a + d)$. Show that R is an equivalence relation.

20. Show that the relation, which is symmetric and transitive, is not necessarily reflexive.

ANSWERS

1. $aRb = \{(1, 4), (1, 5), (2, 4), (3, 4), (2, 5), (3, 5), (4, 5)\}$,
$R^{-1} = \{(4, 1), (5, 1), (4, 2), (5, 2), (4, 3), (5, 3), (5, 4)\}$

2. Domain $(R) = \{2, 3, 5\}$, Range $(R) = \{3, 6, 10\}$, $R^{-1} = \{(6, 2), (10, 2), (3, 3), (6, 3), (10, 5)\}$

3. (i) $\{2, 3, 4, 5, 6\}$, $\{1, 2, 3, 4, 5\}$, (ii) ϕ, ϕ **4.** (iii) **5.** (iv) **6.** (i) Domain $(R) = \{1, 2, 3, 4, 5, 6\}$, Range $(R) = \{5, 6, 7, 8, 9, 10\}$ (ii) Domain $(R) = \{2, 3, 5, 7\}$, Range $(R) = \{8, 27, 125, 243\}$ (iii) Domain $(R) = \{1, 2, 3, 4\}$, Range $(R) = \{4\}$ (iv) Domain $(R) = \{0, -1, -2, -3, 1, 2, 3\}$, Range $(R) = \{1, 2, 3, 4, 0, 1, 2\}$ **11.** R_1 = Equivalence relation, R_2 = Not equivalence **14.** (i), (ii) **16.** Domain $(R) = \{1, 2, ..., 19, 20\}$, Range $(R) = \{39, 37, 35, ..., 5, 3, 1\}$ **18.** $\{(1, 2), (2, 1), (2, 3), (3, 2), (1, 3), (3, 1), (1, 1), (2, 2), (3, 3), (4, 4), ...\}$

1.4 FUNCTIONS

Definition. *Let A and B be two sets, then a rule or correspondence, which associates each element of A to a unique element of B, is called a function from set A to set B.*

If a general element of set A is denoted by x, and of set B is denoted by y, then we say that y is a function of x if, for every $x \in A$, one and only one value of $y \in B$ can be determined.

Symbolically: If f is a function from a set A to a set B, then we write $f : A \to B$, read as f is a function from A to B or f maps A to B.

1.4.1 RANGE AND DOMAIN OF A FUNCTION

Let an element $y \in B$ be corresponded by an element $x \in A$, then y is called the image of x and is denoted by $f(x)$. Here, x is defined as the pre-image of y.

The set A is called the domain and the set B is called the co-domain of the function f.

The set of all f-images of the elements of A, is called image set or the range of f and is denoted by

$$f(A) \quad \text{or} \quad \{f(x) : x \in A\}$$

Evidently, $f(A) \subseteq B$.

Thus, a mapping $f : A \to B$ is the set of ordered pairs $\{(a, b) : a \in A, b \in B\}$, so that no two ordered pairs have the same finite element.

$$f = \{(a, b) : a \in A, b \in B, b = f(x) \; \forall \; a \in A\}$$

For example : Let $A = \{-2, -1, 0, 1, 2\}$ and B is the set of natural numbers for every $x \in A$, $f(x) \in B$ and $f(x) = x^2$.

Here, A is the domain and B is the co-domain.

$f(a)$ is the value of the function $f(x)$, when x takes the value a, i.e., when x is replaced by a.

The elements of the co-domain which is equal to $f(x)$ form the range.

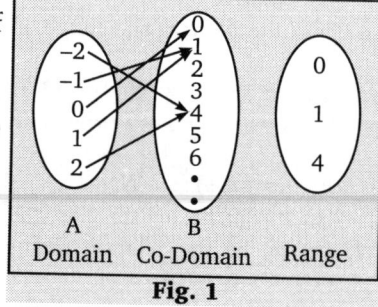

When $x = -2$, $f(-2) = (-2)^2 = 4$

When $x = -1$, $f(-1) = 1$

When $x = 0$, $f(0) = 0$

When $x = 1$, $f(1) = 1$

When $x = 2$, $f(2) = 4$.

Which can be illustrated in the figure 1.

A
Domain

B
Co-Domain

Range

Fig. 1

☞ **REMARKS**

- If $f: A \to B$ then a single element in A cannot have more than one image in B. However, two or more elements in A may have the same image in B.
- Every element in A must have its image in B, but every element in B may not have it pre-image in A.
- To each element x in A, there exists a unique element y in B such that $y = f(x)$.
- The unique element y of B is called the value of f at x (the image of f under x), and written as $y = f(x)$.
- The range of f consist of those elements in B which appear as the image of at least one element in A.
- Range of a function is the image of its domain.
- Range is a subset of co-domain.

1.5 TYPE OF FUNCTIONS

(a) **One-One function:** A function f from A to B, *i.e.*, $f: A \to B$ is said to be one-one (or injective) iff distinct elements of A have distinct images.

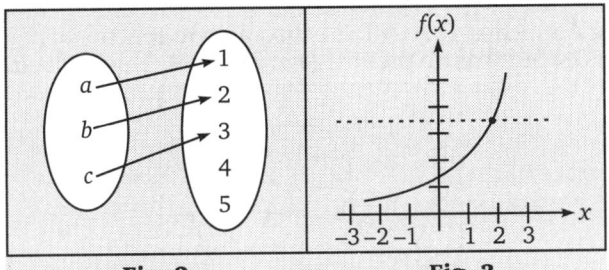

| Fig. 2 | Fig. 3 |

Symbolically: f is one-one if for $x_1, x_2 \in A$, we have

$$x_1 \neq x_2 \quad \Rightarrow \quad f(x_1) \neq f(x_2) \; \forall \; x_1, x_2 \in A$$

or $\qquad f(x_1) = f(x_2) \Rightarrow \quad x_1 = x_2 \; \forall \; x_1, x_2 \in A$

It is also called Univalent function.

Graphically, a function is one-one if and only if no line parallel to x-axis meets the graph of the function at more than one point.

(b) **Many-One Function:** A function $f: A \to B$ is called many-one, if at least one element of co-domain B has two or more than two pre-images in domain A.

Symbolically: f is many-one if for $x_1, x_2 \in A$, we have $x_1 \neq x_2 \Rightarrow f(x_1) = f(x_2)$

This can be illustrated in the following figures.

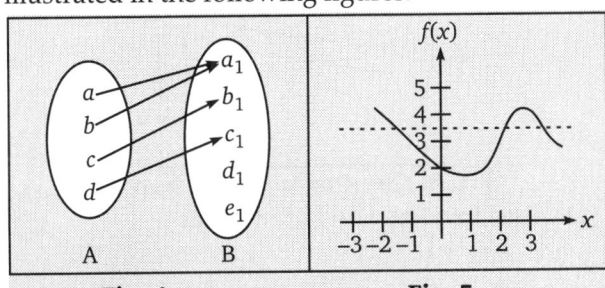

| Fig. 4 | Fig. 5 |

Graphically, a function is many-one if and only if a line parallel to x-axis meets the graph of the function at more than one point.

☞ REMARK

• One-many function does not exist.

(c) **Onto function:** A function $f : A \to B$ is called an onto function, if there is no element of B which is not an image of some element of A, *i.e.*, every element of B appears as the image of at least one element of A. This is illustrated in Figure 6.

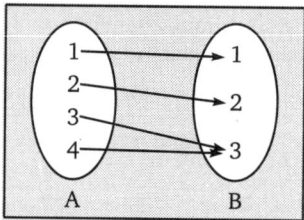

Fig. 6: Onto Function

☞ REMARKS

• In an onto function, Range = Co-domain
• Onto function is also called surjective.

(d) **Into function:** A function $f : A \to B$ is called an into function, *i.e.*, if there is at least one element of set B which has no pre-image in the set A. This is illustrated in Figure 7.

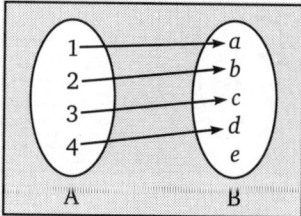

Fig. 7: Into Function

☞ REMARK

• In an into function, Range $\subset$ Co-domain.

(e) **One-One Into Function:** A function $f : A \to B$ is called a one-one into function, if it is both one-one and into, *i.e.*, the different points in A are joined to different points in B and there are some points in B which are not joined to any point in A. This is illustrated in Figure 8.

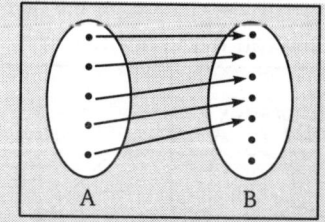

Fig. 8: One-One Into Function

Symbolically : One-one into function is defined as

(i) Range $\subset$ Co-domain.

(ii) $f(x_1) \neq f(x_2) \Rightarrow x_1 \neq x_2$.

(f) **One-One Onto Function:** A function $f : A \to B$ is both one-one and onto, *i.e.*, the different points in A are joined to different points in B and no point in B is left vacant. This is illustrated in Figure 9.

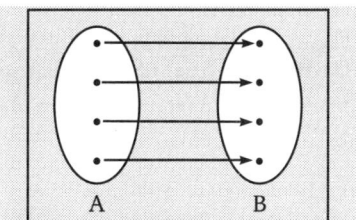

Fig. 9: One-one Onto Function

☞ REMARKS

- One-one onto mapping is also known as bijective.

- For a one-one onto function

  Range = Co-domain, and $x_1 \neq x_2 \Rightarrow f(x_1) \neq f(x_2)$ or $f(x_1) = f(x_2) \Rightarrow x_1 = x_2$

(g) Many-One Into Function: A function $f : A \to B$ which is both many-one and into function is called a many-one into function, *i.e.*, two or more points in A are joined to same points in B and there are some point in B which are not joined to any point in A. Therefore, for many-one into function.

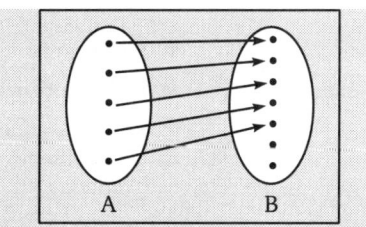

Fig. 10: Many-One Into Function

(i) Range $\subset$ Co-domain.

(ii) $x_1 \neq x_2 \Rightarrow f(x_1) = f(x_2)$

(h) Many-One Onto Function: If function $f : A \to B$ is both many-one and onto function is called a many one onto function, *i.e.*, in B one point is joined to at least one point in A and two or more points in A are joined to some points in B. Therefore, for many-one onto function.

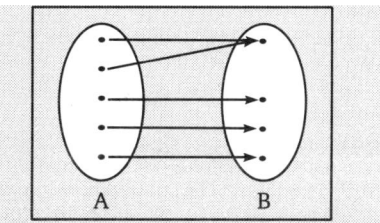

Fig. 11: Many-One Onto Function

(i) Range = Co-domain.

(ii) $x_1 \neq x_2 \Rightarrow f(x_1) = f(x_2)$

WORKING PROCEDURE

1.	**For checking the Injectivity (One-One) of the function**	
	Let x and y be two arbitrary elements in the domain of f.	
Step 1.	Take $f(x) = f(y)$	
Step 2.	If we get $x = y$, after solving $f(x) = f(y)$. Then, $f : A \to B$ is one-one.	
2.	**For checking the surjectivity (Onto) of a function**	
Step 1.	Take an arbitrary element y in the co-domain.	
Step 2.	Put $f(x) = f(y)$	
Step 3.	Solve $f(x) = y$ for x and obtain x in terms of y.	
Step 4.	Get the equation of the form $x = g(y)$	
Step 5.	If $x = g(y)$ belongs to domain f, for all values of y, then f is onto.	

 ## Recapitulations

♦ For a function $f : A \to B$, A = domain,
   B = co-domain.

♦ **For one-one function:** $x_1 \neq x_2$
   $\Rightarrow f(x_1) \neq f(x_2) \; \forall \; x_1, x_2 \in A$
   or $f(x_1) = f(x_2) \Rightarrow x_1 = x_2 \; \forall \; x_1, x_2 \in A$

♦ **For many-one function:**
   $x_1 \neq x_2 \Rightarrow f(x_1) = f(x_2), x_1, x_2 \in A$

♦ **For onto function:** Range = co-domain

♦ **For into function:** Range $\subseteq$ co-domain

♦ **For one-one into function:**
   (i) Range $\subseteq$ co-domain
   (ii) $f(x_1) \neq f(x_2) \Rightarrow x_1 \neq x_2$

♦ **For one-one onto function:**
   (i) Range = codomain
   (ii) $x_1 \neq x_2 \Rightarrow f(x_1) \neq f(x_2)$
   or $f(x_1) = f(x_2) \Rightarrow x_1 = x_2$

♦ **For many-one into function:**
   (i) Range = co-domain
   (ii) $x_1 = x_2 \Rightarrow f(x_1) = f(x_2)$

♦ **For many-one onto function:**
   (i) Range = co-domain
   (ii) $x_1 \neq x_2 \Rightarrow f(x_1) = f(x_2)$

 ## Solved Examples

EXAMPLE 1. Let $f : R \to R$ be a function defined by

$$f(x) = \begin{cases} 3x - 1 & when \quad x > 3 \\ x^2 - 1 & when \; -2 \leq x \leq 3 \\ x + 3 & when \quad x < -2 \end{cases}$$

Find (i) $f(2)$, (ii) $f(4)$, (iii) $f(-1)$, (iv) $f(-3)$

SOLUTION.   (i) $f(2) = (2)2 - 2 = 4 - 2 = 2$

(ii) $f(4) = 3(4) - 1 = 12 - 1 = 11$

(iii) $f(-1) = (-1)^2 - 2 = 1 - 2 = -1$

(iv) $f(-3) = 2(-3) + 3 = -6 + 3 = -3$

EXAMPLE 2. For $y = +\sqrt{x}$, say whether it is a function or not. If it is a function, find its domain and range.

SOLUTION. Here we have $y = +\sqrt{x}$ ...(1)

Since y is real if $x \geq 0$ and is unique and finite for each $x \geq 0$.

Therefore, (1) is a function with domain $[0, \infty[$.

Again from (1), $y \geq 0 \ \forall \ x \geq 0$

Hence, range $= [0, \infty [$

EXAMPLE 3. *Find the domain of* $f(x) = \dfrac{x^3 - x^2 + 4x + 2}{3x + 11}$.

SOLUTION. Since f is defined for all real values of x except when $3x + 11 = 0$

i.e., when, $x = -\dfrac{11}{3}$

Hence, domain of $f = R - \left\{ -\dfrac{11}{3} \right\}$

EXAMPLE 4. *Let $f : N - \{1\} \rightarrow N$ be defined by $f(n) =$ the highest prime factor of n. Show that f is neither one-one nor onto. Also, find the range f.*

SOLUTION. Since we have

$f(6) =$ the highest prime factor of $6 = 3$

$f(9) =$ the highest prime factor of $9 = 3$

$f(12) =$ the highest prime factor of $12 = 3$

Therefore, f is a many-one function.

Clearly, image of any $n \in N - \{1\}$ is the largest prime number that divides n. So the range of f consists of prime number only. Consequently, range of $f \neq N$ (Co-domain)

$\Rightarrow$ f is not onto function.

Hence, f is neither one-one nor onto. The range of f is the set of all prime numbers.

EXAMPLE 5. *Let $A = \{1, 2\}$. Find all one-to-one function from A to A.*

SOLUTION. Let $f : A \rightarrow A$ be a one-one function.

Then, for $f(1)$, there are two choices, *i.e.,* 1 or 2.

Let us first suppose $\quad f(1) = 1$.

As $f : A \rightarrow A$ is one-one, $\quad f(2) = 2$

Therefore, we have $\quad f(1) = 1, f(2) = 2$

Now, let $\quad f(1) = 2$

Since, $f : A \rightarrow A$ is one-one, therefore $f(2) = 1$.

Therefore, we have $\quad f(1) = 2$ and $f(2) = 1$.

Hence, we have two one-one function say f and g form A and A given by

$\quad f(1) = 1, f(2) = 2$ and $f(2) = 1$ and $f(1) = 2$.

EXAMPLE 6. *Let $\{x \in R : -1 \leq x \leq 1\} = B$. Show that $f : A \rightarrow B$ given by $f(x) = x \ |x|$ is one-one and onto.*

SOLUTION. Let x, y be any two elements in A, then

$$x \neq y \Rightarrow x|x| \neq y|y| \Rightarrow f(x) \neq f(y).$$

Therefore, f is one-one.

Since, range of $f = f(A) = B$ so $f : A \rightarrow B$ is onto mapping. Hence f is one-one and onto.

EXAMPLE 7. *Find the domain and range of the function.*

$$f(x) = -\sqrt{-5 - 6x - x^2}$$

SOLUTION. Given that, $f(x) = -\sqrt{-5 - 6x - x^2}$

For f to be real, $-5 - 6x - x^2 \geq 0$ $\Rightarrow$ $x^2 + 6x + 5 \leq 0$

$\Rightarrow$ $x^2 + 6x \leq -5$ $\Rightarrow$ $x^2 + 6x + 9 \leq -5 + 9$

$\Rightarrow$ $(x + 3)^2 \leq 4$ $\Rightarrow$ $|x + 3|^2 \leq 4$

$\Rightarrow$ $|x + 3| \leq 2$ $\Rightarrow$ $-2 \leq x + 3 \leq 2$

$\Rightarrow$ $-2 - 3 \leq x \leq 2 - 3$ $\Rightarrow$ $-5 \leq x \leq -1$

Therefore, domain of $f(x)$ = $[-5, -1]$

To find the range of $f(x)$,   put $y = f(x)$

Therefore, $f(x) = -\sqrt{-5 - 6x - x^2}$, $y \leq 0$

$\Rightarrow$ $y^2 = -5 - 6x - x^2$ $\Rightarrow$ $x^2 + 6x + (y^2 + 5) = 0$

For real x, discriminant ≥ 0, *i.e.,* $(6)^2 - 4 \times 1 \times (y^2 + 5) \geq 0$

$\Rightarrow$ $36 - 4y^2 - 20 \geq 0$ $\Rightarrow$ $-4y^2 \geq -16$

$\Rightarrow$ $y^2 \leq 4$ $\Rightarrow$ $|y|^2 \leq 4$

$\Rightarrow$ $|y| \leq 2$ *i.e.,* $-2 \leq y \leq 2$

But $y \leq 0$ therefore, $-2 \leq y \leq 0$.

Hence, Range of f = $[-2, 0]$

1.6 BINARY OPERATION

Let S be a non-empty set. Then any function from $S \times S$ to S is called binary operation. It is usually denoted by any of the following symbols : $*, o, O, \oplus, +, .$ etc.

That is, any function $* : S \times S \rightarrow S$ is said to be binary operation, where $S \times S = \{(a, b) : a, b \in S\}$.

Instead of writting $*(a, b)$, we write $a * b$ for $a, b \in S$. Thus a binary operation $*$ on S is a rule which assign to a pair $a, b \in S$ another element $a*b \in S$.

Illustrations

✦ The addition '+': $Z \times Z \rightarrow Z$ is a binary operation, because for all $a, b \in Z$, we have $a + b \in Z$.

✦ The multiplication '.': $Z \times Z \rightarrow Z$ is binary operation, as $a.b \in Z$ for all $a, b \in Z$.

✦ The subtraction '$-$': $N \times N \rightarrow N$ is not a binary operation, as $3 \in N, 5 \in N$ but $3 - 5 = -2 \notin N$.

✦ The subtraction '$-$': $Z \times Z \rightarrow Z$ is binary operation, as $a - b \in Z$ for all $a, b \in Z$.

✦ Let S be a non-empty set and $P(S)$ be its power set. Then the union opeartion on $P(S)$ is a binary opaeration as $A \cup B \in P(S)$ for all $A, B \in P(S)$.

✦ Addition of the set S of all irrationals is not a binary operation as $2 + \sqrt{3} \in S$ and $2 - \sqrt{3} \in S$ but $2 + \sqrt{3} + 2 - \sqrt{3} \notin S$.

✦ Multiplication on the set S of all irrationals is not a binary operation as $\sqrt{2} \in S, -\sqrt{2} \in S$ but $(\sqrt{2})(-\sqrt{2}) = -2 \notin S$.

☞ REMARKS

• A binary operation combines any two elements a and b of a set to give another element of the same set, this fact is also known as closure property or we can say that the set is closed with respect to binary operation.

• Binary operation is never one-one.

1.7 NUMBER OF BINARY OPERATIONS

Let $f : A \to B$ be a function, where $n(A) = p$ and $n(B) = q$. Then, the total number of functions from A to B is given by $[n(B)]^{n(A)}$.

Let S be a finite set containing n elements, then $S \times S$ will have n^2 elements. Since the binary operation is a function form $S \times S$ to S, so that total number of binary operations on S is $(n)^{n^2}$.

Illustration

✦ If $S = \{1, 2\}$, then the total number of binary operations on $S = (2)^{2^2} = 2^4 = 16$.

1.8 PROPERTIES OF BINARY OPERATION

Let $'*' : S \times S \to S$ and $'o' : S \times S \to S$ be any two binary operations, where S is any non-empty set.

Then we define the following properties.

(i) **Associative property :** A binary operation $*$ on S is said to be associative, if
$$(a*b)*c = a*(b*c) \text{ for all } a, b, c \in S.$$

If $'*'$ denotes addition (+) and multiplication ($\times$), then $'*'$ is always associative on S but if $'*'$ denotes subtraction (–), then $'*'$ is not associative on S.

For example : Addition and multiplication on Z, the set of all integers are always associative, i.e.,
$$(a + b) + c = a+(b+c)$$
and $\quad (a \times b) \times c = a \times (b \times c) \text{ for all } a, b, c \in Z.$

But subtraction is not associative on Z, i.e.,
$$3 - (5 - 4) \neq (3 - 5) - 4$$

(ii) **Commutative property :** A binary opeartion $'*'$ on a set S is said to be *commutative* if
$$a*b = b*a \text{ for all } a, b \in S.$$

If $'*'$ denotes additon (+) and multiplication ($\times$), then $'*'$ is always *commutative* on S but if $*$ denotes subtraction (–), then $'*'$ is not commutative on S.

For example : If $S = Z$, the set of all integers, then
$$a+b = b+a$$
and $\quad a \times b = b \times a \text{ for all } a, b \in Z.$

But subtraction is not commutative as $3{-}5 \neq 5{-}3$ for $3, 5 \in Z$.

(iii) **Distributive property :** A binary opeartion $'*'$ is said to be *distributive* over another binary operation $'o'$ on S if
$$a*(b \text{ o } c) = (a*b) \text{ o } (a*c) \text{ for all } a, b, c \in S$$
and $\quad (b \text{ o } c)*a = (b*a) \text{ o } (c*a) \text{ for all } a, b, c \in S$

Here the first distribution is known as *left distribution* whereas the second is known as *right distribution*. That is,

Left distributive property :
$$a*(b \text{ o } c) = (a*b) \text{ o } (a*c) \text{ for all } a, b, c \in S$$

Right distributive property :

$$(b \text{ o } c)*a = (b*a) \text{ o } (c*a) \text{ for all } a, b, c \in S$$

For example : If $S = Z$, the set of all integers and '*' denotes multiplication, 'o' denotes addition, then '*' is distributive over 'o' on Z, *i.e.*,

$$a \times (b+c) = a \times b + a \times c$$

and

$$(b+c) \times a = b \times a + c \times a$$

But if '*' denotes addition and 'o' denotes multiplication, then '*' is not distributive over 'o' on Z, *i.e.*,

$$5 + (3 \times 2) \neq (5+3) \times (5+2)$$

1.9 ALGEBRAIC STRUCTURE

Let S be a non-empty set and '*' be a binary operation on S, then $(S, *)$ is known as algebraic structure.

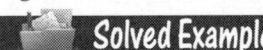 Solved Examples

EXAMPLE 1. *Determine whether the following operations are binary on the given set or not:*

  (i) *'*' on **N** defined by $a*b = ab$ for all $a, b \in N$*

  (ii) *'*' on **N** defined by $a*b = a + b - 2$ for all $a, b \in N$*

  (iii) *'*' on **N** defined by $a*b = a^b + b^a$ for all $a, b \in N$*

  (iv) *'*' on **Z** defined by $a*b = \sqrt{|ab|}$ for all $a, b \in Z$*

  (v) *'*' on **Z** defined by $a*b = \sqrt{a^2 + b^2}$ for all $a, b \in Z$*

  (vi) *'*' on **Z** defined by $a*b = \dfrac{1}{a-b}$ for all $a, b \in Z$*

SOLUTION. (i) For all $a, b \in N$, $ab \in N$.

∴ $a * b \in N$

Hence, $*$ is binary operation on N.

(ii) For all $a, b \in N$, $a + b \in N$

But $a+b-2 \notin N$ for all $a, b \in N$,

For example if $a = b = 1$ then $a + b - 2 = 0 \notin N$.

Hence, $*$ is not binary on N, where $a * b = a + b - 2$.

(iii) For all $a, b \in N$, $a^b \in N$ and $b^a \in N$, then

$$a^b + b^a \in N \Rightarrow a * b \in N$$

Thus $a * b \in N$ for all $a, b \in N$. Hence, $*$ is binary operation on N.

(iv) If $a = 1$ and $b = 2$, then $|ab| = |1 \times 2| = 2$.

Now $\sqrt{|ab|} = \sqrt{2}$

∴ $\sqrt{|ab|} \notin Z$ for all $a, b \in Z$

⇒ $a * b \notin Z$ for all $a, b \in Z$

Hence $*$ is not binary operation on Z.

(v) Since $a * b = \sqrt{a^2 + b^2}$, for all $a, b \in Z$

If $a = b = 1$, then $\sqrt{a^2 + b^2} = \sqrt{1^2 + 2^2} = \sqrt{2} \notin Z$

$$\therefore \qquad \sqrt{a^2 + b^2} \notin \mathbf{Z} \text{ for all } a, b \in \mathbf{Z}$$

$$\Rightarrow \qquad a * b \notin \mathbf{Z} \text{ for all } a, b \in \mathbf{Z}$$

Hence $*$ is not binary operation on $\mathbf{Z}$.

(vi) Since $\qquad a * b = \dfrac{1}{a-b} \text{ for all } a, b \in \mathbf{Z}.$

If $a = 3$ and $b = 1$, then $\dfrac{1}{a-b} = \dfrac{1}{3-1} = \dfrac{1}{2} \notin \mathbf{Z}$

$$\therefore \qquad \dfrac{1}{a-b} \notin \mathbf{Z} \text{ for all } a, b \in \mathbf{Z}$$

$$\Rightarrow \qquad a * b = \dfrac{1}{a-b} \notin \mathbf{Z} \text{ for all } a, b \in \mathbf{Z}$$

Hence $*$ is not binary operation on $\mathbf{Z}$.

EXAMPLE 2. *Let S be a set having more than one element. Let '$*$' $S \times S \rightarrow S$ be binary operation defined by $a * b = a$ for all $a, b \in S$. Is $(S, *)$ associative or commutative?*

SOLUTION. Since S has more than one elenment, so if $a, b \in S$, then $a \neq b$.

Now, $\qquad\qquad a * b = a$ and $b * a = b$

$\therefore \qquad\qquad a + b \neq b * a \qquad\qquad$ for all a, b

Thus $*$ is not commutative on S.

Again, $\qquad\qquad a * (b * c) = a * b = a$

and $\qquad\qquad (a * b) * c = a * c = a$

$\therefore \qquad\qquad a * (b * c) = (a * b) * c \qquad$ for all $a, b, c \in S$

Thus $*$ is associative on S.

EXAMPLE 3. *Let '$*$' be a binary opeararion on $\mathbf{Q}$ the set of all rational numbers. Find which of the binary opeartions are commutative.*

(i) $a * b = a - b \qquad$ for all $a, b \in \mathbf{Q}$

(ii) $a * b = a^2 + b^2 \qquad$ for all $a, b \in \mathbf{Q}$.

SOLUTION. (i) $a * b = a - b = -(b - a) = -b * a$

$\therefore \qquad\qquad a * b \neq b * a \text{ for all } a, b \in \mathbf{Q}.$

Thus $*$ is not commutative on $\mathbf{Q}$.

(ii) $a^2 \in \mathbf{Q}, b^2 \in \mathbf{Q}$ for all $a, b \in \mathbf{Q}$. Then

$$a * b = a^2 + b^2$$
$$= b^2 + a^2 \text{ [}\because \text{Addition is always commutative on } \mathbf{Q}\text{]}$$
$$= b * a$$

$\therefore \qquad\qquad a * b = b * a \text{ for all } a, b \in \mathbf{Q}$

Thus $*$ is commutative on $\mathbf{Q}$.

1.10 IDENTITY ELEMENT

Let $(S, *)$ be an algebraic structure. If there exists an element $e \in S$ such that $a*e = a = e * a$ for all $a \in S$ then e is called on identity element of S with respect to binary operation '$*$'.

Illustrations

✦ Let $S = \mathbf{Z}$, the set of all integers and addition $(+)$ is a binary operation on $\mathbf{Z}$. Then we know that $0 \in \mathbf{Z}$ such that

$$0 + a = a = a + 0 \text{ for all } a \in \mathbf{Z}.$$

Thus, 0 is the identity element for addition on $\mathbf{Z}$.

✦ If $S = \mathbf{N}$, the set of all natural numbers and multiplication '$*$' is binary operation on $\mathbf{N}$. Then we know that $1 \in \mathbf{N}$ such that

$$1 \cdot a = a = a \cdot 1 \text{ for all } a \in \mathbf{N}.$$

Thus, 1 is the identity element for multiplication on $\mathbf{N}$.

✦ Let $P(S)$ denote the power set of a non-empty set S. Then we know that
$$A \cup \phi = A = \phi \cup A \text{ for all } A \in P(S)$$
Thus, ϕ is the identity element for the union of sets on $P(S)$.

✦ Let $P(S)$ denotes the power set of a non-empty set S. Then we know that
$$A \cap S = A = S \cap A \text{ for all } A \in P(S)$$

☞ REMARK

• '0' is not an identity element for multiplication on N.

1.11 INVERSE OF AN ELEMENT

Let $(S, *)$ be an algebraic structure, and e be the identity element of S. Then an element $a \in S$ is said to be invertible element, if there exists an element $b \in S$ such that
$$a*b = e = b*a$$
The element b is called an inverse of a.

Illustrations

✦ Let $(Z, +)$ be an algebraic structure. Then $0 \in Z$ is the identity element for addition. Now corresponding to each element $a \in Z$, there exists $-a \in Z$ such that
$$a + (-a) = 0 = (-a) + a$$
Thus, $-a$ is the additive inverse of a.

✦ Let $(R, *)$ be an algebraic structure. Then $1 \in R$ is the multiplicative identity. If $a \neq 0 \in R$, then correspondig to each non-zero element $a \in R$, then exists an element $\frac{1}{a} \in R$, such that
$$a.\frac{1}{a} = 1 = \frac{1}{a}.a. \text{ Thus } \frac{1}{a} \text{ is the multiplicative inverse of } a.$$

☞ REMARK

• The inverse of an element a (if it exists) with respect to the addition (or multiplication) binary operations is generally is denoted by $a^{-1} \left(\text{or } \frac{1}{a} \right)$

THEOREM 1.

Let $(S, *)$ be an algebraic structure. If S has the identity element for '*', then it is unique.

PROOF.   Let e_1 and e_2 be two identities for '*' on S. Then by definition of identity, we have,
$$e_1 * e_2 = e_2, \text{ as } e_1 \text{ is the identity} \qquad \text{... (1)}$$
and $\qquad e_1 * e_2 = e_1, \text{ as } e_2 \text{ is the identity} \qquad \text{... (2)}$
From equations (1) and (2), we get
$$e_1 = e_2$$
Hence, the identity, if exists, is unique.

THEOREM 2.

Let $(S, *)$ be algebraic structure with identity element e. Then every element $a \in S$ has unique inverse in S, if '*' is associative.

PROOF.   Let b and c be two inverses of an element $a \in S$ in S. Then we have
$$a*b = e = b*a$$
and $\qquad a*c = e = c*a$
Now, $\qquad (b*a)*c = e*c$
$$= c \qquad \qquad (\because b*a = e)$$
$$\text{[By the definition of identity]}$$
and $\qquad b*(a*c) = b*e$
$$= b \qquad \qquad (\because a*c = e)$$
$$\text{[By the definition of identity]}$$
Since '*' is associative on S, so that $(b*a)*c = b*(a*c)$ for all $a, b, c \in S$

$$\Rightarrow \qquad\qquad c=b$$

Hence, $a \in S$ has unique inverse in S.

THEOREM 3.

Let $(S,*)$ be an algebraic structure and '$*$' be an associative binary operation on S. If a be an invertible element of S, then

$$(a^{-1})^{-1} = a$$

PROOF. Let e be the identity element of S for '$*$' and a be an invertible element of S, then

$$a * a^{-1} = e = a^{-1} * a$$

$$\Rightarrow \qquad a^{-1}* a = e = a * a^{-1}$$

$$\Rightarrow \qquad a \text{ is the inverse of } a^{-1}$$

$$\Rightarrow \qquad (a^{-1})^{-1} = a$$

☞ **REMARK**

- For identity element e, we have $e = e^{-1}$

THEOREM 4.

Let $(S, *)$ be an algebraic structure and $*$ be an associative binary operation on S. If each element of S has inverse in S. Then $(a * b)^{-1} = b^{-1} * a^{-1}$.

PROOF. Let e be the identity element of S for '$*$'. Now for $a, b \in S$, we have

$$(a * b)*(b^{-1} * a^{-1}) = a* (b * b^{-1})*a^{-1} \qquad \text{(By associativity)}$$

$$= a* e * a^{-1} \qquad\qquad (\because b*b^{-1} = e)$$

$$= a * a^{-1} \qquad\qquad (\because a*e = a)$$

$$= e \qquad\qquad (\because a * a^{-1} = e)$$

Similarly, $\quad (b^{-1} * a^{-1}) * (a * b) = e$

$$\therefore \qquad (a *b)*(b^{-1} *a^{-1}) = e = (b^{-1} *a^{-1})*(a*b)$$

$$\Rightarrow \quad b^{-1} * a^{-1} \text{ is the inverse of } a*b$$

$$\Rightarrow \qquad (a * b)^{-1} = b^{-1} * a^{-1}$$

1.12 COMPOSITION TABLE FOR BINARY OPERATION ON FINITE SETS

Let $S = \{a_1, a_2,... a_n\}$ be a finite set and '$*$' be a binary operation on S. Then we construct a composition table by means of following instructions:

First we write down the elements $a_1, a_2, ..., a_n$ of S in a top horizontal row and in a left vertical column as shown below. Now we write down the element $a_i * a_j$ at the intersection of row headed by a_i $(1 \leq i \leq n)$ and the column headed by a_j $(1 \leq j \leq n)$ to get the following table:

$*$	a_1	a_2	$\cdots$	a_j	$\cdots$	a_n
a_1	$a_1* a_1$	$a_1* a_2$	$\cdots$	$a_1* a_j$	$\cdots$	$a_1* a_n$
a_2	$a_2* a_1$	$a_2* a_2$	$\cdots$	$a_2* a_j$	$\cdots$	$a_2* a_n$
$\vdots$	$\vdots$	$\vdots$	$\vdots$	$\vdots$	$\vdots$	$\vdots$
a_i	$a_i * a_1$	$a_i *a_2$	$\cdots$	$a_i * a_j$	$\cdots$	$a_i* a_n$
$\vdots$	$\vdots$	$\vdots$	$\vdots$	$\vdots$	$\vdots$	$\vdots$
a_n	$a_n * a_1$	$a_n * a_2$	$\cdots$	$a_n * a_j$	$\cdots$	$a_n* a_n$

From above table, we conclude the following properties:

(i) **Closure property:** If all the entries in the table are the elements of S, then S is closed under binary operation '∗'.

(ii) **Commutative property:** If the entries in every row coincide with the corresponding entries in the coerresponding column, we say that the composition is commutative, otherwise it is said to be non-commutative.

(iii) **Existence of identity:** If the row headed by an element a_i of S just coincides with the top row of the table and the column headed by a_i coincides with column on extreme left of the table, then a_j is the identity element of S for the composition '∗'.

(iv) **Existence of inverse:** Look at the position of the identity element e anywhere in the table except in the top row and in the extreme column. If e is placed at the intersection of the row headed by a_i and the column headed by a_j, then a_i and a_j are the inverse of each other.

 Solved Examples

EXAMPLE 1. Let $S = \{1,2,3,4\}$ and '∗' be a binary operation in S defined by $a∗b = r$, where r is the least non-negative remainder when ab is divided by 5. Construct the composition table for '∗' on S.

SOLUTION. We have

$1∗1$ = least non negative remainder, when 1 is divided by $5 = 1$
$2∗3$ = least non-negative remainder, when 6 is divided by $5 = 1$

Similarly,

$1∗2 = 2,$ $1∗3=3,$ $1∗4 = 4,$
$2∗1 = 2,$ $2∗2 =4,$ $2∗3 =1,$ $2∗4 =3,$
$3∗1 = 3,$ $3∗2 =1,$ $3∗3 =4,$ $3∗4 =2,$
$4∗1 =4,$ $4∗2 =3,$ $4∗3=2,$ $4∗4 =1$

Now, we construct the composition tabel for '∗' on S as follows:

∗	1	2	3	4
1	1	2	3	4
2	2	4	1	3
3	3	1	4	2
4	4	3	2	1

From above composition table, we observe that

(i) All the entries in the table are the elements of S, so S is closed under '∗'.

(ii) The binary operation '∗' is commutative on S, as the composition table is symmetrical about the diagonal starting at the upper left corner and ending at the lower right corner.

(iii) 1 is the identity element for '∗' because the row headed by 1 coincides with the top row and the column headed by 1 coincides with extreme left column of the table.

(iv) Every element of S is invertible with respect to '∗' because the identity element 1 appears in each row headed by 2 and column headed by 3, so 2 and 3 are the inverse of each other. Similarly 4 is the inverse of itself.

EXAMPLE 2. *Construct the composition table for the composition of functions, defined on the set $S = \{f_1, f_2, f_3, f_4\}$ of four functions from **C**, the set of all complex numbers to itself, given by*

$$f_1(z) = z, \ f_2(z) = -z, \ f_3(z) = \frac{1}{z} \ and \ f_4(z) = -\frac{1}{z} \ for \ all \ z \in C.$$

SOLUTION. Since each function is defined from **C** to **C**, so $f_1 \circ f_1, f_1 \circ f_2, f_1 \circ f_3, f_1 \circ f_4$ etc, exist.

So,
$$(f_1 \circ f_1)(z) = f_1(f_1(z)) = f_1(z)$$
$$(f_1 \circ f_2)(z) = f_1(f_2(z)) = f_1(-z) = -z = f_2(z)$$
$$(f_1 \circ f_3)(z) = f_1(f_3(z)) = f_1\left(\frac{1}{z}\right) = \frac{1}{z} = f_3(z)$$

$$(f_1 \circ f_4)(z) = f_1(f_4(z)) = f_1\left(-\frac{1}{z}\right) = -\frac{1}{z} = f_4(z)$$

$$(f_2 \circ f_1)(z) = f_2(f_1(z)) = f_2(z) = -z = f_2(z)$$
$$(f_2 \circ f_2)(z) = f_2(f_2(z)) = f_2(-z) = -(-z) = z = f_1(z)$$
$$(f_2 \circ f_3)(z) = f_2(f_3(z)) = f_2(1/z) = -1/z = f_4(z)$$

Similarly, other compositions can be obtained.

Now we construct the composition table for the composition of functions 'o' as follows:

o	f_1	f_2	f_3	f_4
f_1	$f_1 \circ f_1 = f_1$	$f_1 \circ f_2 = f_2$	$f_1 \circ f_3 = f_3$	$f_1 \circ f_4 = f_4$
f_2	$f_2 \circ f_1 = f_2$	$f_2 \circ f_2 = f_1$	$f_2 \circ f_3 = f_4$	$f_2 \circ f_4 = f_3$
f_3	$f_3 \circ f_1 = f_3$	$f_3 \circ f_2 = f_4$	$f_3 \circ f_3 = f_1$	$f_3 \circ f_4 = f_2$
f_4	$f_4 \circ f_1 = f_4$	$f_4 \circ f_2 = f_3$	$f_4 \circ f_3 = f_2$	$f_4 \circ f_4 = f_1$

1.13 BOUNDEDNESS OF A SUBSET OF REAL NUMBERS

1.13.1 UPPER BOUND OF A SUBSET OF R

A subset S of **R** is said to be bounded above, if there exists a real number u such that $s \leq u \ \forall \ s \in S$. The real number u is said to be upper bound of S.

If there exists no such upper bound, then the set is said to be unbounded above.

For Example:
(1) The set of natural number $\mathbf{N} = (1, 2, 3, ...)$ is not bounded above or unbounded above.
(2) The set of positive integers $\mathbf{Z}^+$ is not bounded above.
(3) The set $S = [1, 2, 3, 4]$ is bounded above by 4.
(4) The set $\left[\dfrac{1}{n} : n \in \mathbf{N}\right]$ is bounded above by 1.
(5) The set of negative integers is bounded above by 0.

1.13.2 LOWER BOUND OF A SUBSET OF R

A subset S of **R** is said to be bounded below if there exists a real number l such that $s \geq l \ \forall \ s \in S$. The real number l is said to be the lower bound of S and if there exists no such lower bound, then the set is said to be unbounded below.

For Example :

(1) The set of natural numbers, **N** is bounded below by 1.

(2) The set $\left[\dfrac{1}{n} : n \in \mathbf{N}\right]$ is bounded below by 0.

(3) The set $S = [1, 2, 3, 4]$ is bounded below by 1.

(4) The set of positive real numbers is bounded below.

1.13.3 BOUNDED SET

A subset S of **R** is said to be a bounded if it is bounded below as well as bounded above *i.e.*, if there exist two real numbers l and u such that

$$l \le s \le u, \ \forall \ s \in S.$$

Equivalently, if there exists an interval $I \ (= [l, u])$ such that $S \subseteq I$

For Example :

(1) Every finite set is bounded.

(2) The set $\left[\dfrac{1}{n} : n \in \mathbf{N}\right]$ is bounded.

1.13.4 UNBOUNDED SET

A subset S of **R**, which is not bounded is called an unbounded set.

For Example :

(1) The sets **N, Z, Q, R** are unbounded sets.

(2) Set of all prime numbers is an unbounded set.

☞ **REMARKS**

- If a set is bounded above, then it has infinitely many upper bounds in as much as every number greater than an upper bound is also an upper bound.
- If a set is bounded below, then it has infinitely many lower bounds in as much as every number smaller than a lower bound is also a lower bound.
- It is not necessary that lower bounds and upper bounds of a set S are the members of S.
- The null set ϕ is bounded but it is neither possesses lower bound nor upper bound.

1.14 SUPREMUM AND INFIMUM OF A SET

1.14.1 LEAST UPPER BOUND (OR SUPREMUM)

A real number u is said to be a least upper bound of a set S if

    (i) u is an upper bound of S

and (ii) if u' is an another upper bound of S then $u \le u'$.

i.e., no real number less than u can be an upper bound of S.

1.14.2 GREATEST LOWER BOUND (OR INFIMUM)

A real number l is called a greatest lower bound of a set S if

    (i) l is a lower bound of S

and (ii) if l' is another lower bound of S, then $l' \le l$

i.e., no real number greater then l can be a lower bound of S.

For Example :

If $S = \left[\dfrac{1}{n} : n \in \mathbf{N}\right]$ then $l.u.b. = 1$ and $g.l.b.$ is 0.

☞ **REMARKS**

- If a real number u is the supremum of a subset S of real numbers then, for every $\varepsilon > 0$, there exists a real number $x \in S$ such that $u - \varepsilon < x < u$.
- If a real number is the infimum of a subset S of real numbers then, for every $\varepsilon > 0$, there exists a real number $x \in S$ such that $l \le x < l + \varepsilon$.
- Supremum is defined only for the bounded above sets and infimum for the subset, which are bounded below.
- The supremum and infimum of a set may or may not belong to the set.
- If supremum of a set belongs to the set, then supremun is the largest element of the set.
- If infimum of a set belongs to the set, then infimum is the smallest element of the set.
- Supremum and infinium of a bounded subset of **R**, are unique.
- In case of singleton set $S = [a]$, $a \in \mathbf{R}$, supremum and infimum coincide.
- If u and l are the supremum and infimum of a non-empty subset S of **R**, then $l \le u$.

THEOREM I.

The supremum of a set $S \subset \mathbf{R}$, if exists, is unique.

PROOF.   Let S be a non-empty subset of **R**.

Let if possible, s_1 and s_2 be two supremum of S.

To show $s_1 = s_2$.

Since we assume that s_1 and s_2 are the supremums of S.

$\Rightarrow$ s_1 and s_2 are the upper bounds of S.   ⎯⎯⎯

Let us first suppose s_1 is a supremum and s_2 is an upper bound of S, then

$$s_1 \le s_2.$$ ...(1)

Now, if s_2 is the supremum and s_1 is the upper bound of S, then

$$s_2 \le s_1.$$ ...(2)

From (1) and (2), $s_1 = s_2$.

Hence, supremum of a set, if exists is unique.

THEOREM 2.

The infimum of a set $S \subset \mathbf{R}$, if exists, is unique.

PROOF.   Proof is similar as theorem 1 and left to the reader.

THEOREM 3.

*If S is a non-empty subset of **R**, then a real number s is the supremum of S if and only if*

(i) $x \le s \ \forall \, x \in S$

and (ii) for each positive real number ε, there exists a real number $x \in S$ such that $x > s - \varepsilon$.

PROOF.   **Necessary Condition** (only if part).

Let us first suppose s be the supremum of the set S.

Let s be the supremum of $S \Rightarrow s$ is an upper bound of S.

By definition $x \le s \ \forall \, x \in S$.

Let $\varepsilon > 0$ be any real number. Then obviously $s - \varepsilon < s$

$\Rightarrow$ $(s - \varepsilon)$ is not an upper bound of S.   ($\because s$ is l.u.b. of S.)

Hence, there must exist some $x \in S$ such that $x > s - \varepsilon$.

Sufficient part (If part)

Let us suppose condition (i) and (ii) holds.

Then, to show $s = \sup S$

By condition (i), we have s is an upper bound of S. To show s is the supremum of S, for this, it is enough to show that no real number less than s can be an upper bound of S.

Let s_1 be any real number less than s

$$\Rightarrow s - s_1 > 0.$$

Let us take $\varepsilon = s - s_1$ $\Rightarrow$ $\varepsilon > 0.$

Then by condition (ii), these exists $x \in S$ such that $x > s - \varepsilon$

$\Rightarrow$ $x > s - (s - s') \Rightarrow x > s', x \in S$

$\Rightarrow$ s' is not an upper bound of S.

Hence, we can say that s is an upper bound of S and no real number less than s is an upper bound of S.

$\Rightarrow$ s is the supremum of S.

THEOREM 4.

Let S be a non-empty subset of $\mathbf{R}$, then a real number t is the infimum of S if and only if

(i) $x \geq t$ for all $x \in S$ and

(ii) For each real number $\varepsilon > 0$, there exists a real number $x \in S$ such that $x < t + \varepsilon$.

PROOF.   Proof is similar as theorem 3.

Solved Examples

EXAMPLE 1. *Show that (i) The set $\mathbf{R}^+$ of positive real numbers, is bounded below and unbounded above.*

(ii) The set $\mathbf{R}^-$ of negative real numbers, is bounded above and unbounded below.

SOLUTION. (i) Since every member of $\mathbf{R}^- \cup [0]$ is lower bound of $\mathbf{R}^+$, therefore $\mathbf{R}^+$ is bounded below.

To prove $\mathbf{R}^+$ is unbounded above.

Let if possible, suppose u is an upper bound of $\mathbf{R}^+$ we have $u \geq 1$ for $1 \in \mathbf{R}^+$. Since $2 \in \mathbf{R}^+$, $2 > 0$ and so $u \geq 1$, $2 > 0$ gives $u + 2 > 1 + 0$ i.e., $u + 1 > 0$. Thus $(u + 1) \in \mathbf{R}^+$ and $(u + 1) > u$ which is a contradiction, that u is an upper bound of $\mathbf{R}^+$.

Hence, $\mathbf{R}^+$ is unbounded above.

(ii) Proof follows in a similar manner.

EXAMPLE 2. *Show that the set of real numbers, $\mathbf{R}$ is an unbounded set.*

SOLUTION. From example 1, we conclude that the set $\mathbf{R}^+$ is unbounded above and $\mathbf{R}^-$ is always unbounded below.

Also $$\mathbf{R} = \mathbf{R}^- \cup [0] \cup \mathbf{R}^+$$

$\Rightarrow$ $\mathbf{R}$ is not bounded.

EXAMPLE 3. *Show that the null set ϕ is neither bounded below nor above, nor unbounded.*

SOLUTION. Since, there is no member in ϕ, we cannot check whether a given real number can be a bound for ϕ or not. Thus, bounds for ϕ do not exists. On the other hand we can as well say that every real number is a lower or upper bound for there is no member in ϕ which does not satisfy the required property of bounds.

EXAMPLE 4. *Show that every non-empty finite subset of* **R** *is bounded.*

SOLUTION. Let S be a non-empty finite subset of **R**.

$\Rightarrow$ S contains a finite number of elements. Then by the properties of the ordered relation in **R**, out of these elements, one element $s \in S$, shall be the smallest element of S and another element $b \in S$, shall be the greatest element of S

$\Rightarrow$ $\qquad\qquad a \le x \le b \ \forall x \in S.$

Hence, S is always bounded.

EXAMPLE 5. *Find the supremum and infimum of the set* $S = [x \in Z : x^2 \le 25]$.

SOLUTION. Since $\qquad\qquad S = [x \in \mathbf{Z} : x^2 \le 25]$

$\qquad\qquad\qquad\qquad = [-5, -4, -3, -2, -1, 0, 1, 2, 3, 4, 5].$

Since S is a finite subset of **R**, the smallest member of S is -5, which is a lower bound of S, and hence infimum of S is -5. Similarly 5 is the supremum of S.

EXAMPLE 6. *Find the supremum and infimum, if they exist, of the following sets*

(i) $\left[\dfrac{1}{n} : n \in \mathbf{N} \right]$ (ii) $\left[x \in \mathbf{Q} : x = \dfrac{n}{n+1}, \ n \in \mathbf{N} \right]$

(iii) $\left[1 + \dfrac{(-1)^n}{n} : n \in \mathbf{N} \right]$ (iv) $\left[\pi + \dfrac{1}{2}, \ \pi + \dfrac{1}{4}, \ \pi + \dfrac{1}{8}, \dots \right]$

SOLUTION. (i) Here we have

$$S = \left[\frac{1}{n} : n \in \mathbf{N} \right] = \left[1, \frac{1}{2}, \frac{1}{3}, \dots \right].$$

The set S is bounded above by 1, also any member less than 1 is not an upper bound of S, therefore $\sup S = 1$.

Also, 0 is a lower bound of S, because $x \ge 0, \ \forall \ x \in S$. Let l be any arbitrary positive small number, then there exists $n \in \mathbf{N}$ such that $\dfrac{1}{n} < l$, which shows that l is not an upper bound of S. Thus 0 is a lower bound of S and no other positive real number is a lower bound of S. Therefore, infimum of $S = 0 \notin S$.

(ii) Let $\qquad\qquad S = \left[\dfrac{n}{n+1} : n \in \mathbf{N} \right] = \left[\dfrac{1}{2}, \dfrac{2}{3}, \dfrac{3}{4}, \dots \right]$

Then, the set S is bounded below by $\dfrac{1}{2}$ and any number greater than $\dfrac{1}{2}$ can not be a lower bound of S, therefore infimum of $S = \dfrac{1}{2}$.

Also, $\left(\dfrac{n}{n+1} \right) < 1, \ \forall \ n \in \mathbf{N}$, therefore 1 is an upper bound of S, and any number less than 1 not be a upper bound of S.

Therefore supremum of $S = 1$.

(iii) Let $\qquad\qquad S = \left[1 + \dfrac{(-1)^n}{n} : n \in \mathbf{N} \right] = \left[0, \dfrac{3}{2}, \dfrac{2}{3}, \dfrac{5}{4}, \dfrac{4}{5}, \dfrac{7}{6}, \dfrac{6}{7}, \dots \right]$

$$= \left[\frac{0}{1}, \frac{2}{3}, \frac{4}{5}, \frac{6}{7}, \frac{8}{9}, \dots, \frac{2n-2}{2n-1} \right] \cup \left[\frac{3}{2}, \frac{5}{4}, \frac{7}{6}, \frac{9}{8}, \dots, \frac{2n+1}{2n} \right].$$

Here, the proper fraction $\frac{0}{1}, \frac{2}{3}, \frac{4}{5}, \frac{6}{7},...$ are increasing and tending to 1, and

the improper fractions begin with $\frac{3}{2}$ are decreasing and tending to 1.

Therefore, infimum of $S = 0$ and supremum of $S = \frac{3}{2}$.

(iv) Let $S = \left[\pi + \frac{1}{2}, \pi + \frac{1}{4}, \pi + \frac{1}{8},... \right]$.

Here, we have $x \le \pi + \frac{1}{2} \ \forall \ x \in S$

$\Rightarrow \quad \pi + \frac{1}{2}$ is an upper bound for S.

Since, $\pi + \frac{1}{2} \in S$, therefore no real number less than $\pi + \frac{1}{2}$ can be upper

bound for S. Thus, $\pi + \frac{1}{2}$ is the least upper bound. Therefore, supremum of

$S = \pi + \frac{1}{2}$.

Similarly, we can show that π is the infimum of S.

Exercise 1.2

1. Find the supremum and infimum, if exist of the following sets.

(i) $\left[\frac{1}{5n} : n \in Z, n \ne 0 \right]$

(ii) $\left[x : x = 1 + \frac{1}{n} : n \in N \right]$

(iii) $[x \in R : x = 2^n : n \in N]$

(iv) $[3, 8, 14, 20]$

(v) $\left[-\frac{1}{n} : n \in N \right]$

(vi) $\left[m + \frac{1}{n} : m, n \in N \right]$

(vii) $\left[x \in Q : x = \frac{(-1)^n}{n} : n \in N \right]$

(viii) $S = \left[\left(1 - \frac{1}{n} \right) \sin \frac{n\pi}{2} : n \in N \right]$

(ix) $\left[x = (-1)^n \left(\frac{1}{4} - \frac{4}{n} \right) : n \in N \right]$

2. Find the supremum and infimum of the set
$S = \left[\frac{2n+1}{3n+3} : n \in N \right]$.

3. Prove that every subset of a bounded above (below or both) set is bounded above (below

or both).

4. If A and B are subsets of R, then prove that the set $A + B = [x + y : x \in A, y \in B]$ is also bounded and
   $$\inf (A + B) = \inf (A) + \inf (B).$$

5. If $A \ne \phi$ is bounded below and $-A$ denotes the set of all $-x$ for which $x \in A$, then prove that $-A \ne \phi$, that $-A$ is bounded above and that $-\sup(-A) = \inf (A)$.

6. If $A \ne \phi$, $B \ne \phi$ and $x \le y \ \forall \ x \in A$ and $y \in B$, then show that
   (i) sup $A \le y \ \forall \ y \in B$
   (ii) sup $(A) \le \inf (B)$.

7. If $A \subseteq B$ and B is bounded, then show that
   $$\sup B \ge \sup A \ge \inf A \ge \inf B.$$

8. If A and B are two bounded subset of R, then $A \cup B$ and $A \cap B$ ($\ne \phi$) are also bounded and
   (i) sup $(A \cup B) = \max (\sup A, \sup B)$
   (ii) inf $(A \cup B) = \min (\inf A, \inf B)$
   (iii) sup $(A \cap B) = \min(\sup A, \sup B)$
   (iv) inf $(A \cap B) = \max (\inf A, \inf B)$.

9. Give an example of a set in which supremum is equal to infimum.

10. Show that the set $[x : x \in Q, x > 0$ and $x^2 < 3]$ does not have any supremum in Q.

11. For a real number λ and a subset A of $\mathbf{R}$, let λA be the set defined by $\lambda A = [\lambda x : x \in A]$. Prove that if A is bounded, then λA is also bounded and

$$\inf(\lambda A) = \begin{cases} \lambda \inf(A) & \text{if } \lambda \geq 0 \\ \lambda \sup(A) & \text{if } \lambda \leq 0. \end{cases}$$

12. Give an example of a set which is
    (i) bounded above but not below.
    (ii) bounded below but not above.
    (iii) neither bounded above nor bounded below.
    (iv) both bounded above and below.

13. Find the supremum and infinium of the sets

(i) $S = [x \in \mathbf{Z} : x^2 \leq 16]$

(ii) $S = \left\{ 2 + \dfrac{1}{n} : n \in \mathbf{N} \right\}$

14. Check the boundedness of the following sets:
    (i) $[-1, -2, -3, ...]$
    (ii) $[1, 2, 3, 4, 5, ...]$
    (iii) $[2, 2^2, 2^3, ..., 2^n, ...]$
    (iv) $\left[1, \dfrac{1}{4}, \left(\dfrac{1}{4}\right)^2, \left(\dfrac{1}{4}\right)^3, ..., \left(\dfrac{1}{4}\right)^n, ... \right]$
    (v) $\left[x : x = (-1)^n \dfrac{1}{n} : n \in \mathbf{N} \right]$
    (vi) $[x : x = (-2)^n : n \in \mathbf{N}]$

ANSWERS

1. (i) $\inf = -\dfrac{1}{5}$, $\sup = \dfrac{1}{5}$ (ii) $\sup = 2$, $\inf = 1$ (iii) $\inf = 2$, sup, does not exist (iv) $\inf = 3$, $\sup = 20$
   (v) $\sup = 0$, $\inf = -1$ (vi) $\inf = 1$, sup, does not exist (vii) $\inf = -1$, $\sup = 1/2$
   (viii) $\inf = -1$, $\sup = 1$ (ix) $\sup = 15/4$, $\inf = -7/4$

2. $\sup = \dfrac{2}{3}$, $\inf = \dfrac{3}{5}$

9. Singlton set 12. (i) $[-1, -2, -3, ...]$ (ii) N (iii) Z, Q or R (iv) Any finite set.

14. (i) Bounded above but not below   (ii) Bounded below but not above
    (iii) Bounded below but not above   (iv) Bounded below and above, both
    (v) Bounded below and above both   (vi) Neither bounded below nor above.

1.15 SEQUENCES

Let N be the set of natural numbers and S be any set of real numbers. A function, whose domain is the set of natural numbers and range is a subset of S, is called a sequence in S.

Symbolically. If we define a function $f : N \to S$, then f is a sequence. We shall denote a sequence in a number of ways as follows :

(i) Usually, a sequence is denoted by its images. For a sequence f, the image corresponding to $n \in N$ is denoted by f_n or $<f(n)>$ and $f(n)$ is called the nth term of the given sequence. For example $<1, 4, 9, ...>$ is the sequence whose n^{th} term is n^2.

(ii) Using in order, the first few element of a sequence, here the rule for writing down different elements becomes clear. For example, $<1, 2, 3, ...>$ is the sequence whose n^{th} term is n.

(iii) Defining a sequence by a recurrence formula, i.e., by a rule which express the nth term by $(n-1)^{\text{th}}$ term. For example, let $a_1 = 1, a_{n+1} = 2a_n \quad \forall n \geq 1$.

These above relations define a sequence whose n^{th} term is 2^{n-1}.

☞ REMARKS
- A sequence is represented as $<s_n>$ or $\{s_n\}$, when s_n is the nth term of the sequence. The set of all distinct terms of a sequence is called the range set of that sequence.
- A sequence, whose range is a subset of real numbers R is called a real sequence or a sequence of real numbers.

1.15.1 CONSTANT SEQUENCES

A sequence $<s_n>$ defined by $s_n = a,\ \forall n \in N$, is called a constant sequence.

1.15.2 EQUALITY OF SEQUENCES

Two sequence $<s_n>$ and $<t_n>$ are said to be equal, if $s_n = t_n\ \forall n \in N$.

1.15.3 OPERATION ON SEQUENCES

Since, the sequence are real valued functions, therefore, the sum, difference, product etc. of two sequence are defined as follows :

(i) If $<s_n>$ and $<t_n>$ be any two sequences, then the sequence, whose n^{th} terms are $s_n + t_n,\ s_n - t_n$ and $s_n.t_n$ are respectively known as the sum, difference and product of the sequence $<s_n>$ and $<t_n>$ and are denoted by $<s_n + t_n>, <s_n - t_n>$ and $<s_n.t_n>$ respectively.

(ii) If $s_n \neq 0\ \forall n \in N$, then the sequence, whose n^{th} term is $\dfrac{1}{s_n}$ is called reciprocal of the sequence $<s_n>$ and is denoted by $<\dfrac{1}{s_n}>$.

(iii) The sequence, whose n^{th} term $s_n / t_n (t_n \neq 0\ \ \forall n \in N)$ is known as the quotient of the sequence $<s_n>$ by the sequence $<t_n>$ and is denoted by $<\dfrac{s_n}{t_n}>$.

(iv) The sequence, whose n^{th} term is ks_n, where $k \in R$ is known as the scalar multiple of the sequence $<s_n>$ by k and is denoted by $<ks_n>$.

1.15.4 BOUNDED SEQUENCE

(i) Bounded below sequence. A sequence $<s_n>$ is said to be bounded below if there exists a real number l such that $s_n \geq l\ \ \forall n \in N$.

The number l is known as the lower bound of the sequence $<s_n>$.

(ii) Bounded above sequence. A sequence $<s_n>$ is said to be bounded above if there exists a real number u such that
$$s_n \leq u\ \ \forall n \in N.$$
The number u is said to be upper bound of the sequence $<s_n>$.

(iii) Bounded sequence. A sequence $<s_n>$ is said to be bounded if it is bounded above as well as bounded below.

(iv) Unbounded sequence. A sequence $<s_n>$ is said to be unbounded if it is not bounded.

(v) Least upper bound. If a sequence $<s_n>$ is bounded above, then there exists a number u_1 such that
$$s_n \leq u_1\ \ \forall n \in N. \hspace{2cm} ...(1)$$
This number u_1 is called an upper bound of the sequence $<s_n>$. If $u_1 < u_2$. Then from (1), we find that
$$s_n < u_2\ \ \forall n \in N$$
which implies, u_2 is also an upper bound of the sequence $<s_n>$. Hence, we can say that any number greater than u_1 is an upper bound of $<s_n>$.

Hence, a sequence has an infinite number of upper bounds, if it is bounded above. Let u be the least of all the upper bound of the sequence $<s_n>$. Then u is defined as the least upper bound (l.u.b) or supremum of the sequence $<s_n>$.

(vi) Greatest lower bound. If a sequence $< s_n >$ is bounded below, then there exists a number $l_1 \in \mathbf{R}$ such that

$$l_1 \le s_n \quad \forall n \in \mathbf{N} \qquad\qquad …(2)$$

This number l_1 is known as the lower bound of $< s_n >$. If $l_2 < l_1$, then from (2)

$$l_2 \le s_n \quad \forall n \in \mathbf{N}$$

which implies, l_2 is also a lower bound of the sequence $< s_n >$. Hence, we can say that any number less than l_1 is a lower bound of $< s_n >$.

Hence, a sequence has infinite number of lower bounds, if it is bounded below. Let l be the greatest of all the lower bounds of the sequence $< s_n >$. Then l is known as greatest lower bound (*g.l.b*) or infimum of the sequence $< s_n >$.

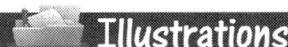 **Illustrations**

✦ The sequence $<n^2>$ is bounded below by 1 but not bounded above.

✦ The sequence $<\dfrac{n}{n+1}>$ is bounded as

$$\frac{1}{2} \le \frac{n}{n+1} < 1 \quad \forall n \in N.$$

✦ The sequence $<\dfrac{1}{n}>$ is bounded since $\left|\dfrac{1}{n}\right| \le 1 \ \forall n \in N$.

✦ The sequence $<2^n>$ is bounded below and has smallest term as 2. Every member of $]-\infty\ 2]$ is a lower bound of the sequence and the sequence is not bounded above.

1.15.5 LIMIT POINT OF THE SEQUENCE

A real number l is called a limit point of a sequence $< s_n >$ if every nbd of l contains infinite number of terms of the sequence.

Thus, $l \in \mathbf{R}$ is a limit point of the sequence $< s_n >$ if for given $\varepsilon > 0, s_n \in \ ]l-\varepsilon, l+\varepsilon]$ for infinitely many points.

Here it must be noted that

(i) limit point of a sequence need not be a member of the sequence.

(ii) A limit point of a sequence may or may not be a limit point of the range of the sequence but the limit point of the range of a sequence is always a limit point of the sequence.

(iii) In case of real numbers, limit points of a sequence may also be called accumulation, cluster or condensation points.

Illustrations

✦ The sequence $<\dfrac{1}{n}>$ has one limit point, *i.e.*, 0.

✦ The sequence $<(-1)^n>$ has two limit points 1 and –1.

✦ The sequence $<n>$ has no limit point.

✦ The sequence $<1+\dfrac{(-1)^n}{n}>$ has one limit point, *i.e.*, 1.

1.15.6 SUFFICIENT CONDITIONS FOR NUMBER l TO BE OR NOT BE A LIMIT POINT OF THE SEQUENCE $<s_n>$

(i) If for every $\varepsilon > 0, \exists m \in \mathbf{N}$ such that $s_n \in \ ]l-\varepsilon, l+\varepsilon[\ \forall n \ge m$ or equivalently $|s_n - l| < \varepsilon \ \forall n \ge m$, then l is the limit point of the sequence $< s_n >$.

(ii) If for any $\varepsilon = 0, s_n \in \ ]l-\varepsilon, l+\varepsilon[$ for only a finite number of values of n, then l is not a limit point of the sequence $< s_n >$. Such a condition is also necessary for a number l not to be limit point of the sequence $< s_n >$.

1.15.7 BOLZANO-WEIRSTRASS THEOREM FOR SEQUENCE

[KANPUR–2000]

Statement. *Every bounded sequence has at least one limit point.*

Proof. Let $S = \{s_n : n \in N\}$ be the range set of the bounded sequence $< s_n >$.

Then, S is a bounded set. Now, there may be two cases :

(i) Let S be a finite set. Then $s_n = p$ for infinitely many indices n. Here $p \in R$. Obviously p is a limit point of $< s_n >$.

(ii) Let S be an infinite set. Since, S is bounded, then by Bolzano-Weirstrass theorem for set of real numbers, S has a limit point say p. Therefore, every nbd of p contains infinity many distinct points of S, *i.e.*, infinitely many term of $< s_n >$ and hence p is a limit point of the sequence $< s_n >$.

1.15.8 LIMIT SUPERIOR AND LIMIT INFERIOR

The greatest limit point of a bounded sequence is called the upper limit or limit superior and is denoted by $\overline{\lim} \ s_n$ and the smallest limit point of a bounded sequence is called the lower limit or limit inferior and is denoted by $\underline{\lim} \ s_n$

- By definition, it is obvious that $\underline{\lim} \ s_n \leq \overline{\lim} \ s_n$.
- A bounded sequence $< s_n >$ for which the upper limit and lower limit coincide with real number l is said to converge to l.

1.15.9 LIMIT OF A SEQUENCE

A sequence $< s_n >$ is said to have a limit l if for a given $\epsilon > 0$ $\exists$ a positive integer m such that

$$\left| s_n - l \right| < \epsilon \quad \forall n \geq m$$

1.15.10 CONVERGENT SEQUENCE

A sequence $< s_n >$ is said to converge to a number l, if for a given $\epsilon > 0$ there exists a positive integer m such that

$$\left| s_n - l \right| < \epsilon \quad \forall n \geq m$$

☛ REMARK

- A sequence $<s_n>$ is said to be convergent iff it is bounded and has exactly one limit point.

1.15.11 DIVERGENT SEQUENCE

A sequence, which is not convergent, is known as divergent sequence.

1.15.12 OSCILLATORY SEQUENCE

A sequence $< s_n >$ is said to be an oscillatory sequence if it is neither convergent nor divergent.

An oscillatory sequence is said to be oscillate finitely or infinitely according as it is bounded or unbounded.

In other words, we can say

(i) a bounded sequence, which is not convergent is said to be oscillate finitely.

(ii) an unbounded sequence, which does not diverge, is said to be oscillate infinitely.

(iii) a bounded sequence, which does not converge and has at least two limit points is said to be oscillate finitely.

Illustrations

+ The sequence $\langle 1+(-1)^n \rangle$ oscillate finitely.

+ The sequence $\langle (-1)^n \rangle$ oscillate finitely.

+ The sequence $< (-1)^n \left(1+\dfrac{1}{n}\right) >$ oscillate finitely.

+ The sequence $<n(-1)^n>$ oscillate infinitely.

1.16 BASIC CONCEPTS OF TOPOLOGY

1.16.1 TOPOLOGICAL SPACES

Let $X \ne \phi$ and ζ be the collection of all those subsets of X which satisfy the following three conditions :

   (i) $\phi \in \zeta$, $X \in \zeta$

   (ii) If $G_1 \in \zeta$ and $G_2 \in \zeta$, then $G_1 \cap G_2 \in \zeta$.

   (iii) If $\{G_\lambda : \lambda \in \Delta\} \in \zeta$, then $\bigcup_{\lambda \in \Delta} [G_\lambda] \in \zeta$

Then ζ is called a topology on X and (X, ζ) is called a topological space.

1.16.2 TYPES OF TOPOLOGIES

   (i) Stronger and Weaker Topologies. Let ζ_1 and ζ_2 be two topologies defined on X. If $\zeta_1 \subset \zeta_2$, then ζ_1 is said to be coarser or weaker or smaller than ζ_2 and ζ_2 is said to be finer or stronger or larger than ζ_1.

   (ii) Discrete Topology. Given a non-empty set X and D be a family of all subset of X so that (X, D) is a topological space, D is called the discrete topology for X.

  (iii) Indiscrete Topology. For $X \ne \phi$ and $I = \{\phi, X\}$, I is said to be the indiscrete topology for X and (X, I) is called indiscrete topological space.

  (iv) Non-trivial Topology. A topology defined on X other than the two trivial topologies is said to be non-trivial topology.

   (v) Usual Topology. If U be the family of subsets of **R** (set of real numbers) defined such that a subset $a < r < b$ and $[\, x : x \in \mathbf{R}, a < x < b\,] \subset A$, then U is called a usual topology.

  (vi) Cofinite or Finite Compliment Topology. Given a non-empty set X, if ζ is the family of subset of X defined such that a subset A of $X \in \zeta \Leftrightarrow A = \phi$ or $X - A = A'$ is finite, then the topology is known as cofinite topology.

1.16.3 PRODUCT AND QUOTIENT SPACES

   (1) If (X_1, ζ_1) and (X_2, ζ_2) be two topological spaces and we define

$$X = X_1 \times X_2$$

and

$$\beta = (G_1 \times G_2 : G_1 \in \zeta_1, G_2 \in \zeta_2)$$

such that β is a base for same topology ζ on X, then ζ is said to be the product topology and (X, ζ) is known as product of topological spaces.

   (2) If (X, ζ) be a topological space, Y is a set and f is a mapping of X and Y, then the largest topology say ζ^* for Y such that $\zeta \to \zeta^*$ is continuous is said to be quotient topology for Y relative to f and T.

1.17 COMPACTNESS

1.17.1 COVER

Let (X, ζ) be a topological space and $A \subset X$, then a class $C^* = [G_i : i \in \Delta]$ of subset of X is said to be the cover or covering of A if and only if $A \subset \bigcup_i G_i$ or $A \subset \bigcup [G_i : i \in X]$

1.17.2 OPEN COVER

If each G_i is open, then the cover defined above is called an open cover, *i.e.*, X is said to be an open cover if each $x \in A \subset X$ there exists at least one G_i, *i.e.*, $\bigcup G_i = A$ such that $x \in G_i$.

1.17.3 SUB COVER

A subclass of an open cover which is itself an open cover is said to be a subcover.

1.18 CONNECTEDNESS

1.18.1 SEPARATED SETS

Let (X, ζ) be a topological space. Two non-empty subsets A and B of X are said to be separated if and only if

$$A \cap \bar{B} = \phi \quad \text{and} \quad \bar{A} \cap B = \phi$$

or equivalently

$$(A \cap \bar{B}) \cup (\bar{A} \cap B) = \phi$$

Therefore, A and B are separated if and only if A and B are disjoint and neither of them contains limit point of the other.

☞ REMARK
- Any two separated sets are disjoint. But two disjoint sets are not necessarily separated.

1.18.2 CONNECTED AND DISCONNECTED SETS

Let (X, ζ) be a topological space. A subset A of X is said to be disconnected iff it is the union of two non-empty separated sets, *i.e.*, if there exist two non-empty sets C and D such that $C \cap \bar{D} = \phi$, $\bar{C} \cap D = \phi$ and $A = C \cup D$.

☞ REMARK
- A is said to be connected if and only if it is not disconnected.

1.18.3 GENERAL RESULTS (TO BE USED DIRECTLY)

(1) A topological space X is disconnected if and only if there exists a non-empty proper subset of X which is both open and closed in X.

(2) A topological space X is connected if and only if every non-empty proper subset of X has a non-empty frontier.

(3) If connected subset E of X such that $E \subset A \cup B$, where A and B are separated sets. Then either $E \subset A$ or $E \subset B$, *i.e.*, E can not intersect both A and B.

(4) Let E be a connected subset of X. If F is a subset of X such that $E \subset F \subset \bar{E}$, then F is connected. In particular $\bar{E}$ is connected.

(5) A subset E of R is connected if and only if it is an interval.

(6) Continuous image of a connected space is connected.

(7) A topological space X is disconnected iff there exists a continuous mapping of X onto the discrete two point space $[0, 1]$.

(8) A maximal connected subset of a topological space X is called a component of a space.

(9) A topological space X is said to be locally connected at a point x iff every open neighbourhood of x contains a connected open neighbourhood of x.

(10) A topological space X is locally connected if and only if the components of every open subset of X are open in X.

(11) The image of a locally connected space under a mapping which is both continuous and open is locally connected.

1.18.4 SUMMARY OF RESULTS ON COMPACTNESS (TO BE USED DIRECTLY)

(1) Every compact subset A of a T_2-space X is closed.

(2) Closed subsets of compact sets are compact.

(3) A topological space X is compact if and only if every basic open cover of X has a finite subcover.

(4) A topological space X is compact iff every collection of closed subsets of X with the finite intersection property is fixed, *i.e.*, has a non-empty intersection.

(5) Every compact space has Bolzano Weirstrass property.

(6) A subset A of R is compact if and only if A is bounded and closed (Heine-Borel Theorem).

(7) A topological space X is said to be countably compact iff every countable open cover of X has a finite subcover.

(8) A topological space X is said to be locally compact if and only if every point in X has at least one neighbourhood whose closure is compact.

(9) A T_2-space is locally compact if and only if each of its points is an interior point of some compact subspace of X.

(10) In a T_2-space, any locally compact subspace A is the intersection of an open set and a closed set and that in a locally compact space X, the intersection of an open set and a closed set is a locally compact subspace of X.

(11) The intersection of two locally compact subsets of X is locally compact.

(12) Let f be a continuous mapping of a compact topological space X into a topological space Y. Then $f(X)$ is compact, *i.e.*, continuous image of a compact space is compact.

Exercise 1.3

1. Let $A = \{-2, -1, 0, 1, 2\}$ and $f : A \rightarrow Z$ given by $f(x) = x^2 - 2x - 3$. Find :
   (i) the range of f,
   (ii) pre-image of 6, –3 and 5.

2. Find the domain and range of the following function $f(x) = \sqrt{(x-1)(3-x)}$

3. Find the range of the following function $f(x) = \dfrac{1}{(2x-3)(x+1)}$

4. Find the domain and range of the following functions :

   (i) $f(x) = \dfrac{x^2 - 1}{x - 1}$ (ii) $y = -|x|$

   (iii) $f(x) = \dfrac{|x-1|}{x-1}$ (iv) $y = \sqrt{x-3}$

5. If $A = \{-1, 0, 2, 5, 6, 11\}$, $B = \{-2, -1, 0, 18, 25, 108\}$ and $f(x) = x^2 - x - 2$, find $f(A)$.

6. Let A be the set of two positive integers. Let $f : A \rightarrow Z^+$, set of positive integers be defined by $f(n) = p$, where p is the highest prime factor of n. If range of $f = \{3\}$, find A.

7. Find the domain for which the function $f(x) = 2x^2 - 1$ and $g(x) = 1 - 3x$ are equal.

8. Let $f_1 : R \to R$ and $f_2 : C \to C$ be two functions defined as $f_1(x) = x^3$ and $f_2(x) = x^3$. Show that they are not equal.

9. Let $A = \{p, q, r, s\}$ and $B = \{1, 2, 3\}$. Which of the following relations from A to B not a function?

  (i) $R_1 = \{(p, 1), (q, 2), (r, 1), (s, 2)\}$
  (ii) $R_2 = \{(p, 1), (q, 1), (r, 1), (s, 1)\}$
  (iii) $R_3 = \{(p, 1), (q, 2), (r, 2), (s, 3)\}$
  (iv) $R_4 = \{(p, 2), (q, 3), (r, 2), (s, 2)\}$

10. Write the following relations as sets of ordered pairs and find which of them are functions :

  (i) $\{(x, y) : y = 3x, x \in (1, 2, 3), y \in (3, 6, 9, 12)\}$
  (ii) $\{(x, y) : y > x + 1, x = 1, 2 \text{ and } y = 2, 4, 6\}$
  (iii) $\{(x, y) : x + y = 3 \ x, y \in (0, 1, 2, 3)\}$

11. Express the following functions as sets of ordered pairs, and find their range :

  (i) $f_1 : A \to R : f_1(x) = x^2 + 1$
  where $A = \{-1, 0, 2, 4\}$
  (ii) $f_2 : A \to N : f_2(x) = 2x$
  where $A = \{x : x \in N, x \le 10\}$

12. Let $f : R \to R$ be a function such that $f(x) = 2^x$. Determine :

  (i) range of f (ii) $\{x : f(x) = 1\}$
  (iii) whether $f(x + y) = f(x) \cdot f(y)$ holds

13. Let $f : R^+ \to R$, be a function such that $f(x) = \log x$. Determine :

  (i) the image set of domain of f
  (ii) $\{x : f(x) = -2\}$
  (iii) whether $f(xy) = f(x) + f(y)$ holds

14. Give an example of a map which is :

  (i) one-to-one but not onto
  (ii) not one to one, but onto
  (iii) neither one-to-one nor onto

ANSWERS

1. (i) $f(A) = \{-4, -3, 0, 5\}$, (ii) ϕ, $\{1, 2\}$, -2 **2.** Domain $= [1, 3]$, Range $= [-1, 1]$

3. $\left]-\infty, \dfrac{-8}{25}\right] \cup [0, \infty[$

4. (i) $R - \{1\}$, $R - \{2\}$, (ii) $R : R - R^+$, (iii) $R - \{1\}$, $\{-1, 1\}$, (iv) $[3, \infty[$, $[0, \infty]$

5. $f(A) = \{1, -2, 18, 28, 108\}$ **6.** $A = \{3, 6\}$ or $(3, 9)$ or $[3, 12]$ etc. **7.** $(-2, 1/2)$ **9.** (iii)

10. (i) $\{(1, 3), (2, 6), (3, 9)\}$, function, (ii) $\{(1, 4), (1, 6), (3, 4), (3, 6)\}$, not function
  (iii) $\{(0, 3), (1, 2), (2, 1), (3, 0)\}$, function

11. (i) $f_1 = \{x, f(x) : x \in A\} = \{(-1, 2), (0, 1), (2, 5), (4, 17)\}$
  (ii) $f_2 = \{(x, g(x)) : x \in A\} = \{(1,2),(2,4), (3, 6), ..., (10, 20)\}$

12. (i) Range of $f = R^+$, the set of positive real numbers, (ii) $(x : f(x) = 1) = \{0\}$,
  (iii) $f(x+y) = f(x) \cdot f(y)$ holds for all $x, y \in R$

14. (i) $n \to n^2 : N \to N$ (ii) $n \to |n| : Z \to N \cup \{0\}$ (iii) $n \to |n|^2 : Z \to N \cup \{0\}$

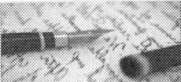
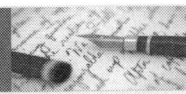

CHAPTER Summary

KEY TERMS

- **RELATION:** Let A and B be two sets, then a relation R from A to B is a subset of $A \times B$.
- **SEQUENCE :** A function whose domain is the set of natural numbers and range is the subset of real numbers is called sequence.
- **CONVERGENT SEQUENCE :** A sequence $<s_n>$ is said to be convergent if its limit exists.
- **METRIC SPACE :** Let $X \neq \phi$. Then a mapping $\phi : X \times X \to R^+ \cup \{0\}$ is said to be metric if
  (i) $d(x, y) \geq 0 \ \forall \ x, y \in X$
  (ii) $d(x, y) = d(y, x) \ \forall \ x, y \in X$
  (iii) $d(x, y) = 0 \Leftrightarrow x = y \ \forall \ x, y \in X$
  (iv) $d(x, y) \leq d(x, z) + d(z, y) \ \forall \ x, y, z \in X$

- **COMPLETE METRIC SPACE :** A metric space (X, d) is said to be complete if every Cauchy sequence in X is convergent.
- **TOPOLOGY :** Let $X \neq \phi$ and ζ be the collection of all those subsets of X which satisfy the following three conditions :
  (i) $\phi \in \zeta, \ X \in \zeta$
  (ii) If $G_1 \in \zeta$ and $G_2 \in \zeta$, then $G_1 \cap G_1 \in \zeta$
  (iii) If $\{G_\lambda : \lambda \in \Delta\} \in \zeta$, then $\bigcup_{\lambda \in \Delta} [G_\lambda] \in \zeta$

  Then ζ is called a topology on X and (X, ζ) is called a topological space.

RESULTS

- If R is a relation from A to B, then A is called the domain and B the range of R.
- If R is a relation from a non-empty set A to a non-empty set B and if $(a, b) \in R$, then we write aRb, read as "a is related to b by the relation R." On the other hand, if $(a, b) \notin R$, we write $a\cancel{R}b$ and say that 'a is not related to b by the relation R'.
- Any subset $A \times A$ defined on a relation in A, known as Binary relation.
- For a non-empty set A, $\phi \in A \times A$, therefore it is a relation on A, called void or empty relation on A.
- The void relation ϕ and the universal relation $A \times B$ are called trivial relations from A to B.
- The void and universal relation on set A respectively the smallest and the largest relation on A.
- Sometimes, the inverse of a relation coincides with the relation itself.
- The identity relation R on a set A is an anti – symmetric relation.
- If $(x, y) \in R$ and $(y, x) \notin R$, then it may be noted that $x = y$.
- The universal relation on a set A containing at least two elements is not anti – symmetric.
- $R_1 o R_2 \neq R_2 o R_1$
- $(R_2 o R_1)^{-1} = R_1^{-1} o R_2^{-1}$
- The intersection of two equivalence relations on a set is an equivalence relation.
- The union of two equivalence relations on a set is not necessarily an equivalence relation.
- If R is an equivalence relation, then R^{-1} is also an equivalence relation.
- Every subset of a well ordered set is well ordered.
- A well ordered set can not be similar to one of its initial segment.
- Every set of ordinal numbers is a well ordered set.
- If $f : A \to B$ then a single element in A cannot have more than one image in B. However, two or more elements in A may have the same image in B.
- Every element in A must have its image in B, but every element in B may not have it pre-image in A.
- To each element x in A, there exists a unique element y in B such that $y = f(x)$.
- The unique element y of B is called the value of f at x (the image of f under x), and written as $y = f(x)$.
- The range of f consist of those elements in B which appear as the image of at least one element in A.
- Range of a function is the image of its domain.
- Range is a subset of co-domain.
- One-many function does not exist.
- In an onto function, Range = Co-domain
- Onto function is also called surjective.
- In an into function, Range $\subset$ Co-domain.
  One-one onto mapping is also known as bijective or one-to-one.

- For a one-one onto function
  Range = Co-domain, and $x_1 \neq x_2 \Rightarrow f(x_1) \neq f(x_2)$
  or $f(x_1) = f(x_2) \Rightarrow x_1 = x_2$
- A binary operation combines any two elements a and b of a set to give another element of the same set, this fact is also known as closure property or we can say that the set is closed with respect to binary operation.
- Binary operation is never one-one.
- '0' is an identity element for addition on N.
- Let $(S, *)$ be an algebraic structure. If S has the identity element for '$*$', then it is unique.
- Let $(S, *)$ be algebraic structure with identity element e. Then every element $a \in S$ has unique inverse in S, if '$*$' is associative.
- Let $(S, *)$ be an algebraic structure and '$*$' be an associative binary operation of S. If a be an invertible element of S, then $(a^{-1})^{-1} = a$.

- For identity element e, we have $e = e^{-1}$.
- Let $(S, *)$ be an algebraic structure and $*$ be an associative binary operation on S. If each element of S has inverse in S. Then $(a * b)^{-1} = b^{-1} * a^{-1}$.
- A sequence is represented as $<s_n>$ or $\{s_n\}$, when s_n is the nth term of the sequence.
- The set of all distinct terms of a sequence is called the range set of that sequence.
- A sequence, whose range is a subset of real number R is called a real sequence or a sequence of real numbers.
- A sequence $<s_n>$ is said to be convergent iff it is bounded and has exactly one limit point.
- Any two separated sets are disjoint. But two disjoint sets are not necessarily separated.
- A is said to be connected if and only if it is not disconnected.

➤ WORTHY READINGS

☞ The number of distinct elements contained in a finite set is called its cardinality.

☞ The void and universal relation on the set A are respectively the smallest and largest relation.

☞ The universal relation on a set A, containing at least two elements is not anti symmetric.

☞ Range is a subset of codomain.

☞ A sequence whose range is a subset of R, is called real sequence.

☞ Limit point of a sequence may or may not be a limit point of the range of a sequence is always a limit point of the sequence.

☞ An oscillatory sequence is said to be oscillatory finitely or infinitely according as it is bounded or unbounded.

➤ FURTHER READINGS

☞ It is quite possible that the set of points of a sequence may have a limit point, but can not have a limit.

☞ Compact subsets of a metric space are closed.

☞ Closed subsets of compact sets are compact.

☞ The intersection of two locally compact subsets of X is locally compact.

☞ Any open subspace of a separable space is separable.

☞ The sum of a unifomly convergent series

of real valued continuous function is continuous.

☞ If f and g are real valued continuous function then $f \cup g$ and $f \cap g$ are continuous.

☞ The limit superior, limit inferior and limit (if exists) of a sequence of sets are unaltered if a finite number of terms of the sequence are changed.

☞ If $<E_n>$ is a decreasing sequence then $\lim\limits_{n \to \infty} E_n = 0$.

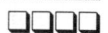

Chapter
2 Countability

2.1 INTRODUCTION

In the previous classes, we have studied about the set and the number of elements in the given set. The number of elements of a set may be finite or infinite. For equality of two sets, they must have the same number of elements. In a finite set, we may count the number of elements, but in case of infinite set, we should know the definition of the sets.

SOME GENERAL DEFINITIONS

(1) **Finite set:** A set consisting of a finite number of elements is called a finite set.

For example $\{1, 2, 3\}$, $\{a, b, c, d\}$, $\{a_1, a_2, ..., a_3\}$ all are finite sets.

(2) **Infinite set:** A set consisting of an infinite number of elements is called an infinite sets.

For example N, Z, Q, ..., etc. all are infinite sets.

☞ REMARK
- Every infinite set is equivalent to a proper subset of itself.

2.2 CARDINALLY EQUIVALENT SETS

A set A is said to be cardinally equivalent to a set B if there exits at least one, one-to-one correspondence from A to B. If A is cardinally equivalent to B, then we write $A \sim B$.

Illustrations

- Two sets $A = \{1, 2, 3, ...\}$ and $B=\{2,4, 6, ...\}$ are cardinally equivalent sets. For this we define a mapping $f : A \to B$ such that $f(x) = 2x, \forall x \in A$

- Any two singlton set are always equivalent.
- The set $P = \{1, 2, 3, ..., 4\}$ and $Q = \{1^3, 2^3, ..., n^3\}$ are cardinally equivalent.

2.3 CARDINAL NUMBER

Let A be any non empty finite set. Then number of elements in the given set A is called the cardinality of the set A.

It is a well known fact that the relation $A \sim B$ is an equivalence relation, and we know that the equivalence relation decompose the family of sets into disjoint equivalence classes. Each equivalence class has a unique cardinal number.

Definition. *A set which is equivalent to the set $\{1, 2, ..., n\}$ is said to have the cardinal number n.*

The Cardinal numbers of the set $A, B, C, \ldots$ etc are denoted by small letter $a, b, c, \ldots$ or $|A|$, $|B|$, $|C|$ ... or Card (A), Card (B), Card (C) ...

☞ **REMARKS**

- The cardinal number of a set is some times called 'power' or 'potency'.
- For a finite set, cardinal number is just the number of elements in the given set.
- The cardinal number of a null set ϕ is always zero.
- The cardinal number of a finite set is called a 'finite cardinal number'.
- The cardinal number corresponding to an infinite set is called a transfinite cardinal number.
- The cardinal number of the set of all real valued functions defined in the interval $[0,1]$ is denoted by f.
- The cardinal numbers of the set $\mathbf{N}$ and the set of real numbers in $[0, 1]$ are respectively denoted by a and c, i.e., $|\mathbf{N}| = a$, $|[0, 1]| = c$.
- Every interval also has cardinal number, because we know that all intervals (open or closed) are equivalent to $[0, 1]$.
- If $P \sim Q$ then $|P| = |Q|$, i.e., Card(P) = Card(Q)
- All transfinite cardinal numbers are always greater than any finite cardinal number.

2.4 ALGEBRA OF CARDINAL NUMBERS

(i) **Sum of Cardinal Numbers:** Let A and B be two disjoint sets then
$$\text{Card}(A) + \text{Card}(B) = \text{Card}(A \cup B)$$
In general $\quad \sum_{\alpha \in \Delta} \text{Card} \cdot A_\alpha = \text{Card} \cdot (\bigcup_{\alpha \in \Delta} A_\alpha)$

where $A_\alpha \cap A_\beta = \phi$, i.e., each $A_\alpha's$ are paisewise disjoint

For example: If $A = \{1, 2\}$, $B = \{3, 4, 5\}$

Then Card$(A) = 2$, Card$(B) = 3$, $A \cap B = \phi$

Now $A \cup B = \{1, 2, 3, 4, 5\} \Rightarrow$ Card$(A \cup B) = 5$

Then clearly,
$$\text{Card}(A \cup B) = \text{Card}(A) + \text{Card}(B)$$

☞ **REMARK**

- The result Card$(A \cup B)$ = Card(A) + Card(B) is true only when $A \cap B = \phi$, i.e., A and B are disjoint.

(ii) **Product of Cardinal Numbers:** Let A and B be any two sets. Then
$$\text{Card}(A) \times \text{Card}(B) = \text{Card}(A \times B),$$
where $A \times B$ denote the cartesian product of two given sets A and B.

In general Card$\cdot P_1 \times$ Card$\cdot P_2 \ldots =$ Card$\cdot$[Cartesian product of sets P_i $(i = 1, 2, 3, \ldots)$]

For example: Let $A = \{a, b\}$, $B = \{1, 2, 3\}$

Then Card$(A) = 2$, Card$(B) = 3$

Now $A \times B = \{(a, 1), (a, 2), (a, 3), (b, 1), (b, 2), (b, 3)\}$

$\Rightarrow$ Card$(A \times B) = 6$

Hence, Card$(A) \times$ Card(B) = Card$(A \times B)$

(iii) **Comparison of Cardinal numbers:** Let A and B be two given sets then

(I) Card$(A) <$ Card(B) if there exist a set $C \subset B$ such that $A \sim C$ and if $A \sim B$ then Card(A) = Card(B).

(II) Card$(A) \le$ Card(B) if there exists a set $C \subseteq B$ such that $A \sim C$, i.e., there exists a one-one onto map $f: A \to C \subseteq B$

☞ REMARKS
- $\text{Card}(A \cup B) \geq \text{Card}(A)$ or $\text{Card}(B)$
- The cardinality of **N**, *i.e.*, *a* is the smallest infinite cardinal number.

2.5 COUNTABLE SETS

A set which can be put in one-to-one correspondence with the set of natural numbers or with its subsets, is called countable set.

For example: A set $A = \{2, 4, 6, \ldots\}$ can be put in one-to-one correspondence with the set of natural numbers by $f(x) = \dfrac{x}{2}$. Therefore, A is countable.

☞ REMARKS
- Every finite set is countable.
- An infinite set may or may not be countable.
- An infinite countable set is also called '**Countably infinite**' or '**enumerable set**' or '**denumerable set**'.
- A set *A* is countable if and only if its elements can be written in the form of a sequence. The fact behind this is that, every element of a countable set can be put in one-to-one correspondence with the set of natural numbers $\mathbf{N} = \{1, 2, \ldots\}$.
  If we denote the element of A corresponding to the natural numbers 1, 2, 3, ... by $a_1, a_2, a_3,$ ... etc. Then we can write $A = \{a_1, a_2, a_3, \ldots\}$
- ✦ For denumerable set A, $|A| = \mathbf{a} = |\mathbf{N}|$

2.5.1 UNCOUNTABLE SET

A set A which is not countable, is called uncountable set, *i.e.*, if A is infinite and A is not cardinally equivalent to **N**, the set of natural numbers.

For example:

The set of real numbers **R** and the set of complex numbers **C** are uncountable sets.

☞ REMARKS
- Uncountable sets are always infinite.
- Infinite sets may or may not be uncountable.
- The words 'Uncountable', 'Non-countable', non-denumerable, non-enumerable have the same meaning.
- A is uncountable $\Rightarrow A \sim (0, 1) \Rightarrow |A| = |[0, 1]| = \mathbf{c}$

2.5.2 POWER OF CONTINUM AND POWER SET

Definition 1. *A set A is said to have the power of continum if $A \sim [0, 1]$, i.e., cardinality of A is* **c**.

Definition 2. *Let A and B be two sets. Define $A^B = \{f : f : B \to A\}$, i.e., A^B is the set of all mapping from B to A. Therefore, the cardinal number of the set of functions from B to A is defined by $|A|^{|B|}$.*

Meaning of Cardinal number $2^{|A|}$: The symbol 2 stands for the cardinal number 2, *i.e.*, the set consisting of two elements say (0, 1).

2.6 ALGEBRAIC NUMBERS

Consider a polynomial $P_n(x) = a_0 x^n + a_{n-1} x^{n-1} + \ldots + a_1 x + a_0 \ (a_n \neq 0)$ where a_i's are integral coefficients. The algebraic numbers are defined as the roots of polynomial $P_n(x) = 0$.

THEOREM 1.

Every subset of a countable set is countable.

[MEERUT–1988, 94, 2003, 10, 17, GARHWAL–2007, ROHILKHAND–2015, KANPUR–2000]

PROOF. Let A be a countable set and B be any subset of A.

Case-I: If A is finite.

We know that every subset of a finite set is finite and we also know that every finite set is countable.

$\Rightarrow$ B is countable.

Case-II: If A is an infinite set.

Since $B \subseteq A$ and A is infinite. Then B may or may not be finite.

If B is finite or empty then obviously it is countable.

But if $B \neq \phi$ and B is infinite.

Since A is countable therefore, A can be written as a sequence such that $A = \{a_1, a_2, \ldots\}$.

Suppose that n_1 be the least positive integer such that $a_{n_1} \in B$. Further let n_2 be the least positive integer with $n_2 > n_1$ such that $a_{n_2} \in B$. Proceeding in the same way we conclude that each element of B can be written in the form of a sequence as $\{a_{n_1}, a_{n_2}, \ldots\}$.

Hence, B is countable.   [$\because$ A is countable if and only if its elements can be written in the form of a sequence]

☞ **REMARK**

- Every super set of a countable set is countable.

THEOREM 2.

The union of enumerable collection of enumerable sets is enumerable.

[KANPUR–2000, BANARAS–2016, MEERUT–2004, DELHI–2008, GARHWAL–1995]

PROOF. Let $A_1, A_2, \ldots$ be the enumerable sets.

Define $A = \{A_1, A_2, \ldots\}$ as an enumerable collection of enumerable sets such that $A_n = \{A_1, A_2, \ldots\} \ \forall \ n \in \mathbf{N}$. To prove that $\cup A_n$ is enumerable.

Now construct a progression of the elements of A_n appears in the following ways:

$$\underset{n \in \mathbf{N}}{\cup} A_n = \{a_{11} \rightarrow \quad a_{12} \quad\quad a_{13} \ \rightarrow \ a_{14} \quad \ldots$$

$$a_{21} \quad\quad a_{22} \quad\quad a_{23} \quad a_{24} \quad \ldots$$

$$a_{31} \quad\quad a_{32} \quad\quad a_{33} \quad a_{34} \quad \ldots$$

$$a_{41} \quad\quad a_{42} \quad\quad a_{43} \quad a_{44} \quad \ldots$$

The path among the above elements has been shown as above. We observe that every element of A lies somewhere on the above path which shows the one-to-one correspondace between $\cup A_n$ and $\mathbf{N}$. Hence A is enumerable. Therefore $\cup An$

$= \{a_{11}, a_{12}, a_{21}, a_{31}, a_{32}, \ldots\}$ can be written as a sequence.

Hence, $\cup A_n$ is enumerable.

DEDUCTIONS. (1) The union of countable collection of countable sets is also countable.

(2) The finite union of enumerable sets is again enumerable.

THEOREM 3.

The set of all real numbers in the open interval $]0, 1[$ *is not enumerable.*

[HIMACHAL–2004, 14, KANPUR–2004, MEERUT–1996, 2012]

PROOF. Let if possible, the set of all real numbers in the open interval $]0, 1[$ is enumerable. Since, we know that the elements of an enumerable set can be written in the form of a sequence, therefore the elements of $]0, 1[$ can be written as a sequence $\{x_1, x_2, x_3, \ldots\}$

Further, using the decimal expansion of the elements of the above sequence in the following manner:

$$x_1 = \cdot a_{11}a_{12}a_{13} \cdots a_{1n} \cdots$$
$$x_2 = \cdot a_{21}a_{22}a_{23} \cdots a_{2n} \cdots$$
$$x_3 = \cdot a_{31}a_{32}a_{33} \cdots a_{3n} \cdots$$
$$\cdots \quad \cdots \quad \cdots \quad \cdots \quad \cdots \quad \cdots \quad \cdots$$
$$x_n = \cdot a_{n1}a_{n2}a_{n3} \cdots a_{nn} \cdots$$
$$\cdots \quad \cdots \quad \cdots \quad \cdots \quad \cdots \quad \cdots \quad \cdots$$

In the above decimal expansion all a_{ij}'s may be any integer from 0 to 9. Now suppose that $x_n = \cdot b_1 b_2 b_3 \cdots$ where each b_i's is the digit from 0 to 9 such that

$$b_1 \neq a_{11}, b_2 \neq a_{22}, b_3 \neq a_{33}, \ldots b_m \neq a_{mm} \ \forall \ m \in \mathbf{N}$$

which implies $x \neq x_1, x \neq x_2, \ldots x \neq x_m$

Clearly $x \in]0, 1[$ and $x \notin \{x_1, x_2, \ldots\}$

Since, $\{x_1, x_2, \ldots\}$ is countable but there exists elements belonging to the interval $]0, 1[$ which is a contradiction.

Hence, the set of all real numbers in the open interval $]0, 1[$ is not enumerable.

DEDUCTION. The set of all real numbers in the closed interval $[0, 1]$ is not enumerable because $]0, 1[$ is a subset of $[0, 1]$ and by above theorem $]0, 1[$ is not enumerable.

THEOREM 4.

The set $\mathbf{R}$ *of all real numbers is not enumerable.*

PROOF. Let if possible $\mathbf{R}$ is enumerable. We know that every subset of enumerable set is enumerable.

Sicne, $]0, 1[$ is a subset of $\mathbf{R}$

$\Rightarrow$ $]0, 1[$ is enumerable [Being the subset of enumerable set]

But in previous theorem, we have proved that the open interval $]0, 1[$ of $\mathbf{R}$ is not enumerable.

$\Rightarrow$ A contradiction.

Hence, the set of real numbers $\mathbf{R}$ is not enumerable.

THEOREM 5.

The set of rational numbers is enumerable.

PROOF. We know that a number which can be expressed in the form of $\frac{p}{q}(q \neq 0), p, q \in \mathbf{Z}$ is called rational number.

i.e.,
$$Q = \left\{ \frac{p}{q} : p, q \in \mathbf{Z}, q \neq 0 \right\}$$

We have to prove that $\mathbf{Q}$ is enumerable.

Let us define a map $f : \mathbf{Q}^+ \to \mathbf{N} \times \mathbf{N}$ such that $f\left(\frac{m}{n}\right) = (m, n)$ where m and n are positive integer, relatively prime to each other.

Clearly, f is one-one and

$$|\mathbf{Q}^+| \leq |\mathbf{N} \times \mathbf{N}| = |\mathbf{N}| = a$$

$\Rightarrow \qquad |\mathbf{Q}^+| \leq a$ ...(1)

Further, we know that $\mathbf{N} \subseteq \mathbf{Q}^+$

$\Rightarrow \qquad |\mathbf{N}| \leq |\mathbf{Q}^+|$

$\Rightarrow \qquad a \leq |\mathbf{Q}^+|$ ...(2)

On combining (1) and (2) we get

$$a \leq |\mathbf{Q}^+| \leq a$$

$\Rightarrow \qquad |\mathbf{Q}^+| = a$

Also, $\qquad |\mathbf{Q}^-| = a$

$\left(\because \mathbf{Q}^+ \text{ is Cardinally equivalent to } \mathbf{Q}^- \text{ under the mapping } \frac{p}{q} \to -\left(\frac{p}{q}\right) \right)$

Finally, $\qquad |\mathbf{Q}| = |\mathbf{Q}^+ \cup \mathbf{Q}^- \cup \{0\}|$

$\qquad\qquad\qquad = a + a + 1 = (a + a) + 1$ (By associativity)

$\qquad\qquad\qquad = a + 1$ $(\because a + a = a)$

$\qquad\qquad\qquad = a$ $(\because a + 1 = a)$

Hence, $\mathbf{Q}$ the set of rationals is enumerable.

THEOREM 6.

The set of all irrational numbers is not enumerable.

PROOF. Let if possible, the set of irrational numbers is enumerable. In previous theorem, we have proved that the set of rational number is enumerable.

$\Rightarrow$ The set of rational and irrational number is enumerable.

$\qquad\qquad\qquad$ ($\because$ union of two enumerable sets is enumerable)

$\Rightarrow$ The set of real number is enumerable.

$\qquad\qquad\qquad$ ($\because$ Union of rational and irrational numbers is the set of reals)

which is a contradiction, because the set of reals is not enumerable.

$\Rightarrow$ Our assumption is wrong.

Hence, the set of irrational numbers is not enumerable.

THEOREM 7.

The set of integers $\mathbf{Z}$ is enumerable.

PROOF. We have to prove that the set of integers $\mathbf{Z}$ is enumerable. For this we shall prove that $|\mathbf{Z}| = a$

Let $\mathbf{Z}^+$ and $\mathbf{Z}^-$ be the set of positive integers and set of integers respectively. Then evidently

$$\mathbf{Z} = \mathbf{Z}^+ \cup \mathbf{Z}^- \cup \{0\}$$

Since, $\mathbf{Z}^+$, $\mathbf{Z}^-$ and $\{0\}$ all are disjoint, therefore

$$|\mathbf{Z}| = |\mathbf{Z}^+| + |\mathbf{Z}^-| + |\{0\}| \qquad \qquad \qquad ...(1)$$

Now, since $\mathbf{Z}^+ \sim \mathbf{N}$ under the mapping $n \to n$
and $\mathbf{Z}^- \sim \mathbf{N}$ under the mapping $-n \to n$

$\Rightarrow \qquad \qquad |\mathbf{Z}^+| = |\mathbf{N}|$ and $|\mathbf{Z}^-| = |\mathbf{N}|$

$\Rightarrow \qquad \qquad |\mathbf{Z}^+| = |\mathbf{Z}^-| = |\mathbf{N}| = a$

and $\qquad \qquad |\{0\}| = 1$

Putting all these values in (1) we get

$$|\mathbf{Z}| = a + a + 1 = (a + a) + 1$$
$$= a + 1 = a \qquad \qquad (\because a + a = a \text{ and } a + 1 = a)$$

Hence, the set of integers is enumerable.

THEOREM 8.

Every infinite subset of an enumerable set is enumerable.

PROOF.   Let A be an enumerable set and B be any infinite subset of A.

We have to prove that B is enumerable.

Since, A is enumerable

$\Rightarrow$ A can be written in the form of a sequence such that $A = \{a_n : n \in \mathbf{N}\}$

Since, $B \subseteq A$, we may assume that the element $a_{n_1}, a_{n_2}, a_{n_3}, ...$ $(n_1 < n_2 < n_3 ...)$ of A belongs to B.

Then we have the following conditions:

  (i) B has a first element n_1.

  (ii) Each element of B has a definite (fixed) place in the set.

$\Rightarrow$ The elements of B can be written in the form of a sequence.

$\Rightarrow$ B is a sequence.

Hence, B is enumerable.

THEOREM 9.

Every infinite set contains an enumerable subset.

PROOF.   Let A be any infinite set.

We have to prove that $B \subset A$ is enumerable.

Let $a_1 \in A$. Then clearly $A - \{a_1\} \neq \phi$ $\qquad \qquad (\because A$ is an infinite set$)$

Now let $a_2 \in A - \{a_1\}$, $a_1 \neq a_2$. Then $A - \{a_1, a_2\} \neq \phi$ $\qquad (\because A$ is an infinite set$)$

Similarly, let $a_3 \in A - \{a_1, a_2\}$, $a_1 \neq a_2 \neq a_3$. Then $A - \{a_1, a_2, a_3\} \neq \phi$

$\qquad \qquad \qquad \qquad \qquad \qquad \qquad \qquad \qquad \qquad (\because A$ is an infinite set$)$

Proceeding in the same manner we picked the elements $a_1, a_2, ..., a_n$ from A such that $A - \{a_1, a_2, ..., a_n\} \neq \phi$ and all a_i's are distinct.

Repeating this process again and again we can find

$$A - \{a_1, a_2, a_3, ...\} \neq \phi$$

If we write $B = \{a_1, a_2, a_3, ...\}$

Then clearly $B \subset A$. It is also clear that B is expressible in the form of a sequence.

Hence, B is enumerable.

THEOREM 10.

The set of all algebraic numbers is enumerable.   [MEERUT–1996, 2009, GARHWAL–2003, 04, 05]

PROOF.   Let $a_0x^n + a_1x^{n-1} + \dots + a_n \ (a_0 \neq 0)$ be an algebraic equation of degree n. Then we define the rank of this equation as follows

$$|a_0| + |a_1| + \dots |a_n| = m \text{ (say)}$$

Obviously, rank is a positive integer and a_i's all are integers.

Therefore, ranks is an integer ≥ 1.

Further, for a given rank, the roots of the equation will be finite and hence enumerable.

Now since, a one-one correspondance can be put in the set of natural number with the algebraic equation arranged with respect to rank.

$\Rightarrow$ The set of all algebraic equations is enumerable.

Further, since each algebraic equation has enumerable number of roots therefore, the set of all algebraic numbers is the enumerable collection of enumerable sets.

Hence, the set of all algebraic numbers is enumerable.

THEOREM II.

If A_i is enumerable set then $\bigcup\limits_{i=1}^{n} A_i$ is enumerable.

PROOF.   Let A_i is an enumerable set.

$\Rightarrow$ A_i is countably infinite set.

Let us write $A = \bigcup\limits_{i=1}^{n} A_i$

We have to prove that A is enumerable.

Write the elements of A_i in the form given below

$$A_1 : a_{11}a_{12}a_{13} \dots a_{1n} \dots$$
$$A_2 : a_{21}a_{22}a_{23} \dots a_{2n} \dots$$
$$A_3 : a_{31}a_{22}a_{33} \dots a_{3n} \dots$$
$$\dots \quad \dots \quad \dots \quad \dots \quad \dots \quad \dots$$
$$\dots \quad \dots \quad \dots \quad \dots \quad \dots \quad \dots$$

Let us write $B = \{a_{11}, a_{12}, \dots, a_{1n}, \dots, a_{21}, a_{22}, \dots, a_{n1}, a_{n2}, \dots\}$

Clearly, B, the set of distinct elements is countably infinite.

So, $|B| = a$

Now, if $A_i \cap A_j = \phi$ for $i \neq j$. Then $|A| = |B| = a$

and if $A_i \cap A_j \neq \phi$ for $i \neq j$. Then $|A| \leq |B| = a \Rightarrow |A| \leq a$

But $A_i \subset A$ and $|A_i| = a$. Therefore, $a = |A_1| \leq |A| \Rightarrow a \leq |A|$

Combining above two results, i.e., $|A| \leq a$ and $a \leq |A|$

We conclude that $|A| = a$

DEDUCTION.   Using above theorem we can deduce $n \cdot a = a$ as follows:

Assume that $A_i \cap A_j = \phi$ for $i \neq j$ and $i, j = 1, 2, \dots, n$

By above theorem $|A| = a$

$\Rightarrow \qquad \left| \bigcup\limits_{i=1}^{n} A_i \right| = a \text{ or } \sum\limits_{i=1}^{n} |A_i| = a$

$\Rightarrow \quad a + a + \dots \text{ upto } n \text{ terms } = a$

$\Rightarrow \qquad\qquad n \cdot a = a$

THEOREM 12.

(i) If A_i is non-enumerable set for $1 \le i \le n$ then $\bigcup\limits_{i=1}^{n} A_i$ is non-enumerable and hence

$$\mathbf{c} + \mathbf{c} + \dots \text{ to } n \text{ terms} = \mathbf{c}$$

(ii) If A_i is non-enumerable $"i \in N$ then $\bigcup\limits_{i=1}^{\infty} A_i$ is non-enumerable and hence

$$\mathbf{c} + \mathbf{c} + \dots \text{ to } n \text{ terms} = \mathbf{c}$$

PROOF. (i) Since, each A_i is non-enumerable for $1 \le i \le n$

Then Card $A_i = \mathbf{c}$ for $1 \le i \le n$

$\Rightarrow \qquad A_i - [a_i, a_{i+1}[, a_i, a_{i+1} \in \mathbf{R}$ for $i = 1, 2, 3, \dots, n$

Then $\qquad A_1 \sim [a_1, a_2[$

$\qquad\qquad A_2 \sim [a_2, a_3[$

$\qquad\qquad \dots \quad \dots \quad \dots \quad \dots$

$\qquad\qquad \dots \quad \dots \quad \dots \quad \dots$

$\qquad\qquad A_n \sim [a_n, a_{n+1}[$

Now, we have the following two cases:

Case-I: If $A_i \cap A_j = \phi$ for $i \ne j$

Clearly, $\bigcup\limits_{i=1}^{n} A_i$ is equivalent to some set of $[a_1, a_{n+1}[$

Then $\quad \text{Card} \left[\bigcup\limits_{i=1}^{n} A_i \right] \le \mathbf{c}$ $\qquad\qquad\qquad \dots(1)$

By set theory, we have

$$A_i \subseteq \bigcup\limits_{i=1}^{n} A_i$$

$\Rightarrow \qquad \text{Card}(A_i) \le \text{Card} \left[\bigcup\limits_{i=1}^{n} A_i \right]$

$\Rightarrow \qquad \mathbf{c} \le \text{Card} \left[\bigcup\limits_{i=1}^{n} A_i \right]$ $\qquad\qquad\qquad \dots(2)$

Form (1) and (2) we conclude that

$$\mathbf{c} \le \text{Card} \left[\bigcup\limits_{i=1}^{n} A_i \right] \le \mathbf{c}$$

$\Rightarrow \qquad \text{Card} \left[\bigcup\limits_{i=1}^{n} A_i \right] = \mathbf{c}$

$\Rightarrow \qquad \bigcup\limits_{i=1}^{n} A_i$ is non-enumerable.

Case-II: If $A_i \cap A_j \ne \phi$ for $i \ne j$

$\Rightarrow \qquad \text{Card} \left[\bigcup\limits_{i=1}^{n} A_i \right] = \text{Card} [a, a_{n+1}[$

Clearly, $\qquad \bigcup\limits_{i=1}^{n} A_i \sim [a_i, a_{n+1}[$

$\Rightarrow \qquad \text{Card} \left[\bigcup\limits_{i=1}^{n} A_i \right] = \mathbf{c}$

DEDUCTION: We have already proved that

$$\text{Card}\left[\bigcup_{i=1}^{n} A_i\right] = \mathbf{c}$$

$\Rightarrow \quad \mathbf{c} + \mathbf{c} + \dots \text{ to } n \text{ terms} = \mathbf{c}$

(ii) Let us write $A = \bigcup_{i=1}^{n} A_i$, where $\text{Card } A_i = \mathbf{c} \ \forall \ i \in \mathbf{N}$

Now $\text{Card}(A_i) = \mathbf{c}$ implies $A_i \sim \left[1 - \dfrac{1}{2^{i-1}}, 1 - \dfrac{1}{2^i}\right[$

Then we have

$$A_1 \sim \left[0, \frac{1}{2}\right[$$

$$A_2 \sim \left[\frac{1}{2}, \frac{3}{4}\right[$$

$$A_3 \sim \left[\frac{3}{4}, \frac{7}{8}\right[$$

... ...

$$A_i \sim \left[1 - \frac{1}{2^{i-1}}, 1 - \frac{1}{2^i}\right[$$

Now consider the following two cases:

Case-I: If $A_i \cap A_j = \phi$ **for** $i \neq j$

Then clearly $\bigcup_{i=1}^{\infty} A_i \sim [0, 1[$

$\Rightarrow \quad \text{Card}\left[\bigcup_{i=1}^{\infty} A_i\right] = \text{Card}([0, 1[)$

$$= \text{Card}(A) = \mathbf{c}$$

Case-II: If $A_i \cap A_j \neq \phi$ **for** $i \neq j$

Then $\bigcup_{i=1}^{\infty} A_i$ is cardinally equivalent to some subset of $[0, 1[$

Therefore $\text{Card}\left[\bigcup_{i=1}^{\infty} A_i\right] \leq \mathbf{c}$ ...(1)

By set theory, we have

$$A_i \subseteq \bigcup_{i=1}^{\infty} A_i$$

$\Rightarrow \quad \text{Card}(A_i) \leq \text{Card}\left(\bigcup_{i=1}^{\infty} A_i\right)$

$\Rightarrow \quad \mathbf{c} \leq \text{Card}\left(\bigcup_{i=1}^{\infty} A_i\right)$ ...(2)

From (1) and (2) we conclude that

$$\mathbf{c} \leq \mathrm{Card}\left(\bigcup_{i=1}^{\infty} A_i \right) \leq \mathbf{c}$$

$$\Rightarrow \quad \mathrm{Card}\left(\bigcup_{i=1}^{\infty} A_i \right) = \mathbf{c}$$

Hence, $\bigcup_{i=1}^{\infty} A_i$ is non-enumerable.

DEDUCTION. In the above case-I, we have prove that

$$\mathrm{Card}\left(\bigcup_{i=1}^{\infty} A_i \right) = \mathbf{c}$$

$$\Rightarrow \quad \sum_{i=1}^{\infty} \mathrm{Card}(A_i) = \mathbf{c}$$

$$\Rightarrow \quad c + c + \dots \text{ to } a \text{ terms} = \mathbf{c}$$

THEOREM 13.

If a finite set of elements is added to an enumerable set, the resulting set is also enumerable.

PROOF. Let A be an enumerable set and B be any finite set containing n elements. Then we can write

$$|A| = a \qquad |B| = n$$

Suppose that A and B are disjoint, *i.e.*, $A \cap B = \phi$

We have to prove that $A \cup B$ is enumerable. For this it is sufficient to prove that $|A \cup B| = |\mathbf{N}|$

Let us write the set B as

$$B = \{b_1, b_2, \dots, b_n\}$$

Since, A is enumerable, so it can be expressed in the form of a sequence.

Therefore, $\qquad A = \{a_{n+1}, a_{n+2}, \dots, a_0\}$

Now define a map $f : \mathbf{N} \to A \cup B$ such that

$$f(r) = \begin{cases} b; & \text{if } 1 \leq r \leq n \\ a; & \text{if } r > n \end{cases}$$

Clearly f is one-one onto

$$\Rightarrow \qquad \mathbf{N} \sim A \cup B$$

$$\Rightarrow \qquad |\mathbf{N}| = |A \cup B|$$

$$\Rightarrow \qquad a = n + a$$

☞ **REMARK**
• The above theorem can be restated as $n + a = a$, n being any finite cardinal number.

THEOREM 14.

If a finite set of elements is added to an infinite set, the power of the set is unaffected.

PROOF. Let A be any infinite set with power α and C be any finite set containing n elements such that $A \cap C = \phi$.

We have to prove that $|A \cup C| = |A|$

Since, A is infinite set therefore, $\exists\, B \subset A$ such that $|B| = a$

Let us write $A - B = P$. Then $A \cup C = B \cup P \cup C$

$$\Rightarrow \qquad A \cup C = B \cup C \cup P \qquad \qquad \dots(1)$$

We know that finite union of a finite set and an enumerable set is enumerable, therefore $B \cup C$ is enumerable.

So,　　　　　　　$B \cup C \sim N$

Now,　　　$|B| = a$　　$\Rightarrow$　$B \sim N$

　　　　　　　　　　　$\Rightarrow$　$N \sim B$

　　　　　$B \cup C \sim N, N \sim B$

$\Rightarrow$　　　　$B \cup C \sim B$

Further　　　　　　$P \sim P$　　　　　　　　　(By reflexivity)

Now, $B \cup C \sim B$ and $P \sim P$. Therefore $(B \cup C \cup P) \sim (B \cup P)$

$\Rightarrow$　　　$|B \cup C \cup P| = |A|$　　　　($\because A - B = P$)

$\Rightarrow$　　　　$|A \cup C| = |A|$　　　　　(From (1))

$\Rightarrow$　　　　$\alpha + n = \alpha$

☞ **REMARK**

• The above theorem can be restated as:

$n + \alpha = \alpha \; \forall \; n \in N$ where α is any infinite cardinal number.

THEOREM 15.

If an enumerable set is added to an infinite set then cardinal number of the infinite set is unaffected.

PROOF.　　Let A be any infinite set such that $\text{Card}(A) = \alpha$

Since, A is an infinite set, there exist a subset B of A such that B is enumerable and $\text{Card}(B) = a$.

We have to prove that $|A \cup N| = |A|$　　　　($A \cap N = \phi$)

Now, we can write　　$A = (A - B) \cup B$　　(By set theory)

Then　　$A \cup N = ((A - B) \cup B) \cup N$

　　　　　　$= (A - B) \cup (B \cup N)$　　　　...(1)

Since, B and N are enumerable therefore, $B \cup N$ is enumerable.

So,　　　$B \cup N \sim N$

Now, $B \cup N \sim N$, $N \sim B$. Then by transitivity $B \cup N \sim B$

Also, $B \cup N \sim B$ and $A - B \sim A - B$

$\Rightarrow (A - B) \cup (B \cup N) \sim (A - B) \cup B$　　　...(2)

From (1) and (2) we conclude that

　　　　$A \cup N \sim (A - B) \cup B$

$\Rightarrow$　　　$A \cup N \sim A$　　　　($\because (A - B) \cup B = A$)

$\Rightarrow$　　$|A \cup N| \sim |A|$

$\Rightarrow$　　　$\alpha + n = \alpha$

THEOREM 16.

If we subtract an enumerable set from a non-enumerable set, then remaining set is non-enumerable.

PROOF.　　Let A be a non-enumerable and B be an enumerable set.

Let us write　$A - B = C$

We have to prove that C is a non-enumerable set.

Let if possible C be an enumerable set.

Since, $A - B = C$, therefore, $A = B \cup C$

Also, since B and C both are enumerable set therefore, being the union of two enumerable sets, $B \cup C$ is enumerable.

$\Rightarrow$　A is enumerable.

Which is a contradiction. So, our assumption is wrong. Thus, C is non-enumerable.

THEOREM 17.

If an enumerable set is subtracted from another enumerable set then remaining set is also enumerable.

PROOF.   Let A and B be two enumerable sets. We have to prove that $A - B$ is enumerable.

Let us write $A - B = C$

Let if possible C is not enumerable.

Now, $A - B = C \Rightarrow A = B \cup C$ (By set theory)

Also, B and C both are non-enumerable, therefore, $B \cup C$ is also non-enumerable.

$\Rightarrow$ A is non-enumerable.

which is a contradiction. Thus our assumption is wrong.

Therefore C and hence $A - B$ is enumerable.

THEOREM 18. (Dedekind-Peirce Theorem)

Every infinite set is equivalent to its proper subset.

PROOF.   Let A be an infinite set. We have the following two cases:

Case-I: If A is countably infinite

We know that every countably infinite set can be written in the form of a sequence. Thus, we can write

$$A = \{a_1, a_2, \ldots\}$$

Clearly, the function $f(a_n) = a_{n+1}$ set a one-to-one correspondance between the set A and $A - \{a_1\}$, which is clearly a proper subset of A.

i.e., $A \sim [A - \{a_1\}]$

Case-II: If A is uncountably infinite.

In this case A has an enumerable subset say B

where $B = \{a_1, a_2, \ldots\}$

($\because$ Every enumerable set can be written in the form of a sequence)

Now, we shall prove that

$$A \sim (A - \{a_i\})$$

Let us write $C = A - B$ so $A = B \cup C$ and $B \cap C = \phi$

and $A - \{a_i\} = (B - \{a_i\}) \cup C$

Further, let $e(x)$ be the identity mapping which associates each $x \in A$ onto itself and f be a function such that $f(a_n) = a_{n+1}$

Then define a function h such that

$$h(x) = \begin{cases} e(x) & : & x \in C \\ f(x) & : & x \in B \end{cases}$$

Clearly, the range of h is $(B - \{a_i\}) \cup C$, which is clearly a proper subset of $B \cup C (= A)$

Hence, we conclude that every infinite set is equivalent to its proper subset.

THEOREM 19. (Galeleo's Paradox)

Any enumerable set can be put in a one-to-one correspondence with a proper subset of itself.

PROOF.   Let A be any enumerable set. Then by definition A can be expressed in the form of a sequence as

$$A = \{a_1, a_2, a_3, \ldots\}$$

Let us define $B = A - \{a_1\} = \{a_2, a_3, \ldots\}$

Clearly, B is a proper subset of A.

Now, define a map $f : A \to B$ such that $f(a_n) = a_{n+1}, n \in \mathbf{N}$

Clearly, f is one-one and onto mapping.

Hence, any enumerable set can be put in a one-to-one correspondence with a proper subset of itself.

THEOREM 20.

$c \cdot c = c$

[GARHWAL–2003, 05]

PROOF.   Let $A = \{x : 0 \le x \le 1\}$. Then clearly, Card$(A) = \mathbf{c}$

Further let $B = \{(0, x) : x \in A\}$

Clearly, $B \subseteq A \times A$

$\Rightarrow$ Card$(B) \le$ Card$(A \times A)$ ...(1)

Further $A \sim B$ under the mapping such that $f(x) = (0, x) \ \forall \ x \in A$

$\Rightarrow$ Card$(A) \le$ Card(B) ...(2)

From (1) and (2) we have,

Card$(A) \le$ Card$(A \times A)$ ...(3)

If x, y be any two real numbers in the closed interval [0, 1]. Then x and y can be extended uniquely in the form of infinite decimals which contain non-zero digits. Now define a mapping $g : A \times A \to A$ by $g(x, y) = 0 \cdot x_1 y_1 x_2 y_2 x_3 y_3 \ldots$

Clearly g is one-one.

$\Rightarrow$ Card$(A \times A) \le$ Card(A) ...(4)

From (3) and (4) we conclude that

Card$(A \times A) =$ Card(A)

$\Rightarrow$ Card $A \times$ Card $A =$ Card A ($\because$ Card $(A \times B) =$ Card $A \times$ Card B)

$\Rightarrow$ $\mathbf{c \cdot c = c}$

THEOREM 21.

$Card(P \times Q) = Card(Q) + Card(Q) + \ldots P \ terms.$

PROOF.   By definition of $P \times Q$ we can write

$$P \times Q = \{(x, y) : x \in P, y \in Q\}$$
$$= \bigcup_{x \in P} \{(x, y) : y \in Q\} \qquad \ldots(1)$$

Therefore, Card$(P \times Q) =$ Card$\left(\bigcup_{x \in P} \{(x, y) : y \in Q\} \right)$

Now, let $x \in P$ be arbitrary and fixed. Then consider a map
$$f : Q \to \{(x, y) : y \in Q\} \text{ such that } f(y) = (x, y) \ \forall \ y \in Q$$
which is clearly one-one and onto

So,   Card$(Q) =$ Card$\{(x, y) : y \in Q\}$

Hence, from (1)

Card$(P \times Q) =$ Card$(Q) +$ Card$(Q) + \ldots P$ terms

THEOREM 22.

Let P and Q be any two sets. Then

(i)   Card$\cdot P +$ Card$\cdot Q$ is unique

(ii) (Card$\cdot P$)(Card$\cdot Q$) is unique

PROOF.   Let P and Q be two given sets.

Let there exists two sets P_1 and Q_1 such that
$$P \sim P_1, Q \sim Q_1 \text{ and } P_1 \cap Q_1 = \phi$$

(i) Here $P \sim P_1 \Rightarrow$ There exists a one-one mapping $f : P \xrightarrow{\text{onto}} P_1$

Similarly, $Q \sim Q_1 \Rightarrow$ There exists a one-one mapping $g : P \xrightarrow{\text{onto}} Q_1$

Now, define a function $h : P \cup Q \to P_1 \cup Q_1$ such that

$$h(x) = \begin{cases} f(x): & \forall x \in P \\ g(x): & \forall x \in Q \end{cases}$$

Since, f and g both are one-one and onto, therefore $h(x)$ is also one-one and onto.

Therefore, $P \cup Q \sim P_1 \cup Q_1$

$\Rightarrow \text{Card}(P \cup Q) = \text{Card}(P_1 \cup Q_1)$

Hence Card P + Card Q is unique.

(ii) Let $x \in P$, $y \in Q$. Then $(x, y) \in P \times Q$

$\Rightarrow (f(x), g(x)) \in P_1 \times Q_1$

Now define a function $h : P \times Q \to P_1 \times Q_1$ such that

$$h(x, y) = (f(x), g(y)) \; \forall \, x, y \in P \times Q$$

Further, since f and g both are one-one and onto therefore, h is also one-one and onto. Therefore,

$$P \times Q \sim P_1 \times Q_1$$

$\Rightarrow \qquad \text{Card}(P \times Q) = \text{Card}(P_1 \times Q_1)$

Hence, $\text{Card}(P) \cdot \text{Card}(Q)$ is unique.

THEOREM 23.

For any two sets P and Q, $P \times Q$ is cardinally equivalent to $Q \times P$.

PROOF. Let P and Q be two given sets.

Then by definition of cartesian product of two sets,

$$P \times Q = \{(p, q) : p \in P, q \in Q\}$$

Now define a map $f : P \times Q \to Q \times P$ such that $f(p, q) = (q, p)$

Further, suppose that

$$f(p_1, q_1) = f(p_2, q_2)$$

$\Rightarrow \qquad (q_1, p_1) = (q_2, p_2) \qquad\qquad\qquad$ (By definition of f)

$\Rightarrow \qquad q_1 = q_2 \text{ and } p_1 = p_2$

$\Rightarrow \qquad (p_1, q_1) = (p_2, q_2)$

So, f is one-one.

Also, $P \times Q$ and $Q \times P$ both have the same number of elements and f is one-one, therefore, f is onto.

Hence, $P \times Q \sim Q \times P$, i.e., $P \times Q$ is cardinally equivalent to $Q \times P$.

THEOREM 24.

Let $\text{Card}(P) = p$, $\text{Card}(Q) = q$ and $\text{Card}(R) = r$. Then

(i) $p + q = q + p$, i.e., addition of cadinal numbers is commutative.

(ii) $p \cdot q = q \cdot p$, i.e., multiplication of cardinal numbers is commutative.

(iii) $p \cdot (q + r) = p \cdot q + p \cdot r$, i.e., multiplication is distributive over addition.

(iv) $p \cdot (q \cdot r) = (p \cdot q) \cdot r$, i.e., associative law holds for multiplication

(v) $p + (q + r) = (p + q) + r$, i.e., associative law holds for addition

PROOF.　　　Let P, Q and R be three sets such that $\text{Card}(P) = p$, $\text{Card}(Q) = q$ and $\text{Card}(R) = r$.

    (i)　If P and Q are disjoint, i.e., $P \cap Q = \phi$

       Since, order of elements in any set is immaterial

       Therefore,　　$P \cup Q = Q \cup P$

       $\Rightarrow$　　　$\text{Card}(P \cup Q) = \text{Card}(Q \cup P)$

       $\Rightarrow \text{Card}(P) + \text{Card}(Q) = \text{Card}(Q) + \text{Card}(P)$

       $\Rightarrow$　　　　　$p + q = q + p$

   (ii)　Using above theorem, we can write

       　　　$P \times Q \sim Q \times P$

       $\Rightarrow$　　　$\text{Card}(P \times Q) = \text{Card}(Q \times P)$

       $\Rightarrow$　$\text{Card}(P) \cdot \text{Card}(Q) = \text{Card}(Q) \cdot \text{Card}(P)$

       $\Rightarrow$　　　　　$p \cdot q = q \cdot p$

  (iii)　If Q and R are disjoint then

$$p \cdot (q + r) = \text{Card}[P \times (Q \cup R)]$$
$$= \text{Card}[(P \times Q) \cup (P \times R)]$$
$$= \text{Card}(P \times Q) + \text{Card}(P \times R)$$
$$= p \cdot q + p \cdot r$$

  (iv)　Since, $P \times (Q \times R) \sim (P \times Q) \times R$ under the mapping $f(x, (y, z)) = f((x, y), z)$

       Therefore, $\text{Card}[P \times (Q \times R)] = \text{Card}[(P \times Q) \times R]$

       $\Rightarrow$　　　　　$p \cdot (q \cdot r) = (p \cdot q) \cdot r$

   (v)　Let us suppose that P, Q and R are pairwise disjoint sets.

       Also, we know that

       　　$(P \cup Q) \cup R = P \cup (Q \cup R)$

       So,　$\text{Card}[(P \cup Q) \cup R] = \text{Card}[P \cup (Q \cup R)]$

       Hence,　　$(p + q) + r = p + (q + r)$

2.7　TRANSCENDENTAL NUMBER

We know that a real number which is not algebraic is called transcendental number.

For example: The number e and π are transcendental number.

☞ REMARKS

- All rational numbers are algebraic but all irrational are not necessarily transcendental.
- Every transcendental number is irrational.

2.8　CONTINUM HYPOTHESIS

It states that there is no cardinal number between a and c. Therefore, c is assumed to be the second transfinite cardinal number. But this hypothesis does not assert that there exists no set with cardinal number greater than c. However, there are other cardinal numebr greater than **c**. Cantor had proved that the power set $P(A)$ of any set A has cardinal number greater than the cardinality of A. For instance Card $P(\mathbf{R}) > $ **c**.

THEOREM 1.

Every monotonic function in a closed interval is discontinuous at a countable number of points of that interval.

PROOF.   Let $f(x)$ be a function which is monotonic in the closed interval $[a, b]$.

Without loss of any generality, we may assume that $f(x)$ is monotonically increasing.

It is also given that $f(x)$ is discontinuous at countable number of points in $[a, b]$.

Let it be discontinuous at a point x.

Then $f(x) = f(x + 0) - f(x - 0) > 0$

$$(\because f(x) \text{ is not continuous} \Leftrightarrow f(x + 0) \neq f(x - 0))$$

where $f(a) = f(a - 0), f(b) = f(b + 0)$

Let $t_1, t_2, \ldots t_{m-1}$ be numbers in the intervals $x_k < t_k < x_{k+1}$ where $a < x_1 < x_2 < \ldots < x_m < b$

Let us write $t_0 = a$ and $t_m = b$

Then $f(t_k) - f(t_{k-1}) \geq f(x_k + 0) - f(x_k - 0) = \delta(x_k)$

$$\Rightarrow \qquad f(b) - f(a) = \sum_{k=1}^{m} [f(t_k) - f(t_{k-1})] \geq \sum_{k=1}^{m} f(x_k)$$

If we take $\delta(x_k) > \dfrac{1}{n} \forall k.$ Then

$$f(b) - f(a) > \frac{m}{n}$$

$$\Rightarrow \qquad n[f(b) - f(a)] > m$$

$\Rightarrow$ number m, of the point of discontinuity of x with $\delta(x) > \dfrac{1}{n}$ is bounded above.

$\Rightarrow$ The number of points of discontinuity x with $\delta(x) > \dfrac{1}{n}$ are finite in the closed interval $[a, b]$.

Since, every finite set is countable and for every $x \ni n \in \mathbf{N}$, therefore the number of points of discontinuity in the closed interval $[a, b]$ will be enumerable union of countable sets and hence countable.

THEOREM 2. (Cantor's Theorem)

For any set A, Card(A) < Card(P(A)) where P(A) is the power set of A.

[MEERUT–2011, 15, 17, ASSAM–2007, RAJASTHAN–2009, DELHI–2014]

PROOF.   Let A be the given set.

We have to prove that $|A| < |P(A)|$

Let us write a set $B_1 = \{\{x\} : x \in A\}$

Then we have

(i) $B_1 \subset P(A) \quad \Rightarrow \quad |B_1| < |P(A)|$ ...(1)

(ii) $B_1 \sim A$ under the mapping $\{x\} \to x$

$\Rightarrow \qquad |B_1| = |A| \Rightarrow |A| \leq |P(A)|$ ...(2)

(2) $\Rightarrow \qquad$ Card$(A) \leq$ Card$(P(A))$

Here, it remains to prove that $\text{Card}(A) \neq \text{Card}(P(A))$, i.e., A is not cardinally equivalent to $P(A)$. Let if possible $A \sim P(A)$

Then by definition there exists a one-one mapping $f : A \xrightarrow{\text{onto}} P(A)$
Now, let $B = \{x \in A : x \notin f(x)\}$
Clearly, $B \subset A \quad \Rightarrow \quad B \in P(A)$
Since, f is onto, there must exist $x \in A$ such that $f(x) = B$. Further, if $x \in B$. Then by definition of B, $x \in f(x)$, which is not possible. A contradiction arrived. The second possibility that $x \notin B$ then $x \in f(x) = B$ also ruled out.
So, A is not cardinally equivalent to $P(A)$.
Hence, $\text{Card}(A) < \text{Card}(P(A))$.

☞ **REMARK**
- From above theorem, $2^a > a$.

THEOREM 3. (Equivalence Theorem)

If $A_1 \subset B \subset A$ and $A \sim A_1$. Then $A \sim B$.

PROOF.   It is given that $A \sim A_1$ which implies there exist one-one map $f : A \xrightarrow{\text{onto}} A_1$
Also $B \subset A$ therefore, f_B, (the restriction of f to B) is one-one and onto.
$$\Rightarrow \qquad B \sim B_1 \subset A_1$$
In a similar way $\qquad A_1 \sim A_2 \subset B_1$
Continuing in the same manner, we get the sequence of equivalent sets $A, A_1, A_2, \ldots,$ $B, B_1, B_2, \ldots$ such that
$$A \supset B \supset A_1 \supset B_1 \supset A_2 \supset B_2 \supset A_3 \supset B_3 \supset \ldots$$
Let us write $\qquad S = A \cap B \cap A_1 \cap B_1 \cap A_2 \cap B_2 \cap \ldots$
Then $\qquad A = (A - B) \cup (B - A_1) \cup (A_1 - B_1) \cup \ldots \cup S$
and $\qquad B = (B - A) \cup (A_1 - B_1) \cup (B_1 - A_2) \cup \ldots \cup S$
Now define a map $h : A \to B$ such that
$$h(A - B) = A_1 - B_1$$
$$h(A_1 - B_1) = A_2 - B_2$$
$$h(A_2 - B_2) = A_3 - B_3$$
$$\ldots \quad \ldots \quad \ldots \quad \ldots \quad \ldots$$
$$\ldots \quad \ldots \quad \ldots \quad \ldots \quad \ldots$$
$$h(B - A_1) = B - A_1$$
$$h(B_1 - A_2) = B_1 - A_2$$
$$\ldots \quad \ldots \quad \ldots \quad \ldots \quad \ldots$$
$$\ldots \quad \ldots \quad \ldots \quad \ldots \quad \ldots$$
$$h(S) = S$$
Clearly, the mapping h is one-one and onto. Hence, A is cardinally equivalent to B, i.e., $A \sim B$.

☞ **REMARK**
- The above theorem can be restated as follows:
"If $A_1 \subset B \subset A$ and $\text{Card}(A_1) = \text{Card}(A)$, then $\text{Card}(A) = \text{Card}(B)$"

THEOREM 4. (Schorder-Bernstein Theorem)

For any two sets A and B, if Card(A) ≤ Card(B) and Card(B) ≤ Card(A) then Card(A) = Card(B).

PROOF. Let $f: A \to B$ and $g : B \to A$ be two one-one and onto mappings.

Also, let $f(A) = B_1 \subset B$ and $g(B) = A_2$ and $g(B_1) = A_3$

Then $\qquad\qquad\qquad A = A_2 \supset A_3$

and $\qquad\qquad g(B_1) = A_3, f(A) = B_1 \Rightarrow g[f(A)] = A_3$

$\Rightarrow$ (gof) is a one-to-one mapping from A to A_3.

$\Rightarrow$ $\qquad\qquad$ $Card(A) = Card(A_3)$

Then by equivalence theorem $Card(A) = Card(A_2)$ $\qquad\qquad$ ...(1)

Similarly, $g(B) = A_2$ shows that $Card(B) = Card(A_2)$ $\qquad\qquad$ ...(2)

Hence, from (1) and (2) we conclude that

$\qquad\qquad\qquad Card(A) = Card(B)$

THEOREM 5.

The set of all transcendental numbers in any interval is non-enumerable.

[PUNJAB–2002, 17, MEERUT–2003]

PROOF. We know that the set of algebraic numbers and set of transcendental numbers form the set of real numbers, and we have already proved that the set of real numbers is not enumerable and the set of algebraic numbers in an interval is enumerable.

From above it is clear that the set of transcendental number can be obtained from the set of real numbers by removing algebraic numbers and we know that if an enumerable set is removed from a non-enumerable set, the remaining set is non-enumerable..

Hence, the set of transcendental numbers is non-enumerable.

THEOREM 6.

$2^a = c$

PROOF. We know that $Card[0, 1] = \mathbf{c}$

Further, we know that each $x \in [0, 1]$ can be expressed in the form of binary expansion as $x \in 0 \cdot x_1 \cdot x_2 \cdot x_3 \dots$ where each $x_i = 0$ or 1.

Now, selecting each x_i as 0 or 1 (two ways) we can form at most 2^a numbers. Therefore, $Card[0, 1] = 2^a$.

$\Rightarrow$ $\qquad\qquad$ $2^a = \mathbf{c}$

THEOREM 7.

Every non empty open set on real line is the countable union of non-empty disjoint open intervals.

[GARHWAL–2013]

PROOF. Let A be an open set and $x \in A$. Then by definition of open set, there exists an open interval I_x with centre x such that $x \in I_x \subseteq A$.

If C_x be the union of all such type of open intervals then we can write

$$C_x = \cup[I_x : I_x \subset A]$$

Clearly, C_x is the largest open interval containing x such that $x \in C_x \subset A$.

So, we can write $A = \cup C_x$

Now we have two possibilities : Either $C_x \cap C_y = \phi$ or $C_x \cap C_y \neq \phi \ \forall \ x, y \in A$

Consider the cases $C_x \cap C_y \neq \phi$

Then
$$C_x \subset (C_x \cup C_y) \subset A \Big]$$

and
$$C_y \subset (C_x \cup C_y) \subset A \Big] \qquad \ldots(1)$$

Now by definition of C_x and C_y

$$(C_x \cup C_y) \subset C_x \text{ and } (C_x \cup C_y) \subset C_y \qquad \ldots(2)$$

Therefore, from (1) and (2)

$$C_x = C_x \cup C_y \text{ and } C_y = C_x \cup C_y$$

which is possible only when $C_x = C_y$

So for all $x, y \in A$, we have either $C_x = C_y$ or $C_x \cap C_y = \phi$ and $A = \cup C_x$

Hence, A is the union of pairwise disjoint non-empty intervals. Now, we shall prove that the intervals C_x form a countable collection.

Let $G = \{G_n\}$ be a collection of open subsets of $\mathbf{R}$ such that

(i) $G_n \neq \phi \; \forall \, n$

(ii) $G_n \cap G_m = \phi$ for $n \neq m$

Since each G_n contains an infinite number of rational and irrational numbers so let $\mathbf{K} = \{K_n\}$ where K_n is the set of all rational numbers in G_n.

Now, define a map $f : \mathbf{K} \to G$ such that $f(K_n) = G_n$

Also, since for each $K_n \in \mathbf{K}$, there is a unique open set $G_n \in \mathbf{G}$ and conversely. So, f is one-one and onto.

$\Rightarrow$ $\mathbf{K}$ is cardinally equivalent to G.

But since $\mathbf{K}$ is the set of rational numbers therefore, $\cup K_n$ is countable and $\mathbf{K} \subset \mathbf{Q}$. Hence, $\mathbf{G}$ is countable.

☞ **REMARK**

• The above theorem can be restated as follows:

"A bounded set of non-overlapping intervals is countable."

THEOREM 8.

If $\{G_n\}$ be any collection of non-empty disjoint open set in $\mathbf{R}$ then $\{G_n\}$ is countable.

PROOF. Let $\mathbf{G} = \{G_n\}$ be a collection of open subsets of $\mathbf{R}$ such that

(i) $G_n \neq \phi \; \forall \, n$

(ii) $G_n \cap G_m = \phi$ for $n \neq m$

Since each G_n contains an infinite number of rational and irrational numbers so let $\mathbf{K} = \{K_n\}$ where K_n is the set of all rational numbers in G_n.

Now, define a map $f : K \to \mathbf{G}$ such that $f(K_n) = G_n$

Also, since for each $K_n \in \mathbf{K}$, there is a unique open set $G_n \in \mathbf{G}$ and conversely. So, f is one-one and onto.

$\Rightarrow$ $\mathbf{K}$ is cardinally equivalent to G.

But since $\mathbf{K}$ is the set of rational numbers therefore, $\cup K_n$ is countable and $\mathbf{K} \subset \mathbf{Q}$. Hence, $\mathbf{G}$ is countable.

THEOREM 9. ··

A discrete set (set of isolated points) is countable.

PROOF. Let A be a discrete set. We have to prove that A is countable. Let $x \in A$ be arbitrary.

$\Rightarrow$ x is an isolated point of A. 　　　　　　　(By definition of discrete set)

⇒ x is not the limit point of A.

⇒ $x \notin D(A)$, where $D(A)$ is the derived set of A.

By definition of limit point, $x \notin D(A)$ implies there exist an open set G containing x such that $G \cap A = \phi$ or $\{x\}$.

Now, since $x \in A$ and $x \in G$, therefore, $G \cap A = \{x\}$

Also, G is open interval therefore $G = \bigcup_{r=1}^{n} G_r, G_n \cap A = \{x_n\}$

If may be possible that $G_r \cap G_{r'} \neq \phi$ for $r \neq r'$

But we can make these intervals non-overlapping by reducing their length than $G_r \cap G_{r'} \neq \phi$. Also, we know that the set of non-overlapping intervals is enumerable, so G is enumerable.

⇒ $G \sim N$

Now define a map $f : A \to G$ such that $f(x_r) = G_r$

Clearly, f is one-one and onto, therefore, $A \sim G$.

But $G \sim N$

⇒ $A \sim N$

Hence A is enumerable.

THEOREM 10.

Every countable set is a Borel set.

PROOF.   Let A be a countable set. We have to prove that A is a Borel set. We know that a set is said to be Borel if it can be obtained by the formation of countable union and intersection of closed sets and open sets.

Since A is countable, then it can be written as

$$A = \{a_1, a_2, \ldots\}$$

Here, $$\{a_r\} = \{x : x = a_r\}$$

$$= \bigcup_{n=1}^{\infty} \{x : a_r \leq x < a_n + \frac{1}{n}\},$$

which is a countable collection of closed set.

Also, $$A = \bigcup_{r \in N} \{a_r\}$$

⇒ A can be obtained by the formation of countable union of closed sets.

Hence, A is a Borel set.

 Solved Examples

EXAMPLE 1.   *If α be any cardinal number, then show that $\alpha \leq |A| \leq \alpha \Rightarrow |A| = \alpha$*

SOLUTION.   For any cardinal number α, it is given that

$$\alpha \leq |A| \leq \alpha$$

We have to prove that $|A| = \alpha$

Let us suppose ∃ a set B such that $|B| = \alpha$

Here it is sufficient to prove that $|A| = |B|$, *i.e.*, $A \sim B$.

Since, it is given that $\alpha \leq |A|$

⇒ $$|B| \leq |A|$$

$\Rightarrow$ $B \sim$ to a subset of A or $B \sim A$ ...(1)

Now $|A| \le \alpha \Rightarrow |A| \le |B|$

$\Rightarrow$ $A \sim$ to a subset of B or $A \sim B$ ...(2)

From (1) and (2) we conclude that $A \sim B$

$\Rightarrow$ $\qquad\qquad |A| = |B|$

$\Rightarrow$ $\qquad\qquad |A| = \alpha$

EXAMPLE 2. *If α and β are two cardinal numbers such that $\alpha \le \beta$ and $\beta \le \alpha$ then show that $\alpha = \beta$.*

SOLUTION.   Let A and B be two sets such that

$\qquad\qquad$ Card$(A) = \alpha$ and Card$(B) = \beta$

Now, $\qquad \alpha \le \beta \Rightarrow$ Card$(A) \le$ Card(B)

$\qquad\qquad \Rightarrow$ $A \sim$ to a subset of B or $A \sim B$ ...(1)

If $\beta \le \alpha \Rightarrow$ Card$(B) \le$ Card(A)

$\qquad\qquad \Rightarrow$ $B \sim$ to a subset of A or $B \sim A$ ...(2)

From (1) and (2) we conclude that

$\qquad\qquad A \sim B$

$\Rightarrow$ $\qquad$ Card$(A) =$ Card(B)

$\Rightarrow$ $\qquad\qquad \alpha = \beta$

EXAMPLE 3. *Show that for every real number x, the real number in the semi-open interval $[x, x + 1[$ from an uncountable set.*

SOLUTION.   For any arbitrary $x \in R$, define a map

$\qquad\qquad f : [x, x + 1[\to [0, 1[$ such that $f(X) = X - x$

Clearly, $\qquad f(x) = x - x = 0$

and $\qquad f(x + 1) = x + 1 - x = 1$

which shows that f is well defined

Now, $\qquad f(x_1) = f(x_2)$

$\Leftrightarrow$ $\qquad x_1 - x = x_2 - x; x_1, x_2 \in [x, x + 1[$

$\Leftrightarrow$ $\qquad x_1 = x_2$

Thus, f is one-one.

Further, since f is continuous mapping therefore, f is onto also.

$\Rightarrow$ $\qquad [x, x + 1[\sim [0, 1[$

$\Rightarrow$ $\qquad |[x, x + 1[| = |[0, 1[|$

But we know that the set of real numbers in $[0, 1[$ form an uncountable set. Hence, the set of all real numbers in $[x, x + 1[$ form an uncountable set.

EXAMPLE 4. *If α is any transfinite cardinal number then show that $a \le \alpha$.*

SOLUTION.   Let A be any infinite set such that $|A| = \alpha$

We have to prove that $a \le \alpha$

Since A is infinite therefore, $\exists$ a set $B \subset A$ such that $|B| \le |A|$

$\Rightarrow$ $\qquad\qquad a \le \alpha$

EXAMPLE 5. *Prove that $a < c$.*

SOLUTION.   We know that

$\qquad\qquad |N| = a, |R| = c$ and $N \subset R$

Now, $N \subset R$ $\qquad \Rightarrow |N| \le |R|$

$\qquad\qquad \Rightarrow$ $a \le c$ ...(1)

Since, N is not cardinally equivalent to R therefore, $a \ne c$.

Hence, from (1) $a < c$

EXAMPLE 6. *Prove that the set {±1, ±4, ±9, ±16, ...} is countable.* [KANPUR–2004, AGRA–2014]

SOLUTION. Let $A = \{\pm 1, \pm 4, \pm 9, \pm 16, ...\}$

Let us define two sets B and C such that

$$B = \{1, 4, 9, 16, ...\}$$

and $\qquad C = \{-1, -4, -9, -16, ...\}$

Clearly, $A = B \cup C$ and $B \cap C = \phi$.

Then $\mathbf{N} \sim B$ under the mapping $n \to n^2$, *i.e.*, $f : \mathbf{N} \to B$ such that $f(n) = n^2$ is one-one and onto.

Therefore, $\qquad |\mathbf{N}| = |B|$

$\Rightarrow \qquad\qquad |B| = a \qquad\qquad\qquad\qquad\qquad (\because |\mathbf{N}| = \mathbf{a})$

In a similar way $B \sim C$ under the map $n \to -n$

$\Rightarrow \qquad\qquad |B| = |C|$

$\Rightarrow \qquad\qquad |C| = a$

Finally $\qquad\qquad A = B \cup C$

$\Rightarrow \qquad\qquad |A| = |B| + |C| = a + a = a \qquad\qquad (\because a + a = a)$

Hence, A is countable.

EXAMPLE 7. *Show that two enumerable sets are equivalent.*

SOLUTION. Let A and B be two enumerable sets.

We have to prove that $A \sim B$.

Since A and B both are enumerable, therefore by definition

$$A \sim N \text{ and } B \sim N$$

We know that the relation $\sim$ is an equivalence relation.

So, by symmetry $B \sim N \Rightarrow \boldsymbol{N} \sim B$

Hence, by transitivity $A \sim N, N \sim B \Rightarrow A \sim B$.

EXAMPLE 8. *Find the power of an aggregate of number given by* $\dfrac{M}{2^m}$, *M and m are positive integers.*

SOLUTION. Let us define

$$A = \left\{ \frac{M}{2^m} : m, M \in \boldsymbol{N} \right\}$$

Write $\qquad A_m = \left\{ \dfrac{M}{2^m}, m \in \boldsymbol{N} \right\} \forall M \in \boldsymbol{N}$

Then elements of A_m can be written as follows:

$$A_1 : \frac{1}{2^1}, \frac{1}{2^2}, \frac{1}{2^3}, ..., \frac{1}{2^n}, ...$$

$$A_2 : \frac{2}{2^1}, \frac{2}{2^2}, \frac{2}{2^3}, ..., \frac{2}{2^n}, ...$$

$$A_3 : \frac{3}{2^1}, \frac{3}{2^2}, \frac{3}{2^3}, ..., \frac{3}{2^n}, ...$$

$$... \quad ... \quad ... \quad ... \quad ... \quad ...$$

$$A_n : \frac{n}{2^1}, \frac{n}{2^2}, \frac{n}{2^3}, ..., \frac{n}{2^n}, ...$$

We observe that

(1) Each A_i is enumerable.

(2) $A_i \cap A_j = \phi \; \forall \; i, j \in N, i \neq j$

(3) $A = \overset{\infty}{\underset{r=1}{\cup}} A_r$

Since, each A_i is enumerable and we know that enumerable union of enumerable sets is enumerable therefore, from (3) A is enumerable. Therefore,

$$|A| = a$$

Hence, the power of the given set is a.

EXAMPLE 9. *If each a_i (i = 1, 2, ..., n) is a rational number then the rational point $a = (a_1, a_2, ..., a_n) \in R^n$ is enumerable.*

SOLUTION. We have already known that the set of rational numbers is countable. Therefore, varying $a_1, a_2, ..., a_n$ we can form an rational points.

Now since $a \cdot a = a$ therefore $a^n = a$

which shows that the set of all rational points has the same cardinality as that of **N**. Hence, set of rational points is countable.

EXAMPLE 10. *Show that the set of points in the closed interval [2, 4] and in the open interval]1, 2[and cardinally equivalent.*

SOLUTION. Define a map $f: [2, 4] \to [1, 2]$ such that $f(x) = \left(\dfrac{x-2}{2}\right) + 1$

Now, $\qquad\qquad f(x_1) = f(x_2)$

$\Leftrightarrow \qquad \dfrac{x_1 - 2}{2} + 1 = \dfrac{x_2 - 2}{2} + 1$

$\Leftrightarrow \qquad \dfrac{x_1 - 2}{2} = \dfrac{x_2 - 2}{2}$

$\Leftrightarrow \qquad\qquad x_1 = x_2$

Therefore, f is one-one.

Also, since f is continuous, therefore, f is onto.

Now f is one-one onto

$\Rightarrow \qquad\qquad [2, 4] \sim [1, 2]$

$\Rightarrow \qquad\qquad |[2, 4]| = |[1, 2]|$

But we know that $|\,]1, 2[\,| = |[1, 2]|$

Hence, $\qquad |[2, 4]| = |\,]1, 2[\,|$

$\Rightarrow \qquad\qquad [2, 4] \sim \,]1, 2[$

EXAMPLE 11. *Let X be any non-empty set and C be the family of functions $f : X \to [0, 1]$. Show that the family of subsets of X, i.e., the power set of X is equivalent to C.*

SOLUTION. Let $P(X)$ = Power set of X

Further, let $A \in P(X)$

Now define the characteristic function ϕ_A of A relative to X.

Further define a mapping $f : P(X) \to C$ by the formula $f(A) = \phi_A$

Evidently f is one-one and onto.

Hence, $P(X) \sim C$.

EXAMPLE 12. *Prove that $]0, 1] \sim \,]0, 1[$.*

SOLUTION. Let x and y be denotes the points of $]0, 1]$ and $]0, 1[$ respectively. Then define a correspondence

$$y = \frac{3}{2} - x \text{ for } \frac{1}{2} < x \le 1 \text{ then } \frac{1}{2} \le y < 1$$

$$y = \frac{3}{4} - x \text{ for } \frac{1}{4} < x \le \frac{1}{2} \text{ then } \frac{1}{4} \le y < \frac{1}{2}$$

$$y = \frac{3}{8} - x \text{ for } \frac{1}{8} < x \le \frac{1}{4} \text{ then } \frac{1}{8} \le y < \frac{1}{4}$$

Now, we observe that, for every $x \in]0, 1]$ there correspond one and only one y of $]0, 1[$. Hence, $]0, 1] \sim]0, 1[$.

EXAMPLE 13. *Show that the interval $]0, 1[$ is equivalent to the set of real numbers $\mathbf{R}$ and hence show that $Card(]0, 1[) = Card(\mathbf{R})$.*

SOLUTION. Let us define a function $f :]0, 1[\to \mathbf{R}$ such that

$$f(x) = \begin{cases} \dfrac{2x-1}{x}; & x \in \left]0, \dfrac{1}{2}\right[\\ \dfrac{2x-1}{1-x}; & x \in \left[\dfrac{1}{2}, 1\right[\end{cases}$$

We can easily verify that the function f is one-one and onto.

Therefore, $]0, 1[\sim \mathbf{R}$.

Hence, $Card(]0, 1[) = Card(\mathbf{R}) = c$

☞ **REMARKS**
- Since the set $]0, 1[$ is uncountable and $]0, 1[\sim \mathbf{R}$. Therefore, $\mathbf{R}$ is also uncountable.
- If two sets have the same cardinally (as in the above example), then this cardinality is called the **Cardinal number of Continum**.

EXAMPLE 14. *Prove that $a < c < f$ where a, c and f denote the cardinal number of the sets of all natural numbers, real numbers and the set of all real valued function defined over $[0, 1]$ respectively.* [KERALA–2014, CALCUTTA–2006, MEERUT–2009, GARHWAL–1997]

SOLUTION. Since we know that

$$a < c \qquad \qquad \ldots(1)$$

Therefore, it is sufficient to prove that $c < f$

Let F be the set of all real valued functions defined over $[0, 1]$. Define a mapping $f_k : [0, 1] \to \mathbf{R}$ such that $f_k(x) = k \; \forall \; x \in [0, 1]$ where k is a real number in $[0,1]$. Further consider the mapping $f_k : [0, 1] \to \mathbf{R}$ defined as $f_k(x) = k \; \forall \; x \in [0, 1]$ and $k \in [0, 1]$ is a real number.

Since each function f_k is real valued, therefore, the set $F^* = \{f_k : 0 \le k \le 1\}$ is a proper subset of F.

We can easily set up a one-to-one correspondance between $[0, 1]$ and F^* such that $F^* \subset F$.

Hence, $Card[0, 1] = Card \, F^* < Card \, F$

$\Rightarrow$ $c < f$ $\ldots(2)$

Finally, from (1) and (2) we conclude that

$$a < c < f$$

EXAMPLE 15. *If the derived set of a set is countable then show that the original set is also countable.*

SOLUTION. Let A be any set and $D(A)$ be the derived set of A such that $D(A)$ is countable. We have to prove that A is countable.

Now define a set $B = \{x \in A : x \notin D(A)\}$

Then $B \subset A$

Further $B \subset A \Rightarrow D(B) \subset D(A)$

Therefore, $x \notin D(A)$ and $D(B) \subset D(A) \Rightarrow x \notin D(B)$

$\Rightarrow$ x is not the limit point of B

$\Rightarrow$ x is an isolated point of B

$\Rightarrow$ B is an isolated set

And we know that every isolated (Discrete) set is countable.

$\Rightarrow$ B is countable.

Further $A - B = A \cap D(A)$

$\Rightarrow$ $\qquad A = B \cup (A \cap D(A))$ ...(1)

But $A \cap D(A) \subset D(A)$ and $D(A)$ is countable.

$\Rightarrow$ $A \cap D(A)$ is countable.

Then from (1), being the union of two countable sets, A is countable.

EXAMPLE 16. *Let X be any set and A(X) be the family of all the characteristic functions of X, then show that the power set of X is equivalent to A(X).*

SOLUTION. For any set X, $A(X)$ denote the family of all characteristic function of X and $P(X)$ denote the power set of X.

We have to show that $A(X) \sim P(X)$.

For any arbitrary set $B \subset X$, define the chararcterstic function X_B of B relative to X. Then

$$X_B : X \rightarrow \{0, 1\} \text{ such that } X_B(x) = \begin{cases} 1 & \text{if } x \in B \\ 0 & \text{if } x \notin B \end{cases}$$

By definition of $A(X)$, X_B is an arbitrary element of $A(X)$ and B is an arbitrary element of $P(X)$.

Define a map $f : A(X) \rightarrow P(X)$ such that $f(X_B) = B$

$\Rightarrow$ f maps the characteristic function of B relative to X into the set B

Clearly, f is one-one and onto.

Hence, $A(X) \sim P(X)$.

EXAMPLE 17. *Show that the set $\mathbf{N} \times \mathbf{N}$ is countable.*

SOLUTION. Let $\mathbf{N}$ be the set of natural numbers.

We know that $|\mathbf{N}| = a$

In order to prove that $\mathbf{N} \times \mathbf{N}$ is countable, we shall prove that

$\qquad a \cdot a = a$

By definition of cartesian product of two sets, the elements of $\mathbf{N} \times \mathbf{N}$ can be written as follows:

$\qquad$ (1, 1), (1, 2), (1, 3), ..., (1, m), ...

$\qquad$ (2, 1), (2, 2), (2, 3), ..., (2, m), ...

$\qquad$ ... ...

$\qquad$ (n, 1), (n, 2), (n, 3), ..., (n, m), ...

Now, if we write $A_i = \{(i, 1), (i, 2), (i, 3), ...\}$

Then we observe that

(i) $N \times N = \bigcup_{i=1}^{\infty} A_i$

(ii) $A_i \cap A_j = \phi$ for $i \neq j$

(iii) Each A_i is enumerable

$\Rightarrow$ $\bigcup_{i=1}^{\infty} A_i$ is enumerable

(∵ Enumerable union of enumerable sets is enumerable)

$\Rightarrow$ $N \times N$ is enumerable.

Therefore $N \times N \sim N$

$\Rightarrow$ $|N \times N| = |N|$

$\Rightarrow$ $a \times a = a$

Recapitulations

- A is enumerable $\Rightarrow A \sim N \Rightarrow |A| = |N| = a$
- A is uncountable $\Rightarrow A \sim [0, 1] \Rightarrow |A| = |[0,1]|$ $= c$
- $a + n = n + a = a$ for any $n \in N$
- $na = a$, $nc = c$ for $n \in N$

- Cancellation laws does not hold.
- $c^c = 2^c$
- For any transfinite cardinal number α, $a \leq \alpha$.
- Two enumerable sets are equivalent.

Exercise 2.1

1. Show that the set of all real numbers is equivalent to the set of positive real numbers.

2. For any two sets X and Y, prove that $(X \times Y) \sim (Y \times X)$.

3. Show that every quotient set of a countable set is countable.

4. Let $f : A \to B$ be a function. Show that if A is countable then B is also countable.

5. Prove that the continuous image of a countable set is countable.

6. Prove that the set of all finite sequence whose terms are algebraic numbers is countable.

7. Show that the set of all finite sequences of natural numbers is countable.

8. Prove that the set of points of discontinuity of a monotonic function is countable.

9. Prove that the set of all straight line in a plane each of which passes through at least two points (different) with rational coordinates is countable.

10. If Card(A) = Card(C) and Card(B) = Card(D), show that Card($A \times B$) = Card($C \times D$).

11. Show that the set of all sequences of real numbers has cardinal number c.

12. Show that the set of all continuous real valued functions defined on the closed interval [0, 1] has power c.

13. Show that $n < 2^n$ for any cardinal number n.

14. If $f : A \to B$ and range of f is uncountable then prove that domain of f is also uncountable.

15. Prove that the set of complex numbers is uncountable.

16. Prove that the set of all sequences whose elements are the digits 0 and 1, is uncountable.

2.9 CANTOR-LIKE SETS

Cantor-like sets and the functions defined on it are very useful. The most popular example of Cantor-like set is Cantor's ternary set, established by G. Cantor. It is also simply known as Cantor's set.

Definition. *The Cantor's set is a subset of the interval [0, 1] which is left after the removal of a certain specified countable collection of open intervals from [0, 1].*

2.9.1 CONSTRUCTION OF CANTOR'S TERNARY SET

Consider the closed interval [0, 1]. Divide the interval [0, 1] into three equal parts and remove one part (middle).

$$
\begin{array}{c c c c}
0 & 1/3 & 2/3 & 1
\end{array}
$$

Remove the open interval $\left]\dfrac{1}{3}, \dfrac{2}{3}\right[$ of the length $\dfrac{1}{3}$.

Further divide each of the remaining intervals into three equal parts and again remove the middle one, *i.e.*, remove the intervals $\left]\dfrac{1}{3^2}, \dfrac{2}{3^2}\right[$ and $\left]\dfrac{7}{9}, \dfrac{8}{9}\right[$ of the length $\dfrac{1}{3^2}$.

Continuing in the same way infinitely many times, we have at pth step, 2^{p-1} open intervals are removed each of length $\dfrac{1}{3^p}$.

Then remaining sets constitute Cantor's ternary set. Let this set be denoted by F. Then F′ is the enumerable union of mutually disjoint open intervals.

Clearly F′ is open which imply that F is always a closed set.

Now, $F = [0, 1] - F'$ where $F' = \left]\dfrac{1}{3}, \dfrac{2}{3}\right[\cup \left]\dfrac{1}{9}, \dfrac{2}{9}\right[\cup \left]\dfrac{7}{9}, \dfrac{8}{9}\right[\cup \ldots$

We observe that the Cantor-ternary set definitely contains the points $0, 1, \dfrac{1}{3}, \dfrac{2}{3}, \dfrac{1}{9}, \dfrac{2}{9}, \dfrac{7}{9}, \dfrac{8}{9}, \ldots$ etc.

THEOREM I.

Cantor set is a perfect set.

PROOF. Let C be a cantor set. We have to prove that F is perfect, *i.e.*, closed and dense itself. We know that every Cantor set is closed.

$\Rightarrow$ It contains all its limit point (By def. of closed set)

$\Rightarrow$ Every limit point of C belongs to C.

Now, we shall prove that every number of C is a limit point of numbers having terminating ternary expansions.

Let $x_0 \in C$ be arbitrary. Then ternary expansion of x_0 is given by $x_0 = \cdot a_1 a_2 a_3 \ldots a_n \ldots$, where each $a_n = 0$ or 2

Construct a sequence $<x_n>$ of elements of C as given below

$$x_1 = \cdot a_1' a_2 a_3 \ldots a_n \ldots$$
$$x_2 = \cdot a_1 a_2' a_3 \ldots a_n \ldots$$
$$\ldots \quad \ldots \quad \ldots \quad \ldots \quad \ldots$$
$$\ldots \quad \ldots \quad \ldots \quad \ldots \quad \ldots$$
$$x_n = \cdot a_1 a_2 a_3 \ldots a_n' \ldots$$

Clearly for all $n \in \mathbf{N}, a_n' = 0$ if $a_n = 2$ and $a_n' = 2$, if $a_n = 0$. Therefore, $x_n \neq x_0 \ \forall \ n$.

Also, $\qquad \lim\limits_{n \to \infty} x_n = x_0$

$\Rightarrow \quad x_0$ is the limit point of $C \quad \Rightarrow x_0 \in D(C)$. Thus, $C \subseteq D(C)$.

$\Rightarrow \quad C$ is dense-in-itself.

Hence, C is a perfect set.

THEOREM 2.

Cantor's set is uncountable.

PROOF. Let F be a Cantor set. We have to prove that F is uncountable. Let if possible F is countable, then by definition of countable set, the elements of F can be arranged in the form of a sequence as follows

$$F = \{x_n : n \in N\}$$

Now express each x_is in ternary expansion as follows:

$$x_1 = 0 \cdot x_{11} x_{12} x_{13} \cdots x_{1m} \cdots$$
$$x_2 = 0 \cdot x_{21} x_{22} x_{23} \cdots x_{2m} \cdots$$
$$\cdots \quad \cdots \quad \cdots \quad \cdots \quad \cdots \quad \quad \cdots$$
$$\cdots \quad \cdots \quad \cdots \quad \cdots \quad \cdots \quad \quad \cdots$$
$$x_n = 0 \cdot x_{n1} x_{n2} x_{n3} x_{n3} \cdots x_{nm} \cdots$$

such that $x_{nr} = 0$ or 2 $\forall$ r and n

Further construct a real number

$$x = \cdot \alpha_1 \alpha_2 \alpha_3 \cdots$$

such that $\alpha_m = 2$ if $x_{mm} = 0$ and $\alpha_m = 0$ if $x_{mm} = 2$.
In either case $x_{mm} \neq a_m$ for all m giving $x_m \neq n$ $\forall$ $m \in N$.
Since, $\alpha_m = 0$ or 2 for all m, therefore, $x \in F$

$\Rightarrow$ F contains other points also besides x_m

which is a contradiction, so our assumption is wrong.
Hence, the Cantor set is uncountable.

THEOREM 3.

Each point of the Cantor set F is a limit point of F.

PROOF. Let $x_0 \in F$ be arbitrary then ternary expansion of x_0 can be written as follows:

$$x = \cdot a_1 a_2 a_3 \cdots a_n \cdots$$

when $a_n = 0$ or 2
Now construct a sequence $<x_n>$ of points as given below:

$$x_1 = \cdot a_1' a_2 a_3 \cdots a_n \cdots$$
$$x_2 = \cdot a_1 a_2' a_3 \cdots a_n \cdots$$
$$x_3 = \cdot a_1 a_2 a_3' \cdots a_n \cdots$$
$$\cdots \quad \cdots \quad \cdots \quad \cdots \quad \cdots$$
$$\cdots \quad \cdots \quad \cdots \quad \cdots \quad \cdots$$
$$x_n = \cdot a_1 a_2 a_3 \cdots a_n' \cdots$$

where $a_n' = 2$ if $a_n = 2$ and $a_n' = 2$ if $a_n = 0$

$\Rightarrow$ $<x_n>$ is a sequence of points in F such that $x_n \neq x_0$ for any n.

Also, $$\lim_{n \to \infty} x_n = x_0$$

$\Rightarrow$ x_0 is the limit point of F.

Finally, since $x_0 \in F$ be arbitrary. Hence each point of F is the limit point of F.

THEOREM 4.

The Cardinal number of the cantor set is the Cardinal number c of the linear continuum. [MEERUT]

PROOF.   Define a mapping $f : F \to [0, 1]$

Let $x \in F$, then its ternary expansion can be written as follows:
$$x = 0 \cdot x_1 x_2 x_3 \ldots$$
where each $x_i = 0$ or 2

Then clearly we define $f(x)$ as the number whose binary expansion is $0 \cdot k_1 k_2 k_3 \ldots$

where $k_i = \dfrac{1}{2} x_i \; \forall i \in N$

So, $f(0 \cdot x_1 x_2 x_3 \ldots) = 0 \cdot k_1 k_2 k_3 \ldots$, where $k_i = \dfrac{1}{2} x_i \; \forall i \in N$

Then

(i) f is one-one

Let $x = 0 \cdot x_1 x_2 x_3 \ldots$ and $y = 0 \cdot y_1 y_2 y_3 \ldots$ be any two distinct elements of F such that each x_i and $y_i = 0$ or 2.

Now $f(x) = f(y)$

$\Leftrightarrow$ $f(0 \cdot x_1 x_2 x_3 \ldots) = f(0 \cdot y_1 y_2 y_3 \ldots)$

$\Leftrightarrow$ $0 \cdot k_1 k_2 k_3 \ldots = 0 \cdot p_1 p_2 p_3 \ldots, \; k_i = \dfrac{1}{2} x_i$ and $p_i = \dfrac{1}{2} y_i \; \forall i$

$\Leftrightarrow$ $k_i = p_i$ for each i

$\Leftrightarrow$ $x_i = y_i$ for each i

$\Leftrightarrow$ $x = y$

$\Leftrightarrow$ f is one-one.

(ii) f is onto

Let $z \in [0, 1]$. Then its binary expansion be given by
$$z = 0 \cdot l_1 l_2 l_3 \ldots \text{ where each } l_i = 0 \text{ or } 1$$

If $2 l_i = x_i$ then $x_i = 0$ or 2

So the number $x = 0 \cdot x_1 x_2 x_3 \ldots$, where $x_i = 2 l_i$, belongs to the set F such that
$$f(x) = f(0 \cdot x_1 x_2 x_3 \ldots) = 0 \cdot l_1 l_2 l_3 \ldots = z, \; l_i = \dfrac{1}{2} x_i \; \forall i$$

$\Rightarrow$ For each $z \in [0, 1]$ there exists a preimage x in F under the mapping f.

$\Rightarrow$ f is onto.

From (i) and (ii) we conclude that f is one-one and onto.

$\Rightarrow$ $\text{Card}(F) = \text{Card}([0, 1]) = \mathbf{c}$

Hence, $\text{Card}(F) = \mathbf{c}$.

☞ **REMARK**

- The Cantor set can be put into a one-to-one correspondance with [0, 1].

Exercise 2.2

1. Prove that the Cantor's set is monotonic increasing and continuous.

2. Prove that the each point x of the cantor set F can be represented uniquely by a series of the form $x = \sum\limits_{n=1}^{\infty} \dfrac{a_n}{3^n}$ where each a_n is either 0 or 2 and conversely.

3. Prove that Cantor's set can be put into a one-to-one correspondance with the interval [0,1].

4. Show that Canor's set is bounded.

5. Show that Cantor's set contains no open interval.

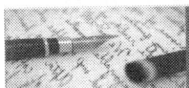
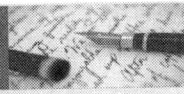

CHAPTER Summary

KEY TERMS

- **COUNTABLE SET :** A set which can be put in one-to-one correspondance with the set of natural numbers or with its subset is called countable set.
- **ENUMERABLE SET:** An infinite countable set is known as enumerable or denumerable or countably infinite set.
- **UNCOUNTABLE SET:** A set which is not countable, is called uncountable.
- **ALGEBRAIC NUMBERS:** The numbers which can be define as a roots of the polynomial are called algebraic numbers.
- **TRANSCENDENTAL NUMBERS:** A number which is not algebraic is called transcendental number.
- **CARDINALLY EQUIVALENT SET:** Two sets P and Q are said to be cardinally equivalent if there exists a one-to-one correspondance between P and Q.
- **CARDINAL NUMBER:** The no. of elements in the given finite set is called Cardinal number.
- **TRANSFINITE CARDINAL NUMBER:** The Cardinal number of an infinite set is called transfinite cardinal number.
- **CANTOR'S SET:** The cantor's set F is the set of all numbers in the interval $[0, 1]$ which have a ternary expansion with digits 0 or 2.

RESULTS

- Every subset of a countable set is countable.
- The union of enumerable collection of enumerable sets is also enumerable.
- Union of countable collection of countable sets is also countable.
- The set of all rational numbers $\mathbf{Q}$ is enumerable.
- The set of all real numbers in $[0, 1]$ or in $]0, 1[$ is not enumerable.
- The set of real numbers $\mathbf{R}$ is not enumerable.
- The set of all irrational numbers is not enumerable.
- The set of all algebraic number is enumerable.
- The set of polynomials with integral coefficients is enumerable.
- The set of all transcendental numbers in any interval is non-enumerable.
- The relation ~ is an equivalent relation.
- Every infinite set has a subset with cardinality $= |\mathbf{N}| = a$.
- If an enumerable set is added to an infinite set, then Cardinal number of the infinite set is unaffected.
- Every monotonic function in a closed interval is discontinuous at a countable number of points of that interval.
- $\mathrm{Card}(A) < \mathrm{Card}(P(A))$ **[Cantor's Theorem]**
- If $A_1 \subset B \subset A$ and $A \sim A_1$ then $A \sim B$ **(Equivalence Theorem)**
- If $\mathrm{Card}(A) \le \mathrm{Card}(B)$ and $\mathrm{Card}(B) \le \mathrm{Card}(A)$ then $\mathrm{Card}(A) = \mathrm{Card}(B)$ **(Schorder-Bernstein theorem)**
- Every superset of an uncountable set is uncountable.
- A countable set is a Borel set.
- Cantor set is a perfect set (dense-in-itself and closed)
- Cantor's set is uncountable.
- Each point of the Cantor's set is its limit point.
- The Cardinal number of the Cantor set is the Cardinal number of the linear continum.

WORTHY READINGS

☞ A cardinal number m is finite if and only if $2^{2^m} + 1 \ne 2^{2^m}$.

☞ A set of cardinality c has 2^c different subsets, each of cardinality c.

☞ $1 + 2^{2^a} = 2^{2^a}$

☞ $1^a = 1 = 1^c$

☞ $(n + 1)^a = c, \mathbf{n} \ge 1$

☞ For two tranfinite cardinal numbers α and β
   $\alpha + \beta = \alpha\beta = \max\{\alpha, \beta\}$

☞ If $A = \cup A_n$ and $|A| = c$ then there is at least one of the sets A_n has cardinality c.

☞ Cantor's set contains no open interval and hence contains no interior point.

☞ Cantor's set is closed and bounded and hence compact.

☞ Between any two points of Cantor set C there exist an open interval which belongs to the complement of C.

☞ Cantor set is no where dense set.

☞ FURTHER READINGS

☞ The set N and E (even natural numbers) are equivalent because if define a function $f : N \to E$ by $f(n) = 2n$, $n \in N$ then f is one-one and onto.

☞ The function $f : Z \to N$ defined by $f(0) = 1$, $f(n) = 2n$ and $f(-n) = 2n + 1$ for $n \in N$ is one-one onto function. So $Z \sim N$.

☞ If $A = \{1, 2, 3, 4\}$ and $B = \{a, b, c, d\}$. Then $A \sim B$ because there exist a function $f : A \to B$ such that $f(1) = a, f(2) = b, f(3) = c$ and $f(4) = d$, which is clearly one-one and onto.

☞ Let $A = \{1, 2, 3\}$ and $B = \{a, b\}$. If we list all the functions defined from A to B, then none of them is one-to-one. Hence, A is not equivalent to B.

☞ The finite interval $\left] -\dfrac{\pi}{2}, \dfrac{\pi}{2} \right[$ is equivalent to the set of real numbers R, because there exist a function $f : \left] -\dfrac{\pi}{2}, \dfrac{\pi}{2} \right[\to R$ defined by $f(x) = \tan x$, which is one-one and onto.

☞ For any cardinal numbers α, β and γ, we have the following results:

(i) $\alpha^\beta \cdot \alpha^\gamma = \alpha^{\beta + \gamma}$

(ii) $(\alpha\beta)^\gamma = \alpha^{\beta\gamma}$

(iii) $(\alpha\beta)^\gamma = \alpha^\gamma \beta^\gamma$

(iv) $\alpha^\gamma \le \beta^\gamma$ if $\alpha \le \beta$

Chapter
3

Lebesgue Measure on Real Line

3.1 INTRODUCTION

In previous classes we have studied about the length of the interval. It is defined as the difference of the end points. Clearly, the length of each of the interval $[a, b]$, $[a, b[$, $]a, b]$ and $]a, b[$ is $b - a$. If I is the interval then length of I is denoted by $|I|$. The concept of measure in an interval is an extension of concept of length. In this chapter we shall discuss the concept of measure with the help of the length of the interval.

3.2 LENGTHS OF OPEN AND CLOSED SETS

We know that the length is an example of a set function, *i.e.,* a function which associates an extended real number to each set in some collection of sets. In case of length, the domain is the collection of all intervals. The set function l satisfying the following conditions:

(i) $l(I) \geq 0$ for all intervals I, *i.e.,* length of any interval is always non-negative.

(ii) If $\{I_i\}$ is a countable collection of mutually disjoint intervals such that $\bigcup_i I_i$ is an interval then

$$l(\bigcup_i I_i) = \sum_i l(I_i)$$

(iii) For any fixed real number x, $l(I) = l(I + x)$.

Thus, we conclude that in the case of length, the domain is the collection of all intervals.

Definition 1. *Let G be an open subset of an interval $[a, b]$ then there exists a countable collection of disjoint open intervals $\{I_n\}$ such that $G = \bigcup_n I_n$. Then length of G, denoted by $|G|$ is defined as the sum of the lengths of the intervals of this family, i.e., $|G| = \sum_n |I_n|$.*

Definition 2. *Let F be any closed subsets of the interval $[a, b]$ then length of F denoted by $|F|$ is defined by*

$$|F| = |G| - |G - F|$$

where G is an open subset of $[a, b]$. Since F is closed, so $G - F$ is open.

We can find the length of G and $G - F$ as discussed in definition (1).

Particularly, if $F \subset [a, b]$ is closed then

$$|F| = (b - a) - |F'|$$

☞ **REMARKS**
- If G_1 and G_2 be two open subsets of $[a, b]$ such that $G_2 \subseteq G_1$ then $|G_1| \geq |G_2|$.
- If G_1 and G_2 are two open subsets of $[a, b]$ then
$$|G_1| + |G_2| = |G_1 \cup G_2| + |G_1 \cap G_2|$$
- If G_1 and G_2 are disjoint, i.e., $G_1 \cap G_2 = \phi$ $(\because |G_1 \cap G_2| = |\phi| = 0)$
  Then $\qquad\qquad |G_1| + |G_2| = |G_1 \cup G_2|$

3.2.1 MEASURE OF AN OPEN AND A CLOSED SET

Let G be an open set contained in the interval $[a, b]$ then measure of G, denoted by $m(G)$ is defined by

$$m(G) \leq b - a$$

Similarly, let F be a closed set contained in the open interval $]a, b[$ then measure of F, i.e., $m(F)$ is given by

$$m(F) = b - a - m(F') \text{ where } F' =]a, b[- F$$

☞ **REMARKS**
- $m[]a, b[] = b - a$
- $m[[a, b]] = b - a$
- Let $R(a < x < b, c < y < d)$ be an open rectangle then $m(R) = (b - a)(d - c)$
- If $V(a < x < b, c < y < d, l < z < m)$ be a parallelopiped then $m(V) = (b - a)(d - c)(l - m)$

3.3 LEBESGUE OUTER MEASURE OF A SET

Let A be any subset of real number R. Then outer measure m^* is a set function defined from the power set $P(R)$ of R into the set of all non-negative extended real numbers such that

$$m^*(A) = \begin{cases} 0 & \text{if } A = \phi \\ \text{infimum } \{y : y = \Sigma \mid I_i \mid, \text{ where } \{I_i\} \text{ is a countable family of} \\ \text{open intervals such that } A \subseteq \cup I_i, A \neq \phi \end{cases}$$

☞ **REMARKS**
- The Lebesgue outer measure of a set is also known as Lebesgue exterior measure or briefly outer measure.
- Other notations of Lebesgue outer measure are $m^e(A)$ or $\bar{m}(A)$.

3.3.1 PROPERTIES OF LEBESGUE OUTER MEASURE

PROP. 1   For all set A, $m^*(A)$ is always non-negative, i.e., $m^*(A) \geq 0$, $\forall A \subseteq R$.

PROP. 2   If $\{I_n\}$ is any countable family of open intervals such that $\bigcup_n I_n \supseteq A$ then $m^*(A) \leq \Sigma_n |I_n|$

PROP. 3   For any set A, $m^*(A)$ is the least length to cover the set A from outside.

PROP. 4   For every set A, $m^*(A)$ is unique.

PROP. 5   If G is an open set of real numbers then $m^*(G) = |G|$.

PROP. 6   For each $\varepsilon > 0$ there exists at least one countable family of open intervals such that $\bigcup_n I_n \supseteq A$ and $m^*(A) + \varepsilon > \Sigma_n |I_n|$. In other words, we can say that, $m^*(A)$ is less than or equal to the length of any family of open intervals but when we add a very small positive number ε to $m^*(A)$, it becomes strictly greater than the length of at least one family of open intervals covering A.

PROP. 7　　　If $A \neq \phi$. Then we can define

$$m^*(A) = \text{infimum}\{|G| : G \text{ is open set such that } A \subseteq G\}$$

THEOREM 1.

If A and B are two sets such that $A \subseteq B$. Then $m^*(A) \leq m^*(B)$.

PROOF.　　　Let A and B be two sets such that $A \subseteq B$.

Define a countable family $\{I_n\}$ of open intervals such that

$$\bigcup_n I_n \supseteq B \qquad\qquad\qquad ...(1)$$

in such a way that $m^*(B) = \sum_n |I_n|$

It is given that $B \supseteq A$　　　　　　　　　　　　　　　...(2)

$\Rightarrow$ 　　　　　　　　$\bigcup_n I_n \supseteq A$ 　　　　　(From (1) and (2))

$\Rightarrow$ 　　　　　　　$m^*(A) \leq \sum_n |I_n| = m^*(B)$

Hence $m^*(A) \leq m^*(B)$.

THEOREM 2.

The outer measure of an interval on the real line is equal to its length.

PROOF.　　　Let I be the given interval.

Let us first suppose I is an open interval such $I =]a, b[$. Then clearly the family $\{]a, b[\}$ of open intervals will be the least length covering I. Therefore,

$$m^*(I) = |(a, b)| = b - a$$

Similar result follows in case of closed interval.

THEOREM 3.

For every singleton A, $m^*(A) = 0$.

PROOF.　　　Let A be the singleton set such that $A = \{a\}$.

Then we can write

$$A = \{a\} = [a, a]$$

$\Rightarrow$ 　　　　　$m^*(A) = \text{length of } \{[a, a]\}$

$$= a - a = 0$$

THEOREM 4.

The Lebesgue measure function m^* is translation invariant.　　　[HPU–2000, 02, 04, 17, KURUKSHETRA–2014]

PROOF.　　　Let $I = [a, b]$ be the given interval. Then we define

$$I + x = \{y + x : y \in I\}$$

Also,　　　　　$l(I + x) = l(I)$　　　　　　　　　　　　　...(1)

Further, let $\varepsilon > 0$ be given, then there exists a countable collection $\{I_n\}$ of open intervals such that $A \subset \bigcup_n I_n$ and

$$\sum_n l(I_n) \leq m^*(A) + \varepsilon \qquad\qquad\qquad ...(2)$$

Now, $A + x \subset U(I_n + x)$

$$\Rightarrow \qquad m^*(A+x) \leq \sum_n l(I_n + x) = \sum_n l(I_n) \leq m^*(A) + \varepsilon \qquad \text{(Using (2))}$$

$$\Rightarrow \qquad m^*(A + x) \leq m^*(A) + \varepsilon$$

Since $\varepsilon > 0$ is arbitrary therefore,

$$m^*(A + x) \leq m^*(A) \qquad \qquad ...(3)$$

Now by assuming $A = (A + x) - x$ and apply the same procedure as above we can find

$$m^*(A) \leq m^*(A + x) \qquad \qquad ...(4)$$

Finally, from (3) and (4), we conclude that

$$m^*(A) = m^*(A + x)$$

Hence, m^* is translation invariant.

THEOREM 5. (Countably Subadditive Property)

*If $\{A_n\}$ is a countable family of subsets of **R**, then* $m^* \left[\bigcup_{i=1}^{\infty} A_n \right] \leq \sum_{n=1}^{\infty} m^*(A_n)$

[GARHWAL–2007, MADRAS–2010, ASSAM–2015, MEERUT–2003, 10, 18, PUNJAB–2003, HPU–2008]

PROOF. Let $\{A_1, A_2, A_3, ...\}$ be a countable family of subsets of **R**. We have to prove that

$$m^* \left[\bigcup_{i=1}^{\infty} A_n \right] \leq \sum_{n=1}^{\infty} m^*(A_n) \qquad \qquad ...(1)$$

Case-I: If one of the sets A_n has an infinite measure. Then RHS of (1) is infinity and (1) hold goods.

Case-II: Consider the case when $m^*(A_n)$ is finite for all A_n. Then, we have a countable family $\{I_{n_k}\}$ of open intervals such that

$$A_n \subseteq \bigcup_k I_{n_k} \quad \text{and} \quad m^*(A_n) + \varepsilon > \sum_{k=1}^{\infty} |I_{n_k}|$$

Let $\varepsilon = \dfrac{\lambda}{2^n} > 0$

Then $\qquad m^*(A_n) + \dfrac{\lambda}{2^n} > \sum_{k=1}^{\infty} |I_{n_k}|$

$$\Rightarrow \qquad \sum_{n=1}^{\infty} m^*(A_n) + \lambda > \sum_{n=1}^{\infty} \left(\sum_{k=1}^{\infty} |I_{n_k}| \right) \qquad \qquad ...(1)$$

$$\left[\begin{array}{l} \text{Sum of Infinite G.P.} = \dfrac{a}{1-r} \\[2mm] \therefore \sum_{n=1}^{\infty} \dfrac{\lambda}{2^n} = \lambda \sum_{n=1}^{\infty} \dfrac{1}{2^n} \\[2mm] \qquad = \lambda \left(\dfrac{1/2}{1 - 1/2} \right) = \lambda \end{array} \right]$$

Now, since each $m^*(A_n)$ is finite, therefore, $\sum_n m^*(A_n)$ is also finite.

$$\Rightarrow \qquad \sum_k \sum_n |I_{n_k}| \text{ is finite.}$$

$$\Rightarrow \qquad \sum \sum |I_{n_k}| \text{ is convergent.}$$

$\Rightarrow$ Terms in the above series can be added in any order.

Further, write the terms (intervals) in the form of a sequence $I_1, I_2, I_3, \ldots$ such that $A = \bigcup_n A_n \subseteq \bigcup I_n$.

$\Rightarrow$ $$m^*(A) \le \Sigma \mid I_n \mid = \Sigma\Sigma \mid I_{n_k} \mid < \Sigma m^*(A_n) + \lambda \qquad \text{(From (1))}$$

Since, λ is arbitrary, therefore
$$m^*(A) \le \Sigma m^*(A_n)$$

$\Rightarrow$ $$m^*\left(\bigcup_{n=1}^{\infty} A_n\right) \le \sum_{n=1}^{\infty} m^*(A_n)$$

THEOREM 6.

The outer Lebesgue measure of a countable set is zero.

[HPU–2000, 02, NAGPUR–2006, GARHWAL–2017, MEERUT–2014, 16, HPU–2002]

PROOF.   Let A be a countable set. We know that every countable set can be written in the form of a sequence. Therefore,
$$A = \{a_1, a_2, a_3, \ldots\}$$

Clearly, $A = \bigcup_i \{a_i\}$

$\Rightarrow$ A is the countable union of singleton sets $\{a_i\}$.

$\Rightarrow$ $$m^*(A) = m^*(\cup\{a_i\})$$

$$\le \sum_{i=1}^{\infty} m^*(\{a_i\}) \qquad \text{(By previous theorem)}$$

$$= 0 \qquad (\because \text{ measure of a singleton set is zero})$$

$\Rightarrow$ $$m^*(\{a_i\}) \le 0 \qquad \ldots(1)$$

But we know that $m^*(\{a_i\}) \ge 0$ $\qquad \ldots(2)$

Hence, from (1) and (2) we conclude that
$$m^*(\{a_i\}) = 0$$

$\Rightarrow$ $$m^*(A) = 0$$

$\Rightarrow$ The measure of a countable set is zero.

☛ **REMARK**

• The converse of the above theorem is not necessarily true, *i.e.*, a set with outer measure zero may or may not be countable.

For example, the Cantor ternary set has the outer measure zero is uncountable.

• A set with outer measure non-zero is uncountable.

Illustrations

✦ Since the sets of rational numbers *Q* natural numbers *N*, irrationals *I* and algebraic numbers *A* all are countable, so outer measure of each set is zero.

THEOREM 7.

*If A and B are any two disjoint subsets of real numbers **R**, then*
$$m^*(A \cup B) = m^*(A) + m^*(B)$$

[GARHWAL–2004, 14, GURUKUL KANGRI–2001, RAJASTHAN–2016, MEERUT–2012, AVADH–2014]

PROOF.   By countable subadditive property we can write
$$m^*(A \cup B) \le m^*(A) + m^*(B) \qquad \ldots(1)$$

Now, it remains to prove that
$$m^*(A \cup B) \geq m^*(A) + m^*(B)$$
Let $G = \{I_n\}$ be the family of open intervals such that $m^*(A \cup B) = \sum_n |I_n|$.

Since, A and B are disjoint (given), therefore, split the family G into two subfamilies G_1 and G_2 such that
$$G_1 = \{I_k' : k \in N\}$$
and
$$G_1 = \{I_k'' : k \in N\}$$
which covers A and B respectively.
Here, it is clear that
$$G = G_1 \cup G_2 \text{ and } G_1 \cap G_2 = \phi \quad (\because A \cap B = \phi)$$
$$\Rightarrow \qquad |G| = \sum_n |I_n| = \sum_k |I_k'| + \sum_k |I_k''| \qquad \qquad \ldots(2)$$
Since, $G_1 = \{I_k' : k \in N\}$ is a family of open intervals covering A therefore, we can write
$$m^*(A) \leq \sum_k |I_k'| \qquad \qquad \ldots(3)$$
and similarly $\quad m^*(B) \leq \sum_k |I_k''| \qquad \qquad \ldots(4)$
From (3) and (4) we have
$$m^*(A) + m^*(B) \leq \sum_k |I_k'| + \sum_k |I_k''|$$
$$= |G| \qquad \qquad \text{(From (2))}$$
$$\Rightarrow \qquad m^*(A) + m^*(B) \leq m^*(A \cup B) \qquad (\because m^*(A \cup B) = \sum_n |I_n| = |G|)$$
$$\ldots(5)$$

Finally from (1) and (5) we conclude that
$$m^*(A \cup B) = m^*(A) + m^*(B)$$

THEOREM 8.

The outer measure of an interval is equal to its length.

[MEERUT–2011, ROHTAK–2002, 03, 17, HPU–2002, RAJASTHAN–2012, NAGPUR–2015]

PROOF.   Here we have the following cases:

Case-I: If Interval I is an open interval.

Let $\qquad \qquad I =]a, b[$

Then by definition $m^*(I) = b - a = $ length of I

Case-II: If Interval I is an closed interval.

Let $I = [a, b]$ be the closed interval. Then for arbitrary $\varepsilon > 0$ we can write
$$I = [a, b] \subset \left] a - \frac{\varepsilon}{2}, b + \frac{\varepsilon}{2} \right[$$
which implies $\quad m^*(I) < \left| \left] a - \frac{\varepsilon}{2}, b + \frac{\varepsilon}{2} \right[\right|$
$$< (b - a) + \varepsilon$$
Since, ε is arbitrary, letting $\varepsilon \to 0$, we get
$$m^*(I) \leq b - a \qquad \qquad \ldots(1)$$

Further, let $\{I'_k\}$ be a countable family of open intervals covering $[a, b]$. Then there exists a finite sub-collection $\{I_n\}$ of open intervals covering I.

$\Rightarrow$ $\qquad\qquad \cup I_n \supseteq I$ $\qquad\qquad\qquad$ (By Heine-Borel's theorem)

Therefore, $\qquad\quad |I| \leq \Sigma |I_n|$

$\Rightarrow$ $\qquad\qquad \Sigma |I_n| \geq (b - a)$ $\qquad\qquad\qquad\qquad\qquad\qquad$ ...(2)

$\qquad\qquad\qquad\qquad\qquad\qquad\qquad\qquad\qquad (\because \; |I| = b - a)$

This result is true for all families $\{I'_k\}$ and hence for all families $\{I_n\}$ such that

$$|I_n| \leq \Sigma_k |I'_k| \text{ which covers } I$$

Therefore, $\min \Sigma |I_n| \geq (b - a)$ $\qquad\qquad\qquad\qquad\qquad$ (From (2))

$\Rightarrow$ $\qquad\qquad \inf\{\Sigma |I_n|\} \geq (b - a)$

$\Rightarrow$ $\qquad\qquad m^*(I) \geq b - a$ $\qquad\qquad\qquad\qquad\qquad\qquad\qquad$ ...(3)

Finally from (2) and (3) we get

$$m^*(I) = m^*[a, b] = b - a$$

Case-III: If $I = \,]a, b]$ is a semi-closed interval

Let $I = \,]a, b]$ and $a > -\infty$

If $a = b$ then $I = \phi$ then $m^*(I) = m^*(\phi) = 0 = b - a$

Further suppose that $a < b$

Now, let $0 < \varepsilon < b - a$ then

$$I' = [a + \varepsilon, b] \subset I$$

$\Rightarrow$ $\qquad\qquad m^*(I') \leq m^*(I)$

Also $m^*(I') = b - a - \varepsilon = |I| - \varepsilon$

Since $I \subset [a, b + \varepsilon]$

$\Rightarrow$ $\qquad\qquad m^*(I) < m^*[a, b + \varepsilon] = |(a, b + \varepsilon)|$

$\Rightarrow$ $\qquad\qquad m^*(I) < b - a + \varepsilon = |I| + \varepsilon$

$\Rightarrow$ $\qquad\qquad |I| - \varepsilon \leq m^*(I) < |I| + \varepsilon$

Since, ε is arbitrary, letting $\varepsilon \to 0$ we get

$$|I| \leq m^*(I) \leq |I|$$

$\Rightarrow$ $\qquad\qquad m^*(I) = |I|$

Case-IV: If I is an infinite interval

Here following four type of intervals may exists :

$$]-\infty, a], \;]-\infty, a[, \;[b, -\infty[\text{ and }]-b, \infty[$$

Let $I = \,]-\infty, a[$

If M is any number (however large) greater than zero, we may get a number $k \leq 0$ such that the interval $[k, k + M[\subseteq I$

$\Rightarrow$ $\qquad\qquad m^*(I) > k + M - k = M$

$\Rightarrow$ $\qquad\qquad m^*(I) > M$

But M is arbitrary chosen larger number, therefore,

$$m^*(I) = \infty = |I| = l(I)$$

Similar result follows for the other three intervals.

3.4 LEBESGUE INNER MEASURE

Let A be a given set. Then Lebesgue inner measure of A, denoted by $m_*(A)$ or $m_i(A)$ is defined as follows:

$$m_*(A) = b - a - m^*(A')$$

where A' is the compliment of A relate to the interval $[a, b]$ such that $A \subseteq [a, b]$

3.4.1 PROPERTIES OF LEBESGUE INNER MEASURE

PROP. 1   For empty set ϕ, $m_*(\phi) = 0$

PROP. 2 $m_*(A) = b - a - m^*(A')$

$= b - a - \inf. \{|G| : G \supseteq A' \text{ and } A' \text{ is open}\}$

$= \sup \{|H| : H \subseteq A \text{ and } A \text{ is closed}\}$

PROP. 3 $m_*(A) \geq 0$

PROP. 4   If $A' \subseteq [a, b]$ therefore $m_*(A') \leq b - a$

PROP. 5   For any closed set H, $m_*(H) = |H|$

PROP. 6   For each $\varepsilon > 0$, we can find a closed set $H \subset A$ and satisfying the condition $|H| > m_*(A) - \varepsilon$

PROP. 7 $m^*(A) \geq m_*(A)$

3.5 LEBESGUE MEASURABLE SET

A set A is said to be Lebesgue measurable set if for each set E

$$m^*(E) = m^*(A \cap E) + m^*(A' \cap E)$$

Alternatively, the set A is said to be Lebesgue measurable if

$$m^*(A) = m_*(A)$$

☞ REMARKS

- The common value $m^*(A) = m_*(A)$ is called the measure of A. It is denoted by $m(A)$.
- If A is Lebesgue measurable then $m^*(A) = m_*(A) = m(A)$.

THEOREM 1.

For any set A, $m^*(A) \geq m_*(A)$.

PROOF.   Let A be any set contained in the open interval $]a, b[$.

Then by definition of exterior measure, there exists open sets G_1 and G_2 containing A and A' respectively such that

$$\left. \begin{array}{l} m(G_1) < m^*(A) + \varepsilon \\ m(G_2) < m^*(A') + \varepsilon \end{array} \right] \qquad \qquad \dots(1)$$

which implies that every point of the interval $]a + \varepsilon, b - \varepsilon[$ is an interior point of an interval contained in G_1 and G_2. Now by Heine-Borel theorem, we can find an open set G from these intervals such that

$]a + \varepsilon, b - \varepsilon[\subseteq G$ ...(2)

and $m(G_1) + m(G_2) \geq m(G)$ ...(3)

From (2) $m(G) \geq m[a + \varepsilon, b - \varepsilon] = b - \varepsilon - a - \varepsilon$

$\Rightarrow$ $m(G) \geq b - a - 2\varepsilon$

and from (1)

$m(G_1) + m(G_2) < m^*(A) + m^*(A') + 2\varepsilon$ ...(4)

Using (3) we get

$$m(G) \leq m(G_1) + m(G_2) < m^*(A) + m^*(A') + 2\varepsilon$$

Using (4) we get

$$b - a - 2\varepsilon < m^*(A) + m^*(A') + 2\varepsilon$$

$$\Rightarrow \quad b - a - m^*(A') < m^*(A) + 4\varepsilon$$

Using $m_*(A) = b - a - m^*(A')$, we get

$$\Rightarrow \quad m^*(A) < m^*(A) + 4\varepsilon$$

Since ε is arbitrary, letting $\varepsilon \to 0$ we get

$$m_*(A) \le m^*(A)$$

THEOREM 2.

A set is Lebesgue measurable if and only if its compliment is measurable. [MEERUT–2016]

PROOF. Let A be the given set contained in $]a, b[$.

By definition, we know that

$$m_*(A) = b - a - m^*(A') \qquad \qquad ...(1)$$

Let us first suppose A is Lebesgue measurable. We have to prove that A' is Lebesgue measurable.

Since A is measurable, therefore

$$m_*(A) = m^*(A) = m(A) \qquad \qquad ...(2)$$

Using (2) in (1) we can write

$$m(A) = b - a - m^*(A')$$

$$\Rightarrow \quad m^*(A') = b - a - m(A) \qquad \qquad ...(3)$$

Replacing A by A' in (1) we get

$$m_*(A') = b - a - m^*(a)$$

Now using (2) in the above equation, we get

$$m_*(A') = b - a - m(A) \qquad \qquad ...(4)$$

From (3) and (4) we conclude that

$$m_*(A') = m^*(A')$$

$\Rightarrow \quad A'$ is Lebesgue measurable.

Conversely, suppose that A' is Lebesgue measurable. We have to prove that A is Lebesgue measurable.

Since, A' is measurable, therefore,

$$m^*(A') = m_*(A') = m(A') \qquad \qquad ...(5)$$

From (1) we can write

$$m_*(A) = b - a - m^*(A')$$

and

$$m_*(A') = b - a - m^*(A)$$

Using (5) in the above equation, we get

$$m_*(A) = b - a - m(A') \qquad \qquad ...(6)$$

and

$$m(A') = b - a - m^*(A) \qquad \qquad ...(7)$$

Using (7) in (6) we get

$$b - a - m_*(A) = b - a - m^*(A)$$

$$\Rightarrow \quad m_*(A) = m^*(A)$$

Hence, A is Lebesgue measurable.

THEOREM 3.

A linear set of outer measure zero is Lebesgue measurable.

PROOF. Let A be the linear set such that $m^*(A) = 0$

By definition $\quad m^*(A) \ge m_*(A) \qquad \qquad ...(1)$

Using $m^*(A) = 0$ in (1) we get

$$m_*(A) \le 0$$

But $\qquad\qquad m_*(A) \ge 0$

and therefore, $m_*(A) = 0$

Hence, $m_*(A) = m^*(A) = 0$

$\Rightarrow$ A is Lebesgue-measurable.

☞ REMARKS

- Any subset of a set whose outer measure is zero is also measurable.
- The necessary and sufficient condition for a set A to be measurable with measure zero is $m^*(A) = 0$

THEOREM 4.

For any two sets A and B such that $A \subset B$, we have

(i) $m_*(A) \le m_*(B)$

(ii) $m^*(A) \le m^*(B)$ $\qquad\qquad$ [ASSAM–2010, AVADH–2009, LUCKNOW–2014]

PROOF. We have $\qquad A \subset B$

(i) We have to prove that $m_*(A) \le m^*(B)$

By definition, we can write

$$m_*(A) = \sup. \{m(F) : F \text{ is closed}, F \subset A\}$$

and $\qquad m_*(B) = \sup. \{m(F) : F \text{ is closed}, F \subset B\}$

Let S and T be the set of numbers consisting of measure of all closed subsets of A and B respectively.

Then, we can write

$$m_*(A) = \sup. S \text{ and } m_*(B) = \sup. T \qquad\qquad ...(1)$$

Since, F is closed in A such that $F \subset A$ and $A \subset B$. Then

$$F \subset A \subset B$$

$\Rightarrow \qquad\qquad F \subset B$

$\Rightarrow \qquad F$ is closed subset of B.

which implies that $m(F) \in S$

$\Rightarrow \qquad\qquad m(F) \in T$

$\Rightarrow \qquad\qquad S \subseteq T$

$\Rightarrow \qquad\qquad \sup(S) \le \sup(T)$

$\Rightarrow \qquad\qquad m_*(A) \le m_*(B)$

(ii) We have to prove that $m^*(A) \le m^*(B)$

By definition of exterior measure, we can write

$$m^*(A) = \inf. [m(G) : G \text{ is open}, G \supset A]$$

and $\qquad m^*(B) = \inf. [m(G) : G \text{ is open}, G \supset B]$

Let S and T be the set of numbers consisting of measures of all open supersets of A and B respectively. Then, we can write

$$m^*(A) = \inf. (S)$$

and $\qquad m^*(B) = \inf. (T)$

Further, since, G is any open set such that $G \supset B$

$\Rightarrow \qquad\qquad G \supset B \supset A \qquad\qquad (\because B \supset A)$

$\Rightarrow \qquad\qquad G \supset A$

$\Rightarrow$ G is an open superset of A

Therefore,

$$m(G) \in T \Rightarrow m(G) \in S$$

$\therefore$ $T \subseteq S$

$\Rightarrow$ inf. $(S) \leq$ inf. (T) [$\because$ Greatest lower bound of a set can not exceed greatest lower bounds of a subset of the set]

Therefore, inf. $(S) \leq$ inf. (T)

$\Rightarrow$ $m^*(A) \leq m^*(B)$

THEOREM 5.

Every bounded open set and bounded closed set are measurable.

[KANPUR–2008, ROHTAK–2012, PUNJAB–2016, MEERUT–1995, 97, 2005]

PROOF.   Let A be a bounded closed set. Then

$$m_*(A) = \sup. \{|F| : F \text{ is closed and } F \subseteq A\}$$

$\Rightarrow$ $m_*(A) \geq |A| = m^*(A)$

$\Rightarrow$ $m_*(A) \geq m^*(A)$ ...(1)

But by definition

$$m_*(A) \leq m^*(A) \qquad \qquad ...(2)$$

From (1) and (2) we conclude that

$$m_*(A) = m^*(A)$$

$\Rightarrow$ A is measurable.

Further, suppose that G be a bounded open set

$\Rightarrow$ G' is bounded and closed set

$\Rightarrow$ G' is measurable   (Using above result)

$\Rightarrow$ G is measurable   ($\because A$ is measurable iff A' is measurable)

Hence, every bounded open and bounded closed sets are measurable.

THEOREM 6.

Any set A is measurable if and only if an open set G containing A and a closed set H contained in A can be so determined that

$$|G| - |H| < \varepsilon$$

where ε is arbitrary positive real number (however small)   [GARHWAL–1992, 2003, ROHILKHAND–2007]

PROOF.   Let us first suppose A be a measurable set.

We have to prove that there exists an open set G containing A and a closed set H contained in A such that $|G| - |H| < \varepsilon$.

By definition of inner and outer measure, for given $\varepsilon > 0$ we can find an open set $G \supseteq A$ and a closed set $H \subseteq A$ such that

$$|G| < m^*(A) + \varepsilon/2 \qquad \qquad ...(1)$$

and $m_*(A) < |H| + \varepsilon/2$ ...(2)

Also, we have assume that, A is measurable, therefore,

$$m^*(A) = m_*(A) \qquad \qquad ...(3)$$

So, from (1) and (2) and using (3) we get

$$|G| - \varepsilon/2 < |H| + \varepsilon/2$$

$\Rightarrow \qquad\qquad |G| - |H| < \varepsilon/2 + \varepsilon/2 = \varepsilon$

Here, $\qquad\qquad |G| - |H| < \varepsilon$

Conversely, let us suppose that $|G| - |H| < \varepsilon$. We have to prove that A is measurable.

Using the definition of outer measure, we can write

$$m^*(A) \le |G| \qquad\qquad\qquad ...(4)$$

Similarly, $\qquad\qquad m_*(A) \ge |H|$

$\Rightarrow \qquad\qquad -m_*(A) \le -|H| \qquad\qquad\qquad ...(5)$

From (4) and (5)

$$m^*(A) - m_*(A) < |G| - |H|$$
$$< \varepsilon \qquad\qquad\qquad \text{(By assumption)}$$

$\Rightarrow \qquad\qquad m^*(A) - m_*(A) < \varepsilon$

Letting $\varepsilon \to 0$ ($\because \varepsilon$ is arbitrary), we get

$$m^*(A) = m_*(A)$$

Hence, A is measurable.

THEOREM 7.

Union of two measurable sets is also measurable.

[MEERUT–2000, 01, 04, 10, 16, 17, 18, ROHTAK–2004, 14, KANPUR–2002, GARHWAL–2004, 05, 07]

PROOF. Let A and B be two measurable sets. We have to prove that $E = A \cup B$ is measurable.

Using above theorem, we can say that, if A is measurable, we can find a closed set H_1 and an open set G_1 such that

$$H_1 \subseteq A \subseteq G_1 \text{ and } |G_1| - |H_1| < \varepsilon/2.$$

In a similar way, for measurable set B, we can find a closed set H_2 and an open set G_2 such that $H_2 \subseteq B \subseteq G_2$ and $|G_2| - |H_2| < \varepsilon$.

Further, since G_1 and G_2 both are open therefore, $G = G_1 \cup G_2$ is open.

Similarly, since H_1 and H_2 are closed, therefore, $H = H_1 \cup H_2$ is closed.

Also, $\quad A \subseteq G_1, B \subseteq G_2 \quad \Rightarrow \quad A \cup B \subseteq G_1 \cup G_2 = G$

$\qquad\qquad\qquad\qquad\qquad \Rightarrow \quad A \cup B \subseteq G$

$\qquad\qquad\qquad\qquad\qquad \Rightarrow \quad E \subseteq G \qquad (\because E = A \cup B) \qquad\qquad ...(1)$

Similarly, $\quad H_1 \cup H_2 \subseteq A \cup B = E$

$\Rightarrow \qquad\qquad H_1 \cup H_2 \subseteq E$

$\Rightarrow \qquad\qquad H \subseteq E \qquad\qquad\qquad\qquad\qquad\qquad ...(2)$

Combining (1) and (2) we get

$$H \subseteq E \subseteq G$$

$\Rightarrow \qquad m_*(H) \le m_*(E) \text{ and } m^*(E) \le m^*(G)$

Now, since G and H both are measurable, therefore

$$m^*(H) = m_*(H) = m(H) \qquad\qquad\qquad ...(3)$$
$$m^*(G) = m^*(G) = m(G) \qquad\qquad\qquad ...(4)$$

$\Rightarrow \qquad\qquad m(H) \le m_*(E)$

$\Rightarrow \qquad\qquad -m_*(E) \le -m(H) \qquad\qquad\qquad ...(5)$

and $\qquad\qquad m^*(E) \le m(G) \qquad\qquad\qquad\qquad ...(6)$

Adding (5) and (6) we get

$$m^*(E) - m_*(E) \le m(G) - m(H) \qquad\qquad\qquad ...(7)$$

Again $\qquad G = (G - H) \cup H$ such that $(G - H) \cap H = \phi$

Therefore, $\qquad m(G) = m(G - H) + m(H)$

$\Rightarrow \qquad m(G - H) = m(G) - m(H)$ $\hfill ...(8)$

Using (8) in (7) we get

$$m^*(E) - m_*(E) \le m(G - H)$$
$$= m[(G_1 - H_1) \cup (G_2 - H_2)]$$
$$\le m(G_1) - m(H_1) + m(G_2) - m(H_2)$$
$$= |G_1| - |H_1| + |G_2| - |H_2| \qquad ...(9)$$

But $|G_1| - |H_1| \le \varepsilon/2$ and $|G_2| - |H_2| < \varepsilon/2$

Then from (9)

$$m^*(E) - m_*(E) < \varepsilon/2 + \varepsilon/2 = \varepsilon$$

Since ε is arbitrary, letting $\varepsilon \to 0$ we get

$$m^*(E) = m_*(E)$$

$\Rightarrow \quad E$ is measurable.

Hence, $A \cup B$ is measurable.

☞ **REMARK**
- The above result can be extended to a countable number of measurable sets, *i.e.*, the countable union of measurable sets is measurable.

CORROLLARY 1.

Intersection of two measurable sets is also measurable. [MEERUT–2004, 13, GARHWAL–2014]

PROOF. Let A and B be two measurable sets. We have to prove that $A \cap B$ is measurable.

Since, A and B both are measurable. Therefore, A' and B' are also measurable.

($\because$ Compliment of a measurable sets is again measurable)

Further A' and B' are measurable

$\Rightarrow \quad A' \cup B'$ is measurable $\qquad$ ($\because$ Union of two measurable sets is measurable)

$\Rightarrow \quad (A \cap B)'$ is measurable. $\qquad$ ($\because A' \cup B' = (A \cap B)'$ By Demorgan's law)

$\Rightarrow \quad [(A \cap B)']'$ is measurable. $\qquad$ ($\because A$ is measurable iff A' is measurable)

$\Rightarrow \quad A \cap B$ is measurable. $\qquad$ ($\because (A \cap B) = [(A \cap B)']'$)

Hence, intersection of two measurable sets is also measurable.

☞ **REMARK**
- Using the above result, we can easily prove that finite intersection of measurable sets is measurable.

CORROLLARY 2.

Difference of two measurable sets is measurable. [KUMAON–2007, GARHWAL–2007]

PROOF. Let A and B be two measurable sets. We have to prove that $A - B$ is measurable.

Since B is measurable $\Rightarrow B'$ is measurable.

$\hfill$ ($\because A$ is measurable $\Leftrightarrow A'$ is measurable)

$\hfill$ (By set theory)

Now, $A - B = A \cap B'$

Since, A and B' both are measurable.

$\Rightarrow \quad A \cap B'$ is measurable. $\hfill$ (By Corrollary-1)

$\Rightarrow \quad A - B (= A \cap B')$ is measurable.

Hence, difference of two measurable sets is again measurable.

CORROLLARY 3.

The symmetric difference of two measurable sets is also measurable.

PROOF. Let A and B be two measurable sets. We have to prove that $A \Delta B$ is measurable. By definition of symmetric difference of two sets, we have

$$A \Delta B = (A - B) \cup (B - A) \qquad \qquad ...(1)$$

Since A and B both are measurable, therefore $A - B$ and $B - A$ both are measurable.

($\because$ Difference of two measurable sets is again measurable)

$\Rightarrow \quad A - B$ and $B - A$ both are measurable.

$\Rightarrow \quad (A - B) \cup (B - A)$ is measurable.

$\qquad \qquad \qquad$ [$\because$ Union of two measurable sets is measurable]

$\Rightarrow \quad A \Delta B$ is measurable. $\qquad \qquad$ (From (1))

Hence, symmetric difference of two measurable sets is also measurable.

THEOREM 8.

The Lebesgue measure is finitely additive, i.e., the union of finite number of measurable sets is also measurable.

[AMRITSAR–1998, 2011, GARHWAL–2011, KANPUR–2003]

PROOF. Let $E_1, E_2, ..., E_n$ are measurable sets.

We have to prove that $E = \bigcup\limits_{r=1}^{n} E_r$ is measurable.

Since, each E_r is measurable, therefore for given $\varepsilon > 0$ $\exists$ closed sets H_r and open sets G_r such that $H_r \subseteq E_r \subseteq G_r$

and $m(G_r) - m(H_r) < \varepsilon/n$ $\qquad \qquad ...(1)$

Let us write $H = \bigcup\limits_{r=1}^{n} H_r$ and $G = \bigcup\limits_{r=1}^{n} G_r$

Then clearly, H is closed and G is open set such that

$$H \subseteq E \subseteq G$$

which shows that

$$m_*(H) \leq m_*(E) \text{ and } m^*(E) \leq m^*(G) \qquad \qquad ...(2)$$

Now since H is closed and G is open therefore, both G and H are measurable, so

$$m^*(H) = m_*(H) = m(H)$$

and $\qquad \qquad m^*(G) = m_*(G) = m(G)$

Therefore, $m(H) \leq m_*(E)$ and $m^*(E) \leq m(G)$

which implies $- m_*(E) \geq - m(H)$ and $m^*(E) \leq m(G)$

On adding, we get

$$m^*(E) - m_*(E) \leq m(G) - m(H) \qquad \qquad ...(3)$$

Using set theory, we can write $G - H = G \cap H'$

Here, G and H' both are measurable and so $G \cap H'$ is measurable.

$\Rightarrow \quad G - H$ is measurable.

Now, $\qquad \qquad G = (G - H) \cup H$ and $(G - H) \cap H = \phi$

$\Rightarrow \qquad \qquad m(G) = m(G - H) + m(H)$

$\Rightarrow \qquad \qquad m(G - H) = m(G) - m(H)$

In general, we can write

$$m(G_r - H_r) = m(G_r) - m(H_r)$$

Further, since $\quad G - H \subset \bigcup\limits_{r=1}^{n} (G_r - H_r)$

$\Rightarrow \qquad \qquad m(G - H) = \bigcup\limits_{r=1}^{n} m(G_r - H_r)$

$$\Rightarrow \quad m(G) - m(H) \le \sum_{r=1}^{n} [m(G_r) - m(H_r)]$$

$$< n \cdot \frac{\varepsilon}{n}$$

$$\Rightarrow \quad m(G) - m(H) < \varepsilon \qquad \qquad \qquad ...(4)$$

Using (4) in (3) we get

$$m^*(E) - m_*(E) < m(G) - m(H) < \varepsilon$$

$$\Rightarrow \quad m^*(E) - m_*(E) < \varepsilon$$

Since, ε is arbitrary small positive number, letting $\varepsilon \to 0$ we get

$$m^*(E) - m_*(E) \le 0$$

$$\Rightarrow \quad m^*(E) \le m_*(E)$$

But we know that $m^*(E) \ge m_*(E)$

Thus we conclude that

$$m^*(E) = m_*(E)$$

$\Rightarrow \quad E$ is measurable.

$$\Rightarrow \quad \bigcup_{r=1}^{n} E_r \text{ is measurable.}$$

Hence, union of finite number of measurable sets is measurable.

☞ **REMARK**
  • The arbitrary union of measurable sets is also measurable.

THEOREM 9.

If a measurable set E_1 contains another measurable set E_2 then $E_1 - E_2$ is also measurable and

$$m(E_1 - E_2) = m(E_1) - m(E_2)$$

PROOF.   Let E_1 and E_2 be two measurable sets such that

$$E_1 \supseteq E_2$$

We have to prove that $E_1 - E_2$ is also measurable.

Since, E_1 and E_2 both are measurable.

$\Rightarrow E_1'$ and E_2' both are measurable.

                            [∵ Complement of a measurable set is again measurable]
                                                                              (By set theory)

We can write $E_1 - E_2 = E_1 \cap E_2'$

Since, E_1 and E_2' both are measurable.

$\Rightarrow \quad E_1 \cap E_2'$ is measurable. [∵ Intersection of two measurable sets is measurable]

Therefore, $E_1 - E_2$ is measurable.

Further, $E_1 = (E_1 - E_2) \cup E_2$ such that $(E_1 - E_2) \cap E_2 = \phi$

$$\Rightarrow \quad m(E_1) = m(E_1 - E_2) + m(E_2)$$

Hence, $m(E_1) - m(E_2) = m(E_1) - m(E_2)$

THEOREM 10. (First Fundamental Theorem)

Lebesgue measure is countably additive. In other words Let E_1, E_2, ... are pairwise disjoint

measurable sets and $E = E_1 \cup E_2 \cup ...$ then E is measurable and $m(E) = \sum_{r=1}^{\infty} m(E_r)$ [MADRAS–1999,

DELHI–2004, KANPUR–2005, GARHWAL–2001, 11, 14, MEERUT–2003, 06, 08, 14, 17, 18, BHU–2008, ROHTAK–2005]

PROOF.   Let $E_1, E_2, \ldots$ are pairwise disjoint measurable sets, *i.e.,*

$$E_i \cap E_j = \phi \quad \forall\, i \neq j \qquad \ldots(1)$$

By countable subadditive property of m^*, we can write

$$m^*\left[\bigcup_r E_r\right] \leq \sum_r m^*(E_r)$$

$$\Rightarrow \qquad m^*\left[\bigcup_{r=1}^{\infty} E_r\right] \leq \sum_{r=1}^{\infty} m(E_r) \qquad \ldots(2)$$

We know that the arbitrary union of measurable sets is measurable. Therefore, $\cup E_r$ is measurable and hence E is measurable.

Now, $$\bigcup_{r=1}^{\infty} E_r \supseteq \bigcup_{r=1}^{n} E_r \quad \forall n$$

$$\Rightarrow \qquad m\left[\bigcup_{r=1}^{\infty} E_r\right] \geq m\left[\bigcup_{r=1}^{n} E_r\right] \qquad \ldots(3)$$

Also, since each E_i is pairwise measurable set, therefore,

$$m\left[\bigcup_{r=1}^{n} E_r\right] = \sum_{r=1}^{n} m(E_r)$$

Using this in equation (3) we get

$$m\left[\bigcup_{r=1}^{\infty} E_r\right] \geq \sum_{r=1}^{n} m(E_r) \quad \forall n$$

Letting $n \to \infty$, we get

$$m\left[\bigcup_{r=1}^{\infty} E_r\right] \geq \sum_{r=1}^{\infty} m(E_r) \qquad \ldots(4)$$

From (2) and (4) we conclude that

$$m\left[\bigcup_{r=1}^{\infty} E_r\right] = \sum_{r=1}^{\infty} m(E_r) \qquad \ldots(5)$$

$$\Rightarrow \qquad m(E) = \sum_{r=1}^{\infty} m(E_r)$$

Hence, Lebesgue measure is countable additive for pairwise disjoint sets.

THEOREM II.

Let $E_1, E_2, E_3, \ldots$ *are measurable sets of real numbers then* $\bigcup\limits_{n=1}^{\infty} E_n$ *is measurable and*

$m\left(\bigcup\limits_{n=1}^{\infty} E_n\right) \leq \sum\limits_{n=1}^{\infty} m(E_n).$ [MEERUT–2009, 10, LUCKNOW–2014, AVADH–2011, BHOPAL–2010, GARHWAL–2012]

PROOF.   It is given that $E_1, E_2, \ldots$ are pairwise disjoint measurable sets. We have to prove that $\bigcup\limits_{n=1}^{\infty} E_n$ is measurable. We can write

$$\bigcup_{n=1}^{\infty} E_n = E_1 \cup [E_2 - E_1] \cup [E_3 - (E_1 \cup E_2)] \cup$$

$$\ldots \cup [E_n - (E_1 \cup E_2 \cup \ldots \cup E_{n-1})] \cup \ldots$$

It is evident that each E_1, $E_2 - E_1$, $(E_3 - (E_1 \cup E_2))$ ... are disjoint measurable sets and we know that arbitrary union of measurable sets is measurable and hence $\overset{\infty}{\underset{n=1}{\cup}} E_n$ is measurable.

Further, by equation (5) of previous theorem, we get

$$m\left(\overset{\infty}{\underset{n=1}{\cup}} E_n \right) \le \overset{\infty}{\underset{n=1}{\sum}} m(E_n)$$

Hence, $$m^*\left[\overset{\infty}{\underset{n=1}{\cup}} E_n \right] \le \overset{\infty}{\underset{n=1}{\sum}} m(E_n)$$

THEOREM 12. (Second Fundamental Theorem)

If E_1, E_2, ... are measurable sets then the set $\overset{\infty}{\underset{r=1}{\cap}} E_r$ is measurable.

[MEERUT–2001, 04, 07, 11, 14, 15, 17, 18, GARHWAL–2001, CALCUTTA–2016, ASSAM–2012]

PROOF.   Let E_1, E_2, E_3, ... are measurable sets.

We have to prove that $\overset{\infty}{\underset{r=1}{\cap}} E_r$ is measurable.

Let us write $G = \overset{\infty}{\underset{r=1}{\cap}} E_r$ and $E = \overset{\infty}{\underset{r=1}{\cup}} E_r$

Since each E_i is measurable, therefore $\overset{\infty}{\underset{r=1}{\cup}} E_r$ is measurable.

(By First fundmental theorem)

$\Rightarrow$ E is measurable.

Further, since each E_i is measurable.

$\Rightarrow$ E_i' is measurable   ($\because$ Compliment of a measurable sets is measurable)

$\Rightarrow$ $\overset{\infty}{\underset{r=1}{\cup}} E_r'$ is measurable   [By first fundamental theorem]

$\Rightarrow$ $\left[\overset{\infty}{\underset{r=1}{\cap}} E_r \right]'$ is measurable.   [By Demorgan's law]

$\Rightarrow$ G' is measurable

$\Rightarrow$ G is measurable   [$\because$ A is measurable if and only if A' is measurable]

Hence, $\overset{\infty}{\underset{r=1}{\cap}} E_r$ is measurable.

THEOREM 13.

Let $<E_n>$ be a monotonically increasing sequence of measurable sets and $E = \overset{\infty}{\underset{r=1}{\cup}} E_r$ then $m(E) = \underset{n \to \infty}{\lim} m(E_n)$.

[MEERUT–2010, 14, 15, ROHTAK–2003, PUNJAB–2008, MADRAS–2009, HPU–2001, 02, 03, 04, 14, 18, GARHWAL–2003, 14]

PROOF.   Let $<E_n>$ be a monotonically increasing sequence of measurable sets such that

$E = \overset{\infty}{\underset{r=1}{\cup}} E_r$. We have to prove that

$$m(E) = \underset{n \to \infty}{\lim} m(E_n)$$

Since, $<E_n>$ is monotonically increasing, *i.e.*,
$$E_1 \subseteq E_2 \subseteq E_3 \subseteq ...$$

So, we can write

$$E = E_1 \cup (E_2 - E_1) \cup (E_3 - E_2) \cup ... \cup [E_r - E_{r-1}] \cup ...$$

$$= E_1 \overset{\infty}{\underset{r=1}{\cup}} (E_{r+1} - E_r)$$

Clearly, $(E_{r+1} - E_r)$ is measurable

$$(\because \text{Difference of two measurable sets is measurable})$$

$$\Rightarrow \quad \overset{\infty}{\underset{r=1}{\cup}} (E_{r+1} - E_r) \text{ is measurable} \qquad \text{(By first fundamental theorem)}$$

Also, E is a disjoint union of measurable sets, then

$$m(E) = m(E_1) + \sum_{r=1}^{\infty} m(E_{r+1} - E_r)$$

$$= m(E_1) + \sum_{r=1}^{\infty} [m(E_{r+1}) - m(E_r)] \qquad [\because E_r \subseteq E_{r+1}]$$

$$= m(E_1) + \lim_{n \to \infty} [\{m(E_2) - m(E_1)\} +$$

$$... + \{m(E_n) - m(E_{n-1})\}]$$

$$= m(E_1) + \lim_{n \to \infty} [-m(E_1) + m(E_n)]$$

$$= m(E_1) - \lim_{n \to \infty} m(E_1) + \lim_{n \to \infty} m(E_n)$$

$$(\because \text{limit of the difference of two functions is equal}$$
$$\text{to difference of their limits})$$

$$= m(E_1) - m(E_1) + \lim_{n \to \infty} m(E_n)$$

Hence, $\qquad m(E) = \lim_{n \to \infty} m(E_n)$

THEOREM 14.

If E_1 and E_2 are any two subset of $[a, b]$ then

$$m^*(E_1) + m^*(E_2) \geq m^*(E_1 \cup E_2) + m^*(E_1 \cap E_2)$$

and
$$m_*(E_1) + m_*(E_2) \leq m_*(E_1 \cup E_2) + m_*(E_1 \cap E_2)$$

PROOF. Let E_1 and E_2 be any two subsets of $[a, b]$

Then for given $\varepsilon > 0$, we can find two open sets G_1 and G_2 such that $G_1 \supset E_1$ and $G_2 \supset E_2$.

and $\qquad |G_1| < m^*(E_1) + \varepsilon/2$ ...(1)

$$|G_2| < m^*(E_2) + \varepsilon/2 \qquad ...(2)$$

On adding (1) and (2) we get

$$|G_1| + |G_2| < m^*(E_1) + m^*(E_2) + \varepsilon \qquad ...(3)$$

Since G_1 and G_2 both are open, therefore,

$$|G_1| + |G_2| = |G_1 \cup G_2| + |G_1 \cap G_2| \qquad ...(4)$$

Using (4) in (3) we get

$$|G_1 \cup G_2| + |G_1 \cap G_2| < m^*(E_1) + m^*(E_2) + \varepsilon \qquad ...(5)$$

Further, since $G_1 \cup G_2$ and $G_1 \cap G_2$ are open set containing $E_1 \cup E_2$ and $E_1 \cap E_2$ respectively, therefore

$$m^*(E_1 \cup E_2) \le |G_1 \cup G_2|$$

and $$m^*(E_1 \cap E_2) \le |G_1 \cap G_2|$$

Using these values in (5) we get

$$m^*(E_1 \cup E_2) + m^*(E_1 \cap E_2) < m^*(E_1) + m^*(E_2) + \varepsilon$$

Since, ε is arbitrary, letting $\varepsilon \to 0$ we get

$$m^*(E_1 \cup E_2) + m^*(E_1 \cap E_2) \le m^*(E_1) + m^*(E_2) \qquad \ldots(6)$$

Now since (6) is true for all $E_1, E_2 \subseteq [a, b]$, therefore for $E_1', E_2' \subset [a,b]$
We have

$$m^*(E_1' \cup E_2') + m^*(E_1' \cap E_2') \le m^*(E_1') + m^*(E_2')$$

$$\Rightarrow m^*[(E_1 \cap E_2)'] + m^*[(E_1 \cup E_2)'] \le m^*(E_1') + m^*(E_2') \qquad \text{(By Demorgan's law)}$$

$$\Rightarrow [b - a - m_*(E_1 \cap E_2)] + [b - a - m_*(E_1 \cup E_2)]$$
$$\le [b - a - m_*(E_1)] + [b - a - m_*(E_2)]$$

$$\Rightarrow -[m_*(E_1 \cap E_2) + m_*(E_1 \cup E_2)] \le -[m_*(E_1) + m_*(E_2)]$$

$$\Rightarrow m_*(E_1 \cap E_2) + m_*(E_1 \cup E_2) \ge m_*(E_1) + m_*(E_2)$$

☛ **REMARK**

- If G_1 and G_2 are two open sets in $[a, b]$, then

$$m(G_1) + m(G_2) = m(G_1 \cup G_2) + m(G_1 \cap G_2)$$

and $$m(G_1) + m(G_2) = m(G_1 + G_2) + m(G_1 G_2)$$

THEOREM 15.

If E_1 and E_2 are measurable subsets of $[a, b]$ then

$$m(E_1) + m(E_2) = m(E_1 \cup E_2) + m(E_1 \cap E_2)$$

[MEERUT–2001, 05, 06, 08; GARHWAL–2007, SHIMLA–2000, 02, 12]

PROOF.   Let E_1 and E_2 be two measurable subsets of $[a, b]$.
We have to prove that

$$m(E_1) + m(E_2) = m(E_1 \cup E_2) + m(E_1 \cap E_2)$$

Since, E_1 and E_2 are measurable, therefore

$$m_*(E_1) = m^*(E_1) = m(E_1) \qquad \ldots(1)$$

and $$m_*(E_2) = m^*(E_2) = m(E_2) \qquad \ldots(2)$$

Further $E_1 \cup E_2$ being the union of two measurable sets, is measurable. Therefore,

$$m_*(E_1 \cup E_2) = m^*(E_1 \cup E_2) = m(E_1 \cup E_2) \qquad \ldots(3)$$

Similarly, $E_1 \cap E_2$, being intersection of two measurable sets, is measurable. So,

$$m_*(E_1 \cap E_2) = m^*(E_1 \cap E_2) = m(E_1 \cap E_2) \qquad \ldots(4)$$

Using previous theorem, we have

$$m^*(E_1) + m^*(E_2) \ge m^*(E_1 \cup E_2) + m^*(E_1 \cap E_2) \qquad \ldots(5)$$

and $$m_*(E_1) + m_*(E_2) \le m_*(E_1 \cup E_2) + m_*(E_1 \cap E_2) \qquad \ldots(6)$$

Using (1) to (4) inequality (5) and (6) becomes

$$m(E_1) + m(E_2) \ge m(E_1 \cup E_2) + m(E_1 \cap E_2) \qquad \ldots(7)$$

and $$m(E_1) + m(E_2) \le m(E_1 \cup E_2) + m(E_1 \cap E_2) \qquad \ldots(8)$$

From (7) and (8) we conclude that

$$m(E_1) + m(E_2) = m(E_1 \cup E_2) + m(E_1 \cap E_2)$$

THEOREM 16.

A subset E of $[a, b]$ is measurable if and only if for given $\varepsilon > 0$ (however small) there exist open sets G_1 and G_2 such that $G_1 \supseteq E$, $G_2 \supseteq E'$ and $|G_1 \cap G_2| < \varepsilon$.

PROOF.   Let $E \subseteq [a, b]$

By definition of exterior measure $\exists$ open sets G_1 and G_2 such that

$$G_1 \supset E, \, G_2 \supset E' \text{ and } m(G_1) < m^*(E) + \varepsilon/2, \, m(G_2) < m^*(E') + \varepsilon/2$$

Therefore, $m(G_1) + m(G_2) < m^*(E) + m^*(E') + \varepsilon$

$\Rightarrow \quad m(G_1 \cup G_2) + m(G_1 \cap G_2) < m^*(E) + m^*(E') + \varepsilon$ (By previous theorem)...(1)

Further, since $G_1 \supset E$, $G_2 \supset E'$, therefore $G_1 \cup G_2 \supset E \cup E' = [a, b]$

$\Rightarrow \qquad\qquad\qquad G_1 \cup G_2 \supset [a, b]$

But $\qquad\qquad\qquad G_1 \cup G_2 \subset [a, b]$

$\Rightarrow \qquad\qquad\qquad G_1 \cup G_2 = [a, b]$

$\Rightarrow \qquad\qquad m(G_1 \cup G_2) = m\{[a, b]\} = b - a$

Using this value in (1) we get

$$b - a + m(G_1 \cap G_2) < m^*(E) + m^*(E') + \varepsilon \qquad\qquad\qquad\qquad ...(2)$$

Now, first suppose that E is measurable.

We have to prove that $m(G_1 \cup G_2) < \varepsilon$

Since E is measurable, therefore $m^*(E) = m_*(E)$

We know that

$$m_*(E) = b - a - m^*(E')$$

$\Rightarrow \qquad m_*(E) + m^*(E') = b - a$

Using all these values in equation (2) we get

$$b - a + m(G_1 \cap G_2) < b - a + \varepsilon$$

$\Rightarrow \qquad\qquad m(G_1 \cap G_2) < \varepsilon$

Conversely, let us suppose $m(G_1 \cap G_2) < \varepsilon$. We have to prove that E is measurable.

Since, $G_1 \supset E \Rightarrow m^*(E) \leq m(G_1)$

Similarly, $\qquad m^*(E') \leq m(G_2)$

On adding, we get

$$m^*(E) + m^*(E') \leq m(G_1) + m(G_2)$$

$\Rightarrow \qquad m^*(E) + m^*(E') \leq m(G_1 \cup G_2) + m(G_1 \cap G_2)$

$$[\because m(G_1 \cup G_2) + m(G_1 \cap G_2) = m(G_1) + m(G_2)]$$

$\Rightarrow \qquad m^*(E) + m^*(E') \leq b - a + \varepsilon \qquad\qquad [\because G_1 \cup G_2 \supset [a, b] \Rightarrow m(G_1 \cup G_2) = b - a$

$$\text{and also by our assumption in } (G_1 \cap G_2) < \varepsilon]$$

$\Rightarrow \qquad\qquad m^*(E) \leq b - a - m^*(E') + \varepsilon$

$\Rightarrow \qquad\qquad m^*(E) \leq m_*(E) + \varepsilon$

Letting $\varepsilon \to 0$ we get

$$m^*(E) \leq m_*(E)$$

But we know that

$$m^*(E) \geq m_*(E)$$

$\Rightarrow \qquad\qquad m^*(E) = m_*(E)$

Hence, E is measurable.

THEOREM 17.

Let A, B, C be three measurable subsets of [a, b] then

$$m(A) + m(B) + m(C) = m(A \cup B \cup C) + m(B \cap C) + m(C \cap A) + m(A \cap B) - m(A \cap B \cap C).$$

PROOF. Let A, B, C be measurable subsets of $[a, b]$. Then for measurable sets A and B, we have

$$m(A) + m(B) = m(A \cup B) + m(A \cap B) \qquad \qquad ...(1)$$

Since A and B are measurable, therefore $A \cup B$ is also measurable, therefore from (1)

$$m(A \cup B) + m(C) = m(A \cup B \cup C) + m[(A \cup B) \cap C] \qquad ...(2)$$

From (1)

$$m(A \cup B) = m(A) + m(B) - m(A \cap B) \qquad \qquad ...(3)$$

Put this value in (2) we get

$$m(A) + m(B) - m(A \cap B) + m(C)$$
$$= m(A \cup B \cup C) + m[(A \cup B) \cap C]$$
$$= m[A \cup B \cup C] + m[(A \cap C) \cup (B \cap C)]$$

[By distributive property]

$$= m[A \cup B \cup C] + m(A \cap C) + m(B \cap C) - m(A \cap B \cap C)$$

(By (3))

Therefore, $m(A) + m(B) + m(C)$
$$= m(A \cup B \cup C) + m(A \cap C) + m(B \cap C) + m(A \cap B)$$
$$- m(A \cap B \cap C)$$

THEOREM 18.

If A is any measurable set and $A_1, A_2, ... A_n$ are pairwise disjoint measurable sets, then

$$m\left[A \cap \left[\bigcup_{i=1}^{n} A_i \right] \right] = \sum_{i=1}^{n} m(A \cap A_i) \ \forall n \qquad \qquad ...(1)$$

[ROHTAK–2001, 14, 16, HPU–2000, 02, MEERUT–2004, GARHWAL–2006, AVADH–2014]

PROOF. We shall prove this theorem by the mathematical induction
If $i = 1$ then both sides of (1) becomes, identical.
$\Rightarrow$ Result is true for $n = 1$.

If $i = 2$ then $\qquad$ LHS $= m\left[A \cap \left[\bigcup_{i=1}^{2} A_i \right] \right]$

$$= m[A \cap A_1 \cup A_2]$$
$$= m[(A \cap A_1) \cup (A \cap A_2)]$$
$$= m(A \cap A_1) + m(A \cap A_2)$$

($\because (A \cap A_1)$ and $(A \cap A_2)$ are pairwise disjoint)

$$= \sum_{i=1}^{n} m(A \cap A_i)$$

$\Rightarrow$ Result is true for $n = 2$
If $i = n - 1$ Let the result be true for $i = n - 1$
i.e., result is true for the sets $A_1, A_2, ... A_{n-1}$

$$\Rightarrow \quad m\left[A \cap \left[\bigcup_{i=1}^{n-1} A_i \right] \right] = \sum_{i=1}^{n-1} m(A \cap A_i) \qquad \qquad ...(2)$$

where $A_i \cap A_j = \phi$ for $i = j = 1, 2, ..., n-1$

Now $A_n \cap A_i = \phi \ \forall \ i = 1, 2, ..., n - 1$

Therefore, $A_n \cap \left[\bigcup_{i=1}^{n-1} A_i \right] = \phi$

So, by applying the result for $n = 2$, we get

$$m\left[A \cap \left[\bigcup_{i=1}^{n-1} A_i \cup A_n \right] \right] = m\left[A \cap \left[\bigcup_{i=1}^{n-1} A_i \right] \right] + m(A \cap A_n)$$

Therefore, $m\left[A \cap \left[\bigcup_{i=1}^{n} A_i \right] \right] = \sum_{i=1}^{n-1} m(A \cap A_i) + m(A \cap A_n)$

Hence, $m\left[A \cap \left[\bigcup_{i=1}^{n} A_i \right] \right] = \sum_{i=1}^{n} m(A \cap A_i)$

3.6 F_σ AND G_δ-SETS

3.6.1 F_σ-sets

A set A is said to be a F_σ-set if it can be written as a countable union of closed sets.

i.e., $A = \bigcup_{i \in N} F_i$, where each F_i is closed.

3.6.2 G_δ-sets

A set A is said to be a G_δ-set if it can be written as countable intersection of open sets.

i.e., $A = \bigcap_{i \in N} G_i$, where each G_i is open.

3.7 BOREL SET

The set which can be obtained by taking countable union or intersection of open and closed sets is called Borel set.

For example: F_σ and G_δ sets are always Borel set.

Illustrations

♦ An open interval $]a, b[$ is F_σ-set, because
$$]a,b[= \bigcup_{n=1}^{\infty}\left[a+\frac{1}{n},b-\frac{1}{n}\right]$$
= a countable union of closed sets

♦ A closed interval $[a, b]$ is a G_δ-set because
$$[a,b]= \bigcap_{n=1}^{\infty}\left(\left]a-\frac{1}{n},b+\frac{1}{n}\right[\right)$$
= a countable intersection of open sets

☞ **REMARK**
• Compliment of a G_δ-set is F_σ and vice-versa.

3.8 REGULARITY OF MEASURE

An extended real valued non-negative countable additive set function m defined on a σ-ring R, i.e., $R \to R^+$ is said to be regular measure if for every $\varepsilon > 0$ and $E \in R$ ∃ and open set $O \supseteq E$ and a closed set $G \subseteq E$ in R such that $m|O - E| \le \varepsilon$ and $m(E - G) \le \varepsilon$.

THEOREM I.

The set of the type F_σ and G_δ are measurable sets.

PROOF. Let E be a set of F_σ-type.

Then by definition of F_σ-set, we can write

$$F_\sigma = \bigcup_{k=1}^{\infty} F_k, \text{ where each } F_k \text{ is a closed set.}$$

Since we know that every closed set is measurable.

$\Rightarrow$ Each F_k is measurable.

$\Rightarrow$ $\bigcup\limits_{k=1}^{\infty} F_k$ is measurable.

($\because$ Enumerable union of measurable sets is measurable)

$\Rightarrow$ E is measurable.

Hence, each F_σ-type set is measurable.

Now, it remains to prove that the set of G_δ-type is also measurable.

Let E be the set of G_δ-type.

Then by definition we can write

$$E = \bigcap\limits_{k=1}^{\infty} G_k \text{ where each } G_k \text{ is open set.}$$

Since, we know that every open set is measurable.

$\Rightarrow$ Each G_k is measurable.

$\Rightarrow$ $\bigcap\limits_{k=1}^{\infty} G_k$ is measurable.

($\because$ Enumerable intersection of measurable sets is measurable)

Hence, E is measurable.

THEOREM 2.

Every Borel set is Lebesgue measurable.   [MEERUT–2005, 06, 14, 17, GARHWAL–2003, 13, KANPUR–2008]

PROOF.   Let E be a Borel measurable set. We have to prove that E is Lebesgue measurable set. Since E is Borel set, so by definition

$$E = \left(\bigcup\limits_{k} G_k \right) \cap \left(\bigcap\limits_{k} F_k \right)$$

where each G_K is an open set and F_k is closed set.

Also, being the Borel measurable set, E is bounded.

Now, E is bounded therefore, each G_k and F_k are bounded.

Also, G_k is open and F_k is closed.

$\Rightarrow$ G_k and F_k both are Lebesgue measurable sets.

$\Rightarrow$ $\bigcup\limits_{k} G_k$ and $\bigcap\limits_{k} F_k$ are Lebesgue measurable sets.

[$\because$ Countable union or intersection of measurable sets is measurable]

$\Rightarrow$ $\left(\bigcup\limits_{k} G_k \right) \cap \left(\bigcap\limits_{k} F_k \right)$ is Lebesgue measurable.

($\because$ Intersection of two measurable sets is measurable)

$\Rightarrow$ E is Lebesgue measurable.

Hence, every Borel set is Lebesgue measurable.

THEOREM 3.

Let E be any set and $\varepsilon > 0$ arbitrary small positive number.

(i) Then there exist an open set $O \supset E$ such that

$$m^*(O) < m^*(E) + \varepsilon$$

or $m^*(O - E) < \varepsilon$

(ii) $\exists$ *a* G_δ-*set* $G \supset E$ *such that* $m^*(E) = m^*(G)$

   or $m^*(G - E) = 0$ [NAGPUR–2007, ROHTAK–2000, 14, AMRAVATI–2002, ASSAM–2008]

PROOF.   (i) For given $\varepsilon > 0$ there will exist at least one countable family $\{I_n\}$ of open intervals such that $\bigcup_n I_n \supset E$ and

$$m^*(E) + \varepsilon > \sum_n |I_n|$$

Let us write $O = \bigcup_n I_n$. Now, being the union of open intervals, O is an open set and

$$m^*(O) = m^*\left(\bigcup_n I_n\right) \le \sum_{n=1}^\infty |I_n| < m^*(E) + \varepsilon$$

$\Rightarrow m^*(O) - m^*(E) < \varepsilon$

But $E \subseteq \bigcup_n I_n = O$

$\Rightarrow m^*(O - E) = m^*(O) - m^*(E) < \varepsilon$. Hence, $m^*(O) < m^*(E) + \varepsilon$ or $m^*(O - E) < \varepsilon$

(ii) Taking $\varepsilon = \dfrac{1}{n}, n \in N$ in (i), we will get an open set $O_n \supset E$ such that

$$m^*(O_n) < m^*(E) + \frac{1}{n}$$

Further, let us write $G = \bigcap_{n=1}^\infty O_n$

Since, $E \subset O_n \ \forall \ n \in N$, therefore $E \subset \bigcap_{n=1}^\infty O_n$

$\Rightarrow \quad E \subset G$

Again, being the countable intersection of open sets, G is a G_δ-set and

$$m^*(E) \le m^*(G) \le m^*(O_n) < m^*(E) + \frac{1}{n} \ \forall \ n \in N.$$

Letting $n \to \infty$, we get

$$m^*(E) \le m^*(G) \le m^*(E)$$

Hence, $m^*(E) = m^*(G)$

3.9 NON-MEASURABLE SETS

Most of the sets in analysis are measurable. But there are some sets which are not measurable. In this section we discuss some examples of non-measurable sets.

3.9.1 SUM MODULO 1

For real numbers x, y in [0, 1] the sum modulo 1 (addition modulo 1), denoted by $\overset{\circ}{+}$ is defined by

$$x \overset{\circ}{+} y = \begin{cases} x+y; & x+y < 1 \\ x+y-1; & x+y \ge 1 \end{cases}$$

For example:

(i) $\dfrac{1}{2} \overset{\circ}{+} \dfrac{1}{4} = \dfrac{3}{4}$ because $\dfrac{1}{2} + \dfrac{1}{4} < 1$

(ii) $\dfrac{2}{3} \overset{\circ}{+} \dfrac{1}{2} = \dfrac{2}{3} + \dfrac{1}{2} - 1 = \dfrac{1}{6}$ because $\dfrac{2}{3} + \dfrac{1}{2} > 1$

3.9.2 TRANSLATE MODULO 1

Let E be any subset of $[0, 1[$ then translate modulo 1 of E by y denoted by $E \overset{\circ}{+} y$ is defined by

$$E \overset{\circ}{+} y = \{x + y : x \in E\}$$

3.9.3 PROPERTIES OF ADDITION MODULO 1

1. **Closure property:** $\overset{\circ}{+}$ is closed in $[0, 1[$, *i.e.*, if $x, y \in [0, 1[$ then $x \overset{\circ}{+} y \in [0, 1[$
2. **Commutativity:** $\overset{\circ}{+}$ is commutative, *i.e.*,
$$x \overset{\circ}{+} y = y \overset{\circ}{+} x$$
3. **Associativity:** $\overset{\circ}{+}$ is associative, *i.e.*,
$$(x \overset{\circ}{+} y) \overset{\circ}{+} z = x \overset{\circ}{+} (y \overset{\circ}{+} z)$$

THEOREM 1.

Lebesgue measure is invariant under the operation "translation modulo 1".

PROOF. Let E be any subset of $[0, 1[$. Then by definition of translation modulo 1.
$$E \overset{\circ}{+} y = \{x + y : x \in E\}$$
We have to prove that $m[E \overset{\circ}{+} y] = m(E)$
Let us take $\qquad E_1 = E \cap [0, 1 - y[$
and $\qquad E_2 = E \cap [1 - y, 1[$ for any measurable subset E of $[0, 1[$
Clearly, E_1 and E_2 both are measurable such that $E_1 \cap E_2 = \phi$ and $E_1 \cup E_2 = E$
So we can write
$$m(E) = m(E_1) + m(E_2)$$
Now, $\qquad x \in E_1 \qquad \Rightarrow \quad 0 \le x < 1 - y$
$\qquad\qquad\qquad\qquad \Rightarrow \quad 0 + y \le x + y < 1 - y + y = 1$
$\qquad\qquad\qquad\qquad \Rightarrow \quad y \le x + y < 1$
Therefore, $\qquad E_1 \overset{\circ}{+} y = \{x \overset{\circ}{+} y : x \in E_1\}$
$\qquad\qquad\qquad\qquad = \{x + y : x \in E_1\}$
$\qquad\qquad\qquad\qquad = E_1$
$\Rightarrow \quad E_1 \overset{\circ}{+} y$ is measurable
Now if $\qquad x \in E_2 \qquad \Rightarrow \quad 1 - y \le x < 1$
$\qquad\qquad\qquad\qquad \Rightarrow \quad 1 - y + y \le x + y < 1 + y$
$\qquad\qquad\qquad\qquad \Rightarrow \quad 1 \le x + y < 1 + y$
$\qquad\qquad\qquad\qquad \Rightarrow \quad x \overset{\circ}{+} y = x + y - 1$
Therefore, $\qquad E_2 \overset{\circ}{+} y = \{x \overset{\circ}{+} y : x \in E_2\}$
$\qquad\qquad\qquad\qquad = E_2 \overset{\circ}{+} (y - 1)$
$\Rightarrow \quad E_2 \overset{\circ}{+} y$ is also measurable and $m(E_2 \overset{\circ}{+} y) = m(E_2 + y - 1) = m(E_2)$
$\qquad\qquad\qquad\qquad\qquad\qquad$ ($\because$ Lebesgue measure is translation invariant)

Further, $E \overset{\circ}{+} y = (E_1 \cup E_2) \overset{\circ}{+} y = (E_1 \overset{\circ}{+} y) \cup (E_2 \overset{\circ}{+} y)$

But, since $E_1 \overset{\circ}{+} y$ and $E_2 \overset{\circ}{+} y$ are disjoint measurable sets.

Therefore, $\quad m(E \overset{\circ}{+} y) = m(E_1 \overset{\circ}{+} y) + m(E_2 \overset{\circ}{+} y)$
$$= m(E_1) + m(E_2)$$
$$= m(E)$$

Hence, m is invariant under $\overset{\circ}{+}$.

THEOREM 2.

There exists a non-measurable set in the interval $[0, 1[$.

PROOF.　　Let us define relation ~ in the set $[0, 1[$ such that

$$x \sim y \text{ if and only if } x - y \text{ is a rational number.}$$

We can easily verify that the relation '~' is an equivalence relation. Then we can say that relation ~ partitions the set $[0, 1[$ into disjoint equivalence classes such that any two elements of the class differ by a rational number while two elements taken from different classes will differ by an irrational number. Let us form the set P by choosing one element from each equivalence class induced by the relation ~ in the set $[0, 1[$. Then clearly $P \subset [0, 1[$

Now we shall show that P is non-measurable.

Define a sequence $< r_i >_{i=0}^{\infty}$ of rationals in $[0, 1[$ with $r_0 = 0$

Now, define $P_i = P \overset{\circ}{+} r_i \, \forall \, i = 0, 1, 2, ..., \infty$

Then $P_0 = P \overset{\circ}{+} r_0 = P \overset{\circ}{+} 0 = P$

Step-1 Firstly we shall prove that each P_i is pairwise disjoint, i.e., $P_i \cap P_j = \phi$ if $i \neq j$

If $x \in P_i \cap P_j \, (i \neq j)$. Then $x \in P + r_i$ and $x \in P + r_j$
$\Rightarrow \qquad\qquad x = p_i + r_i$ and $x = p_j + r_j, \, p_i, p_j \in P$
$\Rightarrow \qquad\qquad p_i \overset{\circ}{+} r_i = p_j \overset{\circ}{+} r_j$
$\Rightarrow \qquad\qquad p_i - p_j = r_j - r_i,$ which is rational
$\Rightarrow \qquad\qquad p_i \sim p_j$
$\Rightarrow \quad p_i$ and p_j are the elements of P belonging to the same equivalence class, which is a contradiction, because P contains only one element from each equivalence class.
$\Rightarrow \quad P_i$ and P_j are pairwise disjoint.

Step-2 We shall prove that $\overset{\infty}{\underset{i=0}{\cup}} P_i = [0,1[$

Since each $P_i \subseteq [0, 1[$, therefore, $\underset{i}{\cup} P_i = [0,1[$ 　　　　　　　　　　...(1)

Also each element $x \in [0, 1[$ is in same equivalence class and so is related to same element y of P.

If x differ from y by rational number r_j. Then $x \in P_i$ and hence $[0, 1[\subseteq \cup P_i$ ...(2)

Finally from (1) and (2) we conclude that

$$\overset{\infty}{\underset{i=0}{\cup}} P_i = [0,1[$$

Step-3 We shall prove that P is non-measurable

Let if possible, P is a measurable set

We know that each P_i is a "translation modulo 1" of P.

Therefore, each P_i is also measurable.

$$\Rightarrow \qquad m(P_i) = m(P)$$

$$\Rightarrow \qquad m[\cup P_i] = \sum_{i=0}^{\infty} m(P_i) = \sum_{i=0}^{\infty} m(P)$$

$$= \begin{cases} 0, & \text{if} \quad m(P) = 0 \\ \infty, & \text{if} \quad m(P) > 0 \end{cases} \qquad \qquad ...(3)$$

Further, $\qquad m\left[\bigcup_{i=0}^{\infty} P_i \right] = m([0,1[) = 1$

which contradict (3).

Hence, P is a non-measurable set.

☛ REMARK

• Every set of positive measure contains a non-measurable subset.

🗂 Solved Examples

EXAMPLE 1. *If $A \subset]a, b[$ is a Lebesgue measurable set then prove that $m(A) + m(A') = b - a$.*

SOLUTION. By definition, we have

$$m_*(A) = b - a - m^*(A'), \text{ if } A \subset]a, b[\qquad \qquad ...(1)$$

Since A is measurable $\Rightarrow A'$ is measurable, so by definition

$$\left. \begin{array}{l} m_*(A) = m^*(A) = m(A) \\ \text{and} \qquad m_*(A') = m^*(A') = m(A') \end{array} \right] \qquad \qquad ...(2)$$

From (1) and (2) we have

$$m(A) = b - a - m(A')$$

$$\Rightarrow \qquad m(A) + m(A') = b - a = \text{length of the interval }]a, b[$$

EXAMPLE 2. *Show that the Cantor's set is measurable and its measure is zero.*

SOLUTION. Let F be the Cantor's set, then clearly F' is open.

So, F is a closed set. Further, we know that every open subset of $[0, 1]$ is measurable, so $F' (= [0, 1] - F)$ is measurable and so F is measurable.

Now, $\qquad F' = \left]\dfrac{1}{3}, \dfrac{2}{3}\right[\cup \left]\dfrac{1}{9}, \dfrac{2}{9}\right[\cup \left]\dfrac{7}{9}, \dfrac{8}{9}\right[\cup ...$

$$\Rightarrow \qquad m(F') = m\left(\left]\dfrac{1}{3}, \dfrac{2}{3}\right[\right) + m\left(\left]\dfrac{1}{9}, \dfrac{2}{9}\right[\right) + m\left(\left]\dfrac{7}{9}, \dfrac{8}{9}\right[\right) + ...$$

$$= \dfrac{1}{3} + \dfrac{2}{3^2} + \dfrac{2^2}{3^3} + ... + \dfrac{2^{p-1}}{3^p} + ...$$

$$= \dfrac{1}{3}\left[1 + \dfrac{2}{3} + \left(\dfrac{2}{3}\right)^2 + ...\right]$$

$$= \frac{1}{3} \left(\frac{1}{1 - \frac{2}{3}} \right)$$

$$\left(\because S = \frac{a}{1-r}, \text{ sum of infinite G.P.} \right)$$

$$= 1$$

= length of the interval [0, 1]

But we have $\quad m(F') = b - a - m(F)$ (See example 1)

$\Rightarrow \qquad m(F') + m(F) = b - a = 1 - 0 = 1$

$\Rightarrow \qquad 1 + m(F) = 1$ $\qquad (\because m(F)' = 1)$

$\Rightarrow \qquad m(F) = 0$

EXAMPLE 3. *If E_1, E_2 are measurable subsets of [2, 3] such that $m(E_1) = 1$. Then prove that $m(E_1 \cap E_2) = m(E_2)$.*

SOLUTION. We know that

$$m(E_1 \cap E_2) + m(E_1 \cup E_2) = m(E_1) + m(E_2) \qquad \ldots(1)$$

Using set theory, we know that

$$E_1 \subseteq E_1 \cup E_2$$

$\Rightarrow \qquad m(E_1) \le m(E_1 \cup E_2)$

But $\qquad m(E_1) \ge 1$

Therefore, $m(E_1 \cup E_2) \ge 1$

$\Rightarrow \qquad m(E_1 \cup E_2) \ge 1 \qquad \ldots(2)$

Further $E_1 \subseteq [2, 3]$, $E_2 \subseteq [2, 3]$

$\Rightarrow \qquad E_1 \cup E_2 \subseteq [2, 3]$

$\Rightarrow \qquad m(E_1 \cup E_2) \le m\{[2, 3]\} = 3 - 2 = 1$

$\Rightarrow \qquad m(E_1 \cup E_2) \le 1 \qquad \ldots(3)$

From (2) and (3), we conclude that

$$m(E_1 \cup E_2) = 1 \qquad \ldots(4)$$

It is also given that $m(E_1) = 1$ $\qquad \ldots(5)$

Using (4) and (5) in (1) we get

$$m(E_1 \cap E_2) + 1 = 1 + m(E_2)$$

$\Rightarrow \qquad m(E_1 \cap E_2) = m(E_2)$

EXAMPLE 4. *If $m^*(A) = 0$ then prove that $m^*(A \cup B) = m^*(B)$* [ROHTAK–2002, HPU–2000, 02, 13, 17]

SOLUTION. For any two sets A and B, we have

$$m^*(A \cup B) \le m^*(A) + m^*(B) \qquad \ldots(1)$$

It is given that $m^*(A) = 0$, then from (1)

$$m^*(A \cup B) \le m^*(B) \qquad \ldots(2)$$

By set theory we have

$$B \subseteq A \cup B$$

$\Rightarrow \qquad m^*(B) \le m^*(A \cup B) \qquad \ldots(3)$

From (2) and (3) we conclude that

$$m^*(A \cup B) = m^*(B)$$

EXAMPLE 5. *If A is Lebesgue measurable set and $m^*(A \Delta B) = 0$, then show that B is also measurable and $m^*(B) = m^*(A)$.*

SOLUTION. By definition of symmetric difference of two sets, we have
$$A \triangle B = (A - B) \cup (B - A)$$
It is given that $m^*(A \triangle B) = 0$
$\Rightarrow$ $A \triangle B, A - B$ and $B - A$ all are measurable.
Since, $A \cap B = A - (A - B)$
Clearly, $A \cap B$ is measurable. ($\because A$ and $A - B$ are measurable and
difference of two measurable sets is again measurable)
Therefore, $B = (A \cap B) \cup (B - A)$, being the union of two measurable sets is measurable.

Now, it remains to prove that $m^*(B) = m^*(A)$

Since, $m^*(A \triangle B) = 0$ (Given)

$\Rightarrow$ $m^*[(A - B) \cup (B - A)] = 0$

$\Rightarrow$ $m^*(A - B) + m^*(B - A) = 0$ ($\because A - B$ and $B - A$ both are disjoint)

which is possible only when $m^*(A - B) = 0$ and $m^*(B - A) = 0$ ...(1)

Also, since $B = (A \cap B) \cup (B - A)$, therefore,

$$m^*(B) = m^*[(A \cap B) \cup (B - A)]$$
$$= m^*(A \cap B) + m^*(B - A) \quad (\because (A \cap B) \text{ and } B - A \text{ are disjoint})$$
$$= m^*(A \cap B) + 0 \quad \text{(By (1))}$$

$\Rightarrow$ $m^*(B) = m^*(A \cap B)$ ...(2)

Similarly, we may prove that
$$m^*(A) = m^*(A \cap B) \qquad \qquad \text{...(3)}$$

Finally, from (2) and (3) we conclude that
$$m^*(A) = m^*(B)$$

EXAMPLE 6. *If M is a measurable set, then for any set E, prove that*
$$m^*(E) = m^*(EM) + m^*(E - EM)$$
where $EM = E \cap M$

SOLUTION. Using set theory, we can write
$$E = EM \cup (E - EM)$$
$\Rightarrow$ $m^*(E) = m^*(EM) + m^*(E - EM)$ ($\because EM$ and $E - EM$ are disjoint)

EXAMPLE 7. *Let us define a set $\{x \in \mathbf{R} : 0 < x < 1$ and x has a decimal expansion not using the digit 7\}*
Show that the Lebesgue measure of this set is zero.

SOLUTION. The given interval is $]0, 1[$. Divide this interval into 10 equal parts, each of length $\frac{1}{10}$. Then remove the interior of 8th part (which contain the digit 7). At the next step divide the remaining 9 intervals into 10 equal parts each of length $\frac{1}{10^2}$ and remove the interior of 8th part of each interval. Continue this process infinite number of times. Then remaining subset of $]0, 1[$ is the required set. Let it be denoted by A. This process will be clear from the following table:

No. of steps	No. of intervals deleted	No. of remaining intervals	Length of each deleted intervals	Total length of deleted open intervals
1	1	9	$\dfrac{1}{10}$	$\dfrac{1}{10}$
2	9	9^2	$\dfrac{1}{10^2}$	$\dfrac{9}{10^2}$
3	9^2	9^3	$\dfrac{1}{10^3}$	$\dfrac{9^2}{10^3}$
⋮	⋮	⋮	⋮	⋮
⋮	⋮	⋮	⋮	⋮
⋮	⋮	⋮	⋮	⋮

Clearly A' denote the deleted intervals of $]0, 1[$

$\therefore$
$$m(A') = \frac{1}{10} + 9 \cdot \frac{1}{10^2} + 9^2 \cdot \frac{1}{10^3} + \dots$$

$$= \frac{1/10}{1 - 9/10} = 1$$ (Sum of infinite GP, $S = \dfrac{a}{1-r}$)

Finally using

$$m(A) + m(A') = 1$$

We get $\qquad m(A) = 1 - m(A') = 1 - 1 = 0$

EXAMPLE 8. *Let x be a number in the interval $]0, 1[$ written in the scale of 10 as $x = 0 \cdot x_1 x_2 x_3 \dots$ where x_i's is 3 or 5. Find the measure of the set so defined.*

SOLUTION. Here the given interval is $]0, 1[$.

Since, the decimal expansion of x does not contains the digit 3 or 5. Therefore, we have to delete two subintervals (*i.e.,* interior or 4th and 6th parts). Clearly if the required set is A then removed intervals will be A'. The process of deletion will be clear from the following table:

No. of steps	No. of intervals deleted	No. of remaining intervals	Length of each deleted interval	Total length of deleted open intervals
1	2	8	$\dfrac{1}{10}$	$2 \times \dfrac{1}{10}$
2	2×8	8^2	$\dfrac{1}{10^2}$	$2 \times \dfrac{8}{10^2}$
3	2×8^2	8^3	$\dfrac{1}{10^3}$	$2 \times \dfrac{8}{10^3}$
⋮	⋮	⋮	⋮	⋮
⋮	⋮	⋮	⋮	⋮

Clearly A' is an open set such that

$$m(A') = 2 \times \frac{1}{10} + 2 \times \frac{8}{10^2} + 2 \times \frac{8^2}{10^3} + \dots, \text{ which is a G.P.}$$

$$= \frac{\frac{2}{10}}{1 - \frac{8}{10}} \qquad\qquad (\because S = \frac{a}{1-r})$$

$$= 1$$

Now, using
$$m(A) = |]0, 1[| - m(A')$$
$$= (1-0) - 1$$
$$= 1 - 1 = 0$$

EXAMPLE 9. *Construct a non-dense perfect set in the interval* $[0, 1]$ *whose measure is* $\frac{1}{2}$.

[MEERUT–2003, 14, 15, GARHWAL–2011, ROHILKHAND–2006, DELHI–2015]

SOLUTION. Consider the interval $[0, 1]$. Let $a \in [0, 1]$.

Now proceed same as in example (7) and (8), remove from the interval $[0, 1]$ and also in succession from the remaining subintervals, a part of length $l_n = (n = 1, 2, 3, \dots)$ which satisfies.

$$l_1 + 2l_2 + 2^2 l_3 + \dots + 2^{n-1} l_n = a - \frac{a}{n+2}$$

If A denote the remaining set, then it is clearly a perfect and non-dense set (being the Cantor's ternary set)

Now, limiting sum of the dropped intervals

$$= \lim_{n \to \infty} \left[a - \frac{a}{n+2} \right] = a$$

$$\Rightarrow \qquad m(A') = a$$
$$\therefore \qquad m(A) = m([0, 1]) - m(A')$$
$$= (1 - 0) - a$$
$$= 1 - a$$

Finally choosing $a = \frac{1}{2} \in [0,1]$, we have

$$m(A) = 1 - a$$
$$= 1 - \frac{1}{2} = \frac{1}{2}$$

EXAMPLE 10. *If* $<E_n>$ *is a sequence of measurable sets, all contained in a set of finite measure and limit of* E_n *exists then show that* $lim(E_n)$ *is measurable and* $m(lim(E_n)) = lim(m(E_n))$.

SOLUTION. We know that

$$\overline{\lim} E_n = \bigcap_{n=1}^{\infty} \left(\bigcup_{k=n}^{\infty} E_k \right)$$

and
$$\underline{\lim} E_n = \bigcup_{n=1}^{\infty} \left(\bigcap_{k=n}^{\infty} E_k \right)$$

Since, E_n is measurable (given). Then, being the countable union and intersection of measurable sets, $\underline{\lim}\, E_n$ and $\overline{\lim}\, E_n$ both are measurable.

Also, since $\lim(E_n)$ exist, therefore, we have

$$\underline{\lim}(E_n) = \overline{\lim}(E_n) = \lim(E_n)$$

$\Rightarrow$ $\lim(E_n)$ is also measurable.

Now, it remains to prove that

$$m(\lim E_n) = \lim(m(E_n))$$

Let us suppose

$$\overset{\infty}{\underset{k=n}{\cup}} E_k = A_n \text{ and } \overset{\infty}{\underset{k=n}{\cap}} E_k = B_n$$

Then clearly, $<A_n>$ is a monotonically decreasing sequence of measurable sets, then

$$m(\overline{\lim\, E_n}) = m\left(\overset{\infty}{\underset{n=1}{\cap}} A_n\right) = \lim_{n\to\infty} m(A_n) = \lim_{n\to\infty}(E_n)$$

Similarly, $<B_n>$ is a monotonically increasing sequence of measurable sets then

$$m(\underline{\lim\, E_n}) = m\left(\overset{\infty}{\underset{n=1}{\cap}} B_n\right) = \lim_{n\to\infty} m(B_n) = \lim_{n\to\infty}(E_n)$$

Since, limit exists, therefore, we get

$$\underline{\lim}(E_n) = \overline{\lim}(E_n) = \lim(E_n)$$

Hence, $m(\lim E_n) = \lim(m(E_n))$.

EXAMPLE 11. *Show that m^* is translation invariant.*   [HPU–2004, 14, DELHI–2010]

SOLUTION. Let E be any subset of R. We have to prove that m^* is translation invariant. For this it is sufficient to prove that

$$m^*(E + p) = m^*(E), p \in R$$

By definition $m^*(E) = \underset{n}{\Sigma} |I_n|$

where $<I_n>$ is a family of open intervals such that $\underset{n}{\cup} I_n \supseteq E$ and whose length is minimum.

Now suppose that

$$I_n = \,]a_n, b_n[$$

Then clearly, $E + p$ covered by the family $<I'_n>$ where $I_n = \,]a_n + p, b_n + p[$

Here, $|I'_n| = (b_n + p) - (a_n + p) = b_n - a_n = |I_n|$

$\Rightarrow$ $\Sigma |I'_n| = \Sigma |I_n|$

Also, since $\Sigma |I_n|$ is of minimum length, therefore $\Sigma |I'_n|$ is also of minimum length such that $\cup I'_n = E + p$.

Therefore, $m^*(E + p) = \Sigma |I'_n| = \Sigma |I_n| = m^*(E)$

$\Rightarrow$ $m^*(E + p) = m^*(E)$

Hence, m^* is translation invariant.

EXAMPLE 12. *If E_1, E_2 are any subsets of real numbers such that the measure of $E_1 \triangle E_2$ (symmetric difference of E_1 and E_2) is zero and E_1 is measurable, then show that E_2 is measurable and $m(E_2) = m(E_1)$.*   [PUNJAB–2002, 14, ROHTAK–2009]

SOLUTION. By set theory, we can write
$$E_2 = [E_1 \cup (E_2 - E_1)] - (E_1 - E_2)$$
It is given that $m(E_1 \Delta E_2) = 0$
$\Rightarrow \quad m[(E_1 - E_2) \cup (E_2 - E_1)] = 0$
$\Rightarrow \quad m(E_1 - E_2) + m(E_2 - E_1) = 0 \qquad (\because (E_1 - E_2) \text{ and } (E_2 - E_1) \text{ are disjoint})$
$\Rightarrow \quad m(E_1 - E_2) = 0 \text{ and } m(E_2 - E_1) = 0 \qquad \qquad \ldots(1)$
Further, since $E_1 \cap (E_2 - E_1) = \phi$
Therefore, $\quad m[E_1 \cup (E_2 - E_1)]$
$$= m(E_1) + m(E_2 - E_1) \qquad (\because E_1 \text{ and } E_2 - E_1 \text{ are disjoint})$$
$$= m(E_1) + 0 \qquad (\because m(E_2 - E_1) = 0)$$
$$= m(E_1)$$
$\Rightarrow \quad E_1 \cup (E_2 - E_1)$ is measurable.
$\Rightarrow \quad [E_1 \cup (E_2 - E_1)] - (E_1 - E_2)$ is measurable.
$\qquad \qquad (\because$ difference of two measurable sets is measurable$)$
$\Rightarrow \quad E_2$ is measurable.
Also, $\qquad m(E_2) = m[E_1 \cup (E_2 - E_1)] - m(E_1 - E_2)$
$$= m(E_1) + m(E_2 - E_1) - m(E_1 - E_2)$$
$$= m(E_1) + 0 - 0 = m(E_1) \qquad \qquad \text{(By (1))}$$

EXAMPLE 13. *Let A be any subset of* **R**. *Define* $cA = \{x : c^{-1}x \in A\}$, $c > 0$. *Then prove the following:*

(i) $m^*(A) = cm^*(A)$

(ii) *A is measurable if and only if cA is measurable.*

SOLUTION. (i) Clearly, for given $\varepsilon > 0$ $\exists$ a family $\{I_n\}$ of open intervals such that
$$cA \subseteq \bigcup_i I_i$$
and $\qquad m^*(cA) \le \sum_i |I_i| - \varepsilon$

which implies $A \subseteq \bigcup_i c^{-1} I_i$

$\Rightarrow \qquad m^*(A) \le \sum_i |c^{-1} I_i| = c^{-1} \sum_i |I_i|$

$\Rightarrow \qquad m^*(A) \le c^{-1}[m^*(cA) + \varepsilon]$

$\Rightarrow \qquad cm^*(A) \le m^*(cA) \qquad \qquad \ldots(1)$

Replacing A by cA and c by c^{-1} in (1) we get
$$c^{-1}m^*(cA) \le m^*(c^{-1}(cA))$$
$\Rightarrow \qquad m^*(cA) \le cm^*(A) \qquad \qquad \ldots(2)$

From (1) and (2) we conclude that
$$m^*(A) = cm^*(A)$$

(ii) A is measurable $\quad \Leftrightarrow \quad m^*(A) = m^*(A) = m(A)$

$\Leftrightarrow \quad m_*(cA) = b - a - m^*(cA)' = b - a - m^*(cA')$

$\Leftrightarrow \quad m_*(cA) = b - a - cm^*(A')$
$$= b - a - cm(A') = cm(A)$$

$\Leftrightarrow \quad m_*(cA) = cm(A) = m^*(cA) \qquad \qquad \text{(Using (1))}$

$\Leftrightarrow \quad cA$ is measurable.

☛ **REMARK**

- In particular, if we take $c = -1$ in (i) and (ii), we can deduce the following result:
  "$A = \{x = -x \in A\}$ is measurable iff A is measurable and $m^*(-A) = -m^*(A)$"

EXAMPLE 14. *Show that the set of all irrational numbers in* [0, 1] *is measurable and has measure* 1.

[GARHWAL–2004, DELHI–2013]

SOLUTION.   Let us have the following notations:

$$A = \text{set of rationals in } [0, 1]$$
$$B = \text{set of irrationals in } [0, 1]$$

Clearly, A and B are disjoint such that $A \cup B = [0, 1]$

i.e., $A \cap B = \phi$ and $A \cup B = [0,1]$

Now, $A \cup B = [0, 1]$

$\Rightarrow$ $m(A \cup B) = m\{[0, 1]\}$

$\Rightarrow$ $m(A) + m(B) = 1 - 0 = 1$ $(\because A \cap B = \phi)$ ...(1)

Further, we know that, the set of rational numbers Q is countable and $A \subseteq Q$.

$\Rightarrow$ A is countable   [$\because$ Any subset of countable set is countable]

$\Rightarrow$ $m(A) = 0$ [$\because$ Measure of a countable set is zero]

Using $m(A) = 0$ in (1) we get

$$m(B) = 1$$

EXAMPLE 15. *Let* $<E_i>$ *be the sequence of sets of real numbers, then prove that*

$$m^*(E_1 + E_2 + \ldots) \le m^*(E_1) + m^*(E_2) + \ldots$$

But if the sets E_i *are pairwise disjoint then*

$$m_*(E_1 + E_2 + \ldots) \ge m_*(E_1) + m_*(E_2) + \ldots$$ [KANPUR–2006, BHOPAL–2009]

SOLUTION.   Let $E_1, E_2, \ldots$ be a sequence of real numbers. We have to prove that

$$m^*\left(\sum_i E_i\right) \le \sum_i m^*(E_i)$$

For given $\varepsilon > 0$ $\exists$ an open set G_n such that

$$E_n \subset G_n, \; m(G_n) < m^*(E_n) + \frac{\varepsilon}{2^n}$$ ...(1)

Since, we know that arbitrary union of open sets is open.

Therefore, $\sum_{r=1}^{\infty} G_r$ is an open set such that

$$\sum_{r=1}^{\infty} E_r \subseteq \sum_{r=1}^{\infty} G_r$$ ...(2)

$\Rightarrow$ $E_n \subset G_n \; \forall n$

Now, from (2)

$$\sum_{r=1}^{\infty} E_r \subseteq \sum_{r=1}^{\infty} G_r$$

$\Rightarrow$ $m^*\left(\sum_{r=1}^{\infty} E_r\right) \le m^*\left(\sum_{r=1}^{\infty} G_r\right) = m\left(\sum_{r=1}^{\infty} G_r\right) \le \sum_{r=1}^{\infty} m(G_r)$

$$\Rightarrow \qquad m^*\left(\sum_{r=1}^{\infty} E_r\right) \le \sum_{r=1}^{\infty} m(G_r) < \sum_{r=1}^{\infty}\left[m^*(E_r)+\frac{\varepsilon}{2^r}\right]$$

$$= \sum_{r=1}^{\infty} m^*(E_r)+\varepsilon \qquad \text{(Using (1))}$$

$$\Rightarrow \qquad m^*\left(\sum_{r=1}^{\infty} E_r\right) \le \sum_{r=1}^{\infty} m^*(E_r)+\varepsilon$$

Letting $\varepsilon \to 0$ we get

$$m^*\left(\sum_{r=1}^{\infty} E_r\right) \le \sum_{r=1}^{\infty} m^*(E_r)$$

Further if $E_1, E_2, \ldots$ are pairwise disjoint such that $E_m \cap E_n = \phi$, $n \ne m$.

Therefore, $m_*(E_m \cap E_n) = 0 = m^*(E_m \cap E_n)$ if $m \ne n$ \qquad ...(3)

Also, we know that

$$m_*(E_1) + m_*(E_2) \le m_*(E_1 \cup E_2) + m_*(E_1 \cap E_2) \qquad ...(4)$$

From (3) and (4) we get

$$m_*(E_1) + m_*(E_2) \le m_*(E_1 \cup E_2)$$

$$\Rightarrow \qquad m_*(E_1 \cup E_2) \ge \sum_{r=1}^{2} m_*(E_r)$$

$$\Rightarrow \qquad m_*\left(\sum_{r=1}^{2} E_r\right) \ge \sum_{r=1}^{2} m_*(E_r)$$

In general (by induction)

$$m_*\left(\sum_{r=1}^{n} E_r\right) \ge \sum_{r=1}^{n} m_*(E_r) \qquad ...(5)$$

Further, since $\displaystyle\bigcup_{r=1}^{\infty} E_r \supseteq \bigcup_{r=1}^{n} E_r$

$$\Rightarrow \qquad m_*\left(\bigcup_{r=1}^{\infty} E_r\right) \ge m_*\left(\bigcup_{r=1}^{n} E_r\right) \ge \sum_{r=1}^{n} m_*(E_r) \qquad \text{(Using (5))}$$

$$\Rightarrow \qquad m_*\left(\bigcup_{r=1}^{\infty} E_r\right) \ge \sum_{r=1}^{n} m_*(E_r)$$

Letting $n \to \infty$ we get

$$m_*\left(\bigcup_{r=1}^{\infty} E_r\right) \ge \sum_{r=1}^{\infty} m_*(E_r)$$

or $\qquad m_*\left(\sum_{r=1}^{\infty} E_r\right) \ge \sum_{r=1}^{\infty} m_*(E_r)$

Exercise 3.1

1. Prove that an enumerable set is measurable and its measure is zero.

2. Prove that a continuous function defined in a closed interval is measurable.

3. Let $<E_i>$ be a monotonically increasing sequence of measurable sets. If $E = \sum\limits_{k=1}^{\infty} E_k$ is bounded set then prove that

$$m(E) = \lim_{n \to \infty} m(E_n)$$

4. If O_1 and O_2 are any two open sets then prove that

$$m(O_1 + O_2) + m(O_1 \cdot O_2) = m(O_1) + m(O_2)$$

5. Prove that a set E of real numbers is measurable if and only if for given $\varepsilon > 0 \; \exists$ set t, e_1, e_2 such that $E = t + e_1 + e_2$, where t is the sum of a finite number of intervals and

$$m^*(e_1) < \varepsilon, \; m^*(e_2) < \varepsilon$$

6. Show that the Lebesgue measure of the Cantor subset of the unit interval is zero.

7. If E_1 is a measurable set and $m^*(E_1 \triangle E_2) = 0$ then show that E_2 is a measurable set.

8. Show that every compact set in R is measurable.

9. Show that if A is any set with $m^*(A) = 0$ then there is a non-measurable set E contained in A.

10. Show that $m^*(S) = \inf.\{m(T) \cdot S \subset T\}$ for all measurable set T containing S.

11. Show that the Lebesgue measure is finitely additive.

12. Show that the necessary and sufficient condition for the set E to be measurable and of measure zero is that $m^*(E) = 0$.

13. Show that the Cantor set can be put into a one-to-one correspondance with the interval $[0, 1]$.

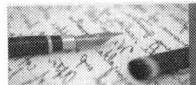 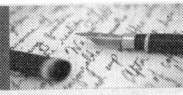

CHAPTER Summary

🕮 KEY TERMS

- **OUTER LEBESGUE MEASURE:** The outer measure of a set $A \subseteq R$ is defined as

$$m^*(A) = \begin{cases} 0 & \text{if} \quad A = \phi \\ \inf.\{y : y = \sum_i |I_i|\} \end{cases}$$

where $\{I_i\}$ is a countable family of open intervals such that $\cup I_i \supseteq A$.

- **LEBESGUE INNER MEASURE:** The inner measure of a set A, denoted by $m_*(A)$ defined by

$$m_*(A) = b - a - m^*(A')$$

- **LEBESGUE MEASURABLE SET:** A set A is said to be Lebesgue measurable for each set E,

$$m^*(E) = m^*(A \cap E) + m^*(A' \cap E)$$

- **BOREL SET:** The set which can be obtained by taking countable union or intersection of open and closed sets is called Borel set.

- **F_σ-SET:** A set which can be written as the countable union of closed sets is called F_σ-set

- **G_δ-SET:** A set which can be written as countable intersection of open sets is called G_δ-set.

- **REGULAR MEASURE:** An extended real-valued non-negative countable additive set function on R is said to be regular measure if for every $\varepsilon > 0$ and $E \subseteq R \; \exists$ an open set $O \supseteq E$ and a closed set $G \subseteq E$ such that

$$m(O - E) \leq \varepsilon \text{ and } m(E - G) \leq \varepsilon$$

🕮 RESULTS

- The function m^* is a set function which is defined from the power set of R into the set of all non-negative extended real numbers.

- The outer measure of an interval is equal to its length.

- For a countable set E, $m^*(E) = 0$

- The set $[0, 1]$ is uncountable.

- Any set with outer measure non-zero is uncountable.

- The Cantor set is uncountable.

- A is measurable iff A' is measurable.

- If E has the outer measure zero, then E is measurable.

- Every subset of a measurable set is measurable.

- Union, intersection and difference of two measurable sets is also measurable.

- For measurable sets E_1 and E_2

$$m(E_1 \cup E_2) + m(E_1 \cap E_2) = m(E_1) + m(E_2)$$

- A countable union of measurable sets is measurable.

- If E_1, E_2 and E_3 are measurable sets then

$$m(E_1) + m(E_2) + m(E_3) + m(E_1 \cap E_2 \cap E_3)$$
$$= m(E_1 \cup E_2 \cup E_3) + m(E_1 \cap E_2)$$

$$+ m(E_1 \cap E_3) + m(E_2 \cap E_3)$$

- There are 2^c measurable sets in every interval.

- Every Borel set is measurable.

- Every interval (open or closed) is measurable.

- If $<E_i>$ is a sequence of measurable sets then the sets $\overline{\lim} E_i$ and $\underline{\lim} E_i$ are also measurable.

- If E is a measurable set then there exist Borel sets B_1 and B_2 such that $B_1 \subseteq E \subseteq B_2$ and $m(B_1) = m(E) = m(B_2)$.

- There exists a non-measurable set in the interval $[0, 1[$.

- Every set of positive measure contains a non-measurable set.

- **FIRST FUNDAMENTAL THEOREM:** If E_1, E_2, ... are pairwise disjoint measurable sets and $E = E_1 \cup E_2 \cup ...$ then E is measurable and

$$m(E) = \sum_{i=1}^{\infty} m(E_i)$$

- **SECOND FUNDAMENTAL THEOREM:** If E_1, E_2, ... are measurable sets and $E = E_1 \cap E_2 \cap ...$ Then E is measurable.

☞ WORTHY READINGS

☞ The set ϕ and R are measurable sets.

☞ Every countable set is measurable and its measure is zero.

☞ There are 2^c measurable sets in every interval.

☞ Every Borel set in R is measurable.

☞ If E_1 and E_2 be measurable sets each having finite measure then following statements are equivalent:

   i) $m(E_1 \Delta E_2) = 0$

   ii) $m(E_1 - E_2) = 0 = m(E_2 - E_1)$

   iii) $m(E_1) = m(E_1 \cap E_2) = m(E_2)$

☞ The set of all irrational numbers in $[0, 1]$ is measurable.

☞ FURTHER READINGS

☞ Every countable set is a Borel set of measure zero.

☞ If G be the class of all open sets then for every E in X

$$m^*(E) = \inf.\{m(U) : E \subset U \subset G\}$$

☞ Let T be a one-to-one transformation of the entire real line onto itself defined by $T(x) = ax + b$, $a, b \in R$, $a \neq 0$. If for every subset E of X, $T(E) = \{ax + b : x \in E\}$. Then $T(E)$ is a Borel set or a Lebesgue measurable set, if and only if E is a Borel set or a Lebesgue measurable set respectively.

☞ To every Lebesgue measurable set E, there correspond two Borel sets A and B such that $A \subset E \subset B$, $m(B - A) = 0$.

☞ Every bounded set has finite outer-measure.

☞ The set of those points in the closed unit interval in which binary expansion all the digits in the even places are 0 is a Lebesgue measurable set of measure zero.

☞ If E is a Lebesgue measurable set such that for every number x in an everywhere dense set $m^*(E \Delta (E + x)) = 0$

Then either $m^*(E) = 0$ or $m^*(E') = 0$.

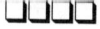

Chapter 4
Outer Measure and Measurability

4.1 INTRODUCTION

In this chapter we shall study the general procedure for defining an outer measure based on some algebra of sets. Some important topics discuss in this chapters include Boolean ring, Boolean algebra, σ-ring, σ-algebra, ideal measure function. Caratheodory's postulates for outer measure and monotone class etc. We shall also confirm the results obtained in the previous chapter for the outer measurable sets.

4.2 RING AND ALGEBRA

4.2.1 BOOLEAN RING

A non-empty class of sets which is closed under the formation of union and differences is called Boolean ring.

i.e., a non-empty class B of sets is called Boolean ring if

(i) $A, B \in B \quad \Rightarrow \quad A \cup B \in B$

(ii) $A, B \in B \quad \Rightarrow \quad A - B \in B$

PROPERTIES

(1) A Boolean ring is closed under the formation of symmetric difference, *i.e.*, Δ.

$$\because \qquad A \Delta B = (A - B) \cup (B - A)$$

Using above definition $A - B$ and $B - A$ both belongs to B.

Also, $\qquad (A - B) \cup (B - A) \in B$ $\qquad$ (Again by definition of Boolean Ring)

$$\Rightarrow \qquad A \Delta B \in B$$

(2) If $A, B \in B$. Then $A \cap B \in B$

$$\because \qquad A \cap B = A - (A - B) \qquad \text{(By set theory)}$$

Clearly, $A, A - B \in B \qquad \Rightarrow \qquad A - (A - B) \in B$

$$\Rightarrow \qquad A \cap B \in B$$

(3) $\phi \in B$ for $A, A \in B$ because $A - A \in B$

$$\Rightarrow \qquad \phi \in B$$

(4) The class $\{\phi\}$ and the class of all subsets of whole set are the trivial example of Boolean ring.

☞ REMARK

• Boolean ring is also called **rings of sets** or finitely additive class.

4.2.2 BOOLEAN ALGEBRA

A non-empty family B of sets is called an Boolean algebra if it is closed under the formation of union and complimentations.

i.e., a non-empty family B of sets is called Boolean algebra if

   (i) $A \in B$ $\Rightarrow$ $A' \in B$

   (ii) $A, B \in B$ $\Rightarrow$ $A \cup B \in B$

☞ REMARKS

- Boolean algebra is also called 'algebra of sets' or a 'field'.
- Boolean algebra B is closed under the formation of finite unions.

4.2.3 σ-RING

A non-empty class S of sets is called a σ-ring if it is closed under the formation of countable union and differences.

i.e., S is said to be σ-ring if

   (i) $A, B \in S$ $\Rightarrow$ $A - B \in S$

   (ii) $A_1, A_2, \ldots \in S$ $\Rightarrow$ $\overset{\infty}{\underset{i=1}{\cup}} A_i \in S$

PROPERTIES

   (1) A σ-ring is also closed under the formation of countable intersection. For

$$\overset{\infty}{\underset{i=1}{\cap}} A_i = A - \overset{\infty}{\underset{i-1}{\cup}} (A - A_i), \text{ where } A = \overset{\infty}{\underset{i-1}{\cup}} A_i$$

   (2) For any finite set X, the power set $P(X)$ and class of all finite subsets of X is a σ-ring.

   (3) Every σ-ring is a Boolean ring.

4.2.4 σ-ALGEBRA

A non-empty class S of sets is called σ-algebra if it is closed under the formation of complement and countable unions.

i.e., A non-empty class S is called σ-algebra, if

   (i) $A \in S$ $\Rightarrow$ $A' \in S$

   (ii) $A_i : i \in N \in S$ $\Rightarrow$ $\cup A_i \in S$

PROPERTIES

   (1) Every σ-algebra is a σ-ring but not conversely.

   (2) Every σ-algebra is closed for the formation of countable intersections.

      For: $A, B \in S$ $\Rightarrow$ $A', B' \in S$

                       $\Rightarrow$ $A' \cup B' \in S$

                       $\Rightarrow$ $(A \cap B)' \in S$

                       $\Rightarrow$ $A \cap B \in S$

   (3) Every σ-algebra is closed for the formation of differences.

      Let $A, B \in S$

      Now, $A - B = A \cap B' \in S$

   (4) $\phi \in S$, For $A - A \in S$ $\Rightarrow$ $\phi \in S$

☞ REMARK

- The class of sets defined above is called a completely additive class.

4.2.5 SEMI-RING

A family $\mathcal{A}$ of subsets of X is called a semi-ring if

(i) $\phi \in \mathcal{A}$

(ii) $A, B \in \mathcal{A} \quad \Rightarrow \quad A - B \in \mathcal{A}$

(iii) $A_i \in \mathcal{A}, A_i \cap A_j = \phi, i \neq j \quad \Rightarrow \quad \exists\, A \in \mathcal{A}$ such that $A = \bigcup_i A_i$

4.3 CLASSES

4.3.1 MONOTONE CLASS

A non-empty class of sets $\mathcal{A}$ is called a monotone class if for every monotonic sequence $<A_i>$ of sets in $\mathcal{A}$, we have $\lim A_n \in \mathcal{A}$.

4.3.2 ADDITIVE CLASS

Let X be the given space and $\mathcal{A}$ be a class of subsets of X. Then $\mathcal{A}$ is said to be finitely additive class of sets if

(i) $\phi \in \mathcal{A}$

(ii) $A, B \in \mathcal{A} \quad \Rightarrow \quad A - B \in \mathcal{A}, A \cup B \in \mathcal{A}.$

☞ REMARK

• Every ring of sets is finitely additive and vice-versa.

4.3.3 COMPLETELY ADDITIVE CLASS

Let X be the given space and $\mathcal{A}$ be the class of subsets of X. Then $\mathcal{A}$ is said to be completely additive class if

(i) $\phi \in \mathcal{A}$

(ii) $A \in \mathcal{A} \Rightarrow A' \in \mathcal{A}$

(iii) If $<A_n>$ is any sequence in $\mathcal{A}$ then $\bigcup_n A_n \in \mathcal{A}$.

☞ REMARK

• Every completely additive class is a σ-field or field and vice-versa.

4.3.4 SOME MORE DEFINITIONS

Let μ be an extended real valued set function on a σ-ring $\mathcal{A}$. Then

(1) μ is non-negative if $\mu(A) \geq 0 \ \forall \ A \in \mathcal{A}$

(2) μ is called additive if for all $A, B \in \mathcal{A}, A \cap B = \phi$

$\Rightarrow \qquad \mu(A \cup B) = \mu(A) + \mu(B)$

(3) μ is called finitely additive if

$A_i \in \mathcal{A}$, for $i = 1, 2, ..., n \ A_i \cap A_j = \phi, i \neq j$

$$\mu\left(\bigcup_{i=1}^{n} A_i\right) = \sum_{i=1}^{n} \mu(A_i)$$

(4) μ is called countably additive if $\mu\left(\bigcup_{i=1}^{\infty} A_i\right) = \sum_{i=1}^{\infty} \mu(A_i)$

(5) μ is called countably subadditive if $\mu\left[\bigcup_{i=1}^{\infty} A_i\right] \leq \sum_{i=1}^{\infty} \mu(A_i)$

(6) μ is called finitely subadditive if $\mu\left[\bigcup_{i=1}^{n} A_i\right] \leq \sum_{i=1}^{n} \mu(A_i)$

(7) μ is called regular if $A \in \mathcal{A}, \varepsilon > 0 \Rightarrow \exists\, G$ and F in $\mathcal{A}$ such that $\mu(G) - \varepsilon \leq \mu(A) \leq \mu(F) + \varepsilon$.

4.4 FUNCTIONS

4.4.1 SET FUNCTIONS

A function is said to be the set function if its domain consists of a family of sets.

4.4.2 REAL VALUED SET FUNCTIONS

A function is said to be real valued set function if its domain is a family of sets and its codomain is the set of real numbers R.

☛ REMARKS

- A real valued set function f is said to be finitely additive if $f\left(\bigcup_{r=1}^{n} A_r\right) = \bigcup_{r=1}^{n} f(A_r)$

- A real valued set function is said to be countably additive, if $f\left(\bigcup_{r=1}^{\infty} A_r\right) = \bigcup_{r=1}^{\infty} f(A_r)$

4.4.3 EXTENDED REAL VALUED SET FUNCTION

An extended real valued set function is a real valued set function which also takes either of the values $+\infty$ or $-\infty$.

4.4.4 COMPLETELY ADDITIVE SET FUNCTION

An extended real valued set function f is said to be completely additive set function if $f : \mathcal{A} \to [-\infty, \infty]$ such that

(i) $\mathcal{A}$ is completely additive class

(ii) $f(\phi) = 0$

(iii) There exists a sequence $<A_n>$ of disjoints sets in $\mathcal{A}$ such that

$$f\left(\bigcup_{i=1}^{\infty} A_i\right) = \bigcup_{i=1}^{\infty} f(A_i)$$

4.4.5 CONTINUOUS FUNCTION

A set function f defined on a ring A is said to be continuous from below if $<f(E_n)> \to f(E)$ where $<E_n>$ is a monotonically increasing sequence converging to E. Further, f is said to be continuous from above if $<f(E_n)> \to f(E)$ where $<E_n>$ is a monotonically decreasing sequence converging to E.

THEOREM 1.

A non-empty collection of sets is a B-ring if it is closed under the formation of intersection and symmetric difference.

PROOF. Let B be a non-empty collection of sets and $A, B \in B$

It is given that $A, B \in B \implies A \cap B \in B$ and $A \Delta B \in B$ ...(1)

We have to show that B is a B-ring.

Since, $A \in B, A \cap B \in B \implies A \Delta (A \cap B) \in B$ (By (1))

But by set theory, we have

$$A \Delta (A \cap B) = A - B$$

Therefore, $A - B \in B$

$\implies B$ is closed under the function of the difference of the sets.

Again by (1), we can say that

$$(A \cap B) \Delta (A \Delta B) \in B$$

But by set theory, we have

$$(A \cap B) \Delta (A \Delta B) = (A \cup B)$$

$\Rightarrow \qquad\qquad A \cup B \in B$

$\Rightarrow \quad B$ is closed under the formation of the unions.

Hence, B is a B-ring.

THEOREM 2.

A B-ring containing whole space X is an algebra.

PROOF.   Let B be a B-ring such that $X \in B$.

We have to prove that B is an algebra. For this it is sufficient to prove that for all $A \subset X, A' \in B$.

$\because \quad A, X \in B$ and B is a B-ring, therefore

$$A, X \in B \qquad \Rightarrow \qquad X - A \in B$$
$$\Rightarrow \qquad A' \in B$$

Hence B is an algebra.

THEOREM 3.

Intersection of two B-rings is a B-ring.

PROOF.   Let B_1 and B_2 be two B-rings. We have to prove that $B_1 \cap B_2$ is a B-ring.

Let $A, B \in B_1 \cap B_2$. Here, we shall prove that $A - B \in B_1 \cap B_2$ and $A \cup B \in B_1 \cap B_2$.

Now, $A, B \in B_1 \cap B_2 \qquad \Rightarrow \quad A, B \in B_1$ and $A, B \in B_2$

So, $A, B \in B_1$ and B_1 is a B-ring therefore, $A - B \in B_1$ and $A \cup B \in B_1$

Similarly, $A, B \in B_2$ and B_2 is a B-ring therefore $A - B \in B_2$ and $A \cup B \in B_2$

Finally, $A - B \in B_1$ and $A - B \in B_2 \quad \Rightarrow \quad A - B \in B_1 \cap B_2$ \qquad (By set theory)

and $A \cup B \in B_1$ and $A \cup B \in B_2 \quad \Rightarrow \quad A \cup B \in B_1 \cap B_2$ \qquad (By set theory)

Hence, $B_1 \cap B_2$ is a B-ring.

THEOREM 4.

Every algebra is a ring.

PROOF.   Let $\mathcal{A}$ be an algebra. We have to prove that $\mathcal{A}$ is a ring. For this we shall prove that for $A, B \in \mathcal{A}, A - B \in \mathcal{A}$ and $A \cup B \in \mathcal{A}$.

Since, $\mathcal{A}$ is an algebra, therefore, $A, B \in \mathcal{A} \quad \Rightarrow \quad A \cup B \in \mathcal{A}$

Now, $A, B \in \mathcal{A} \qquad \Rightarrow \qquad A', B \in \mathcal{A}$ \qquad ($\because \mathcal{A}$ is an algebra)

$\Rightarrow \qquad A' \cup B \in \mathcal{A}$ \qquad ($\because \mathcal{A}$ is an algebra)

$\Rightarrow \qquad (A' \cup B)' \in \mathcal{A}$ \qquad ($\because \mathcal{A}$ is an algebra)

$\Rightarrow \qquad A'' \cap B' \in \mathcal{A}$ \qquad (By Demorgan's law)

$\Rightarrow \qquad A \cap B' \in \mathcal{A}$ \qquad ($\because A'' = A$)

$\Rightarrow \qquad A - B \in \mathcal{A}$ \qquad ($\because A \cap B' = A - B$)

Hence, $\mathcal{A}$ is a ring.

THEOREM 5.

A monotone ring is a σ-ring.

PROOF.   Let $\mathcal{A}$ be a monotone ring and $A_i \in \mathcal{A}$

By definition of $\mathcal{A}$, $\mathcal{A}$ is closed under the formation of finite unions.

Therefore, $A_1, A_1 \cup A_2, \dots \overset{n}{\underset{i=1}{\cup}} A_i \in \mathcal{A}$.

Let us write $B = \overset{n}{\underset{i=1}{\cup}} A_i$

Then $B \in \mathcal{A}$

Further, since $<B_n>$ is an increasing sequence and $\overset{\infty}{\underset{n=1}{\cup}} B_n = \overset{\infty}{\underset{n=}{\cup}} A_n$.

Also, $\mathcal{A}$ is a monotone class, therefore $\lim B_n \in \mathcal{A}$

$$\Rightarrow \qquad \overset{\infty}{\underset{n=1}{\cup}} A_n \in \mathcal{A} \qquad\qquad \left(\because \lim B_n = \overset{\infty}{\underset{n=1}{\cup}} B_n = \overset{\infty}{\underset{n=1}{\cup}} A_n \right)$$

Hence, $\mathcal{A}$ is a σ-ring.

THEOREM 6.

A σ-field is monotone and monotonic field is a σ-field.

PROOF.   Let $\mathcal{A}$ be a σ-field and $<A_n>$ be a monotonic sequence in $\mathcal{A}$.

If $<A_n>$ is an increasing sequence then $\lim A_n = \overset{\infty}{\underset{n=1}{\cup}} A_n \in \mathcal{A}$ (By def. of σ-field)

$\Rightarrow$ $\mathcal{A}$ is a monotone class.

On the other hand, if $<A_n>$ is a decreasing sequence then

$$\lim_{n \to \infty} A_n = \overset{\infty}{\underset{n=1}{\cap}} A_n \in \mathcal{A} \qquad\qquad \text{(By def. of } \sigma\text{-field)}$$

$\Rightarrow$ $\mathcal{A}$ is a monotone class.

Conversely let M be a monotone field. We have to prove that M is a σ-field.

Let $<B_n>$ be a sequence in M such that

$$E_n = \underset{k \le n}{\cup} B_k, \text{ if } <B_n> \text{ is an increasing sequence.}$$

and $$F_n = \underset{k \le n}{\cap} B_k, \text{ if } <B_n> \text{ is a decreasing sequence.}$$

But since, M is a monotone class, therefore,

$$\lim E_n \in M$$

and $$\lim F_n \in M$$

Now, $$\overline{\lim} B_n = \underset{n \ge 1}{\cup} B_n = \underset{n}{\cup} \left[\underset{k \le n}{\cup} B_k \right] = \underset{n}{\cup} E_n = \lim E_n$$

$$\underline{\lim} B_n = \underset{n \ge 1}{\cap} B_n = \underset{n}{\cap} \left[\underset{k \le n}{\cap} B_k \right] = \underset{n}{\cap} E_n = \lim F_n$$

Thus, we conclude that

$$\overline{\lim} B_n, \underline{\lim} B_n \in M$$

$$\Rightarrow \qquad \overset{\infty}{\underset{n=1}{\cup}} B_n \in M, \overset{\infty}{\underset{n=1}{\cap}} B_n \in M$$

Hence, M is a σ-field.

THEOREM 7.

A monotonic ring is a σ-ring and a σ-ring is a monotone class.

PROOF.   Let $\mathcal{A}$ be a monotonic ring, and $A_1, A_2, \ldots$ be any subsets belonging to $\mathcal{A}$. Since,

$\mathcal{A}$ is a ring, therefore $\bigcup\limits_{i=1}^{n} A_i \in \mathcal{A}$

If $B_n = \bigcup\limits_{i=1}^{n} A_i$, then $B_n \in \mathcal{A}$. Also, $<B_n>$ is an increasing sequence and $\lim\limits_{n \to \infty} B_n = \bigcup\limits_{n=1}^{\infty} A_n$.

But $\mathcal{A}$ is a monotone class, therefore, $\lim B_n \in \mathcal{A}$.

$\Rightarrow \qquad\qquad \bigcup\limits_{n=1}^{\infty} A_n \in \mathcal{A}$

$\Rightarrow \quad \mathcal{A}$ is a σ-ring.

Conversely, let $\mathcal{A}$ be a σ-ring and let $<A_n>$ be a monotonic sequence in $\mathcal{A}$.

If $<A_n>$ is an increasing sequence then $\lim A_n = \bigcup\limits_{n=1}^{\infty} A_n$

Since, $\mathcal{A}$ is closed for countable unions. Therefore $\bigcup\limits_{n=1}^{\infty} A_n \in \mathcal{A}$.

$\Rightarrow \qquad\qquad \lim A_n \in \mathcal{A}$

$\Rightarrow \quad \mathcal{A}$ is a monotone class.

In a similar way, if $<A_n>$ is a decreasing sequence then

$$\lim\limits_{n \to \infty} A_n = \bigcap\limits_{n=1}^{\infty} A_n \in \mathcal{A}$$

$\Rightarrow \qquad\qquad \lim\limits_{n \to \infty} A_n \in \mathcal{A}$

Hence, $\mathcal{A}$ is a monotone class.

THEOREM 8.

A ring is closed under formation of symmetric difference and intersection.

PROOF.   We know that a family $\mathcal{A}$ of subsets of X is called a ring of sets if $A, B \in \mathcal{A} \Rightarrow A - B \in \mathcal{A}$
and $A \cup B \in \mathcal{A}$.

We have to prove that

(i) $A, B \in \mathcal{A} \qquad\Rightarrow\qquad A \cap B \in \mathcal{A}$

(ii) $A, B \in \mathcal{A} \qquad\Rightarrow\qquad A \Delta B \in \mathcal{A}$

(i) Let $A, B \in \mathcal{A}$

$\Rightarrow \qquad A - B \in \mathcal{A}$

Now, $A \in \mathcal{A}, A - B \in \mathcal{A}$ then $(A - (A - B)) \in \mathcal{A}$

$\Rightarrow \qquad A \cap B \in \mathcal{A} \qquad\qquad\qquad (\because A \cap B = A - (A - B))$

(ii) Let $A, B \in A \qquad\Rightarrow\qquad A - B \in \mathcal{A}$ and $B - A \in \mathcal{A}$

$\Rightarrow \qquad ((A - B) \cup (B - A)) \in \mathcal{A}$

$\Rightarrow \qquad\qquad A \Delta B \in \mathcal{A}$

THEOREM 9.

Let $\mathcal{A}$ be an algebra of subsets of X and $<A_n>$ be a sequence of sets in $\mathcal{A}$. Then there is a sequence
$<B_n>$ of sets in $\mathcal{A}$ such that $B_n \cap B_m = \phi$, $m \neq n$ and $\bigcup\limits_{i=1}^{\infty} B_i = \bigcup\limits_{i=1}^{\infty} A_i$.

PROOF.   Let $\mathcal{A}$ be an algebra of subsets of X. Then by definition

(i) $A, B \in \mathcal{A} \quad\Rightarrow\quad A \cup B \in \mathcal{A}$

(ii) $A \in \mathcal{A} \qquad\Rightarrow\quad A' \in \mathcal{A}$

Now, finally we shall prove that, $A, B \in \mathcal{A} \Rightarrow A - B \in \mathcal{A}$

$$\Rightarrow \quad A', B \in \mathcal{A}$$

$\Rightarrow$	$A' \cup B \in \mathcal{A}$	(By (i))
$\Rightarrow$	$(A' \cup B)' \in \mathcal{A}$	(By (ii))
$\Rightarrow$	$A \cap B' \in \mathcal{A}$	(By Demorgan's law)
$\Rightarrow$	$A - B \in \mathcal{A}$	$(\because A \cap B' = A - B)$

Further, suppose that $<A_n>$ be a sequence of sets in $\mathcal{A}$.

We have to prove that $\exists$ a sequence $<B_n>$ of sets in $\mathcal{A}$ such that $B_n \cap B_m = \phi$, $m \neq n$ and

$$\bigcup_{i=1}^{\infty} B_i = \bigcup_{i=1}^{\infty} A_i \ .$$

Now, for $A_i \in \mathcal{A}$, let us write $B_n = A_n - \bigcup_{i=1}^{n-1} A_i$

Then clearly, we have

$$B_1 = A_1, B_2 = A_2 - A_1, B_3 = A_3 - (A_1 \cup A_2) \dots \text{ etc.} \qquad \dots(1)$$

From (1) we observe that

(a) $\bigcup_{i=1}^{\infty} B_i = \bigcup_{i=1}^{\infty} A_i$

(b) $B_n \cap B_m = \phi$ for $n \neq m$

(c) $B_n \subset A_n \ \forall \ n$

By (i) we have $A_1 \cup A_2 \in \mathcal{A}$, $A_1 \cup A_2 \cup A_3 \in \mathcal{A}$, ... and so on.

In general $\bigcup_{i=1}^{n} A_i \in \mathcal{A}$

$$\Rightarrow \qquad B_n \in \mathcal{A}$$

$\Rightarrow \quad <B_n>$ is a sequence of sets in $\mathcal{A}$ with the property (i) and (ii).

4.5 IDEAL MEASURE FUNCTION

An extended real valued function μ defined on a σ-ring $\mathcal{A}$ of subset of a space X is said to be ideal measure function, if it satisfies the following properties:

(1) $\mu(A) \geq 0 \ \forall \ A \in \mathcal{A}$, In particular $\mu(\phi) = 0$

(2) μ is countably σ-additive, i.e.,

$$\mu\left[\bigcup_{n=1}^{\infty} A_r\right] = \sum_{r=1}^{\infty} \mu(A_r)$$

where $\{A_r : r \in N\}$ is a countable family of subsets of X such that $A_i \cap A_j = \phi$, $i \neq j$. In particular if $A \cap B = \phi$, $A, B \in \mathcal{A}$. Then $\mu(A \cup B) = \mu(A) + \mu(B)$

(3) μ is translation invariant, i.e., $\mu(A + x) = \mu(A) \ \forall \ x \in X$ where $A + x = \{a + x \ \forall \ a \in A\}$, $A \in \mathcal{A}$

If μ is a measure function defined on a σ-algebra $\mathcal{A}$ of subsets of a space X. Then triplet $(X, \mathcal{A}, \mu)$ is called measure space.

(4) $A, B \in \mathcal{A}$ such that $A \subset B$ then $\mu(A) \leq \mu(B)$.

(5) For an interval, I, $\mu(I) = l(I) = $ length of the interval I

☞ **REMARK**

• Ideal measure is a particular case of Lebesgue measure.

4.5.1 MEASURE FUNCTION

Let μ be a measure function on a σ-ring $\mathcal{A}$ of subsets X. Then

(1) μ is said to be complete if $B \in \mathcal{A}$ such that $m(B) = 0$, $A \subset B \Rightarrow A \in \mathcal{A}$
   i.e., if all the subsets of a set of measure zero are measurable.

(2) Any set $A \in \mathcal{A}$ is said to have finite measure if $\mu(A) < \infty$

(3) The measure of any set $A \in \mathcal{A}$ is said to be σ-finite i.e., $\exists$ a sequence $<A_n> \in R$ such that

   (i) $A \subset \overset{\infty}{\underset{n=1}{\cup}} A_n$

   (ii) $\mu(A_n) < \infty \,\, \forall \, n \in N$

(4) The measure function μ is called totally finite or totally σ-finite if

   (i) $X \in \mathcal{A}$

   (ii) $\mu(X)$ is finite

(5) A non-empty collection $\mathcal{A} = \{A_i\}$ of sets is said to have hereditary property if
   $$A_1 \subseteq A_2, A_2 \in \mathcal{A} \quad \Rightarrow \quad A_1 \in \mathcal{A}$$

THEOREM 1.

The ideal measure function μ is finitely additive.

PROOF. Let (X, A, μ) be a measure space. If $A_1, A_2, \dots A_n \in \mathcal{A}$ are pairwise disjoint and $\overset{n}{\underset{i=1}{\cup}} A_i \in X$. Then we have to prove that

$$\mu\left[\overset{n}{\underset{i=1}{\cup}} A_i \right] = \overset{n}{\underset{i=1}{\sum}} \mu(A_i)$$

Let us extend the sequence $<A_1, A_2, \dots, A_n>$ to $<A_n>$ upto ∞ such that $A_i = \phi$ for all $i > n$. Then using the prop. (2) of ideal measure, we have

$$\mu\left[\overset{n}{\underset{i=1}{\cup}} A_i \right] = \mu\left(\overset{\infty}{\underset{i=1}{\cup}} A_i \right) = \overset{\infty}{\underset{i=1}{\sum}} \mu(A_i) = \overset{n}{\underset{i=1}{\sum}} \mu(A_i) \quad (\because \mu(A_i) = 0 \,\, \forall \, i > n)$$

Hence, measure function μ is finitely additive.

THEOREM 2.

The ideal measure function μ is monotonic.

PROOF. Let $(X, \mathcal{A}, \mu)$ be an ideal measure space.
And $A, B \in \mathcal{A}$ such that $A \subseteq B$. We have to prove that
$$m(A) \le m(B)$$
Since A and $B - A$ are disjoint, i.e., $A \cap (B - A) = \phi$ and $B = A \cup (B - A)$
Then by finitely additive property of μ
$$\mu(B) = \mu(A \cup (B - A)) = \mu(A) + \mu(B - A) \qquad \dots(1)$$
Since, $\mu(B - A) \ge 0$. Therefore, from (1)
$$\mu(B) \ge \mu(A)$$
Hence, μ is monotonic.

4.6 CARATHEODORY'S POSTULATES FOR OUTER MEASURE

Let $\mathcal{A}$ be a σ-ring of the subsets A_i. Then extended real valued set function m_0 having the following properties:

(1) $m_0(A_r) \ge 0$ and $m_0(A_r) = 0$ if $A_r = \phi$

(2) $A_r \subset A_s \Rightarrow m_0(A_r) \le m_0(A_s)$

(3) $m_0\left(\bigcup_{r \in N} A_r\right) \le \sum_{r \in N} m_0(A_r)$, i.e., m_0 is σ-subadditive.

(4) $m_0(A_r \cup A_s) = m_0(A_r) + m_0(A_s)$, provided $A_r \cap A_s = \phi$.

These properties are called Caratheodory's postulates for outer measure.

4.6.1 MEASURABLE SET

Let m_0 be an outer measure function defined on a σ-ring $\mathcal{A} = \{A_i : i \in N\}$ then any member $A \in \mathcal{A}$ is said to be measurable (outer measurable) if

$$m_0(E) = m_0(A \cap E) + m_0(A' \cap E) \ \forall \ E \subseteq \mathcal{A}$$

 Recapitulations

✦ If E is countable then $m_0(E) = 0$

✦ Any set with outer measure different from zero is uncountable.

✦ The outer measure of an interval is equal to its length.

✦ For any subsets $A, B \in \mathcal{A}$,
$$m_0(A \cup B) \le m_0(A) + m_0(B)$$

THEOREM 1.

A set A is measurable iff A′ is measurable.

PROOF. A is measurable

$\Leftrightarrow$ $\exists \ E \subseteq R$ such that

$$m_0(E) = m_0(A \cap E) + m_0(A' \cap E)$$

$\Leftrightarrow$ $m_0(E) = m_0((A')' \cap E) + m_0(A' \cap E)$

$\Leftrightarrow$ A' is measurable.

THEOREM 2.

The union of two outer measurable sets is also outer measurable.

[MEERUT–2003, 04, 05, 07, 08, 14, 16, ROHTAK–2006, GARHWAL–1996, 2006, DELHI–2012, RAJASTHAN–2013]

PROOF.   Let A and B be two outer measurable sets. We have to prove that $A \cup B$ is also outer measurable.

Since, A is outer measurable therefore by definition for any set $E \subseteq R$ we have

$$m_0(E) = m_0(A \cap E) + m_0(A' \cap E) \qquad \qquad ...(1)$$

Similarly, for measurable set B, $\exists \ F \le R$ such that

$$m_0(F) = m_0(B \cap F) + m_0(B' \cap F) \qquad \qquad ...(2)$$

In particular, let us take $F = E \cap A'$ then from (2)

$$m_0(E \cap A') = m_0(E \cap A' \cap B) + m_0(E \cap A' \cap B')$$

$\Rightarrow$ $m_0(E \cap A') = m_0(E \cap A' \cap B) + m_0(E \cap (A \cup B)')$ (By Demorgan's law)

$$...(3)$$

Similarly for $E = E \cap (A \cup B)$, equation (1) becomes

$$m_0(E \cap (A \cup B)) = m_0[A \cap E \cap (A \cup B)] + m_0[A' \cap E \cap (A \cup B)]$$

$\Rightarrow$ $m_0(E \cap (A \cup B)) = m_0(A \cap E) + m_0(E \cap A' \cap B)$ $\qquad ...(4)$

$$(\because (A \cup B) \cap A = A$$
$$\text{and } (A \cup B) \cap A' = (A \cap A') \cup (B \cap A')$$
$$= \phi \cup (B \cap A') = B \cap A' = A' \cap B)$$

From (3)

$$m_0(E \cap A' \cap B) = m_0(E \cap A') - m_0(E \cap (A \cup B)')$$

Using this value in (4) we get

$$m_0[E \cap (A \cup B)] = m_0(A \cap E) + m_0(E \cap A') - m_0(E \cap (A \cup B)')$$

$$\Rightarrow \quad m_0(E \cap (A \cup B)) + m_0(E \cap (A \cap B)')$$
$$= m_0(A \cap E) + m_0(A' \cap E) = m_0(E) \qquad \text{(Using (1))}$$
$$\Rightarrow \quad (A \cup B) \text{ is measurable.}$$

Hence, union of two outer measurable sets is again outer measurable.

☞ REMARK

- The above theorem can be extended up to the union of a finite number of measurable sets, i.e.,

if $A_1, A_2, ..., A_n$ are outer measurable sets then $\bigcup\limits_{r=1}^{n} A_r$ is also measurable.

THEOREM 3.

If the outer measure of a set is zero, then set is outer measurable.

[MEERUT–2004, 07, 09, 11, KUMAUN–2014, DELHI–2008, BANGLORE–2010]

PROOF. Let A be the given set such that $m_0(A) = 0$. We have to prove that A is measurable. For this it is sufficient to prove that for any set $E \subseteq R$

$$m_0(E) \geq m_0(E \cap A) + m_0(E \cap A')$$

By set theory, we know that

$$E \cap A' \subseteq E$$
$$\Rightarrow \quad m_0(E \cap A') \leq m_0(E) \qquad \qquad ...(1)$$
Further, since $\quad E \cap A < A$
$$\Rightarrow \quad m_0(E \cap A) \leq m_0(A)$$
$$\Rightarrow \quad m_0(E \cap A) \leq 0 \qquad \qquad (\because m_0(A) = 0 \text{ (given)})$$
But we have $m_0(E \cap A) \geq 0$
Thus $m_0(E \cap A) = 0 \qquad \qquad ...(2)$
Equation (1) can be written as
$$m_0(E) \geq m_0(E \cap A') + 0$$
$$= m_0(E \cap A') + m_0(E \cap A) \qquad \text{(Using (2))}$$
$$\Rightarrow \quad m_0(E) \geq m_0(E \cap A) + m_0(E \cap A')$$

Hence A is outer measurable.

THEOREM 4.

Let A be an outermeasurable set and B be any set then

$$m_0(A \cup B) + m_0(A \cap B) = m_0(A) + m_0(B)$$

[NAGPUR–2006, ASSAM–2008, MEERUT–2004, 06, 13, 14, KANPUR–2003]

PROOF. Let A be an outer measurable set and B be any set.
If $m_0(B) = \infty$ then result is obvious.
So, let us take $m_0(B)$ is finite.
Since, A is measurable, therefore, for any set $E \subseteq R$, we have
$$m_0(E) = m_0(E \cap A) + m_0(E \cap A') \qquad \qquad ...(1)$$
In particular, let us take $E = A \cup B$
Then (1) reduces to
$$m_0(A \cup B) = m_0[(A \cup B) \cap A] + m_0[(A \cup B) \cap A']$$
$$= m_0(A) + m_0(B \cap A') \qquad \qquad ...(2)$$
$$(\because (A \cup B) \cap A = A$$
$$\text{and } (A \cup B) \cap A' = (A \cap A') \cup (A' \cap B)$$
$$= \phi \cup (A' \cap B) = A' \cap B)$$

If we take $E = B$ in (1) then we get

$$m_0(B) = m_0(A \cap B) + m_0(A' \cap B)$$
$$\Rightarrow \quad m_0(A' \cap B) = m_0(B) - m_0(A \cap B)$$

Putting this value in (2) we get

$$m_0(A \cup B) = m_0(A) + m_0(B) - m_0(A \cap B)$$
$$\Rightarrow \quad m_0(A \cup B) + m_0(A \cap B) = m_0(A) + m_0(B)$$

☞ REMARK

- The above result is also holds good if B is also outer measurable. If A and B both are outer measurable then

$$m_0(A \cup B) = m_0(A) + m_0(B)$$

THEOREM 5.

If A and B are two disjoint measurable set then
$$m_0(A \cup B) = m_0(A) + m_0(B)$$

PROOF. Let A and B are two disjoint measurable sets.

Then using previous theorem

$$m_0(A \cup B) + m_0(A \cap B) = m_0(A) + m_0(B) \qquad \text{(give proof)} \qquad ...(1)$$

Since, A and B are disjoint (given)

$$\Rightarrow \qquad A \cap B = \phi$$
$$\Rightarrow \qquad m_0(A \cap B) = m_0(\phi) = 0$$

Using this value in the above equation (1), we get

$$m_0(A \cup B) + 0 = m_0(A) + m_0(B)$$
$$\Rightarrow \qquad m_0(A \cup B) = m_0(A) + m_0(B)$$

☞ REMARK

- The above result can be extended up to a finite number of sets, *i.e.,*

$$m_0\left[\bigcup_{i=1}^{n} A_i\right] = \sum_{i=1}^{n} m_0(A_i)$$

such that each A_i is pairwise disjoint, *i.e.,* $A_i \cap A_j = \phi$, $i \neq j$

THEOREM 6.

If $<A_i>$ is a sequence of pairwise disjoint measurable subsets of $\mathbf{R}$, then

$$m_0\left[\bigcup_{r=1}^{\infty} A_r\right] = \sum_{i=1}^{\infty} m_0(A_r)$$

PROOF. Let $<A_i>$ be a sequence of pairwise disjoint measurable subsets of R. We have to prove that

$$m_0\left[\bigcup_{r=1}^{\infty} A_r\right] = \sum_{i=1}^{\infty} m_0(A_r)$$

We know that $\quad \bigcup_{r=1}^{n} A_r \subseteq \bigcup_{r=1}^{\infty} A_r$

$$\Rightarrow \qquad m_0\left(\bigcup_{r=1}^{n} A_r\right) \leq m_0\left(\bigcup_{r=1}^{\infty} A_r\right)$$

$$\Rightarrow \qquad \sum_{r=1}^{n} m_0(A_r) \leq m_0\left(\bigcup_{r=1}^{\infty} A_r\right) \qquad \text{(Using above remark)}$$

Letting $n \to \infty$ we get

$$\sum_{r=1}^{\infty} m_0(A_r) \le m_0 \left(\bigcup_{r=1}^{\infty} A_r \right) \qquad \qquad \dots(1)$$

Now, by countable σ-subadditive property of m_0, we have

$$m_0 \left[\bigcup_{r=1}^{\infty} A_r \right] \le \sum_{i=1}^{\infty} m_0(A_r) \qquad \qquad \dots(2)$$

From (1) and (2) we conclude that

$$m_0 \left[\bigcup_{r=1}^{\infty} A_r \right] = \sum_{i=1}^{\infty} m_0(A_r)$$

THEOREM 7.

Let A and B be two outer measurable subsets of R such that $A \subseteq B$ then $m_0(A) \le m_0(B)$, i.e., m_0 is monotonic.

PROOF.   It is given that $A \subseteq B$

$\therefore$ By set theory, we can write

$$B = (B - A) \cup A \text{ such that } (B - A) \cap A = \phi$$

$\Rightarrow \qquad m_0(B) = m_0(B - A) + m_0(A)$

$\Rightarrow \qquad m_0(B) \ge m_0(A) \qquad \qquad (\because m_0(B - A) \ge 0)$

Hence, we conclude that if $A \subseteq B$ then $m_0(A) \le m_0(B)$.

☛ REMARK

• If $A \subset B \subset C \subset D$ ... Then $m_0(A) \le m_0(B) \le m_0(C) \le m_0(D) \le \dots$

THEOREM 8.

Let T be a subset of the set of real numbers such that $0 < m_0(T) < \infty$ and if $\mu(A) = m_0(A \cap T)$ $\forall A \subseteq R$. Then μ is also outer measurable.

PROOF.   Let $A, B \le R$ be arbitrary and $T \subseteq R$ is fixed such that

$$m_0(T) < \infty$$

Let us define $m(A) = m_0(A \cap T) \forall A \subseteq R$

We have to prove that μ is an outer measure.

(I) $\mu(A) \ge 0$

Since, $\mu(A) = m_0(A \cap T)$ and $m_0(A \cap T) \ge 0$

$\Rightarrow \quad \mu(A) \ge 0$

Also if $A = \phi$. Then $m_0(\phi \cap T) = m_0(\phi) = 0$

$\Rightarrow \quad \mu(A) = 0$ if $A = \phi$

(II) If $A \subseteq B$ then $\mu(A) \le \mu(B)$

If $A \subseteq B \qquad \Rightarrow \qquad A \cap T \subseteq B \cap T$

$\qquad \qquad \Rightarrow \qquad m_0(A \cap T) \le m_0(B \cap T)$

$\qquad \qquad \Rightarrow \qquad \mu(A) \le \mu(B)$

(III) If $A \cap B = \phi$ then $\mu(A \cup B) = \mu(A) + \mu(B)$

If $A \cap B = \phi$ then $(A \cap T) \cap (B \cap T) = \phi$

$\Rightarrow \quad m_0[(A \cap T) \cup (B \cap T)] = m_0(A \cap T) + m_0(B \cap T)$

$\Rightarrow \quad \mu(A \cup B) = \mu(A) + \mu(B)$

(IV) $\mu\left[\bigcup_n A_n\right] \leq \sum_n \mu(A_n)$

Consider $\mu\left[\bigcup_n A_n\right] = m_0\left[\mu\left(\bigcup_n A_n\right) \cap T\right] = m_0[\cup(A_n \cap T)]$

$$\leq \sum_n m_0(A_n \cap T) = \sum_n \mu(A_n)$$

$\Rightarrow \qquad \mu\left(\bigcup_n A_n\right) \leq \sum_n \mu(A_n)$

Hence, from (I), (II), (III) and (IV) we conclude that μ is an outer measure.

THEOREM 9.

Let $<A_n>$ be a monotonically increasing (or decreasing) sequence of outer measurable sets then

$$m_0(A) = \lim_{r \to \infty} m_0(A_r), \text{ where } A = \bigcup_{r=1}^{\infty} A_r$$

[MEERUT–2001, 14, KURUKSHETRA–2008, DELHI–2009]

PROOF. Let $<A_n>$ be a monotonically increasing sequence of outer measurable sets.
If $m_0(A_i) = \infty$, the result is hold good automatically.
So, suppose that $m_0(A_i) < \infty$
Since, $<A_n>$ is monotonically increasing therefore, we can write

$$A_1 \subseteq A_2 \subseteq A_3 \subseteq \dots$$

We can write $A = A_1 \cup (A_2 - A_1) \cup (A_3 - A_2) \cup \dots$
such that

$$(A_2 - A_1) \cap A_1 = \phi$$
$$(A_3 - A_2) \cap (A_2 - A_1) = \phi \dots \text{etc}$$

Since, we already prove that

$$m_0\left(\bigcup_{r=1}^{\infty} A_r\right) = \sum_{r=1}^{\infty} m_0(A_r)$$

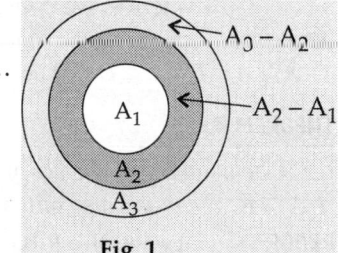

Fig. 1

Therefore

$$m_0\left[\bigcup_{r=1}^{\infty} A_r\right] = m_0(A_1) + m_0(A_2 - A_1) + m_0(A_3 - A_2) + \dots$$

$$= \lim_{r \to \infty}\left[m_0(A_1) + \sum_{i=1}^{r-1} m_0(A_{i+1} - A_i)\right] \qquad \dots(1)$$

$$= \lim_{r \to \infty}\left[m_0(A_1) + \sum_{i=1}^{r-1}[m_0(A_{i+1}) - m_0(A_i)]\right]$$

$$= \lim_{r \to \infty}[m_0(A_1) + \{-m_0(A_1) + m_0(A_r)\}]$$

$$= \lim_{r \to \infty} m_0(A_r)$$

Hence, $\qquad m_0\left(\bigcup_{r=1}^{\infty} A_r\right) = \lim_{r \to \infty} m_0(A_r)$

THEOREM 10.

Let X be a space of at least two points and $x_0 \in X$. For each $A \subset X$, we define

$$\mu(A) = \begin{cases} 0 & \text{if} \quad x_0 \notin A \\ 1 & \text{if} \quad x_0 \in A \end{cases}$$

Then μ is an outer measure. [KANPUR–2010]

PROOF. Let us suppose that $A, B \subseteq X$. Define

$$\mu(A) = \begin{cases} 0 & \text{if} \quad x_0 \notin A \\ 1 & \text{if} \quad x_0 \in A \end{cases} \qquad \text{...(1)}$$

(I) $\mu(A) \geq 0$: By definition of μ, it is clear that

$$\mu(A) \geq 0$$

(II) $\mu(\phi) = 0$ $\because x_0 \notin \phi$. Therefore $\mu(\phi) = 0$ (By (1))

(III) $A \subseteq B \Rightarrow \mu(A) \leq \mu(B)$:

Let $A \subseteq B$ then following possibilities will occur

(1) $x_0 \in B$ if $x_0 \in A$, $x_0 \in B$ if $x_0 \notin A$

and (2) $x_0 \notin B$ if $x_0 \notin A$

If $x_0 \in B$ then $\mu(B) = 0 = \mu(A)$ $(\because x_0 \in A)$

If $x_0 \in B$ and $x_0 \notin A$ then $\mu(B) = 1$ and $\mu(A) = 0$

In both the cases $\mu(A) \leq \mu(B)$

Now, if $x_0 \notin B$ if $x_0 \notin A$

Then $\mu(B) = \mu(A) = 0$

$\Rightarrow \mu(A) \leq \mu(B)$

(IV) $\mu(A \cup B) = \mu(A) + \mu(B)$ if $A \cap B = \phi$:

There are two possibilites, i.e., $x_0 \in A \cup B$ or $x_0 \notin A \cup B$

If $x_0 \notin A \cup B$ then $x_0 \notin A$ and $x_0 \notin B$

$$\mu(A \cup B) = 0, \mu(A) = 0 \ \mu(B) = 0$$

$\Rightarrow \mu(A \cup B) = \mu(A) + m(B)$

If $x_0 \in A \cup B$ then $x_0 \in A$ and $x_0 \notin B$ or $x_0 \in B$ and $x_0 \notin A$ $(\because A \cap B = \phi)$

$\Rightarrow \mu(A \cup B) = 1$

$\Rightarrow \mu(A) = 1, \mu(B) = 0$ or, $\mu(B) = 1, \mu(A) = 0$

In each situations

$$\mu(A \cup B) = \mu(A) + \mu(B)$$

(V) $\mu\left[\bigcup_n A_n\right] \leq \sum_n \mu(A_n)$ where $A_n \subseteq X$:

We have $x_0 \notin \cup A_n$ or $x_0 \in \cup A_n$

If $x_0 \notin \cup A_n$ then $x_0 \notin A_n \ \forall \ n$

$\Rightarrow \mu[\cup A_n] = 0$ and $\mu(A_n) = 0 \ \forall \ n$

$\Rightarrow \mu[\cup A_n] = \sum \mu(A_n)$ $[\because \mu(\cup A_n) = 0 + 0 + \ldots = 0]$

Now, if $x_0 \in \cup A_n$ then $x_0 \in A_{n_0}$ for at least one value of n_0 of n.

$\Rightarrow \mu(A_{n_0}) = 1$ or $\mu(A_n) = 1 \ \forall \ n$

Therefore, if $\mu[\cup A_n] = 1$

Then $$\sum_{n=0}^{\infty} \mu(A_n) = 0+1+0+...+0 = 1 \left.\right]$$

...(1)

$$\sum_{n=1}^{\infty} \mu(A_n) = 1+1+1+...+1 = \infty \left.\right]$$

which implies $\mu(\cup A_n) = \Sigma\mu(A_n) = 1$ or $\mu(\cup A_n) < \Sigma\mu(A_n)$ (From (1))

$\Rightarrow \qquad \mu(\cup A_n) \leq \Sigma\mu(A_n)$

Finally from (I), (II), (III) and (IV) μ is an outer measure function.

THEOREM 11.

Let $<A_n>$ be a monotonically decreasing sequence of outer measurable sets such that $m_0(A_n) < \infty$ for at least one n then

$$m_0\left(\bigcap_{n=1}^{\infty} A_n\right) = \lim_{n\to\infty} m_0(A_n)$$

[MEERUT–2001, 09]

PROOF. Let $<A_n>$ be a monotonically decreasing sequence of outer measurable sets such that $m_0(A_k) < \infty$ (*i.e.*, for $n = k$)

Then we have to show that

$$m_0\left(\bigcap_{n=1}^{\infty} A_n\right) = \lim_{n\to\infty} m_0(A_n)$$

Since, $<A_n>$ is monotonically decreasing sequence of outer measurable sets, *i.e.*,

$$A_1 \supseteq A_2 \supseteq A_3 \supseteq A_4 \supseteq ... \supseteq A_K \supseteq A_{K+1} \supseteq ...$$

We have $m_0(A_r) < \infty \; \forall \; r > k$

$\Rightarrow \qquad \lim_{n\to\infty} m_0(A_n) < \infty$

Let us write $A_k = E \cup (A_k - A_{k+1}) \cup (A_{k+1} - A_{k+2}) \cup ...$

where $E = \bigcap_{n=1}^{\infty} A_n$ and $(A_k - A_{k+1}) \cap (A_{k+1} - A_{k+2}) = \phi$ ... etc

Therefore, we can say that A_k is the union of pairwise disjoint outer measurable sets. Then by theorem-9

$$m_0(A_k) = m_0(E) + \sum_{r=k}^{\infty} m_0(A_r - A_{r+1})$$

$$= m_0(E) + \lim_{h\to\infty} \sum_{r=k}^{h} m_0(A_r - A_{r+1})$$

$$= m_0(E) + \lim_{h\to\infty} \sum_{r=k}^{h} [m_0(A_r) - m_0(A_{r+1})]$$

$$= m_0(E) + \lim_{h\to\infty} \sum_{r=k}^{h} [m_0(A_r) - m_0(A_{r+1})]$$

$\Rightarrow \; m_0(A_k) = m_0(E) + m_0(A_k) - \lim_{h\to\infty} m_0(A_{h+1})$

$\Rightarrow \quad m_0(E) = \lim_{h\to\infty} m_0(A_{h+1})$

$\Rightarrow \; m_0\left(\bigcap_{n=1}^{\infty} A_n\right) = \lim_{n\to\infty} m_0(A_n)$

☛ REMARK
- If we take $m_0(A_n) = \infty \ \forall \ n$. Then above theorem does not hold.

THEOREM 12.

Let $<A_n>$ is a sequence of outer measurable sets then

$$m_0[\underline{\lim} A_n] \le \underline{\lim} m_0(A_n)$$

PROOF.　　Let $<A_n>$ be a sequence of outer measurable sets. Let us write

$$B_n = \bigcup_{k=n}^{\infty} A_k$$

Then $<B_n>$ is monotonically increasing sequence. Then by Theorem-9

$$m_0\left[\bigcup_{n=1}^{\infty} B_n\right] = \lim_{n\to\infty} m_0(B_n)$$

By definition of limit inferior, we have

$$\underline{\lim} A_n = \bigcup_{n=1}^{\infty}\left(\bigcap_{k=n}^{\infty} A_k\right) = \bigcup_{n=1}^{\infty} (B_n)$$

Therefore, $m_0[\underline{\lim} A_n] = \lim_{n\to\infty} m_0(B_n)$ 　　　　　...(1)

Further, we can write

$$B_n \subseteq A_{n+r} \ \forall \ n$$

Therefore, $m_0(B_n) \le m_0(A_{n+r}) \ \forall \ r = 1, 2, 3, \ldots$

$\Rightarrow \qquad m_0(B_n) \le \underline{\lim_{r\to\infty}} m_0(A_{n+r})$

$\Rightarrow \qquad m_0(B_n) \le \underline{\lim_{r\to\infty}} m_0(A_n)$

Letting $n \to \infty$, we get

$$\lim_{n\to\infty} m_0(B_n) \le \underline{\lim_{r\to\infty}} m_0(A_r) \qquad\qquad ...(2)$$

☛ REMARKS
- In the above theorem, if we take $m_0[A_k \cup A_{k+1} \cup \ldots] < \infty$ for at least k, then by the same procedure we can prove that

$$m_0[\overline{\lim} A_n] \le \overline{\lim} m_0(A_n)$$

- If $<A_n>$ is a convergent sequence of outer measurable sets, then $m_0[\lim A_n] = \lim[m_0(A_n)]$ if $m_0(A_K) < \infty$ for at least one.

THEOREM 13.

If $<E_i>$ is a sequence of pairwise disjoint outer measurable sets then for any set A

$$m_0(A \cap E) = \sum_{i=1}^{\infty} m_0(A \cap E_i), E = \bigcup_{i=1}^{\infty} E_i$$

[MEERUT–2003, DELHI–2002, BANGLORE–2007]

PROOF.　　For any set A, let us write

$$A \cap E = A \cap \left[\bigcup_{i=1}^{\infty} E_i\right] = \bigcup_{i=1}^{\infty} (A \cap E_i)$$

which implies that

$$m_0[A \cap E] \le \sum_{i=1}^{\infty} m_0(A \cap E_i)$$

$$\Rightarrow \qquad m_0\left[A \cap \left(\bigcup_{r=1}^{n} E_r\right)\right] = \sum_{r=1}^{n} m_0(A \cap E_r) \qquad \text{(By induction)}$$

Further, $\qquad A \cap E = \bigcup_{i=1}^{\infty}(A \cap E_i) \supseteq \bigcup_{i=1}^{n}(A \cap E_i)$

$$\Rightarrow \qquad m_0(A \cap E) \geq m_0\left[\bigcup_{i=1}^{n}(A \cap E_i)\right] \qquad (\because m_0 \text{ is } \sigma\text{-subadditive})$$

But since $E_i \cap E_j = \phi$, therefore, $(A \cap E_i) \cap (A \cap E_j) = \phi$

Therefore, $\qquad m_0(A \cap E) \geq \sum_{i=1}^{n} m_0(A \cap E_i)$

$$\Rightarrow \qquad m_0(A \cap E) \geq \sum_{i=1}^{\infty} m_0(A \cap E_i) \qquad \text{(By letting n} \to \infty)$$
$$\dots (2)$$

Finally, from (1) and (2) we conclude that

$$m_0(A \cap E) = \sum_{i=1}^{\infty} m_0(A \cap E_i) \text{ where } E = \bigcup_{i=1}^{\infty} E_i$$

THEOREM 14.

Let $\mathcal{A}$ be an algebra of subsets of a space X and let $<E_n>$ be a sequence of sets in $\mathcal{A}$, then there exists a sequence $<B_n>$ of pairwise disjoint sets in $\mathcal{A}$ such that

$$\bigcup_{n=1}^{\infty} B_n = \bigcup_{n=1}^{\infty} E_n \qquad \text{[GARHWAL–2006, HPU–2008, MEERUT–2009, RANCHI–2015]}$$

PROOF. Define a sequence $<B_n>$ such that

$$B_n = E_n - \bigcup_{i=1}^{n-1} E_i$$

$\Rightarrow \quad B_1 = E_1, B_2 = E_2 - E_1, B_3 = E_3 - (E_1 \cup E_2) \dots$

Then clearly

(1) $B_n \subseteq E_n \ \forall \ n \in N$

(2) $B_n \in \mathcal{A}$, because $\mathcal{A}$ is closed under the formation of compliments and finite intersections

(3) $B_n \cap B_m = \phi$ for $n \neq m$, because

$$B_m \cap B_n = B_m \cap \left[E_n - \bigcup_{i=1}^{n-1} E_i\right] = B_m \cap \left[E_n \cap \left(\bigcup_{i=1}^{n-1} E_i\right)'\right]$$

(By Demorgan's law)

$$= B_m \cap [E_n \cap E_n' \cap \dots \cap E_m' \cap \dots \cap E_{n-1}']$$
$$= (B_m \cap E_m') \cap E_n \cap E_n' \cap \dots \cap E_{n-1}'$$
$$= \phi \cap E_n \cap E_n' \cap \dots \cap E_n^{-1} \qquad (\because B_m \subseteq E_m \Rightarrow B_m \not\subseteq E_m'$$
$$= \phi \qquad\qquad\qquad\qquad \Rightarrow B_m \cap E_m' = \phi)$$

(4) $B_n \subseteq E_n \ \forall \ n$

$$\Rightarrow \qquad \bigcup_{n=1}^{\infty} B_n \subseteq \bigcup_{n=1}^{\infty} E_n$$

Because, if $y \in \bigcup\limits_{n=1}^{\infty} E_n$

$\Rightarrow \quad y \in E_n$ for at least one n.

Suppose $n = k$ be the least value of n such that $y \in E_n$. Then $y \in E_i$ for $i = 1, 2, \ldots, k-1$ and

$$y \in E_k \qquad \Rightarrow \quad y \in B_k$$

$$\Rightarrow \quad y \in \bigcup\limits_{n=1}^{\infty} B_k$$

$$\Rightarrow \quad \bigcup\limits_{n=1}^{\infty} E_n \subseteq \bigcup\limits_{n=1}^{\infty} B_k \qquad \text{(Since } y \text{ is arbitrary)}$$

Also, $B_m \subseteq E_n \qquad \Rightarrow \quad \bigcup\limits_{n=1}^{\infty} B_n \subseteq \bigcup\limits_{n=1}^{\infty} E_n$

Thus, we conclude that

$$\bigcup\limits_{n=1}^{\infty} E_n = \bigcup\limits_{n=1}^{\infty} B_n$$

THEOREM 15.

A σ-additive set function is a continuous set function.

PROOF. Let $\mathcal{A}$ be a σ-additive class and μ be a σ-additive function defined on $\mathcal{A}$. We have to prove that μ is continuous.

Let us first suppose that $<E_n>$ be an increasing sequence in $\mathcal{A}$.

Then $\qquad\qquad \bigcup\limits_{n=1}^{\infty} E_n \in \mathcal{A}$

Define a new sequence $<B_n>$ such that

$$B_1 = E_1, B_n = E_n - E_{n-1} \text{ for } n > 1$$

Then for $n \neq m$, $B_n \cap B_m = \phi$ and $\bigcup\limits_{n=1}^{\infty} B_n = \bigcup\limits_{n=1}^{\infty} E_n$

Also, $\qquad E_r \subseteq \bigcup\limits_{n=1}^{r} B_n \qquad \Rightarrow \quad \mu(E_r) = \sum\limits_{n=1}^{r} \mu(B_n)$

$$\Rightarrow \qquad \mu\left[\bigcup\limits_{n=1}^{\infty} E_n \right] = \mu\left[\bigcup\limits_{n=1}^{\infty} B_n \right] = \sum\limits_{n=1}^{\infty} \mu(B_n) = \lim\limits_{r \to \infty} \sum\limits_{n=1}^{r} \mu(B_n)$$

$$= \lim\limits_{r \to \infty} \mu(E_r) \qquad \qquad \ldots(1)$$

Since, $<E_n>$ is an increasing sequence, so $E_1 \subset E_2 \subset E_3 \subset \ldots E_r \subset \ldots$

Therefore, $\qquad\qquad \bigcup\limits_{n=1}^{r} E_n = E_r$

$$\Rightarrow \qquad \lim\limits_{r \to \infty} \bigcup\limits_{n=1}^{r} E_r = \lim\limits_{r \to \infty} E_r$$

$$\Rightarrow \qquad \lim\limits_{r \to \infty} E_r = \lim\limits_{r \to \infty} \bigcup\limits_{n=1}^{r} E_r = \bigcup\limits_{n=1}^{\infty} E_r$$

Put this value in (1) we get

$$\mu\left[\lim\limits_{r \to \infty} E_r \right] = \lim\limits_{r \to \infty} \mu(E_r)$$

Thus, if $<E_n> \to E$ then $\lim_{r\to\infty} \mu(E_r) = \mu(E)$

Hence, μ is a continuous function from below.

In a similar manner, if $<E_n>$ is a decreasing sequence, we can show that μ is a continuous function from above.

Hence, μ is a continuous function.

THEOREM 16.

The class of m_0-measurable sets is a σ-algebra.

PROOF.   Let $\mathcal{A}$ be the class of m_0-measurable sets.

We have to prove that $\mathcal{A}$ is σ-algebra.

For this we shall prove that

  (i) $A \in \mathcal{A}$ then $A' \in \mathcal{A}$

  (ii) $\overset{\infty}{\underset{i=1}{\cup}} E_i \in \mathcal{A}$ when each $E_i \in \mathcal{A}$

Let us define a sequence $<B_n>$ of sets of $\mathcal{A}$ such that

$$B_n = \overset{n}{\underset{i=1}{\cup}} E_i$$

Since, each E_i is outer measurable, so B_n is also outer measurable.

Then for any set A

$$m_0(A) = m_0(B_n \cap A) + m_0(B'_n \cap A) \qquad \ldots(1)$$

Also, if $B_n = \overset{\omega}{\underset{i=1}{\cup}} E_i$ then clearly $B \supseteq B_n$

$\Rightarrow$ $B'_n \supseteq B'$

$\Rightarrow$ $B' \subseteq B'_n$

$\Rightarrow$ $A \cap B' \le A \cap B'_n$

$\Rightarrow$ $m_0(A \cap B') \le m_0(A \cap B'_n)$

Then from (1)

$$m_0(A) \ge m_0(A \cap B_n) + m_0(A \cap B') \qquad \ldots(2)$$

Also, since E_n is outer measurable, therefore,

$$m_0(A) = m_0(A \cap E_n) + m_0(A \cap E'_n)$$

$\Rightarrow$ $m_0(A \cap B_n) = m_0(A \cap B_n \cap E_n) + m_0(A \cap B_n \cap E'_n)$

We have $B_n = \overset{n}{\underset{i=1}{\cup}} E_i \supset E_n$

$\Rightarrow$ $B_n \cap E_n = E_n$

and $B_n \cap E'_n = B_{n-1}$

Therefore, $m_0(A \cap B_n) = m_0(A \cap E_n) + m_0(A \cap B_{n-1}) \qquad \ldots(3)$

Now, putting $n = 2, 3, 4, \ldots, n-1, n$ in (3) in succession, we get

$$m_0(A \cap B_2) = m_0(A \cap E_2) + m_0(A \cap B_1)$$
$$m_0(A \cap B_3) = m_0(A \cap E_3) + m_0(A \cap B_2)$$
$$\vdots \qquad\qquad \vdots \qquad\qquad \vdots$$
$$m_0(A \cap B_{n-1}) = m_0(A \cap E_{n-1}) + m_0(A \cap B_{n-2})$$
$$m_0(A \cap B_n) = m_0(A \cap E_n) + m_0(A \cap B_{n-1})$$

Adding all these we get

$$m_0(A \cap B_n) = \sum_{i=1}^{n} [m_0(A \cap E_i) + m_0(A \cap B_1)]$$

$$= \sum_{i=1}^{n} m_0(A \cap E_i) \qquad (\because B_1 = E)$$

Using this value in (2) we get

$$m_0(A) \geq \sum_{i=1}^{n} m_0(A \cap E_i) + m_0(A \cap B')$$

Letting $n \to \infty$, we get

$$m_0(A) \geq \sum_{i=1}^{\infty} m_0(A \cap E_i) + m_0(A \cap B') \qquad \dots(4)$$

Now,

$$A \cap B = A \cap \left(\bigcup_{i=1}^{\infty} E_i \right) = \bigcup_{i=1}^{\infty} (A \cap E_i)$$

$$\Rightarrow \qquad m_0(A \cap B) = m_0 \left[\bigcup_{i=1}^{\infty} (A \cap E_i) \right]$$

$$= \sum_{i=1}^{\infty} m_0(A \cap E_i)$$

Putting this value in (4) we get

$$m_0(A) \geq m_0(A \cap B) + m_0(A \cap B') \qquad \dots(5)$$

Further, we know that

$$A = (A \cap B) \cup (A \cap B')$$

$$\Rightarrow \qquad m_0(A) \leq m_0(A \cap B) + m_0(A \cap B') \qquad \dots(6)$$

From (5) and (6) we conclude that

$$m_0(A) = m_0(A \cap B) + m_0(A \cap B')$$

$\Rightarrow \quad B$ is outer measurable.

$\Rightarrow \quad \bigcup_{i=1}^{\infty} E_i$ is measurable.

$\Rightarrow \quad \bigcup_{i=1}^{\infty} E_i \in \mathcal{A}$

Hence, $\mathcal{A}$ is a σ-algebra.

THEOREM 17.

An open set in a metric space is measurable w.r.t. any outer measure. [MEERUT–2003, KANPUR–2011]

PROOF. Let $[X, d]$ be a metric space and G be an open set of X.
We have to show that G is an outer measurable set.

Let E be any subset of G. Then define $E_n = \left\{ x \in E : d(x, G') \geq \dfrac{1}{n} \right\}$. Clearly, $<E_n>$ is

monotonically decreasing sequence and $\lim_{n \to \infty} E_n = E$.

We know that

$$m_0(B) \leq m_0(B \cap G) + m_0(B \cap G') \ \forall \ B \in \mathbf{R} \qquad \dots(1)$$

Let $B \cap G = E$, then

$$B = E \cup (B \cap G') \supset E_n \cup (B \cap G')$$

$$\Rightarrow \qquad m_0(B) \geq m_0[E_n \cup (B_n \cap G')]$$

By definition of E_n, we have
$$d(E_n, B \cap G') = 0$$
$$\Rightarrow \quad E_n \cap (B \cap G') = \phi$$
$$\Rightarrow \quad m_0(B) \geq m_0(E_n) + m_0(B \cap G')$$

Letting $n \to \infty$, we get
$$\lim_{n\to\infty} m_0[E_n \cup (B \cap G')] = \lim_{n\to\infty} m_0(E_n) + \lim_{n\to\infty} m_0(B \cap G')$$

$$= m_0(E) + m_0(B \cap G')$$

$$= m_0(B \cap G) + m_0(B \cap G') \qquad (\because E = B \cap G)$$
$$\Rightarrow \quad m_0(B) \geq m_0(B \cap G) + m_0(B \cap G') \qquad \qquad \ldots(2)$$

From (1) and (2) we conclude that
$$m_0(B) = m_0(B \cap G) + m_0(B \cap G')$$
$$\Rightarrow \quad G \text{ is outer measurable.}$$

THEOREM 18.

Let $<E_n>$ be a monotonic decreasing sequence of measurable sets then the limit set $E = \bigcap\limits_{i=1}^{\infty} E_i$ is measurable and for every A of finite outer measure

$$m_0(A \cap E) = \lim_{n\to\infty} m_0(A \cap E_n)$$

PROOF.   Firstly, we shall prove that $\lim\limits_{n\to\infty} m_0(A \cap E_n)$ exists and

$$m_0(A \cap E) = \lim_{n\to\infty} m_0(A \cap E_n)$$

Since, $<E_n>$ is a decreasing sequence (*i.e.*, $E_1 \supseteq E_2 \supseteq E_3 \supseteq \ldots$) then for any set A of finite measure, we have
$$A \cap E_1 \supseteq A \cap E_2 \supseteq A \cap E_3 \supseteq \ldots$$
$$\Rightarrow \quad m_0(A \cap E_1) \geq m_0(A \cap E_2) \geq m_0(A \cap E_3) \geq \ldots$$
$$\Rightarrow \quad <m_0(A \cap E_n)> \text{ is a monotonic decreasing sequence.}$$
$$\Rightarrow \quad <m_0(AE_n)> \text{ is a monotonic decreasing sequence.}$$
$$\text{(For sake of convenience let us write } A \cap E_n = AE_n)$$
Also, $<m_0(AE_n)>$ is non-negative.

Then by monotonic convergence theorem
$$\lim_{n\to\infty} m_0(AE_n) \text{ exists.}$$

Now, $$E = \bigcap_{n=1}^{\infty} E_n \subset E_n$$
$$\Rightarrow \quad E \subset E_n$$
$$\Rightarrow \quad A \cap E \subseteq A \cap E_n$$
$$\Rightarrow \quad AE \subseteq AE_n$$
$$\Rightarrow \quad m_0(AE) \leq m_0(AE_n)$$
$$\Rightarrow \quad \lim_{n\to\infty} m_0(AE) \leq \lim_{n\to\infty} m_0(AE_n) = \lambda \text{ (say)}$$
$$\Rightarrow \quad \lim_{n\to\infty} (AE) \leq \lambda \qquad\qquad \ldots(1)$$

Now the set A can be written as
$$A = AE + AE_1' + E_1 AE_2' + E_2 AE_3' + \ldots + E_{n-1} AE_n'$$

$$\Rightarrow \quad m_0(A) \leq m_0(AE) + m_0(AE_1') + m_0(E_1 AE_2') + \ldots + m_0(E_{n-1} AE_n') \qquad \ldots(2)$$

Further, since each E_n is outer measurable, therefore,
$$m_0(A) = m_0(AE_n) + m_0(AE_n')$$
$$\Rightarrow \qquad m_0(A) = m_0(AE_1) + m_0(AE_1') \qquad \qquad \ldots(3)$$
Let us take $A = E_{n-1}A$, then we have
$$m_0(E_{n-1}A) = m_0(E_{n-1}AE_n) + m_0(E_{n-1}AE_n')$$
$$\Rightarrow \qquad m_0(E_{n-1}A) = m_0(E_nA) + m_0(E_{n-1}AE_n') \quad (\because E_n \subseteq E_{n-1} \Rightarrow E_n \cap E_{n-r} = E_n)$$
$$\Rightarrow \qquad m_0(E_{n-1}AE_n') = m_0(AE_{n-1}) - m_0(AE_n) \qquad \qquad \ldots(4)$$
Using (2) and (3) in (4), we get
$$m_0(A) \leq m_0(AE) + [m_0(A) - m_0(AE_1)] + [m_0(AE_1) - m_0(AE_2)]$$
$$+ [m_0(AE_2) - m_0(AE_3)] + \ldots + [m_0(AE_{n-1}) - m_0(AE_n)]$$
$$= m_0(AE) + m_0(A) - m_0(AE_n)$$
$$\Rightarrow \qquad m_0(A) \leq m_0(AE) + m_0(A) - \lambda$$
$$\text{(By taking } n \to \infty \text{ and using } \lim_{n\to\infty} m(AE_n) = \lambda)$$

$$\Rightarrow \qquad \lambda \leq m_0(AE) \qquad \qquad \ldots(5)$$
From (1) and (5) we conclude that
$$\lambda = m_0(AE)$$
Therefore, $\lim_{n\to\infty} m_0(AE_n) = m_0(AE)$ \qquad \qquad \ldots(6)$

Now we shall prove that $E = \bigcap_{n=1}^{\infty} E_n$ is measurable.

We have $\qquad \qquad A = AE + AE' \qquad \qquad \ldots(7)$
$$\Rightarrow \qquad m_0(A) \leq m_0(AE) + m_0(AE') \qquad \qquad \ldots(8)$$
From (7) $\qquad \qquad AE = A - AE \qquad \qquad \text{(By set theory)}$
Now, $\qquad \qquad AE' = AE_1' + E_1AE_2' + E_2AE_3' + \ldots + E_{n-1}AE_n'$

$$\Rightarrow \qquad m_0(AE') \leq m_0(AE_1') + m_0(E_1AE_2') + m_0(E_2AE_3') + \ldots + m_0(E_{n-1}AE_n')$$

Using (3) and (4) in the above equation we get
$$m_0(AE') \leq [m_0(A) - m_0(AE_1)] + [m_0(AE_1) - m_0(AE_2)]$$
$$+ [m_0(AE_2) - m_0(AE_3)] + \ldots + [m_0(AE_{n-1}) - m_0(AE_n)]$$
$$= m_0(A) - m_0(AE_n)$$
Letting $n \to \infty$, we get
$$m_0(AE') \leq m_0(A) - \lim_{n\to\infty} m_0(AE_n)$$
$$\Rightarrow \qquad m_0(A) \geq m_0(AE') + \lim_{n\to\infty} m_0(AE_n)$$
$$\Rightarrow \qquad m_0(A) \geq m_0(AE') + m_0(AE) \qquad \qquad \text{(Using (6))}$$
$$\ldots(9)$$

Finally, from (8) and (9) we conclude that
$$m_0(A) = m_0(AE) + m_0(AE')$$
$$= m_0(A \cap E) + m_0(A \cap E')$$
$$\Rightarrow \qquad E = \bigcap_{i=1}^{\infty} E_i \text{ is outer measurable.}$$

Solved Examples

EXAMPLE 1. *If A and B are outer measurable sets then show that A − B and A Δ B are also outer measurable.*

SOLUTION. Let A and B are outer measurable sets. We have to show that $A − B$ and $A \Delta B$ are also outer measurable.

Since, B is outer measurable.

$\Rightarrow$ B' is also outer measurable.

(∵ Complement of an outer measurable set is also outer measurable)

Further A and B' both are outer measurable.

$\Rightarrow$ $A \cap B'$ is outer measurable.

(Being the intersections of two measurable sets)

$\Rightarrow$ $A − B$ is measurable.   (∵ $A \cap B' = A − B$)

Similarly, we may prove that $B − A$ is outer measurable.

Now, $A \Delta B = (A − B) \cup (B − A)$

              = Union of two outer measurable sets

              = Outer measurable

EXAMPLE 2. *If A and B are outer measurable and if $B \subseteq A$ then prove that*

$$m_0(A − B) = m_0(A) − m_0(B)$$ [MEERUT–2009, 17]

SOLUTION. Since, $B \subseteq A$ (given). Then by set theory, we can write

$$A = (A − B) \cup B \text{ such that } (A − B) \cap B = \psi$$

$$\Rightarrow \quad m_0(A) = m_0(A − B) + m_0(B)$$

$$\Rightarrow \quad m_0(A − B) = m_0(A) − m_0(B)$$

EXAMPLE 3. *Show that the class of m_0-measurable sets is a Boolean algebra.*

SOLUTION. Let M be the class of m_0-measurable sets.

We have to show that M is m_0-measurable.

Let $A, B \in M$. Therefore, by definition of M, A and B are m_0-measurable.

$\Rightarrow$ A' and $A \cup B$ both are m_0-measurable.

(∵ Compliment of a m_0-measurable set and union of two m_0-measurable sets is also measurable)

Hence, M is a Boolean algebra.

EXAMPLE 4. *Show that the intersection of two outer measurable sets is outer measurable.*

[MEERUT–2004, 05, 06, 10, 16]

SOLUTION. Let A and B be two outer measurable sets. We have to prove that $A \cap B$ is outer measurable.

Since, A and B are outer measurable.

$\Rightarrow$ A' and B' are outer measurable.   (∵ Compliment of an outer measurable set is again outer measurable)

$\Rightarrow$ $A' \cup B'$ is outer measurable.

(∵ Union of two outer measurable sets is also outer measurable)

$\Rightarrow$ $(A \cap B)'$ is outer measurable.   (By Demorgan's law)

$\Rightarrow$ $A \cap B$ is outer measurable.   (∵ A is measurable $\Leftrightarrow$ A' is measurable)

Hence, intersection of two outer measurable sets is also outer measurable.

EXAMPLE 5. *Show that every subset of a set of measure zero is outer measurable and its measure is also zero.*

SOLUTION. Let A be a set and B be a subset of A, i.e., $B \subseteq A$ such that $m_0(A) = 0$.

Now, $m_0(A) = 0 \quad \Rightarrow \quad A$ is measurable.

$(\because A$ set with measure zero is always measurable)

Since, $\quad B \subseteq A \quad \Rightarrow \quad m_0(B) \leq m_0(A)$

$\Rightarrow \quad m_0(B) \leq 0 \qquad\qquad (\because m_0(A) = 0 \text{ (given)})$

But we know that $m_0(B) \geq 0$

Thus we conclude that $m_0(B) = 0$

Finally, since $m_0(B) = 0$ therefore, B is outer measurable.

$(\because A$ set with measure zero is always measurable)

EXAMPLE 6. *If A is a μ-non-measurable set then show that there exists a subset A with a positive finite μ-measure.*

SOLUTION. Let E be a set of finite measure.

Since A is μ-non-measurable therefore

$$\mu(E) < \mu(A \cap E) + \mu(A' \cap E)$$

If $\mu(A \cap E) = 0$ then $\mu(E) < \mu(A' \cap E)$ which is a contradiction because $A' \cap E \subseteq E$ and $\mu(A' \cap E) \leq \mu(E)$.

Also, if $\mu(A \cap E) = \infty$

$\Rightarrow \quad \mu(E) \geq \infty$, which is again a contradiction.

Thus, neither $\mu(A \cap E) = 0$ nor $\mu(A \cap E) = \infty$

But $\mu(A \cap E) \geq 0$

$\Rightarrow \quad 0 < \mu(A \cap E) < \infty$

$\Rightarrow \quad$ Measure of $A \cap E$ is finite.

Hence, we conclude that $\exists$ a subset $A \cap E$ of A of positive finite μ-measure.

EXAMPLE 7. *If a set function f on a ring R is countably additive and there exists a set A and sequence $<A_n> \in R$ such that $A_r \subset A_{r+1}$ and $A = \bigcup\limits_{n=1}^{\infty} A_n$, then prove that $f(A_n) \to f(A)$ as $n \to \infty$.*

SOLUTION. It is given that

(i) $A_n \subset A_{n+1}$ $\qquad$ (ii) $A = \bigcup\limits_{n=1}^{\infty} A_n$ $\qquad$ (iii) f is countably additive

We have to prove that

$$\lim_{n \to \infty} f(A_n) = f(A)$$

Let us define $B_1 = A_1 \quad B_n = A_n - A_{n-1}$ for $n > 1$

Then $B_n \cap B_m$ for $n \neq m$.

and $\qquad \bigcup\limits_{n=1}^{\infty} B_n = \bigcup\limits_{n=1}^{\infty} A_n, A_k = \bigcup\limits_{n=1}^{k} B_n$

$\Rightarrow \qquad f(A_k) = \sum\limits_{n=1}^{k} f(B_n)$ $\qquad\qquad (\because f$ is countably additive)

$\Rightarrow \qquad f(A) = f\left[\bigcup\limits_{n=1}^{\infty} A_n \right] = f\left[\bigcup\limits_{n=1}^{\infty} B_n \right]$

$$= \sum_{1}^{\infty} f(B_n) = \lim_{k \to \infty} f(B_n).$$

$$= \lim_{k \to \infty} f(A_k) = \lim_{n \to \infty} f(A_n) \qquad \text{(From (1))}$$

Hence, $\quad \lim_{n \to \infty} f(A_n) = f(A)$

EXAMPLE 8. *Let A be a m_0-measurable subset of B and C be any set with $m_0(C) < \infty$, $A \subset B$ then show that $m_0[C \cap B \cap A'] = m_0(C \cap B) - m_0(C \cap A)$*

SOLUTION. Let A be an outer measurable set, then by definition

$$m_0(E) = m_0(A \cap E) + m_0(A' \cap E) \; \forall \; E \subseteq R$$

Let us take $E = C \cap B$ then

$$m_0(C \cap B) = m_0(C \cap B \cap A) + m_0(C \cap B \cap A')$$

$$\Rightarrow \quad m_0(C \cap B) - m_0(C \cap A) = m_0(C \cap B \cap A') \qquad (\because A \subset B \Rightarrow A \cap B = A)$$

EXAMPLE 9. *If A is a m_0-measurable subset with $m_0(A) < \infty$ and B is any set containing A, then show that $m_0(B \cap A') = m_0(B) - m_0(A)$*

SOLUTION. Let A be an outer measurable set and $A \subset B$

Since A is outer measurable, therefore

$$m_0(E) = m_0(A \cap E) + m_0(A' \cap E)$$

In particular, let us take $E = B$ then

$$m_0(B) = m_0(A \cap B) + m_0(A' \cap B)$$

$$\Rightarrow \quad m_0(A' \cap B) = m_0(B) - m_0(A \cap B) \qquad \qquad \dots(1)$$

Now, since $A \subseteq B \Rightarrow A \cap B = A$

$$m_0(A \cap B) = m_0(A)$$

Put this value in (1) we get

$$m_0(A' \cap B) = m_0(B) - m_0(A)$$

Exercise 4.1

1. Show that every finitely additive measusre is monotonic.

2. Let X be any set and $S = P(X)$. Prove that the set function $\mu : S \to [0, \infty]$ is defined as

$$\mu(A) = \begin{cases} \infty, \text{if } A \text{ is an infinite subset of } X \\ \text{number of elements in } A, \text{if } A \text{ is} \\ \qquad\qquad\qquad\qquad\qquad \text{finite} \end{cases}$$

is measurable funtion.

3. Consider the set function $\mu : P(N) \to [0, \infty]$ defined by $\mu(\phi) = 0$ and $\mu(A) = \sum_{n \in A} a_n$

where $A \in P(N)$ and $<a_n>$ is a sequence of non-negative real numbers. Show that μ is a measurable function.

4. Let $<A_n>$ be a sequence of Lebesgue measurable subsets of R such that

$\sum_{n=1}^{\infty} \mu(A_n) < \infty$ and let $B = \bigcap_{k=1}^{\infty} \bigcup_{n=k}^{\infty} A_n$, then show that B is measurable and $\mu(B) = 0$.

5. Let $<p_i>$ is a sequence of non-negative real numbers and X be an infinite sets and $x_n \in X$ for $n = 1, 2, \dots$ Define a set function μ such that for $A \subseteq X$

$$\mu(A) = \sum_{x_i \in A} p_i$$

Prove that μ is an outer measure.

6. If $\mu_1, \mu_2, \dots \mu_n$ are n measures on a σ-ring S of subsets of X. Show that the set function μ defined as $\mu(E) = \sum_{i=1}^{n} a_i \mu_i(E)$ is also a measure, where each a_i is a non-negative real number.

7. Show that there exist a set E of real numbers is of measure zero if there exists a sequence of intervals $<I_n>$ such that $E \subset \limsup I_n$ and $\sum |I_n| < \infty$.

8. If μ is a measure function defined on a class E of sets. If $<A_n>$ is any sequence of sets from E for which $\mu(A_n) < \infty$ then show that

$$\mu(\limsup A_n) > \lim(\sup \mu E_n)$$

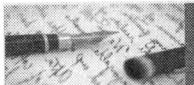 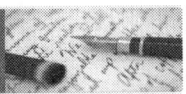

CHAPTER Summary

⇝ KEY TERMS

- **BOOLEAN RING** : A Boolean ring is a non-empty class of sets which is closed under the formation of unions and differences.

- **BOOLEAN ALGEBRA:** A non-empty class A of sets is called an algebra of sets or Boolean algebra if it is closed under the formation of unions and complementations.

- **σ-RING:** A Boolean ring is called σ-ring if it is closed under the formation of countable unions.

- **σ-ALGEBRA:** A non-empty class of sets is called a σ-algebra if it is closed under the formation of countable unions and complementations.

- **MEASURABLE SET:** If μ denote an outer measure function defined on a hereditary σ-ring R then any member $A \in R$ is said to be measurable w.r.t. μ if

$$\mu(E) = \mu(A \cap E) + \mu(A' \cap E) \text{ for all } E \in R$$

- **CARATHEODORY'S OUTER MEASURE:** An extended real valued set function m_0 defined on a ring R is called Caratheodory outer measure if

  (i) $m_0(A_r) \geq 0 \; \forall \; A_i \in R$

  (ii) $m_0(\phi) = 0$

  (iii) $A_r, A_s \in R : A_r \subseteq A_s \Rightarrow m_0(A_r) \leq m_0(A_s)$

  (iv) $m_0 \left[\bigcup_{r \in N} A_r \right] \leq \sum_{r \in N} m_0(A_r)$

⇝ RESULTS

- Every σ-algebra is a σ-ring but not conversely.
- Intersection of two B-rings is a B-ring.
- A monotone ring is a σ-ring and conversely.
- A is m_0-measurable if and only if A' is m_0-measurable.
- If $<A_n>$ is a convergent sequence of outer measurable sets, then

  $$m_0(\lim A_n) = \lim(m_0(A_n))$$

  provided $m_0(A_k) < \infty$ for at least one k.
- A σ-additive set function is a continuous function.
- The class A of m_0-measurable sets is σ-algebra.
- If A and B are two measurable sets then

  (i) $A \cap B$ is m_0-measurable

  (ii) $A - B$ and $B - A$ are m_0-measurable
  (iii) $A \Delta B$ is m_0-measurable
  (iv) $A \cup B$ is m_0-measurable
- Every set with measure zero is m_0-measurable.
- Every subset of a set of measure zero is measurable and its measure is also zero.
- An open set in a metric space is measurable w.r.t. any metric outer measure.
- An outer measure is monotonic and σ-subadditive.
- Every finitely additive measure is monotonic.
- An additive set function defined over a ring can not assume both values $+\infty$ and $-\infty$.
- The empty set ϕ and whole set X are measurable.

⇝ WORTHY READINGS

☞ Any σ-ring is a monotone class.

☞ A monotone class is a σ-ring iff it is a ring.

☞ Every ring of sets is finitely additive class and vice-versa.

☞ Every completely additive class might be a field or σ-field and vice versa.

☞ The measure function is called finite or σ-finite according as the measure of every set is finite or σ-finite.

☞ A plane set is said to be an elementary set if it is expressible as a finite union of pairwise disjoint rectangles.

☞ Let $[X, d]$ be a metric space and μ^* be an outer measure on $P(X)$ such that
$$\mu^*(A \cup B) = \mu^*(A) + \mu^*(B),$$
whenever $d(A, B) > 0$
Then μ^* is called outer measure.

☞ A ring is closed under formation of symmetric difference and intersection.

☞ Every monotone field is a σ-field.

🐌 FURTHER READINGS

☞ **DIRAC MEASURE:** Let $X \neq \phi$ and $x_0 \in X$ be a fixed element. Define a set function μ such that

$$\mu(\phi) = 0 \text{ and } \mu(A) = \begin{cases} 0 & \text{if } x_0 \notin A \\ 1 & \text{if } x_0 \in A \end{cases}$$

where A is a non-empty subset of X. This is called Dirac measure.

☞ **COUNTING MEASURE:** Let $X \neq \phi$ be any set then the set function $\mu : P(X) \to [0, \infty]$ defined by

$$\mu(A) = \begin{cases} \infty, \text{if } A \text{ is infinite subset of } X \\ \text{no. of elements in } A, \text{if } A \text{ is} \\ \qquad\qquad \text{finite subset of } X \end{cases}$$

Then μ is called Counting measure.

☞ **DISCRETE MEASURE:** Let $<p_n>$ be a sequence of non-negative real numbers and X be an infinite set and $<x_n> \in X$. Define

$$\mu(A) = \sum_{x_i \in A} p_i$$

Then outer measure μ is called discrete measure.

☞ **DISCRETE PROBABILITY MEASURE:** In the above definition if $\sum_{i=1}^{\infty} p_i = 1$. Then μ is called discrete probability measure.

☞ A necessary and sufficient condition that a class P of subsets of X be an ideal in the Boolean ring of all subsets of X is that P is a hereditary ring.

☞ Let X be a set of 100 points arranged in a square array of 10 columns each with 10 points, P is the class of all subsets of X, $\mu^*(E)$ is the number of columns which contains at least one point of E.

☞ If X is arbitrary, H be the class of all countable subsets of X, $\mu^*(E)$ is the number of points in E. ($= \infty$ if E is infinite)

Chapter

5 Measurable Functions

5.1 INTRODUCTION

The class of measurable functions plays a very important role in Lebesgue theory of integration. In Riemann theory of integration, the class of functions should be bounded and continuous everywhere while in R-S integrals, functions should be of bounded variation. Also, the upper and lower integrals should be equal. But for the existence of Lebesgue integrability function must satisfies less restriction than that of continuity. In many cases, it is easier to examine the measurability of a function then to investigate the upper and lower integrals directly. In this chapter we shall discuss a new class of function, known as measurable functions.

5.2 SOME SPECIAL FUNCTIONS

5.2.1 EQUIVALENT FUNCTIONS

Two functions f and g defined on the same set E are said to be equivalent if $m[E(f \neq g)] = 0$, i.e., f and g are said to be equivalent if $\exists\ A, B$ in E such that

$$E = A \cup B, f = g \text{ on } A, f \neq g \text{ on } B \text{ and } m(B) = 0$$

5.2.2 CHARACTERISTIC FUNCTION

Let A be any subset of E. Then characteristic function χ_A of A is defined as follows:

$$\chi_A(x) = \begin{cases} 0 & \text{if} \quad x \in A \\ 1 & \text{if} \quad x \in E - A, i.e., \text{if } x \notin A \end{cases}$$

It is also denoted by ϕ_A or ψ_A and some times called indicator functions.

5.2.3 PROPERTIES OF CHARACTERISTIC FUNCTION

(1) $\chi_\phi = 0,\ \chi_E = 1$

(2) $\chi_{A \cap B} = \chi_A \cdot \chi_B$

(3) $\chi_{A \cup B} = \chi_A + \chi_B - \chi_{A \cap B}$

(4) $\chi_{A \cup B} = \chi_A + \chi_B$ if $A \cap B = \chi$

(5) $\chi_{A - B} = \chi_A - \chi_{A \cap B}$

(6) $\chi\left(\bigcup_{i=N} A_i\right) = \sum_{i \in N} \chi_{A_i}$ if $A_i's$ are pairwise disjoint.

5.2.4 SIMPLE FUNCTION

A function is said to be simple if the range of the function is finite, *i.e.*, a real valued function ψ is called simple if it is measurable and assumes only a finite number of values.

If ψ is a simple function and has finite number of values $C_1, C_2, ..., C_n$ then ψ can be expressed as

$$\psi_{(x)} = \sum_{i=1}^{n} C_i \chi_{A_i}$$

where χ_{A_i} is the characteristic function defined on $A_i = \{x : \phi(x) = C_i\}$

☛ REMARKS
- The sum, product and difference of two functions are simple.
- A simple function is always measurable.
- The characteristic functions of a set A is simple function as it takes only two values (0 and 1) on two disjoints sets A and A'.

5.2.5 STEP FUNCTION

A real valued function s defined on an interval $[a, b]$ is said to be step function if there exists a partition $a = x_0 < x_1 < x_2 < ... < x_n = b$ such that the function assumes one and only one values in each interval.

Like simple function, step function also assumes finite number of values, but there are sets $\{x : s(x) = C_i\}$ are intervals for each i.

Illustrations

✦ The function $f : R \to [0, 1[$ such that $f(x) = 5 - [x]$ is a step function where $[x]$ denotes the greater integer $\leq x$.

For, $f(x) = 5 - n$, for $n \leq x \leq n + 1 \ \forall \ n \in Z$

✦ Every step function is also a simple function but converse is not true.
For example, the function

$f : R \to R$ such that
$$f(x) = \begin{cases} 1, & \text{if } x \text{ is rational} \\ 0, & \text{if } x \text{ is irrational} \end{cases}$$
is a simple function but not step, because the set of rational and irrationals numbers are not intervals.

5.2.6 SIGNUM FUNCTION

The signum function is defined as follows:

$$S(x) = \begin{cases} 1 & \text{if } x > 0 \\ 0 & \text{if } x = 0 \\ -1 & \text{if } x < 0 \end{cases}$$

☛ REMARK
- Every signum function is step function.

5.3 LEBESGUE MEASURABLE FUNCTIONS

An extended real valued function f defined over a measurable set E is said to be measurable in the sense of Lebesgue if the set $E[f > a] = \{x \in E : f(x) > a\}$ is measurable for all extended real number a.

The above definition can be written as follows:

The function f is measurable if for every real number a, the inverse image of $]a, \infty]$ under the mapping f, *i.e.*, $f^{-1}(]a, \infty])$ is a measurable set.

☛ **REMARKS**
- $E[f > a]$ may be finite or infinite.
- If $E = R$, the set of real numbers, then the set $E(f > a)$ becomes an open set.
- To handle the function or measure with infinite values in a consistent way, we have the following arithmetic

  i. $a + \infty = \infty \ (a \in R \ \text{or} \ a = \infty)$

  ii. $a \cdot \infty = \infty \ (a > 0)$

  iii. $a \cdot \infty = -\infty \ (a < 0)$

  iv. $\infty \cdot \infty = \infty$

  v. $0 \cdot \infty = 0$

  vi. $0 \cdot (-\infty) = 0$

  vii. $\infty + (-\infty) = \text{Not defined}$

- The domain of the function f defined above, will usually be either R or $R - B$ such that $m(B) = 0$

THEOREM I.

Let f be a measurable function defined over a measurable set $E_i : i \in N$, then f is measurable on E,

where $E = \bigcup_{r=1}^{\infty} E_r$.

PROOF. Let f be a measurable function defined over a measurable set E_i. Let $E = \bigcup_{r=1}^{\infty} E_r$.
We have to prove that f is measurable over E.

Clearly, E is the enumerable union of measurable sets, therefore, E is measurable.

Since, it is given that the set $\{x \in E, f(x) > a\}$ is measurable for all $a \in R$ and $\forall \ r \in N$.

Consider $E(f > a) = \left(\bigcup_{r=1}^{\infty} E_r \right)(f > a)$

$$= \bigcup_{r=1}^{\infty} [E_r(f > a)] \qquad \qquad ...(1)$$

Since, f is measurable on each E_i (given)

$\Rightarrow \quad E_r[f > a]$ is measurable.

Using this result in (1) we get

$\qquad E(f > a) = \text{enumerable union of measurable sets}$

$\qquad \qquad \qquad = \text{measurable}$

$\Rightarrow \quad E(f > a)$ is measurable.

Hence, f is measurable over $E = \bigcup_{i=1}^{\infty} E_i$.

THEOREM 2.

The characteristic function of a set A is measurable if and only if A is measurable.

[MEERUT–2010, KANPUR–2010, AVADH–2014]

PROOF. Let us first suppose, the characteristic function χ_A is measurable.

We have to prove that A is measurable.

Since χ_A is measurable therefore for any $x \in R$, we have $\{x : \chi_A(x) > 0\}$ is measurable.

$\Rightarrow \quad A = \{x : \chi_A(x) > 0\}$ is measurable.

Conversely, let us suppose that A is measurable over a measurable set E.

We have to prove that χ_A is measurable.

Consider, $\quad E[\chi_A > a] = \begin{cases} \phi & \text{if} & a \geq 1 \\ A & \text{if} & 0 \leq a < 1 \\ A \cup A'[= E] & \text{if} & a < 0 \end{cases}$

In the above, every set of RHS is measurable. Therefore, $E[\chi_A > 0]$ is measurable. Hence, χ_A is measurable.

☞ **REMARK**

- The set A and its characteristic function χ_A are both measurable or both are non-measurable, (even if domain set E is measurable).

THEOREM 3.

If f is a measurable function defined over a measurable set E then $\exists$ a sequence $\langle f_n \rangle$ of simple functions which converges pointwise to f on E. If $f \geq 0$ the sequence $\langle f_n \rangle$ can be chosen such that $0 \leq f_n \leq f_{n+1} \; \forall \, n \in N$.

PROOF. Let f be a measurable function defined over a measurable set E. Suppose that $f \geq 0$ on E.

Consider a finite collection of subsets of E defined by

$$E_{n,\alpha} = \left\{ x \in E : \frac{\alpha-1}{2^n} \leq f(x) \leq \frac{\alpha}{2^n} \right\} \text{ for } \alpha = 1, 2, 2^2, \ldots 2^{2n}$$

and

$$E_{n,1+2^{2n}} = \left\{ x \in E : \frac{1+2^{2n}-1}{2^n} \leq f(x) \leq \frac{1+2^{2n}}{2^n} \right\}$$

$$= \left\{ x \in E : 2^n \leq f(x) \leq 2^n + \frac{1}{2^n} \right\}$$

$$= \{ x \in E : f(x) \geq 2^n \}$$

If we define a sequence $\langle f_n \rangle$ of function such that

$$f_n = \sum_{\alpha=1}^{1+2^{2n}} \left(\frac{\alpha-1}{2^n} \right) \chi_{E_{n,\alpha}}$$

$\Rightarrow$ f_n is a simple function and the sequence $\langle f_n \rangle$ is increasing which converges to f on E.

THEOREM 4. (Lusin Theorem)

Let f be a measurable function defined over a measurable set E, then for each $\varepsilon > 0 \; \exists$ a closed set $F \subset E$ with $m(E - F) < \varepsilon$ such that f is continuous on F.

PROOF. Let us first suppose that f is a simple function and $\{a_1, a_2, \ldots, a_n\}$ be a set of non-zero values of f. Then $f = \sum_{n=1}^{m} a_i \chi_{E_i}$.

The sets E_i are measurable and disjoint.

Let us write $\quad E_{m+1} = E - \bigcup_{i=1}^{m} E_i$

Let $\varepsilon > 0$, then corresponding to each E_i ($i = 1, 2, \ldots m + 1$), we can find a closed set $F_i \subset E_i$ such that $m(E_i - F_i) < \dfrac{\varepsilon}{m+1}$.

If
$$F = \bigcup_{i=1}^{m+1} F_i$$

Clearly F is closed ($\because$ Finite union of closed sets is closed)

Also $F \subset E$ and $\quad m(E-F) = \sum_{i=1}^{m+1} m(E_i - F_i) < (m+1) \cdot \dfrac{\varepsilon}{(m+1)}$

$\Rightarrow \qquad\qquad m(E-F) < \varepsilon$

Further, suppose that f is any measurable function defined on a measurable set E, then $\exists$ a sequence $<f_n>$ of simple function converging to f. Then from above, we conclude that for given $\varepsilon > 0$ and for all $n \in N \, \exists$ a measurable set $A_n \subset E$ such that f is continuous on A_n and

$$m(E - A_n) < \frac{\varepsilon}{2^n}$$

Let us set $A = \bigcap_{n=1}^{\infty} A_n$

Since, f_n is continuous so its $\lim\limits_{n\to\infty} f_n = f$ is also continuous in F.

Also, F is measurable set with the condition

$$m(E-F) = m\left[\bigcup_{n=1}^{\infty} (E - A_n)\right]$$

$$\leq \sum_{n=1}^{\infty} m[E - A_n] < \sum_{n=1}^{\infty} \frac{\varepsilon}{2^n}$$

$$= \varepsilon \qquad\qquad \left(\because \sum_{n=1}^{\infty} \frac{1}{2^n} = 1, \text{ sum of infinite G.P.}\right)$$

Hence, $m(E + F) < \varepsilon$

THEOREM 5.

Every monotone sequence of sets is convergent.

PROOF. Let $<A_n>$ be an increasing sequence then

$$A_n \subset A_{n+1} \, \forall \, n \quad \bigcap_{n=k}^{\infty} A_n = A_k \, \forall k$$

Now, by definition

$$\underline{\lim} A_n = \bigcup_{n=1}^{\infty} \left(\bigcap_{m=n}^{\infty} A_m\right) = \bigcup_{n=1}^{\infty} A_n \qquad\qquad \text{...(1)}$$

and $\qquad \overline{\lim} A_n = \bigcap_{n=1}^{\infty}\left[\bigcup_{m=n}^{\infty} A_m\right] \qquad\qquad \text{...(2)}$

Let us take $k = 1$

$\left(\because \text{For any non-decreasing sequence, } \bigcup_{n=k}^{\infty} A_n \text{ is independent of } k\right)$

Then from (2)

$$\overline{\lim} A_n = \bigcap_{n=1}^{\infty}\left[\bigcup_{m=n}^{\infty} A_m\right] = \bigcup_{m=1}^{\infty} A_m = \bigcup_{n=1}^{\infty} A_n$$

$$= \underline{\lim} A_n \qquad \text{(From (1))}$$

$$\Rightarrow \qquad \overline{\lim} A_n = \underline{\lim} A_n = \lim A_n = \bigcup_{n=1}^{\infty} A_n$$

$\Rightarrow$ monotonic increasing sequence is convergent.

Similarly, we may prove that every monotonic decreasing sequence is convergent.

Hence, we conclude that every monotonic sequence of sets is convergent.

THEOREM 6.

A constant fucntion over a measurable set is measurable.

PROOF.   Let f be a constant function defines over a measurable set E. We have to prove that f is measurable. Since, f is constant, therefore,

$$f(x) = c \ \forall \ x \in E$$

For any real number a, consider

$$E[f < a] = \begin{cases} E & \text{if} \quad c > a \\ \phi & \text{if} \quad c \le a \end{cases}$$

In both the above cases $E[f > a]$ is measurable.

Hence, f is measurable over E.

THEOREM 7.

If f is a measurable function over a measurable set E then f is also measurable over any set $A \subset E$, A being a measurable set.   [KANPUR–2011, DELHI–2010]

PROOF.   Let f be a measurable function defined over a measurable set E and $A \subset E$ be any arbitrary measurable set. We have to prove that f is measurable over A.

Since, f is measurable over E.

$\Rightarrow \quad E[f > a]$ is measurable for $a \in \mathbf{R}$

Consider $A[f > a] = E[f > a] \cap A$

$$= \text{Intersection of two measurable sets}$$

$$= \text{measurable}$$

$\Rightarrow \quad A[f > a]$ is measurable.

Hence, f is measurable over A.

THEOREM 8.

A function is simple if and only if it is measurable and assumes a finite number of values.

[MEERUT–2006]

PROOF.   Let us first suppose f is a simple function, *i.e.*,

$$f = \sum_{i=1}^{n} k_i \chi_{A_i} \qquad \qquad ...(1)$$

where A_i are measurable sets and χ_{A_i} are the characteristic function. We have to prove that f is measurable and assumes a finite number of values.

Since, A_i is measurable $\Rightarrow$ χ_{A_i} is measurable   (By theorem-2)

$\Rightarrow \quad k_i \cdot \chi_{A_i}$ is measurable

$\Rightarrow \quad \sum_{i=1}^{n} k_i \chi_{A_i}$ is measurable

$\Rightarrow$ f is measurable (From (1))

Now, it remains to prove that it assume a finite number of values.

If $x \notin A_i$ then $x \notin A_i$ for all $i = 1, 2, ..., n$

Therefore, $f(x) = k_1 \chi_{A_1}(x) + k_2 \chi_{A_2}(x) + ... + k_n \chi_{A_n}(x)$

$= k_1 \cdot 0 + k_2 \cdot 0 + ... + k_n \cdot 0$

$= 0$, which is one value of $f(x)$

Now, $x \in A_j$ (only one set) then $\chi_{A_j}(x) = 1$

$\therefore$ $f(x) = k_1 \chi_{A_1}(x) + k_2 \chi_{A_2}(x) + ... + k_j \chi_{A_j}(x) + ... + k_n \chi_{A_n}(x)$

$= k_1 \cdot 0 + k_2 \cdot 0 + ... + k_j \cdot 1 + ... + k_n \cdot 0$

$= k_j$

Thus, we conclude that if x belongs to a single set A_j, then $f(x)$ can assume at most n values $k_1, k_2, ..., k_n$. So, the number of values of $f(x)$ is at most $^nC_1$.

Now, if $x \in A_j \cap A_p$ then $f(x) = k_j + k_p$, a sum of two numbers, which can be chosen in $^nC_2$ ways out of n.

Similarly, if $x \in A_j \cap A_p \cap A_q$ then $f(x) = k_j + k_p + k_q$, a sum of three numbers which can be chosen in $^nC_3$ ways.

Continuing this process, we observe that $f(x)$ can have

$$1 + {}^nC_1 + {}^nC_2 + ... + {}^nC_n (= 2^n)$$

values in number (finite)

Hence, $f(x)$ assumes only finite number of values.

Conversely, let $f(x)$ be a measurable function which can takes only a finite number of values namely $k_1, k_2, ..., k_n$. We have to prove that f is a simple function. We can write

$$f(x) = \sum_{i=1}^{n} k_i \chi_{A_i}(x)$$

where $A_i = \{x : f(x) = k_i\}$

Since, f is a measurable function, therefore, A_i is measurable.

Hence, f is a simple function.

5.4 LEBESGUE MEASURABLE FUNCTION ON A MEASURABLE SET

An extended real valued function defined over a measurable set E is said to be Lebesgue measurable if any one of the following is measurable:

(i) $E[f > a]$ (ii) $E[f \geq a]$ (iii) $E[f < a]$ (iv) $E[f \leq a]$

for any $a \in R$.

5.4.1 SOME NOTATIONS

(1) $\{x \in E : f(x) \leq a\} = \bigcup_{n=1}^{\infty} \left\{ x \in E : f(x) > a - \frac{1}{n} \right\}$

(2) $E[f \geq a] = \bigcap_{n=1}^{\infty} \left[E\left(f > a - \frac{1}{n} \right) \right]$

(3) $E[f < a] = E - [E(f \geq a)] = \overset{\infty}{\underset{n=1}{\cup}} \left[E\left(f \leq a - \frac{1}{n} \right) \right]$

(4) $E[f \leq a] = \overset{\infty}{\underset{n=1}{\cap}} \left\{ x \in E : f(x) < a + \frac{1}{n} \right\}$

(5) $E[f > a] = E - [E(f \leq a)] = \overset{\infty}{\underset{n=1}{\cup}} \left[E\left(f \geq a + \frac{1}{n} \right) \right]$

(6) $\{ x \in E : f(x) = \infty \} = \overset{\infty}{\underset{n=1}{\cap}} \{ x \in E : f(x) > a \}$

(7) $\{ x \in E : f(x) = -\infty \} = \overset{\infty}{\underset{n=1}{\cap}} \{ x \in E : f(x) < -n \}$

THEOREM 1.

Prove the equivalence of following four definitions of measurable function, i.e., A function f is measurable over E if and only if any one of the following

(1) $E[f > a]$ (2) $E[f \geq a]$ (3) $E[f < a]$ (4) $E[f \leq a]$

is measurable.

PROOF.   **(1) $\Rightarrow$ (2)**

We can write $E[f \geq a] = \overset{\infty}{\underset{n=1}{\cap}} \left[E\left(f > a - \frac{1}{n} \right) \right]$

From (1) $E\left(f > a - \frac{1}{n} \right)$ is measurable.

Therefore, $E[f \geq a]$, being the enumerable intersection of measurable sets, is measurable.

(2) $\Rightarrow$ (1)

Since $E[f > a] = \overset{\infty}{\underset{n=1}{\cup}} \left[E\left(f \geq a + \frac{1}{n} \right) \right]$

From (1) $E\left(f \geq a + \frac{1}{n} \right)$ is measurable.

Therefore, $E[f > a]$, being the enumerable intersection of measurable sets is measurable.

(2) $\Leftrightarrow$ (3)

Clearly, $E(f < a) = \{ E(f \geq a) \}'$

and $E(f \geq a) = [E(f < a)]'$

We know that a set A is measurable if and only if A' is measurable. Therefore, if set of one side is measurable, then the set of other side will also be measurable.

(3) $\Rightarrow$ (4)

We have $E[f \leq a] = \overset{\infty}{\underset{n=1}{\cap}} \left[E\left(f < a + \frac{1}{n} \right) \right]$

From (3) $E\left(f < a + \frac{1}{n} \right)$ is measurable, therefore $E[f \leq a]$, being the enumerable intersection of measurable sets, is measurable.

$\Rightarrow$ $E[f \leq a]$ is measurable.

(4) $\Rightarrow$ (3)

We have $E[f < a] = \overset{\infty}{\underset{n=1}{\cup}} \left[E \left(f \leq a - \dfrac{1}{n} \right) \right]$

From (4) $E \left(f \leq a - \dfrac{1}{n} \right)$ is measurable.

Therefore, $E[f < a]$, being the enumerable union of measurable sets is measurable.

THEOREM 2.

If function f is Lebesgue measurable over a measurable set E then E(f = a) a $\in$ R is measurable.

PROOF.   Let f be a measurable function defined over a measurable set E. We have to prove that $E[f = a]$ is measurable.

Since, we can write

$$E[f = a] = \{E(f \leq a)\} \cap [E(f \geq a)]$$
$$= \text{Union of two Lebesgue measurable sets}$$
$$= \text{measurable}$$

Hence, $E[f = a]$ is measurable.

THEOREM 3.

Let f be a measurable function defined over a measurable set E and c $\in$ R then cf, f + c, |f|, f^2,

$\dfrac{1}{f}(f \neq 0)$ *are measurable.*

[MEERUT–2009, 14, KANPUR–2006, 07, RAJASTHAN–2008, GARHWAL–2004, ROHTAK–1998]

PROOF.   Let f be a measurable function defined over a measurable set E.

(i)   We have to prove that $cf, c \in R$ is measurable.

Consider $E[cf > a]$ which can be written as

$$E[cf > a] = \begin{cases} E\left[f > \dfrac{a}{c} \right]; & \text{if } c > 0 \\[2mm] E\left[f < \dfrac{a}{c} \right]; & \text{if } c < 0 \end{cases}$$

Since, $a, c \in R \Rightarrow \dfrac{a}{c} \in R$, therefore in both the above cases $E[cf > a]$ is measurable. Hence, cf is measurable over E.

(ii)   We have to prove that $c + f, c \in R$ is measurable over E.

Consider $E[c + f > a]$, which can be written as
$$E[c + f > a] = E[f > a - c]$$
Since, $a, c \in R \Rightarrow a - c \in R$, therefore $E[f > a - c]$ is measurable.

$\Rightarrow$ $E[c + f > a]$ is measurable.

Hence, $c + f$ is measurable over E.

(iii) We have to prove that $|f|$ is measurable over E. Consider $E(|f| > a)$, which can be written as

$$E[|f| > a] = \begin{cases} E, & \text{if } a < 0 \\ E[f > a] \cup E[f < -a] & \text{if } a \geq 0 \end{cases}$$

Both the above cases on RHS are measurable because when $a < 0$, $E[|f| > a] = E$, which is given to be measurable and in case of $a \geq 0$, $E[|f| > a]$ is the union of two measurable sets and hence measurable. Therefore, $E[|f| > a]$ is measurable.

Hence, $|f|$ is measurable over E.

(iv) We have to prove that f^2 is measurable over E. Consider $E[f^2 > a]$ which can be written as

$$E[f^2 > a] = \begin{cases} E; & \text{if } a < 0 \\ E[|f| > \sqrt{a}] & \text{if } a \geq 0 \end{cases}$$

$$= \begin{cases} E & \text{if } a < 0 \\ (E(f > \sqrt{a})) \cup (E(f < -\sqrt{a})) & \text{if } a \geq 0 \end{cases}$$

$$[\because E(|f| > \sqrt{a}) = E(f > \sqrt{a}) \cup E(f < -\sqrt{a})]$$

Since, f is measurable over E therefore $E(f > \sqrt{a})$ and $E(f < -\sqrt{a})$ both are measurable, so being the union of two measurable sets, $E(|f| > \sqrt{a})$ is measurable. Therefore, in both the cases, $E[f^2 > a]$ is measurable. Hence, f^2 is measurable over E.

(v) We have to prove that $\frac{1}{f}(f \neq 0 \text{ on } E)$ is measurable. Consider $E\left[\frac{1}{f} > a\right]$ which can be written as

$$E\left[\frac{1}{f} > a\right] = \begin{cases} E[f \geq 0]; & \text{if } a = 0 \\ E(f > 0) \cap E\left(f < \frac{1}{a}\right); & \text{if } a > 0 \\ \left[E(f < 0) \cap E\left(f < \frac{1}{a}\right)\right] \cup [E(f > 0)]; & \text{if } a < 0 \end{cases}$$

The RHS of the above, is measurable in each case (being the intersection and union of measurable sets). Therefore, $E\left[\frac{1}{f} > a\right]$ is measurable.

Hence, $\frac{1}{f}(f \neq 0 \text{ on } E)$ is measurable over E.

DEDUCTION. If f is measurable over E then $-f$ is also measurable over E (We can prove this result by assuming $c = -1$ in the part (i) of the above theorem).

THEOREM 4.

If f and g are measurable functions defined over a measurable set E, then $f + g$, $f - g$ and fg are measurable over E.

[MEERUT–2001, 03, 04, 08, 10, 14, 17, KANPUR–2005, 06, 07, 11, 12, AVADH–2008, MADRAS–2006, NAGPUR–2006, HPU–2000, 03, GARHWAL–2004, ASSAM–2010, ROHTAK–1999, 2007, ROHILKHAND–2002]

PROOF. Let f and g are measurable functions defined over a measurable set E. We have to prove that $f + g$, $f - g$ and fg are measurable over E.

First of all, we shall prove that if f and g are measurable over E then $E[f > g]$ is measurable over E.

Let $f > g$ then obviously there exists a rational number r such that $f > r > g$ then, we can write

$$E[f > g] = \bigcup_{r \in Q} [(E(f > r)) \cap (E(g < r))] \qquad \ldots(1)$$

Since, the set of rational numbers Q is countable, so RHS of (1) is the countable union of measurable sets ($\because E(f > r) \cap E(g < r)$ is measurable, being the intersections of measurable sets)

Therefore, RHS of (1) is measurable ($\because$ Countable union of measurable sets is again measurable)

$\Rightarrow$ $E[f > g]$ is measurable.

(i) We have to prove that $f + g$ is measurable. Consider $E[f + g > a]$ which can be written as

$$E[f + g > a] = E[f > a - g] \qquad \ldots(2)$$

Since, g is measurable $\quad \Rightarrow -g$ is also measurable.

$\qquad\qquad\qquad\qquad\qquad \Rightarrow a - g$ is also measurable.

Now, f and $a - g$ both are measurable, therefore, $E[f > a - g]$ is measurable (By above proved result just before (i))

$\Rightarrow$ $E[f + g > a]$ is measurable over E.

$\Rightarrow$ $f + g$ is measurable over E.

(ii) We have to prove that if f and g both are measurable, then $f - g$ is also measurable.

Since, g is measurable over $E \Rightarrow -g$ is also measurable over E.

Then apply result (i) for f and $-g$ we conclude that $f - g$ is measurable over E.

(iii) We have to prove that fg is measurable over E.

Since, f and g are measurable over E, therefore

$\qquad\qquad f + g$ and $f - g$ are measurable over E $\qquad\qquad$ (By (i) and (ii))

$\Rightarrow \quad (f + g)^2$ and $(f - g)^2$ are measurable

$\qquad\qquad\qquad\qquad\qquad$ ($\because f$ is measurable $\Rightarrow f^2$ is measurable)

$\Rightarrow \quad (f + g)^2 - (f - g)^2$ is measurable $\qquad\qquad\qquad$ (By (ii))

$\Rightarrow \quad \dfrac{1}{4}[(f + g)^2 - (f - g)^2]$ is measurable.

$\qquad\qquad\qquad\qquad\qquad$ ($\because f$ is measurable $\Rightarrow cf$ is measurable)

$\Rightarrow \quad fg$ is measurable over E.

THEOREM 5.

If f and g are measurable functions defined over a measurable set E and if g is vanishes nowhere on the set E then $\dfrac{f}{g}$ is also measurable over E. [MEERUT–2001, 04, 13]

PROOF. Let f and g be two measurable functions defined over a measurable set E and $g(x) \neq 0 \; \forall \; x \in E$.

Now $g(x) \neq 0 \; \forall \; x \in E \Rightarrow \dfrac{1}{g}$ exists.

Since, g is measurable $\Rightarrow \dfrac{1}{g}$ is also measurable   (By Theorem-3(v))

Further f and $\dfrac{1}{g}$ both are measurable over E.

$\Rightarrow \quad f \cdot \dfrac{1}{g}$ is measurable.   (By theorem 4(iii))

$\Rightarrow \quad \dfrac{f}{g}$ is measurable over E.

DEDUCTION.   Using Theorem-4 and 5, we can conclude that the space of measurable functions is closed under the usual operation of arithmetic, *i.e.,* addition, subtraction, multiplication and division.

In other words, we can say that if f and g are measurable functions defined over a measurable set E. Then $f + g, f - g, fg, \dfrac{f}{g} (g \neq 0)$ are also measurable over E.

THEOREM 6.

If f and g are measurable function defined over a measurable set E then $f \cup g$ and $f \cap g$ are measurable over E.   [MEERUT–2010]

PROOF.   Let f and g are measurable functions defined over a measurable set E. We have to prove that $f \cup g$ and $f \cap g$ are also measurable over E. We can write

$$f \cup g = \frac{1}{2}[(f+g) + |\,f - g\,|]$$ ...(1)

and $$f \cap g = \frac{1}{2}[(f+g) - |\,f - g\,|]$$ ...(2)

Since, f and g are measurable, therefore, $f + g$ and $f - g$ both are measurable (By Theorem-4).

Further $f - g$ is measurable over E

$\Rightarrow \quad |f - g|$ is measurable over E (By Theorem-3(iii))

Now $f + g$ and $|f - g|$ both are measurable, therefore, $(f + g) + |f - g|$ and $(f + g) - |f - g|$ both are measurable.

Hence, from (1) and (2) $f \cup g$ and $f \cap g$ are measurable over E.

THEOREM 7.

If $\langle f_n \rangle$ is a sequence of measurable functions defined over a measurable set E then sup.$\langle f_1 f_2 ... \rangle$ and inf.$\langle f_1 f_2 ... \rangle$ are also measurable over E.   [ROHTAK–2008]

PROOF.   Let $\langle f_n \rangle$ be a sequence of measurable function defined over a measurable set E. We have to prove that sup.$\{f_1 f_2 ...\}$ and inf.$\{f_1 f_2 ...\}$ are measurable.

Since, $\langle f_n \rangle$ is measurable over E, therefore, $E[f_n > a]$ is measurable.

$\Rightarrow \quad E[f_n > a]$ is a measurable subset of E for all $n \in N$ and $a \in R$.

Let us define

$$f(x) = \sup. \langle f_n(x) \rangle, \; x \in E, \; n \in N$$

and $\qquad f(x) = \inf<f_n(x)>, x \in E, n \in N$

Firstly, we shall prove that $f(x) = \sup<f_n(x)>$ is measurable over E.

Consider $E[f > a]$, which can be written as

$$E[f > a] = \bigcup_{n=1}^{\infty} E[f_n > a]$$

$\qquad\qquad$ = an enumerable union of measurable sets

$\qquad\qquad$ = measurable

$\Rightarrow$ f is measurable over E.

$\Rightarrow$ $\sup[<f_n(x)>]$ is measurable, $x \in E, n \in N$

Now, we observe that

$$g(x) = -\sup<f_n(x)>, x \in E, n \in N$$

Since each f_n is measurable over $E, n \in N$

$\Rightarrow$ $-f_n$ is measurable over $E, n \in N$ ($\because f$ is measurable $\Rightarrow cf$ is measurable)

Then by above result, $\sup<-f_n(x)>$ is measurable

$\Rightarrow$ $-\sup<-f_n(x)>$ is measurable.

$\Rightarrow$ $g(x)$ is measurable

$\Rightarrow$ $\inf<f_n(x)>, n \in N, x \in E$ is measurable.

THEOREM 8.

Let $<f_n>$ be a sequence of measurable function defined over a measurable sets then $\overline{\lim} f_n$ and $\underline{\lim} f_n$ are measurable over E and hence $\lim f_n$ is measurable, if exists.

[MEERUT–2000, 01, 09, 12, 15, 16, KANPUR–2001, 02, HPU–1998, 2004, AMRAVATI–2007,

GARHWAL–2012, 15, ROHTAK–2001, 02, 04, PUNJAB–2002, 10]

PROOF. $\qquad$ Let $<f_n>$ be a sequence of measurable functions defined over a measurable set E.

Then we have to prove that $\overline{\lim} f_n$ and $\underline{\lim} f_n$ are measurable over E.

Since, we know that if $<f_n>$ is a sequence of measurable function defined over a measurable set E, then $\sup<f_n(x)>$ and $\inf<f_n(x)>$ are also measurable over E (By Theorem-7).

Now, let us define

$$g_k(x) = \sup_{n \geq k} < fn(x) >$$

and $\qquad h_k(x) = \inf_{n \geq k} < fn(x) >$

Clearly, $g_k(x)$ and $h_k(x)$ are measurable (By Theorem-7)

Then by definition of limit superior and limit inferior, we can write

$$\overline{\lim} f_n(x) = \inf_{k \geq 1} < g_k(x) >$$

and $\qquad \underline{\lim} f_n(x) = \sup_{k \geq 1} < h_k(x) >$

Since, $g_k(x)$ and $h_k(x)$ both are measurable.

$\Rightarrow$ $\inf_{k \geq 1} < g_k(x) >$ and $\sup_{k \geq 1} < h_k(x) >$ are measurable.

$\Rightarrow$ $\overline{\lim} f_n$ and $\underline{\lim} f_n$ are measurable.

Now, it remains to prove that $\lim f_n$, if exist is measurable.

Since, limit exists, therefore,

$$\overline{\lim} f_n = \underline{\lim} f_n = \lim f_n$$

We have already proved that $\overline{\lim} f_n$ and $\underline{\lim} f_n$ both are measurable over E. Hence, $\lim f_n$ is also measurable.

THEOREM 9.

If f and g are measurable real valued function defined on X and $F[f(x), g(x)] = h(x) \; \forall \; x \in X$ be real and continuous functions on the Euclidean plane R^2, then h is measurable.

[MEERUT–2001, KANPUR–2003, NAGPUR–2004, PATNA–2006]

PROOF. Let f and g be two measurable functions defined on X.

Let us define $F[f(x), h(x)] = h(x) \; \forall \; x \in X$ which is real and continuous function on R^2. We have to prove that h is measurable.

Define, $\qquad G_a = \{(p, q) : F(p, q) > a\}$

Clearly, G_a is an open subset of R^2 and therefore it can be expressed as countable union of open intervals such that

$$G_a = \bigcup_{n=1}^{\infty} I_n,$$

where $I_n = \{(p, q) : p \in]a_n, b_n[\text{ and } q \in]c_n, d_n[\} \; a_n, b_n \in R$

Since, f is measurable (given) in X, therefore,

$X[f > a_n]$ and $X[f < b_n]$ both are measurable

Therefore, $\{x \in X : f(x) \in]a_n, b_n[\}$

$\qquad = X(f > a_n) \cap X(f < b_n)$

$\qquad =$ intersection of two measurable sets

$\qquad =$ measurable

In a similar way, we can prove that the set $\{x \in X : g(x) \in]c_n, d_n[\}$ is measurable. Therefore, the set

$[x \in X : F(f(x), g(x)) \in I_n]$

$\qquad = \{x \in X : f(x) \in]a_n, b_n[\} \cap \{x \in X : g(x) \in]c_n, d_n[\}$

$\qquad =$ Intersection of two measurable sets

$\qquad =$ a measurable set

Finally, $\{x \in X : h(x) > a\}$

$\qquad = \{x \in X : (f(x), g(x)) \in G_a\}$

$\qquad = \bigcup_{n=1}^{\infty} \{x \in X : (f(x), g(x)) \in I_n\}$

$\qquad =$ measurable $\qquad$ ($\because$ Enumerable union of measurable sets is again measurable)

Hence, $h(x)$ is measurable over X.

THEOREM 10.

A continuous function defined over a measurable set E is measurable.

[MEERUT–2002, 05, 07, 08, KANPUR–2005, GARHWAL–2006, DELHI–2007]

PROOF. Let f be a continuous function defined over a measurable set E. We have to prove that f is a measurable over E.

For any real number a, consider the set $E[f \geq a]$

First we shall prove that $E[f \geq a]$ is a closed set. Here it is sufficient to prove that it contains all its limit points.

Let $A = E[f \geq a]$

$\therefore$ We have to prove that $D(A) \subseteq A$

Let $x_0 \in D(A)$ be arbitrary $\Rightarrow x_0$ is the limit point of A

$\Rightarrow$ $\exists$ a sequence $\langle x_n \rangle$ of elements of A such that $\lim_{n \to \infty} x_n = x_0$.

Since, f is continuous at x_0. Therefore

$$x_n \to x_0 \quad \Rightarrow \quad f(x_n) \to f(x_0)$$

Now, $x_n \in A$

$\Rightarrow \quad f(x_n) \geq a \quad \Rightarrow \quad \lim_{n \to \infty} f(x_n) \geq a$

$\Rightarrow \quad f(x_0) \geq a \qquad\qquad\qquad\qquad (\because \lim f(x_n) = f(x_0))$

$\Rightarrow \quad x_0 \in A$

i.e., $x_0 \in D(A) \quad \Rightarrow \quad x_0 \in A$

Since, x_0 is arbitrary, therefore, $D(A) \subseteq A$

$\Rightarrow \quad A$ is closed.

$\Rightarrow \quad A$ is measurable. $\qquad (\because$ Every closed subset of real number is measurable)

$\Rightarrow \quad E[f \geq a]$ is measurable.

$\Rightarrow \quad f$ is measurable over the measurable set E.

☞ **REMARKS**

• The above theorem can be restated as, "A continuous function defined in a closed interval is measurable."

• Converse of the above theorem is not necessarily true, i.e., a measurable function need not be continuous. **For example:**

(1) A function $f : R \to \{0, 1\}$ defined by $f(x) = \begin{cases} 1; & 0 \leq x \leq 1 \\ 0; & \text{otherwise} \end{cases}$

Clearly, f is measurable but not continuous. The point $x = 0$ is a point of discontinuity.

(2) Consider the function $f(x)$ defined over the closed interval $E = (0, 2)$ such that

$$f(x) = \begin{cases} 1; & x \in [0,1] = A (\text{say}) \\ 2; & x \in]1,2] = A' \end{cases}$$

Then $\qquad E[f > a] = \begin{cases} \phi & \text{if} \quad a \geq 2 \\ A' & \text{if} \quad 1 \leq a < 2 \\ E & \text{if} \quad a < 1 \end{cases}$

Clearly, this function is measurable on $(0, 2)$ but has a sudden jump in the value of $f(x)$ near $x = 1$. Hence, $f(x)$ is discontinuous at $x = 1$.

THEOREM 11.

Let f be a function defined on a measurable set E. Then f is measurable if and only if for any open set $G \subseteq R$, $f^{-1}(G)$ is a measurable set.

PROOF. Let us suppose f is measurable over E. We have to prove that $f^{-1}(G)$ is a measurable set.

Let G be any open subset of R.

$\Rightarrow \quad G$ can be expressed as a countable union of disjoint open intervals, i.e.,

$$G = \bigcup_{n=1}^{\infty} I_n \text{ where } I_n =]a_n, b_n[.$$

Therefore, $f^{-1}(G) = \bigcup_n [x \in E : f(x) \in I_n]$

But $f(x) \in I_n =]a_n, b_n[\qquad \Rightarrow \quad f(x) \in]a_n, b_n[$

$$\Rightarrow \quad a_n < f(x) < b_n$$

$$\Rightarrow \qquad f^{-1}(G) = \bigcup_n [E(f > a_n) \cap (f < b_n)]$$

$$= \bigcup_n [\text{Intersection of two measurable sets}]$$

$$= \bigcup_n [\text{measurable sets}]$$

$$= \text{measurable} \qquad\qquad (\because \text{ enumerable union of measurable sets is measurable})$$

Hence, $f^{-1}(G)$ is measurable.

Conversely, let $f^{-1}(G)$ is measurable. We have to prove that f is measurable.

Let $\qquad\qquad G =]a, \infty[,\ a > 0$

$$\Rightarrow \qquad f^{-1}[G] = \{x \in E : f(x) \in]a, \infty[\}$$

$$= \{x \in E : a < f(x) < \infty\}$$

$$= E[f > a]$$

Since, $f^{-1}(G)$ is measurable (given), therefore, $E[f > a]$ is measurable. Hence f is measurable over a measurable set E.

THEOREM 12.

If f is a measurable function defined over a measurable set E and if f and g are equivalent functions then g is also measurable over E.

PROOF. Let f be a measurable function defined over a measurable set E and $a \in R$. Clearly $E[f > a]$ is measurable.

Suppose f and g are equivalent functions.

$$\Rightarrow \qquad f = g = a \cdot e \text{ on } E$$

We have to prove that g is measurable over E, i.e., $E[g > a]$ is a measurable set.

Since, $f = g = a \cdot e$ therefore, $\exists A \subset E$ such that $m(A) = 0$ and $f(x) = g(x) \ \forall \ x \in E - A = B$ (say)

$\Rightarrow \quad f \neq g$ on A, $f = g$ on B and $m(A) = 0$

$\Rightarrow \quad A \cap B = \phi,\ E = A \cup B$

Now, $m(A) = 0 \quad \Rightarrow \quad A$ is measurable. ($\because$ A set of measure zero is measurable)

$\therefore\ E$ and A both are measurable $\Rightarrow E - A (= B)$ is measurable.

So, f is measurable over E and $B \subseteq E$ is measurable.

$\Rightarrow \quad f$ is measurable over B.

$\Rightarrow \quad B[f > a]$ is measurable.

$\Rightarrow \quad B[g > a]$ is measurable. $\qquad\qquad\qquad (\because f = g \text{ on } B)$

Also, $A[g > a] = \{x \in A : g(x) > a\} \subset A$ and $m(A) = 0$

$\Rightarrow \quad A[g > a]$ is measurable.

Finally, $E[g > a] = [A(g > a)] \cup [B(g > a)] \qquad\qquad (\because E = A \cup B)$

$\qquad\qquad = $ which is a measurable set, being the union of two measurable sets

$\Rightarrow \quad E[g > a]$ is measurable.

$\Rightarrow \quad g$ is measurable.

☞ **REMARK**
- The above theorem can be restated as follows: "If f is measurable function and if $f = g$ almost everywhere ($a \cdot e$) then g is measurable".

THEOREM 13.

A function f is measurable if and only if the set $\{x : f(x) < r\}$ is measurable for every rational number r.

[KANPUR–2010, MEERUT–2001, 04, 12, 16, GARHWAL–2003, ALLAHABAD–2007, BANARAS–2011]

PROOF. Let f be a fucntion defined over a measurable set E and $r \in Q$ be arbitrary.

Let us first suppose f is measurable over $E \Rightarrow E[f < c]$ is measurable.

To prove $\{x : f(x) < r\}$ is measurable.

Since, $E[f < c]$ is measurable $\forall\ c \in R$.

$\Rightarrow\quad E[f < c]$ is measurable for all $c \in Q$ $\hspace{2cm}(\because Q \subseteq R)$

$\Rightarrow\quad E[f < r]$ is measurable for $r \in Q$

$\Rightarrow\quad \{x : f(x) < r\} = \{x \in E : f(x) < r\}$ is measurable.

$\Rightarrow\quad \{x : f(x) < r\}$ is measurable.

Conversely, suppose that $\{x : f(x) < r\}$ is measurable. We have to prove that f is measurable. We have

$$E[f < c] = \{x \in E : f(x) < c\}$$

$$= \bigcup_{r \in Q} \{x \in E : f(x) < r < c\}$$

$$= \bigcup_{r \in Q} \{x \in E : f(x) < r, r < c\}$$

$$= \text{measurable set}$$

$\hspace{2cm}(\because$ enumerable union of measurable sets is measurable$)$

$\Rightarrow\quad E[f < c]$ is measurable.

Hence, f is measurable over E.

THEOREM 14.

If f is a continuous function and g is a measurable function then composite function fog is measurable.

PROOF. Let f be a continuous function and g is a measurable function.

We have to prove that fog is measurable.

Let G be an open set such that

For any real number a

$$A = E[fog > a] = \{x \in E : (fog)x > a\}$$

$$= \{x \in E : f(g(x)) > a\}$$

$$= \{x \in E : g(x) \in G\}$$

We claim that A is a measurable set.

Since, G is an open set, therefore, it can be expressed as the countable union of disjoint open intervals such that

$$G = \bigcup_n I_n \text{ where } I_n =]a_n, b_n[$$

So, $$A = \{x : g(x) \in G\} = \bigcup_n \{x : g(x) \in I_n\}$$

$$= \bigcup_n \{x : g(x) \in]a_n, b_n[\} = \bigcup_n \{x : a_n < g(x) < b_n\}$$

$$= \bigcup_n \{x : g(x) > a_n\} \cap \{x : g(x) < b_n\}$$

$$= \bigcup_n \{\text{Intersection of two measurable sets}\}$$

$$= \text{measurable} \quad \text{(Being the countable union of measurable sets)}$$

$\Rightarrow$ A is measurable.

Hence, fog is measurable over E.

TWO IMPORTANT DEFINITIONS

Definition 1. *Let f_1 and f_2 be two real valued functions with common domain E then the function $f^m = max\{f_1, f_2\}$, and $f_m = min\{f_1, f_2\}$ are defined to be the real valued functions on E such that*

$$f^m(x) = max\{f_1(x), f_2(x)\}$$

and $\qquad f_m(x) = min\{f_1(x), f_2(x)\}$

Definition 2. *Let f be a function then its positive part (f^+) and its negative part (f^-) are defined as follows:*

$$f^+ = max(f, 0) = \frac{1}{2}[f + |f|] \text{ and } f^- = max(-f, 0) = \frac{1}{2}[|f| - f]$$

☛ REMARKS

- $f = f^+ - f^-$
- $|f| = f^+ + f^-$

THEOREM 15.

If f_1 and f_2 are measurable function on E then f^m and f_m are measurable.

PROOF. For any real number a, we can write

$$E[f^m > a] = E[f_1 > a] \cup E[f_2 > a]$$

and $\qquad E[f_m > a] = E[f_1 > a] \cap E[f_2 > a]$

Since, f_1 and f_2 both are measurable over E therefore $E[f_1 > a]$ and $E[f_2 > a]$ both are measurable. Hence, $E[f^m > a]$, being the union of two measurable sets and $E[f_m > a]$, being the intersection of two measurable sets is measurable.

THEOREM 16.

A function f is measurable if and only if both its positive and negative parts are measurable function.

PROOF. For every real valued function f, we may write

$$f^+ = \frac{1}{2}[f + |f|] \text{ and } f^- = \frac{1}{2}[|f| - f]$$

Since f is measurable therefore, $|f|$ is also measurable.

$\Rightarrow$ $(f + |f|)$ and $(|f| - f)$ are measurable.

$\Rightarrow$ $\frac{1}{2}(f + |f|)$ and $\frac{1}{2}(|f| - f)$ are measurable.

$\Rightarrow$ f^+ and f^- both are measurable.

Conversely, let f^+ and f^- both are measurable. To prove f is measurable.

Since, we can write

$$f = f^+ - f^-$$

Clearly f, being the difference of two measurable function is measurable.

5.5 BOREL MEASURABLE FUNCTION

Let f be a function defined on a Borel set E. Then f is said to be Borel measurable or simply Borel function on E if for all $a \in R$ the set $E[f > a]$ is a Borel set.

☛ REMARKS

- Every Borel measurable function is Lebesgue measurable.
- Every measurable function is not necessarily Borel function. For example, the characteristic function of a set of non-Borel Lebesgue measurable set is Lebesgue measurable function but not Borel measurable function.

5.5.1 DIRECT CONSEQUENCE OF BOREL FUNCTION WITH MEASURABLE FUNCTION

If we replace Lebesgue measurable set by a Borel set and Lebesgue measurable function by Borel measurable function, then results obtained in this chapter, will holds for Borel functions also. Some of them are given below :

(1) Let f be an extended real valued function defined on a Borel set E then following are equivalent :

(i) $E[f > a]$ is a Borel set $\forall\ a \in R$

(ii) $E[f \geq a]$ is a Borel set $\forall\ a \in R$

(iii) $E[f < a]$ is a Borel set $\forall\ a \in R$

(iv) $E[f \leq a]$ is a Borel set $\forall\ a \in R$

(2) Let f and g be Borel measurable functions on E and $c \in R$ then each of the following functions is a Borel measurable on E :

(i) $f \pm c$ (ii) cf

(iii) $f \pm g$ (iv) fg

(v) $|f|$ (vi) f^2

(vii) $\dfrac{f}{g}\,(g \neq 0)$

(3) Let $<f_n>$ be a sequence of Borel measurable functions then the function $\max\{f_1, f_2, \ldots, f_n\}$, $\min\{f_1, f_2, \ldots, f_n\}$, $\sup f_n$, $\inf f_n$, and $\overline{\lim}\, f_n$, $\underline{\lim}\, f_n$ are all Borel measurable function.

(4) A continuous function defined on a Borel set is Borel measurable.

(5) If f is a Borel measurable function and B is a Borel set then $f^{-1}(B)$ is a Borel set.

(6) If f and g are Borel measurable functions then fog and gof are also Borel measurable.

(7) If f is a Borel function and g a Lebesgue measurable function then fog (i.e., Borel function of a Lebesgue measurable function) is a Lebesgue measurable function.

(8) To every measurable function f, there correspond a Borel measurable function g such that $g = f$ $a \cdot e$

(9) If f is an increasing function on R then f is a Borel measurable function.

Solved Examples

EXAMPLE I. *Show that every function defined on a set of measure zero is measurable.*

[MEERUT–2009, AMRAVATI–2007]

SOLUTION. Let f be a function defined on a measurable set such that $m(E) = 0$.

We have to prove that f is measurable.

Consider $E[f > a] = \{x \in E : f(x) > a\}$ $a \in R$

Now since $E[f > a] \subseteq E$

$\Rightarrow \qquad m[E(f > a)] \leq m(E) = 0$

$\Rightarrow \qquad m[E(f > a)] \leq 0$

But, we know that $m[E(f > a)] \geq 0$

$\Rightarrow \qquad m[E(f > a)] = 0$

$\Rightarrow \quad f$ is measurable.   ($\because$ Every set of measure zero is measurable)

EXAMPLE 2.   *Show that if f is a measurable function on [a, b] then the inverse image under f of any interval is also a measurable set.*

SOLUTION.   Consider a semi-open interval $[a, b[$. Then we can write

$$[a, b[= [a, \infty[\cap]-\infty, b[$$

$\Rightarrow \qquad f^{-1}([a, b[) = f^{-1}[a, \infty[\cap f^{-1}]-\infty, b[$

$$= E[f \geq a] \cap E[f > b], \; E = [p, q]$$

Now, since f is measurable, therefore, $E[f \geq a]$ and $E[f < b]$ are both measurable. Hence, being the intersection of two measurable sets. $f^{-1}[a, b[$ is a measurable set. Similarly, we may prove that the result for other type of intervals.

EXAMPLE 3.   *If f is a measurable function, then show that for each extended real number a, the set $\{x : f(x) = a\}$ is a measurable set, but converse is not true.*   [HPU–1998, 20003]

SOLUTION.   Let us first suppose that f is a measurable function, then we have to prove that for each extended real number a, the set $\{x : f(x) = a\}$ is a measurable set. Here we have the following cases:

Case-I: If a is finite

Then we can write

$$\{x : f(x) = a\} = [x : f(x) \geq a] \cap [x : f(x) \leq a]$$
$$= \text{intersection of two measurable sets}$$
$$= \text{measurable}$$

$\Rightarrow \quad \{x : f(x) = a\}$ is measurable.

Case-II: If $a = \infty$ or $-\infty$

For $a = \infty$, $\{x : f(x) = \infty\} = \bigcap_{n=1}^{\infty} \{x : f(x) > n\}$

$$= \text{enumerable intersection of measurable sets}$$
$$= \text{measurable}$$

For $a = -\infty$, $\{x : f(x) = -\infty\} = \bigcap_{n=1}^{\infty} \{x : f(x) < -n\}$

$$= \text{enumerable intersection of measurable sets}$$
$$= \text{measurable}$$

Now, we shall prove that, converse of the above is not true.

Let A be non-measurable subset of R and f is defined as

$$f(x) = \begin{cases} x^2, & \text{if } x \in A \\ -x^2, & \text{if } x \in A' \end{cases}$$

Clearly, the set $R(f = a)$ for every $a \in R$ contains exactly two elements and hence measurable.

But $R(f > 0) = A - \{0\}$ which is non-measurable, therefore the function f is not measurable.

EXAMPLE 4. *Let A and B be measurable sets and f is a function with domain A ∪ B. Show that f is measurable iff the restriction to A and B are measurable.* [HPU–2000]

SOLUTION. The restriction of f can be defined as follows:

$$f \mid A(x) = f(x), \ x \in A \text{ and } f \mid B(x) = f(x), \ x \in B \qquad \qquad ...(1)$$

From (1)

$$f(x) > a \text{ iff } f \mid A(x) > a, \ x \in A$$

and

$$f(x) > a \text{ iff } f \mid B(x) > a, \ x \in B$$

$$\Rightarrow \qquad A \cup B(f > a) = A(f \mid A > a) \cup B(f \mid B > a) \qquad \qquad ...(2)$$

Now, first suppose that $f \mid A$ and $f \mid B$ are measurable. We have to prove that f is measurable.

$f \mid A$ and $f \mid B$ are measurable.

$\Rightarrow \quad A(f \mid A > a)$ and $B(f \mid B > a)$ are measurable.

$\Rightarrow \quad A(f \mid A > a) \cup B(f \mid B > a)$ is measurable.

$\Rightarrow \quad A \cup B(f > a)$ is measurable.

$\Rightarrow \quad f$ is measurable over $A \cup B$.

Conversely, suppose that f is measurable over $A \cup B$.

Then clearly f is measurable over A $\qquad\qquad (\because A \subseteq A \cup B)$

$\Rightarrow \quad A[f > a]$ is measurable.

But for all $x \in A$, $f(x) = f \mid A(x)$, therefore

$A[f \mid A > a] = A(f > a)$, which is measurable

$\Rightarrow \quad f \mid A$ is measurable.

Similarly, we may prove that $f \mid B$ is measurable.

EXAMPLE 5. *Let f be a function with measurable domain D. Show that f is measurable if and only if the function g defined by*

$$g(x) = \begin{cases} f(x) & for \quad x \in D \\ 0 & for \quad x \notin D \end{cases}$$

is measurable. [HPU–2000, 01]

SOLUTION. Let f be a measurable function on D.

Now, $\qquad E[g > a] = \begin{cases} D[f > a] & \text{if} \quad a \leq 0 \\ D(f > a) \cup D' & \text{if} \quad a < 0 \end{cases}$

Also, since D is measurable $\Rightarrow D'$ is measurable.

and f is measurable $\quad \Rightarrow \quad D(f > a)$ is measurable.

$\qquad\qquad\qquad\qquad \Rightarrow \quad D(f > a) \cup D'$ is measurable.

Therefore, in both the above cases $E(g > a)$ is measurable.

$\Rightarrow \quad g$ is measurable.

Conversely let us suppose that g is measurable. To prove f is measurable. Since, domain of f is D, we get

$$D(f > a) = D(g > a)$$

which is measurable for all $a \in R$ $\quad (\because g$ is measurable $\Rightarrow D(g > a)$ is measurable)

Hence, f is measurable.

EXAMPLE 6. *Let f be a measurable real valued function, then show that $|f|^p$, $p > 0$ and exp.(ct) are also measurable.*

SOLUTION. Let f be a measurable function. Clearly, we know that $|f|^p, p > 0$ and exp.(ct) both are continuous function and every continuous function is measurable.

Hence, both the functions under considerations are measurable.

EXAMPLE 7. *Show that a necessary and sufficient condition for measurability of a function f is that the set $\{x : a \leq f(x) \leq b\}$ should be measurable for all extended real numbers a and b such that $a < b$ (i.e., a and b can be such that $a = -\infty, b = \infty$).*

SOLUTION. Let us first suppose that f is measurable. We have to prove that the set $\{x : a \leq f(x) \leq b\}$ is also measurable.

Since, f is measurable, therefore, $\{x : f(x) \geq a\}$ and $\{x : f(x) \leq b\}$ both are measurable.

Now, $\{x : a \leq f(x) \leq b\} = \{x : f(x) \geq a\} \cap \{x : f(x) \leq b\}$

$\qquad\qquad\qquad\qquad$ = intersection of two measurable sets

$\qquad\qquad\qquad\qquad$ = measurable

Conversely, suppose that $\{x : a \leq f(x) \leq b\}$ is measurable. To prove that f is measurable.

Since, $\{x : a \leq f(x) \leq b\}$ is measurable

$\Rightarrow \quad \{x : a \leq f(x)\}$ is measurable

$\Rightarrow \quad \{x : f(x) \geq a\}$ is measurable

$\rightarrow \quad f$ is measurable.

EXAMPLE 8. *Show that the set of all measurable function form a vector space over R.*

SOLUTION. Let E be a measurable set and V be the set of all measurable functions defined on E. Then

$$V = \{f : f : E \rightarrow R \text{ is a measurable function}\}$$

We have to prove that $V(R)$ is a vector space.

We know that if f is measurable then cf is measurable and f and measurable

$\Rightarrow f \pm g, fg, -f$ all are measurable.

(1) Firstly we shall prove that $(V, +)$ is an abelian group

$\quad$ (i) $\quad f, g \in V \qquad\qquad \Rightarrow \quad f$ and g are measurable

$\qquad\qquad\qquad\qquad\qquad\quad \Rightarrow \quad f + g$ is measurable

$\qquad\qquad\qquad\qquad\qquad\quad \Rightarrow \quad f + g \in V$

$\quad$ (ii) $\quad \exists\, O \in V$ such that $f + O = O + f = f$

$\qquad\qquad$ where O is the zero function such that $O(x) = 0\ \forall\ x$, clearly O is a special case of constant function.

$\quad$ (iii) $\quad$ Since $(R, +)$ is always an abelian group, therefore,

$$f + g = g + f$$

$\quad$ (iv) $\quad f \in V \Rightarrow -f \in V$

$\quad$ (v) $\quad f + (g + h) = (f + g) + h \qquad\qquad\qquad\qquad (\because (R, +) \text{ is abelian})$

$\qquad\qquad \Rightarrow (V, +)$ is an abelian group.

(2) $\quad f \in V \quad \Rightarrow \quad af \in V$, so

$$(a + b)f = af + bf \text{ and } (a + b)f \in V$$

$$a(f + g) = af + ag$$

and $\qquad\qquad 1 \cdot f = f$

Hence, we conclude that $V(R)$ is a vector space.

EXAMPLE 9. *Determine whether the function defined below is measurable*

$$f(x) = \begin{cases} x+5; & if \quad x<-1 \\ 2; & if \quad -1\le x<0 \\ x^2; & if \quad 0\le x \end{cases}$$

[MEERUT–2004, 05, 09, 15, 16, 17, KANPUR–2007]

SOLUTION. Let $a \in R$. Then $a<0$ and

$$R(f\le a) \quad \Rightarrow \quad x+5 \le a \Rightarrow x\le a-5$$

$$\therefore \quad R[f\le a] = [-\infty, a-5]$$

In view of the above, we can write

$$R[f\le a] = \begin{cases}]-\infty, a-5]; & if \quad a<0 \\ ]-\infty, -5]\cup\{0\}; & if \quad a=0 \\ ]-\infty, a-5]\cup[0,\sqrt{a}]; & if \quad 0<a<2 \\ ]-\infty, a-5]\cup[-1,\sqrt{a}]; & if \quad 2\le a\le 4 \\ ]-\infty, \sqrt{a}]; & if \quad 4\le a \end{cases}$$

All the above sets in RHS are clearly measurable,. So, $R[f\le a]$ is measurable. Hence, f is measurable over R.

EXAMPLE 10. *Let f be a function defined on* $\left[0, \dfrac{1}{\pi}\right]$ *as follows:*

$$f(x) = \begin{cases} 0\cdot 1, & if \quad x=0 \\ 2x\sin\dfrac{1}{x}, & if \quad x>0 \end{cases}$$

Find the measure of the set $\{x : f(x) \ge 0\}$

SOLUTION. Clearly, $f(x) \ge 0$ for $x=0, \dfrac{1}{\pi}$ and in the interval $\left[\dfrac{1}{(2n+1)\pi}, \dfrac{1}{2n\pi}\right], n\in N$.

Therefore, $\{x : f(x)\ge 0\} = \left\{0, \dfrac{1}{\pi}, \left[\dfrac{1}{(2n+1)\pi}, \dfrac{1}{2n\pi}\right], n\in N\right\}$

So, $m\{x : f(x)\ge 0\} = m\left\{0, \dfrac{1}{\pi}\right\} + \sum_{n=1}^{\infty} m\left[\dfrac{1}{(2n+1)\pi}, \dfrac{1}{2n\pi}\right]$

$$= 0 + \sum_{n=1}^{\infty}\left[\dfrac{1}{2n\pi} - \dfrac{1}{(2n+1)\pi}\right] = \dfrac{1}{\pi}\sum_{n=1}^{\infty}\left(\dfrac{1}{2n} - \dfrac{1}{2n+1}\right)$$

$$= \dfrac{1}{\pi}\left[\dfrac{1}{2} - \dfrac{1}{3} + \dfrac{1}{4} - \dfrac{1}{5} + ...\right]$$

$$= \dfrac{1}{\pi}\left[1 - 1 + \dfrac{1}{2} - \dfrac{1}{3} + \dfrac{1}{4} - ...\right]$$

$$= \dfrac{1}{\pi}\left[1 - \log_e 2\right]$$

Exercise 5.1

1. Show that a function which is continuous in an open interval in measurable.

2. Show that the sum, difference and product of two simple functions is a simple function.

3. If I_1, I_2 are intervals of real numbers and f is a measurable function, then show that $f^{-1}[I_1 \cup I_2]$ is a measurable set.

4. If f is an extended real valued function with measurable domain D and $D_1 = \{x : f(x) = \infty\}$ and $D_2 = \{x : f(x) = -\infty\}$ then show that f is measurable on D if and only if D_1, D_2 are measurable sets and restriction of f on $D - (D_1 \cup D_2)$ is measurable.

5. Show that the function $f(x) = [x]$, where $[\cdot]$ is the greatest integer function, is measurable.

6. Show that the function $f : R \to [0, 1]$ defined by $f(x) = 1$, if $0 \le x < 1$ and $f(x) = 0$, otherwise, is a measurable but not continuous.

7. Show that the Cardinality of the class of measurable function is 2^c.

8. Let $\langle f_n \rangle$ be a sequence of measurable function defined in D. Show that the set of points in D where this sequence tends to a limit is measurable.

9. If f is a measurable function on each of the set in a collection $\{E_i\}$ of pairwise disjoint measurable sets then show that f is measurable on $\cup E_i$ also.

10. Let $f : R \to R$ such that

$$f(x) = \begin{cases} \dfrac{1}{x(x-1)}, & x \ne 0, 1 \\ 2, & x = 0, 1 \end{cases}$$

Is f measurable?

11. Let f be a non-negative measurable function and let $\{r_k : k = 1, 2, \ldots\}$ be an enumeration of positive rationals, show that

$$\sqrt{f(x)} = \frac{1}{2} \inf_k \left(\frac{1}{r_k} f(x) + r_k \right)$$

and hence $f^{1/2}$ is a measurable function.

12. Show that the function f defined on $E = [0, 1]$ is measurable where

$$f(x) = \begin{cases} 3; & \text{if} \quad x = 0 \\ 1/x; & \text{if} \quad 0 < x < 1 \\ 5; & \text{if} \quad x = 1 \end{cases}$$

13. Show that an increasing function of a measurable function is also a measurable function.

14. Show that $f(x) = \begin{cases} 1 & \text{if} \quad x \in A \\ -1 & \text{if} \quad x \in A' \end{cases}$

where A is a non-measurable subset of a measurable set E is not measurable while $f^2(x) \ \forall \ x \in E$ is measurable.

15. Let f be a measurable function not almost everywhere infinite. Show that there exists a set of positive measure on which f is bounded.

16. Show that a nowhere dense perfect set can contain a non-measurable set.

17. Show that a measurable function of a continuous function is not necessarily measurable.

18. Show that there exist sets of zero measure which are not Borel set.

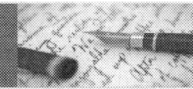

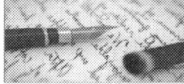

CHAPTER Summary

⪼ KEY TERMS

- **MEASURABLE FUNCTION:** An extended real valued function f defined over a measurable set E is said to be Lebesgue measurable if the set $\{x \in E : f(x) > a\}$ is measurable.

- **ALMOST EVERYWHERE:** A relation which holds in a set of measure zero is said to hold almost everywhere.

- **EQUIVALENT FUNCTIONS:** Two functions f and g defined on the same set E are said to be equivalent if $\exists A, B \subset E$ such that $E = A \cup B$, $f = g$ on A, $f \neq g$ on B, $m(B) = 0$.

- **CHARACTERISTIC FUNCTION:** Let A be a subset of E. The characteristic function χ_A of A is defined by
$$\chi_A(x) = \begin{cases} 0 & \text{if } x \in A \\ 1 & \text{if } x \in A' \end{cases}$$

- **SIMPLE FUNCTION:** A function is said to be simple if the range of the function is finite.

- **STEP FUNCTION:** A real valued function f defined on an interval $[a, b]$ is said to be step function if there exists a partition $a = x_0 < x_1 < x_2 < \ldots < x_n = b$ such that the function assumes one and only one value in each interval.

⪼ RESULTS

- The characteristic function $\chi_A(x)$ is measurable if and only if A is measurable.

- Every monotone sequence of sets is convergent.

- If f is a constant function over a measurable set E then f is measurable.

- If f is measurable over E and $A \subseteq E$ then f is measurable over A also.

- If f and g are measurable over E then $f \pm g$, fg, $cf, c \in R$, $\dfrac{f}{g}(g \neq 0)$ all are measurable. Also $f \cap g$ and $f \cup g$ are measurable.

- The set of all measurable functions form a vector space.

- Let $\langle f_n \rangle$ be a sequence of measurable functions defined over a measurable set E then $\sup \langle f_n \rangle$, $\inf \langle f_n \rangle$, $\varlimsup < f_n >$, $\varliminf < f_n >$ and $\lim f_n$ all are measurable.

- A continuous function defined over a measurable set is measurable.

- The limit of the convergent sequence of measurable function is measurable.

- A continuous function defined over a measurable set is measurable.

- The limit of the convergent sequence of measurable function is measurable.

- If f is a measurable function and $g = f$ a.e. then g is also measurable.

- A function f is measurable iff the set $\{x : f(x) < r\}$ is measurable for every rational number r.

- If f is continuous and g is measurable then $f \circ g$ is measurable.

- Every Borel measurable function is Lebesgue measurable.

- If f is Borel measurable function and A is a Borel set then $f^{-1}(A)$ is Borel measurable.

- The product of two measurable functions is a Borel measurable function.

⪼ WORTHY READINGS

☞ The measure of the set $E[f > a]$ may be finite or infinite.

☞ A constant function with a measurable domain is measurable.

☞ Let f be a function defined over a measurable set E. Then f is measurable if and only if the set $E[f > r]$ is measurable for each rational number r.

☞ Let D be a dense set of real numbers and f be an extended real valued function on R such that $R[f > a]$ is measurable for each $a \in D$. Then f is measurable.

☞ If $\langle f_n \rangle$ is a sequence of measurable function converging to f on E then f is a measurable function.

☞ The set of points on which a sequence $\langle f_n \rangle$ of measurable functions converges is measurable.

☞ The characteristic function of non-measurable sets are non-measurable even though the domain set is measurable.

☞ Each characteristic function of a measurable set is a simple function.

☞ A finite linear combinations of simple function are again simple function.

☞ A continuous function defined on a Borel sets is Borel measurable.

☞ To every measurable function f, there correspond a Borel measurable function g such that $f = g$ a.e.

☞ FURTHER READINGS

☞ A complex valued function is called measurable if both its real and imaginary parts are measurable.

☞ Borel measurable function of a measurable function is a measurable function.

☞ It is not true even if X is measurable, that a Lebesgue measurable function is a measurable function.

☞ There exists a Lebesgue measurable set M, $M \subset \{y : 0 \leq y \leq 1\}$ such that $f^{-1}(M)$ is not Lebesgue measurable.

☞ Let $x \in [0, 1]$ have the expansion to the base l, $x = 0 \cdot x_1 \cdot x_2 \cdot \ldots \cdot x_n \cdot \ldots$ for some integer l, the non-terminating expansion being used in case of ambiguity, then $f_n(x) = x_n$ is a measurable function of x for each n.

☞ Not every measurable set is a Borel set.

☞ Let f be a measurable function on $[a, b]$ and let f be differentiable a.e. then there is a function measurable on $[a, b]$ which equals f' a.e.

☞ There may exists sets of zero measure which are not Borel set.

☞ To every measurable function f, there corresponds a Borel measurable function g such that $f = g$ a.e.

☞ The characteristic function of a set which is Lebesgue measurable and non-Borel is Lebesgue measurable but not a Borel measurable function.

☞ A measurable function of a measurable function may not be measurable.

□□□□

Chapter
6
The Lebesgue Integral of a Function

6.1 INTRODUCTION

In previous classes, we have studied about the Riemann integrals. In Riemann integral, we use subdivison of closed interval $[a, b]$ into subinterval. In present chapter we shall study the Lebesgue integral of a function, in which we use subdivisons of closed interval $[a, b]$ into general kinds of measurable sets. Lebesgue definition of an integral is more general in comparison of Riemann. It enable us to integrate those functions for which Riemann's method fails. The Riemann integral is based on the assumption that f is continuous and bounded function defined on a closed interval $[a, b]$, but Lebesgue integral is defined for both bounded and unbounded functions. It generalize the Riemann integral and hence enlarge the class of integrable functions.

☞ REMARK
- Every Riemann integrable function is Lebesgue integrable but converse is not necessarily true.

6.2 LEBESGUE SUMS

6.2.1 PARTITION

Let $[a, b]$ be the given closed interval. Then by a measurable partition of $[a, b]$, we mean any finite collection $\{P_r : r \in N\}$ of measurable subsets of $[a, b]$ such that

$$\bigcup_{r=1}^{n} P_r = [a, b] \text{ and } m[P_i \cap P_j] = 0, i \neq j$$

Here, the partition of an interval is denoted by P and the sets $P_1, P_2, ..., P_n$ are called the components of the partition P.

Therefore, $P = \{P_1, P_2, ..., P_n\}$

Therefore, a measurable partition P of an interval $[a, b]$ is a finite collection of subsets of $[a, b]$ whose union is the whole $[a, b]$ and whose pairwise intersection have the measure zero.

☞ REMARK
- In case of Riemann subdivision, the components are necessarily intervals while in case of Lebesgue partition, the components are any set.

Illustrations

✦ Many measurable partition do not have interval components. For example, $\{E_1, E_2\}$ is a measurable partition of $[a, b]$ where E_1 and E_2 are respectively the set of all the rationals and irrationals numbers of the interval $[a, b]$.

6.2.2 REFINEMENT OF A PARTITION

Let $[a, b]$ be the closed interval and P be a measurable partition of $[a, b]$. Then another measurable partition P^* of $[a, b]$ is said to be refinement of P if every component of P^* is contained in some components of P. It is written as $P \subset P^*$.

☛ REMARK
- Refinement P^* of P can be constructed by breaking up the components of P.

6.2.3 COMMON REFINEMENT

Let $P = \{P_1, P_2, ..., P_n\}$ and $Q = \{Q_1, Q_2, ..., Q_n\}$ be any two measurable partition of $[a, b]$ then the partition PQ whose components are the sets $P_i \cap Q_j : i \in N, j \in N$ is a common refinement of P and Q, i.e.,

$$PQ = \{P_i = Q_j : i \in N, j \in N\}$$

6.2.4 LOWER AND UPPER LEBESGUE SUMS

Let $P = \{P_1, P_2, ..., P_n\}$ be a measurable partition of the closed interval $[a, b]$ and f be bounded function defined on $[a, b]$ then

(i) Upper Lebesgue sum $= U[f : P] = \sum_{r=1}^{n} M[f : P_r] m(P_r)$

where $m(P_r)$ is the Lebesgue measure of P_r and $M[f, P_r] = \sup\{f(x) : x \in P_r\}$

(ii) Lower Lebesgue sum $= L[f : P] = \sum_{r=1}^{n} m[f : P_r] \cdot m(P_r)$

where, $m[f \cdot P_r] = \inf[f(x) : x \in P_r]$

☛ REMARKS
- $L[f : P] \le U[f : P]$
- $L[-f, P] = -U[f, P]$ and $U[-f : P] = -L[f : P]$

6.2.5 DIRECT CONSEQUENCES OF RIEMANN SUM AND LEBESGUE SUMS

If $P_1, P_2, ..., P_n$ are the internal components of a Riemann subdivison σ of the interval $[a, b]$ then the Upper Lebesgue sum $U[f : P]$ becomes the same as the Upper Riemann sum $U[f : \sigma] = \Sigma M[f : P_r] \cdot l(P_r)$, because in case of interval, length of the interval is equal to Lebesgue measure of the interval. Thus, we conclude that every $U[f, \sigma]$ gives a Lebesgue upper sum $U[f : P]$ and hence the set of numbers $U[f : \sigma]$ for all the Riemann subdivision of $[a, b]$ is a subset of numbers $U[f; P]$ for all measurable partition P of $[a, b]$. Similar result holds for $L[f; \sigma]$ and $L[f; P]$.

6.3 LEBESGUE INTEGRAL OF BOUNDED FUNCTIONS

Let f be a bounded function defined on $[a, b]$. Then we have the following definitions:

6.3.1 LOWER LEBESGUE INTEGRAL

The supremum of $L[f : Q]$ is called the lower Lebesgue integral on $[a, b]$. It is denoted by $L\int_a^b f(x)dx$ or $L\int_a^b f.$, where suprmum is taken over all measurable partitions Q of $[a, b]$, i.e.,

$$L\int_a^b f(x)dx = \sup\{ L[f, Q] : Q \text{ is measurable partition of } [a, b]\}.$$

6.3.2 UPPER LEBESGUE INTEGRAL

The infimum of $U[f : P]$ is called the Upper Lebesgue integral on $[a, b]$. It is denoted by

$L\overline{\int}_a^b f(x)dx$ or $L\overline{\int}_a^b f$

i.e., $L\overline{\int}_a^b f(x)dx = \inf.\{U[f:P] : P$ is a measurable partition of $[a, b]\}$

6.3.3 LEBESGUE INTEGRAL

Let f be a bounded function defined on the interval $[a, b]$. Then f is said to be Lebesgue integrable on $[a, b]$ or L-integrable on $[a, b]$ if

$$L\underline{\int}_a^b f = L\overline{\int}_a^b f$$

6.3.4 AN IMPORTANT SYMBOL

$L[a, b]$ = The class of all bounded functions f which are Lebesgue integrable on $[a, b]$.

INTERPRETATION

   (i) $f \in L[a, b]$ $\Leftrightarrow$ f is integrable on $[a, b]$

   (ii) $\int_a^b f$ exists $\Rightarrow$ f is bounded and integrable over $[a, b]$.

☛ **REMARKS**

- Every bounded function is not necessarily integrable, *i.e.*, there may exists a bounded function f such that $L\underline{\int}_a^b f \neq L\overline{\int}_a^b f$
- The concept of integrbility of a function over an interval as defined here is subject to two limitations:
  - (i) the function is bounded
  - (ii) the interval of integration is finite, *i.e.*, neither of the end points (limits of integration) is infinite.

Recapitulations

♦ $L[f; Q] = -U[f; Q]$

♦ $U[-f, P] = -L[f; P]$

♦ $L\underline{\int}_a^b(-f) = -\left(L\overline{\int}_a^b f\right)$

♦ $L\overline{\int}_a^b(-f) = -\left(L\underline{\int}_a^b f\right)$

♦ $L\underline{\int}_a^b f \geq L[f; Q]$

♦ $L\overline{\int}_a^b f \leq U[f; P]$

♦ For every $\varepsilon > 0$, (however small) there always exists at least one partition P' such that

$$L\overline{\int}_a^b f + \varepsilon > U(f; P')$$

♦ For every $\varepsilon > 0$, (however small) there always exists at least one partition Q' such that

$$L\underline{\int}_a^b f - \varepsilon < L(f; Q')$$

6.4 LEBESGUE INTEGRAL OF BOUNDED FUNCTIONS OVER A SUBSET OF REAL NUMBERS

Let f be a bounded function on $[a, b]$ and E is a measurable subset of $[a, b]$. Then,

$$\int_E f = \int_a^b f \cdot \chi_E$$

where χ_E is the characteristic function of E and if the function f is a simple function and has the Canonical representation $f = \sum_{i=1}^{n} a_i \cdot \chi_{E_i}$ then

$$\int_E f = \sum_{i=1}^{n} a_i m(E_i)$$

where $E = \bigcup_{i=1}^{n} E_i$ and $E_i \cap E_j = \phi, i \neq j$ and $E_i = \{x \in E : f(x) = a_i\}, m(E_i) < \infty.$

☛ **REMARKS**

- Every simple function f is L-integrable and its L-integral is same as the elementary integral and denoted by $\int_a^b f$.
- We can write the elementary integral for a simple function even if its representation is not Canonical.

6.5 GENERAL LEBESGUE INTEGRAL

We are well familiar with the positive part f^+ and negative part f^- of a real valued function f. Clearly, f^+ and f^- both are positive functions. Also, if f is measurable, then f^+ and f^- both are measurable.

Definition. *A measurable function f is said to be Lebesgue integrable over a measurable subset $E \subset [a, b]$ if f^+ and f^- are both L-integrable over E and then*

$$\int_E f = \int_E f^+ - \int_E f^-$$

6.6 INTEGRAL OF NON-NEGATIVE FUNCTION

A non-negative measurable function f defined on a measurable set E is said to be integrable if $\int_E f(x)dx < \infty$ where $\int_E f = \sup_{g \leq f} \int_E g(x)$ and g is a bounded measurable function such that $m[E(x : g(x) \neq 0)] < \infty$.

THEOREM 1.

Let f be a bounded function defined on [a, b] then every upper sum is greater than or equal to every lower sum for f.

PROOF.   Let f be a bounded function defined on a closed interval $[a, b]$. Suppose that P and Q two measurable partitions of $[a, b]$. We have to prove that

$$U[f; P] \geq L[f; Q]$$

Let Q^* be any refinement of Q.

Step 1. First we shall prove that $L[f; Q] \leq L[f; Q^*]$

Let $\{S_r : r \in N\}$ be the components of Q and $S_1 S_2 ... S_i^* S_i^{**} ... S_n$ be the components of Q^* such that $S_i^* \cap S_i^{**} = \phi$ and $S_i = S_i^* \cup S_i^{**}$ (Here, Q^* is obtained from Q by splitting one comonent S_i into two subsets S_i^* and S_i^{**}. We can split S_i into more than two components).

Now, $S_i = S_i^* \cup S_i^{**}$ such that $S_i^* \cap S_i^{**} = \phi$

$\Rightarrow$ $m(S_i) = m(S_i^*) + m(S_i^{**})$

By definition of refinement, we have

$$S_i^* \subseteq S_i \quad \Rightarrow \quad m[f; S_i] \leq m[f; S_i^*] \qquad ...(1)$$

and $S_i^{**} \subseteq S_i \quad \Rightarrow \quad m[f; S_i] \leq m[f; S_i^{**}] \qquad ...(2)$

Here, $m[f, S_i]$ is the minimum value of f on S_i.

Now, $L[f, Q^*] = \sum_{\substack{j=1 \\ j \neq i}}^{n} m[f : S_j] m(S_j) + m[f : S_i^*] m(S_i^*) + m[f; S_i^{**}] m(S_i^{**})$

$$\geq \sum_{\substack{j=1 \\ j \neq i}}^{n} m[f:S_j]m[S_j]+m[f;S_i]\{m(S_i^*)+m(S_i^{**})\}$$

[Using (1) and (2)]

$$\geq \sum_{\substack{j=1 \\ j \neq i}}^{n} m[f:S_j]m(S_j)+m[f;S_j]\cdot m(S_i) = L[f;Q]$$

$\Rightarrow \qquad L[f, Q^*] \geq L[f; Q]$, i.e., $L[f, Q] \leq L[f, Q^*]$ ...(3)

Step 2. Proceeding in the same way as in step (1), we may prove that

$$U[f; P] \geq U[f; P^*] \qquad \qquad \text{...(4)}$$

Step 3. Let $P = [S_1 S_2 ... S_n]$ and $Q = [P_1 P_2 ... P_m]$. Then consider the collection of subsets of the form $S_i \cap P_j \, (i = 1, 2, ..., n, j = 1, 2, ..., m)$ and denote it by PQ. Then clearly PQ is the measurable partition and is refinement of both P and Q.

Therefore, $L[f; Q] \leq L[f; PQ]$ and $U[f; PQ] \leq U[f; P]$

$\Rightarrow \qquad U[f; P] \geq U[f; PQ] \geq L[f; PQ] \geq L[f; Q]$

Hence, $\quad U[f; P] \geq L[f; Q]$

THEOREM 2.

If f is a bounded function on $[a, b]$ and P is a measurable partition of $[a, b]$, then

$$\sup_{Q} . L[f; Q] \leq \inf_{P} . U[f; P]$$

PROOF. Let f be a bounded function on $[a, b]$ and P is a measurable partition of $[a, b]$. Then by theorem-1, we can find

$\qquad U[f; P] \geq L[f; Q]$ for all partitions P and Q of $[a, b]$

$\Rightarrow \qquad L[f; Q] \leq U[f; P]$

$\Rightarrow \quad L[f; Q]$ is a lower bound for the set of upper sums $U[f; P]$

Therefore, $\inf_{P} . U[f; P] =$ greatest lower bound of $U[f; P]$ over P.

$$\geq L[f; Q] \text{ for every } Q$$

$\Rightarrow \qquad \inf_{P} U[f; P] \geq L[f; Q]$ for every Q.

$\Rightarrow \qquad L[f : Q] \leq \text{g.l.b.} \underset{P}{U[f; P]}$

$\Rightarrow \qquad \text{l.u.b.} \underset{Q}{L[f : Q]} \leq \text{g.l.b.} \underset{P}{U[f; P]}$

Hence, $\quad \sup_{Q} . L[f; Q] \leq \inf_{P} . U[f; P]$

☛ REMARK

• From above, we can write $L\underline{\int}_a^b f \leq L\overline{\int}_a^b f$

DEDUCTION. If for some partition P, $U[f; P] = L[f; P]$. Then, since, we have

$$L(f; P) \leq L\underline{\int}_a^b f \leq L\overline{\int}_a^b f \leq U(f; P)$$

Therefore, $\qquad L\underline{\int}_a^b f = L\overline{\int}_a^b f = U(f; P) = L(f; P)$

Hence, f is L-integrable and $L\int_a^b f = U(f; P)$

THEOREM 3.

If f is a bounded function defined on [a b] and f is R-integrable on [a, b] then f is also L-integrable on [a, b] and $L\int_a^b f = R\int_a^b f$.

[MEERUT–2004, 08, 10, 13, 16, 18; KANPUR–1999, 2008; HPU–1999, 2000, 02, 03; ROHTAK–2001, 11; ROHILKHAND–2003; DELHI–2012; AMRITSAR–2011]

PROOF. Let f be a bounded function on $[a, b]$ and σ_1, σ_2 are two Riemann subdivisions of $[a, b]$.

Therefore, $L\underline{\int}_a^b f \le U[f; P_1]$ and $L\overline{\int}_a^b f \ge L[f; P_2]$

$\Rightarrow \qquad L[f; P_2] \le L\underline{\int}_a^b f \le L\overline{\int}_a^b f \le U[f; P_1]$

$\Rightarrow \qquad L[f; \sigma_1] \le L\underline{\int}_a^b f \le L\overline{\int}_a^b f \le U[f; \sigma_2]$

$[\because \sigma_1$ and σ_2 will also give rise to measurable partition P_1 and P_2 of $[a, b]]$

$\Rightarrow \qquad R\underline{\int}_a^b f \le L\underline{\int}_a^b f \le L\overline{\int}_a^b f \le R\overline{\int}_a^b f$ ...(1)

Since, f is R-integrable (given) then $R\underline{\int}_a^b f = R\overline{\int}_a^b f = R\int_a^b f$ ...(2)

Now, from (1) and (2) we get

$$R\underline{\int}_a^b f = L\underline{\int}_a^b f = L\overline{\int}_a^b f = R\overline{\int}_a^b f$$

$\Rightarrow \qquad L\underline{\int}_a^b f = L\overline{\int}_a^b f$

$\Rightarrow$ f is L-integrable over $[a, b]$.

☞ REMARKS

- If both R and L-integrals exists then by above theorem their values are equal. In this situations we may denote the integral by the symbols $\int_a^b f$ or $\int_a^b f(x)dx$.
- Converse of the above theorem is not necessarily true, *i.e.*, every L-integrable function on $[a, b]$ is not necessarily R-integrable.

DEDUCTION. Improper integral of a function may exists without the function being integrable in the sense of Lebesgue.

However, if f is intetgrable then the improper Riemann integral if exist is equal to the L-integral.

FOR EXAMPLE: Let $f : [0, \infty[\to R$ such that $f(x) = \dfrac{(-1)^{n+1}}{n}$ for $n - 1 \le x < n, n \in N$ be a function.

Then $\qquad R\int_0^\infty f(x)dx = \sum_{n=1}^\infty \int_{n-1}^n \dfrac{(-1)^{n+1}}{n} dx = \sum_{n=1}^\infty \dfrac{(-1)^{n+1}}{n}$

Clearly, by Leibnitz's test for alternating series, the above series is convergent, therefore, $R\int_0^\infty f(x)dx$ is finite.

But, being a divergent series $\int_0^\infty |f| dx = \sum_{n=1}^\infty \dfrac{1}{n} = \infty$

$\Rightarrow \quad |f|$ is not L-integrable.

$\Rightarrow \quad f$ is not L-integrable.

THEOREM 4. (First Mean Value Theorem)

Let f be a bounded real valued function such that $a \le f(x) \le b$ on a measurable set $E \subseteq R$, then

$$a \cdot m(E) \le \int_E f(x)dx \le b \cdot m(E)$$

[MEERUT–2012, 13, 17; KANPUR–2001; AMRITSAR–1997; ROHTAK–2002]

PROOF.   Let f be a bounded real valued function such that $a \le f(x) \le b$ on a measurable set $E \subseteq R$.

Sicne, $a \le f(x) \le b$ (given) so for any $m \in N$, we have

$$\left(a - \frac{1}{m}\right) < f(x) < \left(b + \frac{1}{m}\right) \quad \forall x \in E \qquad \qquad \text{...(1)}$$

Let us write $\alpha = a - \dfrac{1}{m}$ and $\beta = b + \dfrac{1}{m}$. Then from (1), we can write

$$\alpha < f(x) < \beta \; \forall \; x \in E$$

Then divide the interval $[\alpha, \beta]$ by means of points y_n such that

$$\alpha = y_0 < y_1 < y_2 < ... < y_n = \beta$$

Now, define $E_0 = \{x \in E : y_0 < f(x) < y_1\}$

and $E_r = \{x \in E : y_r < f(x) < y_{r+1}\}, r = 1, 2, ..., n-1$

Then clearly $E = \displaystyle\bigcup_{r=0}^{n-1} E_r$ and $E_r \cap E_s = \phi, r \ne s$ $\qquad$ ...(1)

Further, since f is measurable over E and each E_r is measurable then from (1) we can write $\qquad m(E) = \displaystyle\sum_{r=0}^{n-1} m(E_r)$ $\qquad \qquad$ ...(2)

Therefore, we found a measurable partition $P = \{E_0, E_1, ..., E_{n-1}\}$ of E.

Also, $\qquad \qquad \alpha \le y_r \le \beta$

$\Rightarrow \qquad \qquad \alpha \cdot m(E_r) \le y_r \cdot m(E_r) \le \beta \cdot m(E_r)$

$\Rightarrow \qquad \displaystyle\sum_{r=0}^{n-1} \alpha \cdot m(E_r) \le \sum_{r=0}^{n-1} y_r m(E_r) \le \sum_{r=0}^{n-1} \beta m(E_r)$

$\Rightarrow \qquad \alpha \cdot \displaystyle\sum_{r=0}^{n-1} m(E_r) \le \sum_{r=0}^{n-1} y_r m(E_r) \le \beta \cdot \sum_{r=0}^{n-1} m(E_r)$

$\Rightarrow \qquad \alpha \cdot m(E) \le \displaystyle\sum_{r=0}^{n-1} y_r \cdot m(E_r) \le \beta \cdot m(E) \qquad$ (Using (2)) $\qquad$ ...(3)

Further, if $\max \{y_{r+1} - y_r\} \to 0 \Rightarrow y_{r+1} \to y_r$, therefore,

$$U[f;P] = \sum_{r=0}^{n-1} y_{r+1} \cdot m(E_r) \text{ and } \sum_{r=0}^{n-1} y_r m(E_r) = L[f;P]$$

$\Rightarrow \qquad \qquad \int_E f = \Sigma y_r m(E_r)$ $\qquad \qquad$ ...(4)

Using (4) in (3) we get

$$\alpha \cdot m(E) \le \int_E f(x)dx \le \beta \cdot m(E)$$

Putting the values of α and β we get

$$\left(a - \frac{1}{m}\right)m(E) \le \int_E f(x)dx \le \left(b + \frac{1}{m}\right)m(E)$$

Letting $m \to \infty$, we get

$$a \cdot m(E) \le \int_E f(x)dx \le bm(E)$$

THEOREM 5. (Necessary and Sufficient Condition of L-integrability)

A bounded function f defined on [a, b] is L-integrable if and only if for each $\varepsilon > 0$, there exists a measurable partition P of [a, b] such that

$$U[f; P] - L[f; P] < \varepsilon$$

[MEERUT–2006, 12; ASSAM–2006]

PROOF.

Necessary Condition: Let us suppose that f is L-integrable. We have to prove that $\exists$ a measurable partition P of $[a, b]$ such that $U[f; P] - L[f; P] < \varepsilon$.

Since f is L-integrable over $[a, b]$, therefore

$$L\overline{\int_a^b} f = \text{g.l.b.}_P U[f;P] = \text{l.u.b.}_Q L[f;Q] = L\underline{\int_a^b} f$$

Now, for $\varepsilon > 0$, we may have partition P and Q such that

$$L\overline{\int_a^b} f + \frac{\varepsilon}{2} > U[f;P] \Rightarrow U[f;P] < L\overline{\int_a^b} f + \frac{\varepsilon}{2} \qquad \ldots(1)$$

and

$$L\underline{\int_a^b} f - \frac{\varepsilon}{2} < L[f;Q] \Rightarrow -L\underline{\int_a^b} f + \frac{\varepsilon}{2} > -L[f;Q]$$

$$\Rightarrow -L[f;Q] < -L\underline{\int_a^b} f + \frac{\varepsilon}{2} \qquad \ldots(2)$$

On adding (1) and (2), we get

$$U[f;P] - L[f;Q] < L\overline{\int_a^b} f - L\underline{\int_a^b} f + \varepsilon$$

$$\Rightarrow U[f; P] - L[f; Q] < \varepsilon \qquad \left[\because L\overline{\int_a^b} f = L\underline{\int_a^b} f\right] \qquad \ldots(3)$$

Further if PQ is the common refinement of P and Q so (3) holds for PQ also, *i.e.*,

$U[f; PQ] - L[f; PQ] < \varepsilon$

Hence, we conclude that, we obtained at least one measurable partition PQ for which

$U[f; P] - L[f; Q] < \varepsilon.$

Sufficient Condition: Let for given $\varepsilon > 0 \exists$ a measurable partition P of $[a, b]$ be such that

$$U[f; P] - L[f; Q] < \varepsilon \qquad \ldots(4)$$

We have to prove that f is L-integrable.

By definition of upper and lower integrals, we can write

$$L\overline{\int_a^b} f \le U[f;P] \text{ and } L\underline{\int_a^b} f \ge L[f;P] \Rightarrow -L\underline{\int_a^b} f \le -L[f;P]$$

On adding the above inequalities, we get

$$\left(L\overline{\int_a^b} f - L\underline{\int_a^b} f\right) < U[f;P] - L[f;P]$$

$$< \varepsilon \qquad \text{(From (4))}$$

$$\Rightarrow L\overline{\int_a^b} f < L\underline{\int_a^b} f + \varepsilon$$

Since ε is arbitrary, letting $\varepsilon \to 0$ we get

$$L\overline{\int_a^b} f \le L\underline{\int_a^b} f \qquad \ldots(5)$$

But we know that

$$L\overline{\int_a^b} f \ge L\underline{\int_a^b} f \qquad \ldots(6)$$

From (5) and (6)

$$L\overline{\int_a^b} f = L\underline{\int_a^b} f$$

Hence, f is L-integrable over $[a, b]$.

☞ **REMARK**

- From the above theorem, we conclude that, if for some function f there exists a measurable partition P such that $U[f; P] = L[f; P]$ then $f \in L[a, b]$.

THEOREM 6.

If f is a bounded function in $L[a, b]$ and $c \in R$ then $cf \in L[a, b]$ and $\int_a^b cf = c\int_a^b f$.

PROOF.   Let f be a bounded function in $L[a, b]$.

Let $c \in R$.

If $c = 0$, then result is obvious. So, let us assume that $c \neq 0$. Let $c > 0$. Now since f is bounded in $L[a, b]$, therefore there exists a partition P of $[a, b]$ such that

$$U[f; P] - L[f; P] < \frac{\varepsilon}{c} \qquad \text{(Using previous theorem)}$$

Further, $c > 0 \Rightarrow (cf)x = cf(x)$

Therefore, $U[cf; P] = cU[f; P]$

and $L[cf; P] = cL[f; P]$

which implies

$$U[cf; P] - L[cf; P] = c[U(f; P) - L(f; P)] < c \cdot \frac{\varepsilon}{c} = \varepsilon$$

$\Rightarrow \qquad U[cf; P] - L[cf; P] < \varepsilon$

Again by previous theorem, $cf \in L[a, b]$

Now, it remains to prove that $c\int_a^b f = \int_a^b cf$

By definition of upper sum, for $\varepsilon > 0$, we have

$$U[f; P] < \int_a^b f + \frac{\varepsilon}{c}$$

$\Rightarrow \qquad cU[f; P] < c\int_a^b f + \varepsilon \qquad \qquad ...(1)$

But $cU[f; P] = U[cf; P] \geq \int_a^b cf \qquad \qquad ...(2)$

From (1) and (2) we conclude that

$$c\int_a^b f + \varepsilon > \int_a^b cf$$

Letting $\varepsilon \to 0$, we get $c\int_a^b f \geq \int_a^b cf \qquad \qquad ...(3)$

Now by replacing f by $-f$ in (3) we get

$$c\int_a^b f \leq \int_a^b cf \qquad \qquad ...(4)$$

Finally, from (3) and (4) we conclude that

$$c\int_a^b f = \int_a^b cf$$

THEOREM 7.

Every bounded measurable function f defined on $[a, b]$ is Lebesgue integrable over $[a, b]$.

[MEERUT–2009; KANPUR–2000, 02; GARHWAL–2006, 17]

PROOF.   Let f be a bounded function defined on $[a, b]$. We have to prove that f is Lebesgue integrable over $[a, b]$.

Since, f is bounded, therefore there exist $c \in N$ such that

$$f(x) \in [-c, c[\quad \forall \, x \in [a, b]$$

$\Rightarrow \quad$ Range of $f(x)$ is $[-c, c[$.

Now divide $[-c, c[$ by means of finite number of points $a_0, a_1, ..., a_n$ such that

$$-c = a_0 < a_1 < a_2 < ... < a_n = c$$

where $a_i - a_{i-1} < \dfrac{\varepsilon}{b-a}, i \in N$ ...(1)

Now, define $E_i = f^{-1}[a_{i-1}, b_i[\ \forall i \in N$

Therefore, $x \in E_i$ which implies that $a_{i-1} \le f(x) \le a_i$

Since, we know that inverse image of any interval under a measurable function is meassurable, therefore E_i is measurable and these $E_i's$ are pairwise disjoint. So, $\{E_1, E_2, ..., E_n\} = P$ is a measurable partition of $[a, b]$.

Clearly, $M[f; E_i] = $ l.u.b. $\{f(x) : x \in E_i\} \le a_i$

Therefore, $U[f; P] = \displaystyle\sum_{i=1}^{n} M[f; Ei] \cdot m(E_i) \le \sum_{i=1}^{n} a_i \cdot m(E_i)$

$\Rightarrow$ $U[f; P] \le \displaystyle\sum_{i=1}^{n} a_i m(E_i)$ ...(2)

Similarly, we may prove that

$$L[f; P] \ge \sum_{i=1}^{n} a_{i-1} m(E_i)$$

$\Rightarrow$ $-L[f; P] \le -\displaystyle\sum_{i=1}^{n} a_{i-1} m(E_i)$ ...(3)

On adding (2) and (3), we get

$$U[f; P] - L[f; P] \le \sum_{i=1}^{n} a_i m(E_i) - \sum_{i=1}^{n} a_{i-1} m(E_i)$$

$$\le \sum_{i=1}^{n} [a_i - a_{i-1}] m(E_i) < \frac{\varepsilon}{b-a} \sum_{i=1}^{n} m(E_i) \qquad \text{(Using (1))}$$

...(4)

Now, since $E_i \cap E_j = \phi$ for $i \ne j$ and $\displaystyle\bigcup_{i=1}^{n} E_i = [a, b]$ therefore,

$$\sum_{i=1}^{n} m(E_i) = m\left(\bigcup_{i=1}^{n} E_i \right) = m([a, b]) = b - a \qquad ...(5)$$

Using (5) in (4) we get

$$U[f; P] - L[f; P] < \varepsilon$$

Hence, f is L-integrable on $[a, b]$.

☛ **REMARK**

• Measurability of the bounded function f is a sufficient condition for a function to be L-integrable.

THEOREM 8.

Let f be a bounded function defined on $[a, b]$ and let f be L-integrable over $[a, b]$. If $a < c < b$. Then f is L-integrable over $[a, c]$, f is L-integrable over (c, b) and

$$\int_a^b f = \int_a^c f + \int_c^b f$$

PROOF.   Let f be a bounded function defined on $[a, b]$ which is L-integrable on $[a, b]$. Let us define two sets E_1 and E_2 such that for $r \in R$,

$$E_1 = \{x \in [a, c] : f(x) > r\}$$

and $E_2 = \{x \in [a, b] : f(x) > r\}$

Then E_2 is measurable and $E = [a, c] \cap E_2$ [$\because f$ is L-integrable $\Rightarrow f$ is measurable]

Further, E_2 is measurable, therefore, $[a, c] \cap E_2$ is measurable.

$\qquad$ [$\because [a, c]$ is an interval $\Rightarrow [a, c]$ is measurable and intersection

$\qquad\qquad\qquad\qquad\qquad\qquad$ of two measurable sets is measurable]

$\Rightarrow \quad E$ is measurable.

$\Rightarrow \quad f$ is bounded and measurable on $[a, c]$.

$\Rightarrow \quad f$ is L-integrable on $[a, c]$.

In a similar way, we may prove that f is L-integrable on $[c, b]$. Further, let $P \cup Q$ be a measurable partitition of $[a, b]$ such that P be partition of $[a, c]$ and Q be partition of $[c, b]$. So,

$$L[f; P] + L[f; Q] = L[f : P \cup Q] \le \int_a^b f$$

$$= \overline{\int_a^b} f = \int_a^b f \qquad\qquad (\because f \text{ is L-integrable over } [a, b])$$

Now, taking supremum over P keeping Q fixed, the last inequality becomes

$$\int_c^a f + L[f : Q] \le \int_a^b f \qquad\qquad [\because \sup L[f : P] = \underline{\int_a^c} f = \int_a^c f = \int_a^c f]$$

Further, taking supremum over all Q, we get

$$\int_a^c f + \int_c^b f \le \int_a^b f \qquad\qquad\qquad ...(1)$$

Similarly, we can establish

$$U[f; P] + U[f; Q] \ge \int_a^b f$$

Now, apply the same procedure (on infinium) as above we get

$$\int_a^c f + \int_c^b f \ge \int_a^b f \qquad\qquad\qquad ...(2)$$

Finally, from (1) and (2) we conclude that

$$\int_a^c f + \int_c^b f = \int_a^b f$$

THEOREM 9.

Let f and g be bounded functions in $L[a, b]$ then $(f + g) \in L[a, b]$ and $\int_a^b (f + g) = \int_a^b f + \int_a^b g$

[MEERUT–2003, 04; KANPUR–1987]

PROOF. $\qquad$ Let f and g be bounded and L-integrable over $[a, b]$.

Therefore, for given $\varepsilon > 0$ ∃ two partitions P_1 and Q such that

$$U[f; P_1] - L[f; P_1] < \varepsilon/2 \qquad\qquad\qquad ...(1)$$

and $\qquad U[g, Q] - L[f; Q] < \varepsilon/2 \qquad\qquad\qquad ...(2)$

Let P be the common refinement of P_1 and Q then from (1) and (2) we can write

$$U[f; P] - L[f; P] < \varepsilon/2$$

and $\qquad U[g; P] - L[g; P] < \varepsilon/2$

On adding above both the inequalities, we have

$$[U[f; P] + U[g; P]] - [L[f; P] + L[f; P]] < \varepsilon \qquad\qquad ...(3)$$

Further, suppose that $P = \{S_1, S_2, ..., S_n\}$. Then we define

$$M_i = \sup\{(f + g)(x) : x \in S_i\}$$

$$m_i = \inf\{(f + g)(x) : x \in S_i\}$$

$$M_i' = \sup\{f(x) : x \in S_i\}$$

$$m_i' = \inf\{f(x) : x \in S_i\}$$

$$M_i'' = \sup\{g(x) : x \in S_i\}$$

$$m_i'' = \inf\{g(x) : x \in S_i\}$$

Clearly, we have $f(x) + g(x) \le M_i' + M_i''$ for all $x \in S_i$

$\Rightarrow$ $\qquad\qquad M_i \le M_i' + M_i''$

Similarly, we may prove that

$$m_i \ge m_i' + m_i''$$

Consider $\qquad U[(f+g); P] = \sum_{i=1}^{n} M_i \cdot m(S_i)$

$$\le \sum_{i=1}^{n} (M_i' + M_i'') m(S_i) = \sum_{i=1}^{n} M_i' \cdot m(S_i) + \sum_{i=1}^{n} M_i'' \cdot m(S_i)$$

But we have $\qquad U[f; P] = \sum_{i=1}^{n} M_i'' \cdot m(S_i)$ and $U[g; P] = \sum_{i=1}^{n} M_i'' \cdot m(S_i)$

Therefore, $\qquad U[(f+g); P] \le U[f; P] + U[g; P]$ $\qquad\qquad$ ...(4)

Similarly, $L[(f+g); P] \ge L[f; P] + L[g; P]$

$\Rightarrow$ $\qquad -L[(f+g); P] \le -L[f; P] - L[g; P]$ $\qquad\qquad$ ...(5)

On adding (4) and (5) we get

$\qquad U[(f+g); P] - L[(f+g); P] \le [U[f; P] + U[g; P]] - [L[f; P] + L[g; P]] < \varepsilon$

$\Rightarrow$ $\quad U[(f+g); P] - L[(f+g); P] < \varepsilon$

Hence, $\qquad\qquad f + g \in L[a, b]$

Further, we have

$\qquad U[f; P] < \int_a^b f + \varepsilon/2$ and $U[g; P] < \int_a^b g + \varepsilon/2$

On adding we get

$\qquad U[f; P] + U[g; P] < \int_a^b f + \int_a^b g + \varepsilon$

Now from (5), we have

$\qquad U[(f+g); P] < \int_a^b f + \int_a^b g + \varepsilon$

$\Rightarrow$ $\qquad U[(f+g); P] \le \int_a^b f + \int_a^b g$ $\qquad\qquad$ (letting $\varepsilon \to 0$)

Taking infimum of both the sides, we have

$\qquad \int_a^b (f+g) \le \int_a^b f + \int_a^b g$ $\qquad\qquad$ ...(6)

Further, since f, g are bounded L-integrable

$\Rightarrow$ $\quad f, g$ are bounded measurable.

$\Rightarrow$ $\quad -f, -g$ are also bounded measurable functions.

$\qquad\qquad\qquad\qquad$ ($\because f$ is measurable $\Rightarrow cf$ is measurable $c \in R$)

$\Rightarrow$ $\quad -f, -g \in L[a, b]$

If we replace f, g by $-f$, $-g$ respectively in (6), then we get

$\qquad \int_a^b [-(f+g)] \le \int_a^b (-f) + \int_a^b (-g)$

$\Rightarrow$ $\qquad -\int_a^b (f+g) \le -\int_a^b f - \int_a^b g$

$\Rightarrow$ $\qquad \int_a^b (f+g) \ge \int_a^b f + \int_a^b g$ $\qquad\qquad$ ...(7)

Finally, from (6) and (7) we conclude that

$$\int_a^b (f+g) = \int_a^b f + \int_a^b g$$

THEOREM 10.

Let f be a bounded function in L[a, b] and if g is a bounded function on [a, b] such that f(x) = g(x) almost everywhere (a·e) in [a, b] then g ∈ L[a, b] and $\int_a^b g = \int_a^b f$.

[MADRAS–2009; ROHILKHAND–2002; GUJRAT–2007; ASSAM–1998]

PROOF.   Let f be a bounded function in $L[a, b]$ and if g is a bounded function on $[a, b]$ such that $f(x) = g(x)$ a.e. in $[a, b]$.

Since $f(x) = g(x)$ a.e. on $[a, b]$ and f is measurable.   ($\because f \in L[a, b] \Rightarrow f$ is measurable)
$\Rightarrow$ g is measurable on $[a, b]$.

For independent proof, we proceed as follows: Since g is bounded (given).
Therefore, $g \in L[a, b]$

Now, it remains to prove that $\int_a^b g = \int_a^b f$

Let us define a set $E = \{x : a \le x \le b\}$ and $E_0 = \{x : x \in E \text{ and } f(x) \ne g(x)\}$ or $M[f-g](x) = 0$ for all $x \in E - E_0$.

which implies $m(E_0) = 0$ and $f(x) = g(x) \ \forall \ x \in E - E_0$

Now let $P = \{E_0, E_1, ..., E_n\}$ be a measurable partition of $[a, b]$. Then

$$U[f-g; P] = M[f-g; E_0] \cdot m(E_0) + M(f-g; E-E_0) \cdot m(E-E_0)$$
$$= M[f-g; E_0] \cdot 0 + 0 \cdot m(E-E_0) = 0$$

$\Rightarrow$ $U[f-g; P] = 0$

Similarly, we may prove that

$$L[f-g; P] = 0$$

Now, $U[f-g; P] = L[f-g; P]$
$\Rightarrow$ $f - g \in L[a, b] \Rightarrow -(f-g) \in L[a, b] \Rightarrow g-f \in L[a, b]$

Since, $f \in L[a, b]$ and $g-f \in L[a, b]$
$\Rightarrow$ $(f + g - f) \in L[a, b]$

Hence, $g \in L[a, b]$.

Now, it remains to prove that $\int_a^b g = \int_a^b f$

Here, we have $L[f-g; P] = 0$ and $U[f-g; P] = 0$

$\Rightarrow$ $0 = L[f-g; P] \le \int_a^b (f-g) \le U[f-g; P] = 0$

$\Rightarrow$ $\int_a^b (f-g) = 0$ or $\int_a^b (g-f) = 0$

Hence, $\int_a^b g = \int_a^b (g-f+f) = \int_a^b (g-f) + \int_a^b f = 0 + \int_a^b f$

$\Rightarrow$ $\int_a^b g = \int_a^b f$

THEOREM 11.

If A and B are two disjoint measurable subset of [a, b] and f is bounded and f ∈ L[a, b] then

$$\int_{A \cup B} f = \int_A f + \int_B f$$

[MEERUT–2001, 07, 08, 14; ROHTAK–2002; HPU–2002; AVADH–2006; BHOPAL–2009]

PROOF.   Let f is bounded and L-integrable over $[a, b]$ and A, B be two disjoint measurable subset of $[a, b]$. We have to prove that $\int_{A \cup B} f = \int_A f + \int_B f$.

Since, A and B are disjoint $\Rightarrow A \cap B = \phi$

Therefore, $\chi_{A \cup B} = \chi_A + \chi_B$

$\Rightarrow$ $\qquad\qquad\qquad f\chi_{A \cup B} = f\chi_A + f\chi_B$ $\qquad\qquad\qquad$ ...(1)

Now, $\qquad\qquad \int_{A \cup B} f = \int_a^b f\chi_{A \cup B} = \int_a^b (f\chi_A + f\chi_B)$ $\qquad\qquad$ (Using (1))

$$= \int_a^b f\chi_A + \int_a^b f\chi_B$$

$$= \int_A f + \int_B f$$

THEOREM 12.

Let f be bounded real valued measurable function defined over a measurable set E of finite measure such that $a \le f(x) \le b$ then

$$a \cdot m(E) \le \int_E f \le b_m(E)$$

PROOF. Define a function $\psi_1(x) = a \ \forall \ x \in E$

$\therefore \quad a \le f(x)$ implies $\psi_1(x) \le f(x) \ \forall \ x \in E$

$\Rightarrow \qquad\qquad f(x) - \psi_1(x) \ge 0 \ \forall \ x \in E$

Then $\qquad\qquad \int_E (f - \psi_1) \ge 0$

$\Rightarrow \qquad\qquad \int_E f - \int_E \psi_1 \ge 0$ i.e., $\int_E f \ge \int_E \psi_1$ $\qquad\qquad$ ...(1)

But we have

$$\int_E \psi_1 = a \cdot m(E)$$

Putting this values in (1) we get

$\qquad\qquad a \cdot m(E) \le \int_E f$ $\qquad\qquad\qquad$ ...(2)

In a similar way, by defining a function $\psi_2(x) = b \ \forall x \in E$, we can find

$\qquad\qquad \int_E f \le b \cdot m(E)$ $\qquad\qquad\qquad$ ...(3)

On combining (2) and (3) we get

$$a \cdot m(E) \le \int_E f \le bm(E)$$

☞ **REMARK**

- The above theorem is a special case of first mean value theorem when the set E is not necessarily an interval, may be any subset of real numbers.

THEOREM 13. (Countable Additive Property of Integrals)

Let $E = E_1 \cup E_2 \cup ... \cup E_n$ be a measurable set where all $E_i's$ are pairwise disjoint and if f is a bounded measurable function (integrable) defined over E then

$$\int_E f = \int_{E_1} f + \int_{E_2} f + ... + \int_{E_n} f$$

[MEERUT–2008; DELHI–2012; GARHWAL–1995, 2008; KANPUR–2002; ROHILKHAND–2004]

Further, it can be generalised for the case when

$$E = \overset{\infty}{\underset{n=1}{\cup}} E_n \text{ such that } E_i \cap E_j = \phi, i \ne j$$

PROOF. Let *f* be a bounded measurable function defined over E. We shall prove this result by principle of mathematical induction.

Step 1. Let $E = E_1 \cup E_2$ and $E_1 \cap E_2 = \phi$

Then using theorem 11, we can write

$\qquad\qquad \int_E f = \int_{E_1} f + \int_{E_2} f$ $\qquad\qquad\qquad$ (give proof)

Step 2. Let the result be true in case

$$E = \overset{n-1}{\underset{k=1}{\cup}} E_k \text{ such that } E_i \cap E_j = \phi, i \ne j$$

Then $\int_E f = \int_{E_1} f + \int_{E_2} f + \ldots + \int_{E_{n-1}} f$

$$= \sum_{k=1}^{n-1} \int_{E_k} f = \sum_{k=1}^{n-1} \int_{E_k} f(x)dx$$

Step 3. Consider the case when $E = \bigcup_{k=1}^{n} E_k$ such that $E_i \cap E_j = \phi, i \neq j$

Then we can write

$$E = \left(\bigcup_{k=1}^{n-1} E_k \right) \cup E_n$$

$\Rightarrow \int_E f(x)dx = \int_{\bigcup_{k=1}^{n-1} E_k} f + \int_{E_n} f$ (By step 1)

$$= \sum_{k=1}^{n-1} \int_{E_k} f + \int_{E_n} f$$ (By step 2)

$$= \sum_{k=1}^{n} \int_{E_k} f(x)dx$$

$\Rightarrow$ Result true for $k = n$.

Hence by principle of mathematical induction result is true for all n, i.e.,

$$\int_E f(x)dx = \sum_{k=1}^{n} \int_{E_k} f(x)dx, E_i \cap E_j = \phi, i \neq j$$

Generalisation

Let us write $E = \left(\bigcup_{k=1}^{n} E_k \right) \cup \left(\bigcup_{k=n+1}^{\infty} E_k \right)$

For sake of convenience, we can write $R_{n+1} = \bigcup_{k=n+1}^{\infty} E_k$. Then

$$E = \left(\bigcup_{k=1}^{n} E_k \right) \cup R_{n+1}$$

Therefore, $\int_E f(x)dx = \sum_{k=1}^{n} \int_{E_k} f(x)dx + \int_{R_{n+1}} f(x)dx$ ...(1)

Also, f is bounded (given) $\Rightarrow \alpha \leq f(x) \leq \beta$ on R_{n+1}

$\Rightarrow$ $\alpha \cdot m(R_{n+1}) \leq \int_{R_{n+1}} f(x)dx \leq \beta \cdot m(R_{n+1})$ (By First mean value theorem)

                                                 ...(2)

Also, $m(R_{n+1}) = m \left(\bigcup_{k=n+1}^{\infty} E_k \right), E_i \cap E_j = \phi, i \neq j$

$\Rightarrow$ $m(R_{n+1}) = \sum_{k=n+1}^{\infty} m(E_k)$

$\Rightarrow$ $\lim_{n \to \infty} m(R_{n+1}) = \lim_{n \to \infty} \left[\sum_{k=n+1}^{\infty} m(E_k) \right]$ (By letting $n \to \infty$)

          $= 0$ (By general principle of convergence of infinite series)

                                                             ...(3)

Further, taking limit $n \to \infty$ in (2) and (3) we get

$$\alpha \cdot 0 \leq \lim_{n \to \infty} \int_{R_{n+1}} f(x)dx \leq \beta \cdot 0$$

$\Rightarrow \lim_{n \to \infty} \int_{R_{n+1}} f(x)dx = 0$

Finally taking $n \to \infty$ in (1) we get

$$\int_E f(x)dx = \lim_{n\to\infty} \sum_{k=1}^{n} \int_{E_k} f(x)dx + 0$$

Hence, $\int_E f(x)dx = \sum_{k=1}^{\infty} \int_{E_k} f(x)dx$

THEOREM 14.

If f is a bounded function in L[a, b] then $|f| \in L[a, b]$ and $\left|\int_a^b f\right| \le \int_a^b |f|$

PROOF. Let f be a bounded function in $L[a, b]$

$f \in L[a, b]$ $\Rightarrow$ f is measurable.

           $\Rightarrow$ $|f|$ is also measurable.

           $\Rightarrow$ $|f| \in L[a, b]$.

Now, it remains to prove that $f(x) \le g(x)$ a.e. on $E \Rightarrow \int_E f \le \int_E g$.

We know that

$$f(x) \le |f(x)| \; \forall x \in [a,b]$$

$\Rightarrow$ $\int_a^b f \le \int_a^b |f|$ ...(1)

Further, we know that

$$-f(x) \le |f(x)| = |f|(x)$$

$\Rightarrow$ $-\int_a^b f \le \int_a^b |f|$ ...(2)

From (1) and (2) we conclude that

$$\left|\int_a^b f\right| \le \int_a^b |f|$$

THEOREM 15.

Let f be a constant function on a measurable set E, i.e., $f(x) = c$ a.e. then $\int_a^b f(x)dx = cm(E)$

PROOF. It is given that $f(x) = c \; \forall \; x \in E'$

Now, $f(x) = c$ $\Rightarrow$ $c \le f(x) \le c$

Then by first mean value theorem

$$c \cdot m(E') \le \int_{E'} f(x)dx \le c \cdot m(E') \qquad ...(1)$$

Further $E - E' = 0$, then again by first mean value theorem

$$0 \le \int_{E-E'} f(x) \le 0$$

$\Rightarrow$ $\int_{E-E'} f(x)dx = 0$ ...(2)

Also, $\int_E f(x)dx = \int_{E'} f(x)dx + \int_{E-E'} f(x)dx = \int_{E'} f(x)dx$ (Using (2))

and $m(E) = m(E') + m(E - E') = m(E')$

Then from (1) $c \cdot m(E) \le \int_E f(x)dx \le c \cdot m(E)$

Hence, $\int_E f(x)dx = c \cdot m(E)$

☞ REMARKS

• The converse of the above theorem is not true. For example consider a real valued function f

defined on the set E = [−2, 2] such that $f(x) = \begin{cases} 1 & \text{if } x \in E, x \ge 0 \\ -1 & \text{if } x \in E, x < 0 \end{cases}$

Then $\int_E f(x)dx = \int_{-2}^{0} f(x)dx + \int_0^2 f(x)dx = -1 \cdot 2 + 1 \cdot 2 \cdot 0$

               $= 0 \cdot m(E) = c \cdot m(E)$ where $c = 0$

• If $m(E) = 0$ or $f = 0$, a.e. then $\int_E f(x)dx = 0$

• If $f(x) = 1$ then $\int_E f(x)dx = m(E)$

THEOREM 16.

If $\int_A f(x)dx = 0$ *for every measurable subset A of a measurable set E then* $f(x) = 0$ *a.e. on E.*

PROOF. Let if possible $m[B \subseteq E(f > 0)] > 0$

Then there exists a closed set $F \subseteq B$ such that $m(F) > 0$

Let $O = B - F$. Also, since $B \subseteq E$ then we get

$$0 = \int_E f(x)dx = \int_F f(x)dx + \int_O f(x)dx$$

$\Rightarrow \qquad \int_O f(x)dx = -\int_F f \neq 0$

Since O is an open set, so it can be written as the countable union of disjoint open intervals $]a_n, b_n[$ and therefore,

$$\int_O f = \sum_{n \in N} \int_{a_n}^{b_n} f$$

Then for at least one $n, \int_{a_n}^{b_n} f \neq 0$, which is a contradiction. So our assumption is wrong. Therefore, $m[E(f > 0)] > 0$ is not true.

In a similar manner, we can show that $m[E(f < 0)] > 0$ is not true.

Thus, $m[E(f \neq 0)] > 0$ is not true.

Hence, $m[E(f \neq 0)] = 0$ implies $f = 0$ a.e. on E.

THEOREM 17.

If $f \in L[a, b]$ *and if* $f(x) \geq 0$ *a.e. in* $[a, b]$ *then* $\int_a^b f \geq 0$.

PROOF. Let f be an L-integrable function on $[a, b]$.

We know that if $f(x) \geq 0 \; \forall \; x \in [a, b]$ then $U[f; P] \geq 0$ for every partition P.

Therefore, $\qquad L\overline{\int}_a^b f = \inf . U[f; P] \geq 0$

Now, since $f \in L[a, b]$ (given) then

$$\int_a^b f = L\overline{\int}_a^b f \geq 0$$

Hence, $\qquad \int_a^b f \geq 0$.

THEOREM 18.

If $f, g \in L[a, b]$ *and if* $f(x) \leq g(x)$ *a.e. on* $[a, b]$ *then*

$$\int_a^b f \leq \int_a^b g \qquad\qquad \text{[HPU–2002; DELHI–2008]}$$

PROOF. Let $f, g \in L[a, b]$

We know that $\qquad f \in L[a, b] \;\Rightarrow\; cf \in L[a, b], c \in R$

In particular $c = -1$, we have

$$f \in L[a, b] \;\Rightarrow\; -f \in L[a, b]$$

Now, $g \in L[a, b], f \in L[a, b] \qquad \Rightarrow\; g - f \in L[a, b]$

Now, it is given that $f(x) \leq g(x)$ a.e. in $[a, b]$, therefore

$$[g(x) - f(x)] \geq 0 \text{ a.e. in } [a, b]$$

$\Rightarrow \qquad \int_a^b [g(x) - f(x)]dx \geq 0 \;\; \forall \; x \in [a, b]$

$\Rightarrow \quad \int_a^b g(x)dx + \int_a^b (-f(x))dx \geq 0 \;\; \forall \; x \in [a, b]$

$\Rightarrow \quad \int_a^b g(x)dx + \int_a^b (-1)f(x)dx \geq 0 \;\; \forall \; x \in [a, b]$

$\Rightarrow \qquad \int_a^b g(x)dx - \int_a^b f(x)dx \geq 0 \;\; \forall \; x \in [a, b]$

Hence, $\int_a^b g(x)dx \geq \int_a^b f(x)dx \quad \forall \, x \in [a, b]$

$\Rightarrow \qquad\qquad\qquad \int_a^b f \leq \int_a^b g$.

THEOREM 19.

Let a simple function f takes the distinct values $a_1, a_2, ..., a_n$, i.e., $f = \sum\limits_{i=1}^{n} a_i \chi_A$ then

(i) $\int fdx = \sum\limits_{i=1}^{n} a_i \cdot m(A_i)$

(ii) $\int_E fdx = \sum a_i m(A_i \cap E)$ for any measurable set E

where $A_i = \{x : f(x) = a_i\}$, $A_i \cap A_j = \phi, i \neq j$ and $\bigcup\limits_{i=1}^{n} A_i = R$

PROOF.   (i) Let $P = \{A_1, A_2, ..., A_n\}$ be a measurable partition such that

$$U[f; P] = \sum\limits_{i=1}^{n} M[f; A_i] \cdot m(A_i) = \sum\limits_{i=1}^{n} a_i m(A_i)$$

and $$L[f; P] = \sum\limits_{i=1}^{n} m[f; A_i] \cdot m(A_i) = \sum\limits_{i=1}^{n} a_i \cdot m(A_i)$$

$\Rightarrow \qquad U[f; P] = L[f; P]$, for the partition P

Hence, $\int fdx = \sum\limits_{i=1}^{n} a_i \cdot m(A_i)$

(ii) We know that $\int_E fdx = \int f \cdot \chi_E dx$

Here, $\int_{\chi_E}$ also assumes the values of $a_1, a_2, ..., a_n$ and hence it is also a simple function.

Now $x \in A_i \cap E \iff x \in A_i$ and $x \in E$

$\iff f(x) = a_i$ and $\chi_E(x) = 1$

$\iff f\chi_E(x) = f(x)\chi_E(x) = a_i \cdot 1 = a_i$

Finally, using the result obtained in (1), we get

$$\int f\chi_E dx = \sum\limits_{i=1}^{n} a_i \cdot m(A_i \cap E)$$

THEOREM 20.

If f is a bounded function and Lebesgue integrable on a measurable subset E of $[a, b]$ then $|f|$ is also L-integrable on E and $\left|\int_E f\right| \leq \int_E |f|$

[MEERUT–2001, 01, 07, 10, 11, 14, 16;
ROHTAK–2000, 03; HPU–2001, 02, 04; NAGPUR–2006; GARHWAL–2006; KANPUR–2010; DELHI–2012]

PROOF.   Let f be a bounded and Lebesgue integrable function over $E \subseteq [a, b]$.

Since, $f \in L[a, b]$ therefore f^+ and f^- also belongs to $L[a, b]$.

Now $|f| = f^+ + f^-$

Clearly, f^+ and f^- both are L-integrable $\Rightarrow |f|$ is also L-integrable.

Also, $\int_E |f| = \int_E f^+ + f^- = \int_E f^+ + \int_E f^-$

Further, since we know that f^+ and f^- are both non-negative, therefore

$\int_E f^+ + \int_E f^- \geq 0$

Now, $\int_E f = \int_E f^+ - \int_E f^- \leq \int_E f^+ + \int_E f^- = \int_E |f|$

$\Rightarrow \qquad \int_E f \leq \int_E |f|$

...(1)

Further, $-\int_E f = -\int_E f^+ + \int_E f^- \le \int_E f^+ + \int_E f^- = \int_E |f|$

$\Rightarrow \qquad -\int_E f \le \int_E |f|$ ...(2)

From (1) and (2) we conclude that

$$\left| \int_E f \right| \le \int_E |f|$$

☞ **REMARK**

- The above inequality will be an equality if either $f \ge 0$ a.e. or $f \le 0$ a.e.

  For, if $\int f \ge 0 \qquad \Rightarrow \qquad \int |f| = \int f \qquad \Rightarrow \qquad \int |f| - f = 0$

  $\qquad\qquad\qquad \Rightarrow \quad |f| = f$ a.e.

  $\qquad\qquad\qquad \Rightarrow \quad f \ge 0$ a.e.

  and if $\int f \le 0$ then $\int |f| = \int (-f) \quad \Rightarrow \quad |f| = -f$ a.e.

  $\qquad\qquad\qquad\qquad\qquad\quad \Rightarrow \quad f \le 0$ a.e.

THEOREM 21.

Let f be a measurable function defined on a measurable set E then f is Lebesgue integrable if and only if |f| is Lebesgue integrable. [MEERUT–2001, 17; ROHTAK–2000, 03, 09; ROHILKHAND–2002]

PROOF. Let us first suppose f is L-integrable over E. Then clearly, f^+ and f^- both are L-integrable over E.

And $|f| = f^+ + f^-$, sum of two integrable functions.

$\Rightarrow \quad |f|$ is L-integrable.

Conversely, let us suppose that $|f|$ is L-integrable. We have to prove that f is also L-integrable.

Since, $|f|$ is L-integrable $\Rightarrow \quad \int_E |f| < \infty$

Also, $\qquad\qquad \int_E |f| = \int_E f^+ + \int_E f^-$

$\Rightarrow \quad \int_E f^+$ and $\int_E f^-$ are both finite.

$\Rightarrow \quad \int_E f^+ < \infty, \int_E f^- < \infty$

$\Rightarrow \quad f^+$ and f^- both are L-integrable.

Finally $f = f^+ + f^-$ is L-integrable,(being the difference of two integrable functions)

THEOREM 22.

Let f be a bounded function defined on a measurable set E with $m(E) < \infty$ then

$$\inf_{f \le \psi} . \int_E \psi(x)dx = \sup_{f \ge \psi} . \int_E \phi(x)dx$$

for all simple function ϕ and ψ if and only if f is measurable.

PROOF. Let us first suppose f is measurable.

It is given that f is bounded therefore, $|f| \le M, M > 0$.

$\Rightarrow \qquad\qquad -M \le f(x) \le M$

Define $\qquad\qquad E_k = \left\{ x \in E : \dfrac{(k-1)M}{n} < f(x) < \dfrac{kM}{n} \right\}, -n \le k \le n$

Clearly, $< E_k >_{k=-n}^{n}$ is a family of disjoint measurable subset of E such that $\cup E_k = E$. Then

$$m(E) = \sum_{k=-n}^{n} m(E_k)$$ ...(1)

Further, define two simple function ψ_n and ϕ_n on E such that

$$\psi_n = \sum_{k=-n}^{n}\left(\frac{M_k}{n}\right)\psi_{E_k} \text{ and } \phi_n = \sum_{k=-n}^{n}\frac{(k-1)M}{n}\psi_{E_k}$$

Then $\qquad \phi_n(x) \le f(x) \le \psi_n(x) \ \forall x \in E$

So, $\qquad \inf_{f \le \psi}.\int_E \psi(x)dx \le \int_E \psi_n(x)dx = \sum_{k=-n}^{n}\frac{M_k}{n}m(E_k) = \frac{M}{n}\sum_{k=-n}^{n}km(E_k)$ ...(2)

and $\qquad \sup_{f \ge \phi}.\int_E \phi(x)dx \ge \int_E \phi_n(x)dx = \frac{M}{n}\sum_{k=-n}^{n}(k-1)m(E_k)$

$\Rightarrow \qquad -\sup_{f \ge \phi}.\int_E \phi(x)dx \le \frac{-M}{n}\sum_{k=-n}^{n}(k-1)m(E_k)$ ...(3)

On adding (2) and (3) we get

$$0 \le \inf.\int_E \psi(x)dx = \sup\int_E \phi(x)dx \le \frac{M}{n}\sum_{k=-n}^{n}m(E_k) = \frac{M}{n}m(E)$$

Finally, letting $n \to \infty$, we get

$$0 \le \inf.\int_E \psi(x)dx - \sup.\int_E \phi(x)dx \le 0$$

$\Rightarrow \qquad \inf_{f \le \psi}\int_E \psi(x)dx = \sup_{f \ge \phi}\int_E \phi(x)dx$ ...(4)

Conversely, let us suppose equation (4) is satisfied. We have to prove that f is measurable.

Now, for every n, $\exists$ simple functions ϕ_n and ψ_n such that

$$\phi_n(x) \le f(x) \le \psi_n(x)$$

and $\int \psi_n(x)dx - \int \phi_n(x)dx < \dfrac{1}{n}$

Define $\psi^* = \inf. <\psi_n>$ and $\phi^* = \sup. <\phi_n>$

Then, being the infimum and supremum of measurable function, ψ^* and ϕ^* both are measurable and $\phi^*(x) \le f(x) \le \psi^*(x)$

Now, define a set $F = \{x : \phi^*(x) \ne \psi^*(x)\} = \{x : \phi^*(x) < \psi^*(x)\}$

Then $\qquad F = \bigcup_{r \in N} F_r, \text{where } F_r = \left\{x : \phi^*(x) < \psi^*(x) - \frac{1}{r}\right\}$

But $\qquad F_r \subseteq \left\{x : \phi_n(x) < \psi_n(x) - \frac{1}{r}\right\} \forall n$

Also, $\qquad m\left[\left[\left\{x : \phi_n(x) < \psi_n(x) - \frac{1}{r}\right\}\right]\right] < \frac{r}{n}$

Therefore, $\qquad m(F_r) \le \dfrac{r}{n}$

Letting $n \to \infty$, we get

$$m(F_r) = 0 \ \forall \ r$$

$\Rightarrow \qquad m(F) = 0 \text{ so } \phi^* = f = \psi^* \text{ a.e.}$

Hence, f is measurable.

THEOREM 23.

Let ϕ and ψ be simple functions which vanish outside a set E of finite measure then for a, b $\in$ R

$$\int (a\phi + b\psi) = a\int\phi + b\int\psi$$

and if $\phi = \psi$ a.e. then $\int\phi = \int\psi$ [HPU–2001, 02, 03, 09, 14]

PROOF.   Let ϕ and ψ are simple functions, then by definition, we can write

$$\phi = \sum_{i=1}^{m} a_i \chi_{A_i} \text{ and } \psi = \sum_{j=1}^{n} b_j \chi_{B_j}$$

where a_i and b_j are non-zero numbers.

Now, $A_i = \{x : \phi(x) = a_i\}$

and $B_j = \{x : \psi(x) = b_j\}$

such that $\bigcup_{i=1}^{m} A_i = \bigcup_{j=1}^{n} B_j = E$

Also, we define two sets

$$A_0 = \{x \notin E : \phi(x) = 0\}$$

and $B_0 = \{x \notin E : \psi(x) = 0\}$

Further, let $<E_k>$ $\{k = 1, ..., N\}$ be the family of sets obtained by the intersection $A_i \cap B_j$. Then $<E_k>$ forms a finite disjoint collection of measurable subsets of the set E.

Now, if p_K is the value assumed by ϕ on E_k and q_k by ψ on E_k. Then, we can write

$$\phi = \sum_{k=1}^{N} p_k \chi_{E_k}, \psi = \sum_{k=1}^{N} q_k \chi_{E_k}$$

Therefore, $a\phi + b\psi = \sum_{k=1}^{N} (ap_k + bq_k) \chi_{E_k}$

which implies $\int (a\phi + b\psi) = \sum_{k=1}^{N} (a_{p_k} + b_{q_k}) m(E_k)$

$$= a\sum_{k=1}^{N} p_k \cdot m(E_k) + b\sum_{k=1}^{N} q_k \cdot m(E_k) = a\int\phi + b\int\psi$$

Further, it is given that $\phi \geq \psi$

$\Rightarrow$ $\phi - \psi \geq 0$

$\Rightarrow$ $\int\phi - \int\psi = 0$

$\Rightarrow$ $\int\phi \geq \int\psi$

THEOREM 24.

If f and g are non-negative measurable function defined on E then $\int_E (f+g) = \int_E f + \int_E g$

                                        [HPU–2003, 11; NAGPUR–2006]

PROOF.   Let f and g be two non-negative measurable functions defined over a measurable set E.

Let us define a functions $h(x)$ and $k(x)$ such that

$$h(x) \leq f(x) \text{ and } k(x) \leq g(x)$$

Then, we have

$$h(x) + k(x) \leq f(x) + g(x) = (f + g)(x)$$

Therefore, $\int_E (h + k) \leq \int_E f + g$

$$\Rightarrow \qquad \int_E h + \int_E k \le \int_E f + g \qquad \qquad \qquad \dots(1)$$

Now, suppose that $F(x)$ be a bounded measurable function such that $F(x) \le (f+g)(x)$ and $F(x)$ vanishes outside a set of finite measure.

Let us take $\qquad h(x) = \min\{f(x), F(x)\}$

and $\qquad k(x) = F(x) - h(x)$

$$\Rightarrow \qquad h(x) + k(x) = F(x) \le f(x) + g(x)$$

$$\Rightarrow \qquad h(x) \le f(x) \text{ and } k(x) \le g(x) \qquad \qquad \dots(2)$$

Also, $\qquad \int_E F = \int_E h + \int_E k \le \int_E f + \int_E g \qquad \qquad$ [From (2)]

which is true for all $F \le (f+g)$, therefore by taking supremum we have

$$\int_E (f+g) \le \int_E f + \int_E g \qquad \qquad \dots(3)$$

Finally, from (2) and (3) we conclude that

$$\int_E f + g = \int_E f + \int_E f$$

THEOREM 25.

If f and g are non-negative measurable functions defined on a measurable set E such that f > g on E and if f is integrable over E then g is also integrable on E.

PROOF. Let f and g be two non-negative measurable function defined on a measurable set E such that $f > g$ on E.

Let f be integrable $\Rightarrow \int_E f < \infty \qquad \qquad \dots(1)$

Now, f and g are non-negative measurable function $\Rightarrow f - g$ is non-negative measurable functions. Therefore,

$$\int_E (f-g) \ge 0 \text{ and } \int_E g \ge 0 \qquad \qquad \dots(2)$$

Now, write $\qquad \int_E f = \int_E (f-g) + g = \int_E f - g + \int_E g$

$$\Rightarrow \qquad \int_E f = \int_E f - g + \int_E g \qquad \qquad \dots(3)$$

Using (1) in (3) we conclude that

$$\int_E f - g < \infty \text{ and } \int_E g < \infty$$

$$\therefore \quad \int_E g < \infty \quad \Rightarrow \quad g \text{ is integrable.}$$

☞ **REMARK**

• From above we conclude that $\int_E f - g = \int_E f - \int_E g$.

THEOREM 26.

Let f be a bounded measurable function defined on a measurable set E such that $f(x) \ge 0$ and $\int_E f(x)dx = 0$. Then $f(x) = 0$ a.e. on E. In other words, we can say that $f(x)$ is equivalent to zero function on E.

[MEERUT–2001, 16; ROHILKHAND–2005; HPU–2004; ROHTAK–2004; NAGPUR–2006]

PROOF. Let us define

$$E_0 = E[f(x) = 0] = \{x \in E : f(x) = 0\}$$

and $\qquad E_r = E\left[\frac{M}{r+1} < f(x) \le \frac{M}{r}\right] \forall r \in N$

Since, $f(x)$ is bounded $\Rightarrow [f(x)] \le M \, \forall \, x \in E, M > 0$

Clearly, $E = \bigcup\limits_{r=0}^{\infty} E_r$ such that $E_i \cap E_j = \phi, i \ne j \qquad \qquad \dots(1)$

We can write

$$E_r = E\left[f(x) \le \frac{M}{r} \right] \cap E\left[f(x) > \frac{M}{r+1} \right]$$

= intersection of two measurable sets

= measurable

$\Rightarrow$ E_r is measurable.

Further, from (1)

$$E - E_0 = \bigcup_{r=1}^{\infty} E_r$$

$\Rightarrow$ $$m(E - E_0) = \sum_{r=1}^{\infty} m(E_r) \qquad \qquad ...(2)$$

Since, $$\frac{M}{r+1} < f(x) \ \forall x \in E, n \in N$$

Therefore, by first mean value theorem, we have

$$\frac{M}{r+1} \cdot m(E_r) < \int_{E_r} f(x)dx \le \sum_{r=0}^{n} \int_{E_r} f(x)dx$$

$$= \int_E f(x)dx = 0 \qquad \text{(given)}$$

$\Rightarrow$ $$\frac{M}{r+1} m(E_r) \le 0 \ \forall r \in N \qquad \qquad ...(3)$$

But $\frac{M}{r+1} \ge 0$ and $m(E_r) \ge 0 \Rightarrow \frac{M}{r+1} m(E_r) \ge 0$ ...(4)

From (3) and (4) we conclude that

$$\frac{M}{r+1} m(E_r) = 0 \ \forall r \in N$$

$\Rightarrow$ $$m(E_r) = 0 \ \forall \ r \in N$$

$\Rightarrow$ $$\sum_{r=1}^{\infty} m(E_r) = 0 \qquad \qquad ...(5)$$

Finally from (2) and (5) we get

$$m(E - E_0) = 0$$

Therefore, $f(x) = 0 \ \forall \ x \in E_0$ and $m(E - E_0) = 0$

Hence, $f(x) = 0$ a.e. on E.

6.7 THE LEBESGUE INTEGRAL OF UNBOUNDED FUNCTIONS

Let $f(x)$ be an unbounded function defined on $[a, b]$, which is measurable and non-negative. Then for an arbitrary $n \in N$, we can define a function $[f(x)]_n$ on $[a, b]$ as follows:

$$[f(x)]_n = \begin{cases} f(x); & \text{if } f(x) \le n \\ n; & \text{if } f(x) > n \end{cases}$$

In other words, we can say that

$$[f(x)]_n = \min\{f(x), n\}$$

Here, we can define

$$\int_E f = \lim_{n \to \infty} \int_E [f_n(x)]_n$$

☞ **REMARK**

- Most of the thorems, which we have proved for bounded measurable functions are also true for unbounded non-negative measurable functions. For example
  (i) $\int_E cf = c\int_E f$
  (ii) $\int_E f - g = \int_E f - \int_E g$ $\qquad c \in R$ etc.

  for non-negative unbounded measurable functions f and g.

THEOREM 1.

The function $[f(x)]_n$ defined above is bounded and measurable over $[a, b]$.

PROOF. Let us define
$$[f(x)]_n = \min[f(x), n]$$
Clearly, $\qquad [f(x)]_n \geq 0$
$\Rightarrow \quad [f(x)]_n$ is bounded over $[a, b]$.
Now for arbitrary $k \in R$, we have

$$\{x \in [a,b] : [f(x)]_n > k\} = \begin{cases} \{x \in [a,b] : f(x) > k\}; & \text{if } n \geq k \\ \phi; & \text{if } n < k \end{cases}$$

Since, $f(x)$ is measurable over $[a, b]$ therefore the set $\{x \in [a, b] : f(x) > k\}$ is measurable. Also, the empty set ϕ is also measurable.
Therefore, $\{x \in [a, b] : [f(x)]_n > k\}$ is measurable.
Hence, $[f(x)]_n$ is measurable over $[a, b]$.

THEOREM 2.

Let f be a non-negative unbounded measurable function defined over a measurable set E of $[a, b]$. Then

$$\int_E f(x)dx = \sum_{r=1}^{\infty} \int_{E_r} fdx, \text{ where } E = \bigcup_{r=1}^{\infty} E_r, E_r \cap E_s = \phi, r \neq s.$$

PROOF. By definition, we can write
$$[f(x)]_n = \begin{cases} f(x); & \text{if } f(x) \leq n \\ n; & \text{if } f(x) > n \end{cases}$$

Also, by definition
$$\int_E f(x)dx = \lim_{n\to\infty} \int_E [f_n(x)]_n dx$$

Using previous theorem, $[f(x)]_n$ is a bounded measurable functions. Therefore,

$$\int_E [f(x)]_n dx = \sum_{r=1}^{\infty} \int_{E_r} [f(x)]_n \qquad \text{(By countable additive property)}$$

$$\geq \sum_{r=1}^{m} \int_{E_r} [f(x)]_n dx$$

Letting $n, m \to \infty$ we get
$$\int_E f(x)dx \geq \sum_{r=1}^{\infty} \int_{E_r} f(x)dx \qquad\qquad \text{...(1)}$$

Further, since $[f(x)]_n \leq f(x)$
$\Rightarrow \qquad \int_{E_r} [f(x)]_n dx \leq \int_{E_r} f(x)dx$

$\Rightarrow \qquad \int_{E_r} [f(x)]_n \, dx \leq \sum_{r=1}^{\infty} \int_{E_r} f(x) \, dx$

$\Rightarrow \qquad \int_E [f(x)]_n \, dx = \sum_{r=1}^{\infty} \int_E [f(x)]_n \, dx \leq \sum_{r=1}^{\infty} \int_{E_r} f(x) \, dx$

Letting $n \to \infty$, we get

$$\int_E f(x) \, dx \leq \sum_{r=1}^{\infty} \int_{E_r} f(x) \, dx \qquad \qquad \dots(2)$$

From (1) and (2) we conclude that

$$\int_E f(x) \, dx = \sum_{r=1}^{\infty} \int_{E_r} f(x) \, dx$$

THEOREM 3.

Let f and g be two non-negative unbounded measurable functions defined over a measurable subset $E \subseteq [a, b]$ then

$$\int_E (f + g) \, dx = \int_E f \, dx + \int_E g \, dx$$

[MEERUT–2001, 04, 12, 15; NAGPUR–2006; KANPUR–1993; GARHWAL–1997, 2012; AVADH–2008]

PROOF. Let us define $h(x) = f(x) + g(x)$

Now it is given that $f(x) \geq 0$, $g(x) \geq 0$

We have $\qquad [h(x)]_n \leq [f(x)]_n + [g(x)]_n \leq [h(x)]_{2n}$ $\qquad \dots(1)$

Further, since $[f(x)]_n$ and $[g(x)]_n$ are bounded and measurable.

Therefore, $\int_E \{[f(x)]_n + [g(x)]_n\} dx = \int_E [f(x)]_n \, dx + \int_E [g(x)]_n \, dx$ $\qquad \dots(2)$

On integrating (1) and then using (2) we get

$$\int_E [h(x)]_n \, dx \leq \int_E [f(x)]_n \, dx + \int_E [g(x)]_n \, dx \leq \int_E [h(x)]_{2n} \, dx$$

Letting $n \to \infty$, we get

$$\int_E h(x) \, dx \leq \int_E f(x) \, dx + \int_E g(x) \, dx \leq \int_E h(x) \, dx$$

$\Rightarrow \qquad \int_E h(x) \, dx = \int_E f(x) \, dx + \int_E g(x) \, dx$

Hence, $\int_E [f(x) + g(x)] \, dx = \int_E f(x) \, dx + \int_E g(x) \, dx$

i.e., $\qquad \int_E f + g = \int_E f + \int_E g$.

THEOREM 4.

If f is a non-negative integrable function defined over a set E, then for given $\varepsilon > 0 \, \exists \, a \, \delta > 0$ such that for every set $A \subset E$ with $m(A) < \infty$, we get $\int_A f < \varepsilon$.

[MEERUT–2010; DELHI–2008; HPU–2003, 04; ROHTAK–2000, 01, 04]

PROOF. Let us first suppose f is a bounded function on E such that $|f(x)| \leq M \quad \forall x \in E$

Then for all $x \in A$ also $|f(x)| \leq M$

Now, choose $\delta = \dfrac{\varepsilon}{M} (> 0)$ for $A \subset E$, $m(A) < \delta$, we get

$$\int_A f \leq M \cdot m(A) < M \cdot \delta = M \cdot \frac{\varepsilon}{M} = \varepsilon$$

$\Rightarrow \qquad \int_A f < \varepsilon$

Now suppose that f is unbounded on E. Then we can define

$$f_n(x) = \begin{cases} f(x) & \text{if } f(x) \leq n \\ n & \text{if } f(x) > n \end{cases}$$

Clearly, $\langle f_n \rangle$ is an increasing sequence of bounded function on E such that $f_n \to f$. Then by monotone convergence theorem, given $\varepsilon > 0$ $\exists$ an integer $n_0 \in N$ such that

$$\int_E f_{n_0} > \int_E f - \frac{\varepsilon}{2}$$

$$\Rightarrow \qquad \int_E f - \int_E f_{n_0} < \frac{\varepsilon}{2} \qquad\qquad\qquad\qquad ...(1)$$

Now since $f > f_{n_0}$ therefore

$$\int_E (f - f_{n_0}) = \int_E f - \int_E f_{n_0} < \frac{\varepsilon}{2} \qquad\qquad \text{(From (1))}$$

$$\therefore \qquad \int_A f = \int_A (f - f_{n_0}) + \int_A f_{n_0}$$

$$\leq \int_E (f - f_{n_0}) + n_0 \cdot m(A) \qquad (\because f_{n_0} \text{ is bounded by } n_0)$$

$$< \frac{\varepsilon}{2} + n_0 \cdot \delta$$

$$< \frac{\varepsilon}{2} + n_0 \cdot \frac{\varepsilon}{2n_0} < \varepsilon \qquad\qquad \text{(letting } \delta < \frac{\varepsilon}{2n_0} \text{)}$$

$$\Rightarrow \qquad \int_A f < \varepsilon$$

THEOREM 5.

If E is any measurable subset of $[a, b]$ and if $f, g \in L[a, b]$ are arbitrary functions such that $f(x) = g(x)$ a.e. on E then $\int_E f = \int_E g$.

PROOF. It is given that $f(x) = g(x)$ a.e. on E.

Also, f, g are non-negative real valued functions in $L[a, b]$.

$$\Rightarrow \qquad [f(x)]_n = [g(x)]_n \text{ a.e. on } E \; \forall \; n \in N \qquad\qquad ...(1)$$

and $[f(x)]_n$ and $[g(x)]_n$ both are bounded function.

Then from (1)

$$\int_E [f(x)]_n = \int_E [g(x)]_n$$

$$\Rightarrow \qquad \int_E \lim_{n \to \infty} [f(x)]_n = \int_E \lim_{n \to \infty} [g(x)]_n$$

$$\Rightarrow \qquad \int_E f = \int_E g$$

Since, $f, g \in L[a, b]$ and $f(x) = g(x)$ a.e. on E.

Therefore $\qquad f^+(x) = g^+(x)$ a.e. on E.

and $\qquad\qquad f^-(x) = g^-(x)$ a.e. on E

$$\Rightarrow \qquad \int_E f^+ = \int_E g^+ \text{ and } \int_E f^- = \int_E g^-$$

Finally, $\int_E f = \int_E f^+ - \int_E f^- = \int_E g^+ - \int_E g^- = \int_E g \qquad (\because f = f^+ - f^-)$

Hence, $\qquad\qquad \int_E f = \int_E g$

Solved Examples

EXAMPLE 1. If f and g are bounded measurable functions defined on a set of infinite measure, show that

(i) $\int_E pf + qg = p\int_E f + q\int_E g$

(ii) If $f = g$ a.e. then $\int_E f = \int_E g$

SOLUTION. (i) Let f and g are bounded measurable function on E.

Then we have already proved that for real numbers p and q, $pf + qg$ is also measurable and bounded.

Now,
$$\int_E (pf + qg) = \int_a^b (pf + qg)\chi_E = \int_a^b pf\chi_E + \int_a^b qg\chi_E$$
$$= p\int_a^b f\chi_E + q\int_a^b g\chi_E$$
$$= p\int_E f + q\int_E g$$

(ii) Since $f = g$ almost everywhere, therefore,
$$\int_E f = \int_a^b f\chi_E = \int_a^b g\chi_E = \int_E g$$

EXAMPLE 2. *Using an example, show that a function which is Lebesgue integrable is not necessarily R-integrable.* [MEERUT–2004, 06, 07, 12, 14, 15, 17; KOHLAPUR–1987, 2009; ROHTAK–2004; KANPUR–2008; ROHILKHAND–1999]

SOLUTION. Let us define a function
$$h(x) = \begin{cases} 1; & \text{if } x \text{ is irrational} \\ 0; & \text{if } x \text{ is rational} \end{cases}$$

We know that $f(x)$ is a discontinuous function and the points of discontinuities form a measurable set. Further, we know that every subinterval of [0, 1] contains both rational and irrationals. (By denseness property of real numbers)

Here, $M_r = 1$, $m_r = 0$

Let us write $0 = x_0 < x_1 < x_2 < \ldots < x_n = 1$ be any mode of subdivision.

Then   lower Riemann sum $= \sum_{r=0}^{n-1} m_r(x_{r+1} - x_r) = 0$ $(\because m_r = 0)$

and   upper Riemann sum $= \sum_{r=0}^{n-1} M_r(x_{r+1} - x_r) = \sum_{r=0}^{n-1} 1 \cdot (x_{r+1} - x_r) = 1 \cdot 1 = 1$

$$\left(\because \sum_{r=0}^{n-1} (x_{r-1} - x_r) = x_n - x_0 = 1 \right)$$

Clearly,   lower Riemann sum $\neq$ upper Riemann sum $\Rightarrow f$ is not R-integrable.

Now, we shall show that the function f defined above is L-integrable.

Define A = set of all points of irrational numebrs in [0, 1]

B = set of all points of rational numbers in [0, 1]

Clearly, $A \cup B = [0, 1]$ and $A \cap B = \phi \Rightarrow m(A \cap B) = m(\phi) = 0$

Here, $P = \{A, B\}$ is a measurable partition of [0, 1]

and f is identically equal to 1 on A and identically equal to 0 on B.

Therefore, $M[f; A] = m[f; A] = 1$

and $M[f; B] = m[f; B] = 0$

Now, $U[f; P] = M[f; A]m(A) + M[f; B]m(B)$
$$= 1 \cdot m(A) + 0 \cdot m(B) = m(A) = 1$$

$(\because B$ is countable $\Rightarrow m(B) = 0$
$$\therefore m(A) = l\{[0, 1] - m(A')\}$$
$$= 1 - 0 - m(B)$$
$$= 1 - 0 = 1 \qquad)$$

In a similar way
$$L[f; P] = m[f; A]m(A) + m[f; B]m(B)$$
$$= 1 \cdot m(A) + 0 \cdot m(B)$$
$$= m(A) = 0$$

which implies that $U[f; P] = L[f; P] = 1$

$\Rightarrow$ $\quad$ $U[f; P] - L[f; P] = 0 < \varepsilon$

$\Rightarrow$ $\quad$ $U[f; P] - L[f; P] < \varepsilon$

$\qquad$ (which is the necessary and sufficient condition of L-integrability)

$\Rightarrow$ $\qquad\qquad$ $f \in L[0, 1]$

Hence, f is L-integrable.

EXAMPLE 3. *If f is a measurable function such that $a \leq f(x) \leq b$, a, $b \in R$ and g is an integrable function, show that there exist a number $c \in R$ such that $a \leq c \leq b$ and*

$$\int f |g| = c \int |g|$$

SOLUTION. Since, $a \leq f(x) \leq b$. Therefore, we can write

$$|fg| \leq (|a| + |b|) |g| \text{ a.e.}$$

Also, fg is L-integrable also.

Again, since $a \leq f \leq b$ a.e.

Therefore, $a|g| \leq f|g| \leq b|g|$ a.e.

$\Rightarrow$ $\qquad$ $a\int|g| \leq \int f|g| \leq b\int|g|$ a.e.

If $\int|g| = 0$ then $g = 0$ a.e., then result is obvious.

If $\int|g| \neq 0$ then we can find a number c such that

$$c = \frac{(\int f |g|)}{\int |g|}$$

$\Rightarrow$ $\qquad\qquad$ $c \cdot \int|g| = \int f|g|$

EXAMPLE 4. *Let $f : [0, 1] \to R$ be a function, defined by $f(x) = \begin{cases} 0; & \text{if } x \text{ is rational} \\ n; & \text{if } x \text{ is irrational} \end{cases}$ and n is the number of zeroes immediately after the decimal sign in the decimal representation of x. Then show that f is measurable and find the value of $\int_0^1 f dx$.*

SOLUTION. Define a function g such that

$$g(x) = n \text{ when } \frac{1}{10^{n+1}} \leq x < \frac{1}{10^n}$$

Clearly, at all the irrational points x in $[0, 1]$, $g(x) = f(x)$ while $m\{x \in [0, 1]\}$ such that

$$f(x) \neq g(x) = m(\text{set of rational no.s in } [0, 1])$$
$$= m[\text{a countable set}]$$
$$= 0$$

$\therefore$ $\qquad\qquad$ $f = g$ a.e.

Further, g is a step function, therefore, measurable.

$\Rightarrow$ f is also measurable.

Now, $\qquad$ $\int_0^1 f(x)dx = \int_0^1 g(x)dx = \sum_{n=0}^{\infty} n\left(\frac{1}{10^n} - \frac{1}{10^{n+1}}\right) = \sum_{n=1}^{\infty} \frac{9^n}{10^{n+1}}$

The R.H.S. of the above equation is a Arithmetic-geometric series.

$\therefore$ $\qquad\qquad$ $S = 9\left(\frac{1}{10^2} + \frac{2}{10^3} + \frac{3}{10^4} + ... \text{to } \infty\right)$

$$\Rightarrow \qquad \frac{1}{10}S = 9\left(\frac{1}{10^3} + \frac{2}{10^4} + \frac{3}{10^5} + \dots \text{to } \infty\right)$$

$$\Rightarrow \qquad S - \frac{1}{10}S = 9\left[\frac{1}{10^2} + \frac{1}{10^3} + \frac{1}{10^4} + \dots \text{to } \infty\right] = 9 \cdot \frac{\dfrac{1}{10^2}}{1 - \dfrac{1}{10}} \qquad \left(\because S = \frac{a}{1-r}\right)$$

$$\Rightarrow \qquad \frac{9}{10}S = 9 \cdot \frac{1}{100} \cdot \frac{10}{9}$$

$$\Rightarrow \qquad S = \frac{1}{9}$$

Hence, $\qquad \int_0^1 f(x)dx = \frac{1}{9}$

EXAMPLE 5. *Give an example of a sequence of Riemann integrable functions on [0, 1] which converges pointwise to a bounded function which is not Riemann integrable. Prove that such an example can not be found if Riemann integral is replaaced by Lebesgue integral.*

SOLUTION. Define a sequence $\langle f_n \rangle$ of functions as follows:

$$f_n(x) = \begin{cases} 1; & \text{if } x \in \{r_1, r_2, \dots, r_n \dots\} \\ 0; & \text{if } x \in [0,1] \sim [r_1, r_2, \dots, r_n \dots] \end{cases}$$

where $\{r_1, r_2, \dots, r_n \dots\}$ be an enumerable set of rational numbers in [0, 1].
Now for all $n \in [0, 1]$ and for subdivision

$$P = \{0, r_1, r_2, \dots, r_n, 1\}$$
$$U[f; P] = L[f; P]$$

$\Rightarrow \quad f_n(x)$ is Riemann integrable.
But in example 2 we have shown that the function

$$\lim_{n \to \infty} f_n(x) = f(x) = \begin{cases} 1 & \text{if } x \text{ is rational} \\ 0 & \text{if } x \text{ is irrational} \end{cases}$$

is not R-integrable.
Also, the R-integrability of f_n ensure the L-integrability of f_n and clearly $\lim_{n \to \infty} f_n(x) = f(x)$ is also L-integrable.

EXAMPLE 6. *If f is a non-negative integrable function, then show that the function $F(x) = \int_{-\infty}^{x} f(t)dt$ is continuous on **R**.*

SOLUTION. In theorem 4 of previous section we have proved that for given $\varepsilon > 0 \, \exists$ a $\delta > 0$ such that for all subsets $A \subseteq R$ such that $m(A) < \infty$ we get $\int_A f < \varepsilon$ and hence $\left| \int_A f \right| < \varepsilon$.

Further, let $x_0 \in R$ be arbitrary then for all $x \in R$ such that $|x - x_0| < \delta$.
We have $\qquad \left| \int_{x_0}^{x} f(t)dt \right| < \varepsilon$
which implies

$$\left| \int_{-\infty}^{x} f(t)dt - \int_{-\infty}^{x_0} f(t)dt \right| < \varepsilon$$

$\Rightarrow \quad |F(x) - F(x_0)| < \varepsilon$ whenever $|x - x_0| < \delta$
$\Rightarrow \quad F(x)$ is continuous at $x_0 \in R$.
Since, x_0 is arbitrary, so we can say that $F(x)$ is continuous on **R**.

EXAMPLE 7. *If the Lebesgue integral of non-negative measurable function f over [0, 1] be zero, show that f = 0 a.e. or we can say $\int f = 0 \Rightarrow f = 0$ a.e.*

SOLUTION. Let f be a non-negative measurable function over [0, 1].

i.e., $\qquad\qquad f(x) \geq 0 \ \forall \ x \in [0, 1]$

It is given that $L\int_0^1 f(x)dx = 0 \Rightarrow \int_0^1 f(x)dx = 0$

Now, $\int_0^1 f(x)dx = \inf_P U[f; P] = U[f; P^*]$ where $P^* = \{A_1, A_2, ..., A_n\}$

which implies $\sum\limits_{i=1}^{n} M[f; A_i] \cdot m(A_i) = 0$ $\qquad\qquad$ ...(1)

But $m(A_i) > 0$ a.e. on P^* and $M[f; A_i]$ is also non-negative.

So, (1) holds good only if $M[f; A_i] = 0$

Thus, maximum value of $f(x)$ is zero on almost each A_i.

$\Rightarrow \qquad\qquad \max[f(x)] = 0$ a.e. on [0, 1]

Hence, $f(x) = 0$ on [0, 1].

EXAMPLE 8. *Show that the function $f(x) = \dfrac{1}{x}, (0 < x \leq 1)$ is not L-inetegrable on [0, 1].*

[MEERUT–2004, 08, 13, 16; KANPUR–2009]

SOLUTION. It is given that $\qquad f(x) = \dfrac{1}{x}, 0 < x \leq 1$

Clearly $f(x)$ is an unbounded function. Then for $m \in N$, we define

$$[f(x)]_n = \begin{cases} f(x); & 0 \leq f(x) \leq m \\ m; & f(x) > m \end{cases}$$

Then clearly, $[f(x)]_m = \dfrac{1}{x}$ if $\dfrac{1}{m} \leq x \leq 1$

and $\qquad\qquad [f(x)]_m = m$, if $0 < x < \dfrac{1}{m}$

Now, $\qquad \int_0^1 [f(x)]_m = \int_0^{1/m} [f(x)]_m + \int_{1/m}^1 [f(x)]_m$

$\qquad\qquad\qquad = \int_0^{1/m} m\,dx + \int_{1/m}^1 \dfrac{1}{x}dx$

$\qquad\qquad\qquad = [mx]_0^{1/m} + [\log x]_{1/m}^1$

$\qquad\qquad\qquad = -\log\dfrac{1}{m} + 1 = \log m + 1$

Letting $m \to \infty$, we have

$$\int_0^1 f(x)dx = 1 + \lim_{m \to \infty} (\log m)$$

But we know that $\lim\limits_{m \to \infty} \log m$ does not exist.

$\Rightarrow \quad f$ is not Lebesgue integrable over [0, 1].

EXAMPLE 9. *Prove that the function*

$$f(x) = \frac{d}{dx}\left(x^2 - \sin\frac{1}{x^2}\right) = 2x\sin\frac{1}{x^2} - \frac{2}{x}\cos\frac{1}{x^2}$$

is not L-integrable over [0, 1].

[MEERUT–2001, 03, 06, 14, 15; KANPUR–2003; GARHWAL–1999, 2009, 13; AVADH–2007, 12]

SOLUTION.   Let $f(x) = 2x \sin \dfrac{1}{x^2} - \dfrac{2}{x} \cos \dfrac{1}{x^2}$

Obviously, the function $2x \sin \dfrac{1}{x^2}$ is bounded and continuous over [0, 1] and

hence measurable over [0, 1].

$\Rightarrow \quad 2x \sin \dfrac{1}{x^2}$ is L-integrable over [0, 1].

Now, we check the L-integrability of the function $-\dfrac{2}{x} \cos \dfrac{1}{x^2}$ over [0, 1].

Let $a_n = \left\{ \left(2n + \dfrac{1}{3} \right) \pi \right\}^{-1/2}$ and $b_n = \left\{ \left(2n - \dfrac{1}{3} \right) \pi \right\}^{-1/2}$ ...(1)

Then, clearly $a_n^2 \le x^2 \le b_n^2$

$\Rightarrow \qquad \left(2n - \dfrac{1}{3} \right) \pi \le \dfrac{1}{x^2} \le \left(2n + \dfrac{1}{3} \right) \pi$

$\Rightarrow \qquad \left| \cos \dfrac{1}{x^2} \right| \ge \dfrac{1}{2}$ ...(2)

So, $\int_0^1 \dfrac{1}{x} \left| \cos \dfrac{1}{x^2} \right| dx = \sum\limits_{n=1}^{\infty} \int_{a_n}^{b_n} \dfrac{1}{x} \left| \cos \dfrac{1}{x^2} \right| dx \ge \sum\limits_{n=1}^{\infty} \int_{a_n}^{b_n} \dfrac{1}{2x} dx$ (By (2))

$= \sum\limits_{n=1}^{\infty} \dfrac{1}{4} \log \dfrac{b_n^2}{a_n^2}$

$= \dfrac{1}{4} \sum\limits_{n=1}^{\infty} \log \left(\dfrac{6n+1}{6n-1} \right)$ (By (1))

$\to \infty$

Therefore, the function $\dfrac{1}{x} \left| \cos \dfrac{1}{x^2} \right|$ is not L-integrable.

EXAMPLE 10.   *Show that the function defined on $E = [0, \infty[$ is as follows:*

$$f(x) = \dfrac{\sin x}{x}, \text{ for } x \ne 0 \text{ and } f(0) = 0$$

is not Lebesgue integrable on E.   [GARHWAL–2003; MEERUT–2008]

SOLUTION.   Consider $\int_0^{n\pi} \left| \dfrac{\sin x}{x} \right| dx = \sum\limits_{r=1}^{n} \int_{(r-1)\pi}^{r\pi} \dfrac{|\sin x|}{x} dx$

$= \sum\limits_{r=1}^{n} \int_0^{\pi} \dfrac{|\sin\{t + (r-1)\pi\}|}{t + (r-1)\pi} dt$

$\ge \sum\limits_{r=1}^{n} \int_0^{\pi} \dfrac{|\sin\{t + (r-1)\pi\}|}{r\pi} dt$

$= \dfrac{1}{\pi} \sum\limits_{r=1}^{n} \dfrac{1}{r} \int_0^{\pi} |\sin t| \, dt$

$$= \frac{1}{\pi}\sum_{r=1}^{n}\frac{1}{r}\int_0^\pi \sin t\, dt = \frac{2}{\pi}\sum_{r=1}^{n}\frac{1}{r}$$

which implies $\lim_{n\to\infty}\int_0^{n\pi}\left|\frac{\sin x}{x}\right|dx \geq \frac{2}{\pi}\sum_{r=1}^{\infty}\frac{1}{r}$

But we know that $\sum_{r=1}^{\infty}\frac{1}{r}$ is a divergent series, therefore $\sum_{r=1}^{\infty}\frac{1}{r}=\infty$

So, $\int_0^\infty |f(x)|\, dx \geq \infty \Rightarrow \int_0^\infty |f(x)|\, dx = \infty$

$\Rightarrow$ $|f|$ is not L-integrable.

Hence, $f(x)$ is not L-integrable.

EXAMPLE 11. *Give an example to show that the integral of a no where zero function can be zero.*

[MEERUT–2008]

SOLUTION.   Let us define a function $f : Q \to R$ such that $f(x) = 1\ \forall\ x \in Q$.

Clearly, the function f defined above is no where zero.

But we know that $m(Q) = 0$.

                 ($\because\ Q$ is a countable set and measure of a countable set is zero)

Then by first mean value theorem

$$1 \cdot m(Q) \leq \int_Q f \leq 1 \cdot m(Q)$$

$\Rightarrow$ $0 \leq \int_Q f \leq 0$

$\Rightarrow$ $\int_Q f = 0$

EXAMPLE 12. *Show that the function f defined by $f(x) = \dfrac{1}{x^{1/3}} : 0 < x \leq 1$ and $f(0) = 0$ is L-integrable over $[0, 1]$.*

SOLUTION.   For $n \in N$, let us define

$$[f(x)]_n = \begin{cases} f(x); & 0 \leq f(x) \leq n \\ n; & f(x) > n \end{cases}$$

Therefore, $[f(x)]_n = \begin{cases} \dfrac{1}{x^{1/3}}, & \text{if } \dfrac{1}{n^3} \leq x \leq 1 \\ n, & \text{if } 0 < x < \dfrac{1}{n^3} \\ 0, & \text{if } x = 0 \end{cases}$ $\begin{array}{l} (\because f(x) \leq n \Rightarrow \dfrac{1}{x^{1/3}} \leq n \\[2mm] \Rightarrow \dfrac{1}{n^3} \leq x) \end{array}$

Then $\int_0^1 [f(x)]_n\, dx = \int_{1/n^3}^1 \frac{1}{x^{1/3}}\, dx + \int_0^{1/n^3} n\, dx$

$$= \frac{3}{2}(x^{2/3})_{1/n^3}^1 + n(x)_0^{1/n^3}$$

$$= \frac{3}{2}\left(1 - \frac{1}{n^2}\right) + \frac{1}{n^2} = \frac{3}{2} - \frac{1}{2n^2}$$

$\Rightarrow$ $\lim_{n\to\infty}\int_0^1 [f(x)]_n\, dx = \frac{3}{2} < \infty$

Hence f is Lebesgue integrable over $[0, 1]$.

EXAMPLE 13. *If $p > 0$, $q > 0$, show that*

$$\int_0^1 \frac{x^{p-1}}{1+x^q} \, dx = \frac{1}{p} - \frac{1}{p+q} + \frac{1}{p+2q} - \frac{1}{p+3q} + \ldots \quad \text{and deduce that}$$

(i) $\log 2 = 1 - \dfrac{1}{2} + \dfrac{1}{3} - \dfrac{1}{4} + \ldots$

(ii) $\dfrac{\pi}{4} = 1 - \dfrac{1}{3} + \dfrac{1}{5} - \dfrac{1}{7} + \ldots$

SOLUTION. Consider

$$\frac{x^{p-1}}{1+x^q} = x^{p-1}(1+x^q)^{-1}$$

$$= x^{p-1}[1 - x^q + x^{2q} - x^{3q} + x^{4q} - \ldots]$$

$$= x^{p-1} \sum_{n=0}^{\infty} [x^{2nq} - x^{(2n+1)q}]$$

$$= \sum_{n=0}^{\infty} [x^{2nq+p-1} - x^{(2n+1)q+p-1}]$$

Therefore,

$$\int \frac{x^{p-1}}{1+x^q} \, dx = \sum_{n=0}^{\infty} \left[\frac{x^{2nq+p}}{2nq+p} - \frac{x^{(2n+1)q+p}}{(2n+1)q+p} \right]_{x=0}^{1}$$

$$= \sum_{n=0}^{\infty} \left[\frac{1}{2nq+p} - \frac{1}{(2n+1)q+p} \right]$$

$$= \frac{1}{p} - \frac{1}{p+q} + \frac{1}{p+2q} - \frac{1}{p+3q} + \ldots \qquad \ldots(1)$$

(i) Put $p = q = 1$ in the above result (1) we get

$$\text{LHS} = \int_0^1 \frac{1}{1+x} \, dx = [\log(1+x)]_0^1 = \log 2$$

Hence, $\log 2 = 1 - \dfrac{1}{2} + \dfrac{1}{3} - \dfrac{1}{4} + \ldots$

(ii) Taking $p = 1$, $q = 2$ in (1), we get

$$\int_0^1 \frac{1}{1+x^2} \, dx = [\tan^{-1} x]_0^1 = \frac{\pi}{4}$$

Hence, $\dfrac{\pi}{4} = 1 - \dfrac{1}{3} + \dfrac{1}{5} - \dfrac{1}{7} + \ldots$

EXAMPLE 14. *Let X be a measurable space in which $\mathcal{M}$ is the O-ring of measurable set and μ is the measure. Suppose f is measurable and non-negative on X and for $A \in \mathcal{M}$ define $\phi(A) = \int_A f d\mu$. Then show that f is countably additive.*

SOLUTION. By countable additive property of integrals, we have

$$\int_E \phi \, dx = \sum_{k=1}^{\infty} \int_{E_k} f d\mu \qquad \ldots(1)$$

Now, $\phi(A) = \int_E f d\mu$, $E = \bigcup_{k=1}^{\infty} E_k = \sum_{k=1}^{\infty} E_k$

Therefore, $\qquad \phi(E) = \sum_{i=1}^{\infty} \phi(E_k)$

$\Rightarrow \qquad \phi\left(\sum_{k=1}^{\infty} E_k\right) = \sum_{k=1}^{\infty} \phi(E_k)$

Hence, ϕ is Countably additive.

EXAMPLE 15. *If E is a measurable subset of [a, b] and f is a bounded measurable function of $f \in L[a, b]$ such that $f(x) \geq 0$ a.e. on E then $\int_E f \geq 0$.*

SOLUTION. We know that $\qquad \int_E f = \int_a^b f\chi_E$, $\qquad \chi_E$ is the characteristic function of E.

It is given that $f \geq 0$ a.e. on E.

Also by definition of characteristic function $\chi_E \geq 0$ on [a, b].

$\Rightarrow \qquad f\chi_E \geq 0$ a.e. on [a, b]

$\Rightarrow \qquad \int_a^b f \cdot \chi_E \geq 0$

$\Rightarrow \qquad \int_E f \geq 0$

Exercise 6.1

1. Prove that two bounded measurable functions which are equal a.c. have the same integral. Also prove that converse is not necessarily true.

2. Prove that if $f(x) = 0$ at every point of Cantor's ternary set and $f(x) = n$ in each of the complimentary interval of length 3^{-n} then $\int_0^1 f(x)dx$ exists in the Lebesgue sense and equal to 3.

3. Prove that a Riemann integral function defined on [a, b] is measurable.

4. Prove that a bounded function f defined on a measurable set E of finite measure is L-integrable if and only if f is measurable.

5. If $E_1 \subset E_2$ then show that $\int_{E_1} f \leq \int_{E_2} f$.

6. Show that $\int_E \chi_E = m(A \cap E)$, where χ_E is the characteristic function of E.

7. If $f(x) = \begin{cases} 0; & \text{if} \quad 0 \leq x < 1 \\ 1; & \text{if} \quad \{1 \leq x < 2\} \cup \{3 \leq x < 4\} \\ 2; & \text{if} \quad \{2 \leq x < 3\} \cup \{4 \leq x < 5\} \end{cases}$

   Show that $\int_0^5 f(x)dx = 6$.

8. Let f be measurable of E and $|f| < g$ and g is measurable on E then show that f is also integrable on E.

9. Prove that the Lebesgue integral is infact a generalisation of the Riemann integral.

10. If E is a set of measure zero, then show that any function f is integrable over E and $\int_E f = 0$.

11. Let $f : R \to R$ be a function defined by

    $f(x) = \begin{cases} 0, & x \notin [0,1] \\ 1, & x \in [0,1] \text{ and rational} \\ -1, & x \in [0,1] \text{ and irrational} \end{cases}$

    Show that f is L-integrable.

12. Show that the function f defined on the interval [a, b] by

    $f(x) = \begin{cases} 0; & \text{if } x \text{ is irrational} \\ 1; & \text{if } x \text{ is rational} \end{cases}$

    is L-integrable but not R-integrable.

13. If a function f is integrable, show that the improper Riemann integral is equal to the Lebesgue integral.

14. If f is L-integrable, show that

    $\int f(x)dx = -\int f(-x)dx$

15. Prove that the integral of the sum of a finite number of bounded measurable function is the sum of integrals of the separate functions.

16. If f is L-integrable, then show that

    $\int_a^b f(t)dt = -\int_{-b}^{-a} f(-t)dt$

17. Show that $f : [0, 1] \to R$ is R-integrable if and only if the discontinuities of f form a set of Lebesgue measure zero.

18. If f is bounded and integrable in the Riemann sense in a closed interval [a, b] then prove that f is measurable and integrable in the Lebesgue sense and the Riemann integral of f over [a, b] is equal to the Lebesgue integral over [a, b].

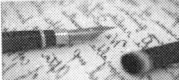
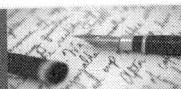

CHAPTER Summary

KEY TERMS

- **LOWER LEBESGUE SUM:** It is defined by
$$L[f;P] = \sum_{r=1}^{n} m[f;S_r] \cdot m(S_r).$$

- **UPPER LEBESGUE SUM:** It is defined by
$$U[f;P] = \sum_{r=1}^{n} M[f;S_r] \cdot m(S_r).$$

- **UPPER LEBESGUE INTEGRAL:** Let f be a bounded function defined on $[a, b]$. Then infimum of $U[f; P]$ is called the upper Lebesgue integral.

- **LOWER LEBESGUE INTEGRAL:** Let f be a bounded function defined on $[a, b]$. Then supremum of $L[f; P]$ is called the lower Lebesgue integral.

- **LEBESGUE INTEGRAL:** A bounded function defined on $[a, b]$ is said to be L-integrable on $[a, b]$ if $L\underline{\int}_a^b f = L\overline{\int}_a^b f$.

- **L-INTEGRAL OF NON-NEGATIVE FUNCTION:** A non-negative function f defined on a measurable set E is said to be integrable if $\int_E f dx < \infty$.

RESULTS

- **(First Mean Value Theorem)** Let f be a bounded measurable real valued function such that $a \le f(x) \le b$ on a measurable set $E \subseteq R$ then
$$a \cdot m(E) \le \int_E f(x)dx \le b \cdot m(E)$$

- **(Necessary and Sufficient Condition for L-integrability)** Let f be a bounded function on $[a, b]$ then the function f is L-integrable if and only if for each $\varepsilon > 0$, $\exists$ a measurable partition such that $U[f; P] - L[f; P] < \varepsilon$

- Every bounded measurable function f defined on $[a, b]$ is L-integrable over $[a, b]$.

- **(First Mean Value Theorem when E is not necessarily an interval)** If f is bounded real valued measurable function defined on a measurable set E of finite measure such that $a \le f(x) \le b$ then

$$a \cdot m(E) \le \int_E f \le b \cdot m(E)$$

- If f measurable on a measurable set E then f is L-integrable if and only if $|f|$ is L-integrable.

- Every R-integrable function is L-integrable. But converse is not necessarily true.

- If $E = \bigcup_{i=1}^{n} E_i, E_i \cap E_j = \phi, i \ne j$ is a measurable set and if f is bounded measurable (integrable) function defined on E, then

$$\int_E f = \sum_{i=1}^{n} \int_{E_i} f$$

- If A and B are disjoint measurable subsets of $[a, b]$ and f is L-integrable function on $[a, b]$ then $\int_{A \cup B} f = \int_A f + \int_B f$.

- If f and g are bounded function in $L[a, b]$ then $f + g \in L[a, b]$ and $\int_a^b (f + g) = \int_a^b f + \int_a^b g$.

WORTHY READINGS

☞ Elementary integral is independent of the choice of the Canonical representation of the simple function.

☞ We can write the elementary integral for a simple function even when its representation is not canonical.

☞ Every simple function f is Lebesgue integrable and its Lebesgue integral is nothing but the same as the elementary integral.

☞ A bounded function defined on an integral may be Lebesgue integral without being R-integrable. Also, if a function is R-integrable, then it is L-integrable too. But in case of improper integral, there are some R-integrable functions which are not L-integrable.

☞ A Riemann integral function defined on $[a, b]$ is measurable.

☞ Lebesgue integral integrates only those measurable function whose absolute value functions are also integrable. But, this is not always true in the case of Riemann integrals.

☞ A Riemann integral may be improper because either the function to be integrated is unbounded on a point(s) in the given interval of integration or the interval of integration itself is unbounded.

⮑ FURTHER READINGS

☞ If f is L-integrable then f is finite valued a.e.

☞ Let f be bounded and measurable on a finite interval $[a, b]$ and let $\varepsilon > 0$ then there exists

  (i) a step function h such that $\int_a^b |f - h| \, dx < \varepsilon$

  (ii) a continuous function g such that g vanish outside a finite interval and $\int_a^b |f - g| \, dx < \varepsilon$.

☞ Let f be a bounded measurable function defined on a finite interval $]a, b[$ then $\lim\limits_{h \to \infty} \int_a^b f(x) \sin(hx) \, dx = 0$.

☞ Let f be integrable, g bounded and measurable and suppose that there exists β such that $g(x + \beta) = - g(x) \ \forall \ x \in R$ then $\lim\limits_{k \to \infty} \int f(x) g(kx) \, dx = 0$.

☞ If an integrable function f is non-negative a.e. then its indefinite integral is monotonic.

☞ The indefinite integral of an integrable function is absolutely continuous.

☞ The indefinite integral of an integrable function is countably additive.

Chapter

7 Convergence of Sequences of Measurable Functions

7.1 INTRODUCTION

The concept of convergence in measure has relevance to the theory of probability when it is often referred to as convergence in probability. In this chapter, we shall discuss some forms of convergence of measurable functions. Convergence in measure is essentially weaker than convergence almost everywhere. We shall also discuss some sequences of measurable functions which are divergent at every point, but convergent in measure.

7.2 CONVERGENCE ALMOST EVERYWHERE

A sequence $<f_n>$ of measurable functions defined on a measurable set E is said to convergence almost everywhere in E if there exists a subset A of E such that

(i) $f_n(x) \to f(x)$ $\forall$ $x \in E - A$ i.e., $<f_n>$ converges pointwise to f on $E - A$, and
(ii) $m(A) = 0$

7.3 POINTWISE CONVERGENCE

A sequence $<f_n>$ of measurable functions defined on a measurable set E is said to be pointwise convergence in E if there exists a measurable function f on E such that

$$f_n(x) \to f(x) \ \forall \ x \in E$$

i.e.,
$$\lim_{n \to \infty} f_n(x) = f(x)$$

In other words, we can define "A sequence $<f_n>$ of measurable functions defined on a measurable set E is said to be pointwise convergent if for arbitrarily chosen positive number ε (however small) $\exists$ a number $n_0 \in N$ such that

$$|f_n(x) - f(x)| < \varepsilon \ \forall \ n \geq n_0$$

☛ REMARK
- The number n_0 defined in the above definition will depend upon ε and x. Therefore, for different values of $x \in E$, we may get different numbers n_0 but we must get n_0 for every $x \in E$.

7.4 CONVERGENCE IN MEASURE

The notation of convergence in measure was first introduced by F. Riesz and E. Fisher in 1906-07. Sometimes it is also called 'approximate convergence' or 'asymptotic convergence'. It is defined as follows:

Let $<f_n>$ be a sequence of measurable functions defined over a measurable set E then the sequence $<f_n>$ is said to convergence in measure to a function f if

    (i) f is measurable over E such that $f(x) < \infty$ a.e. on E.

    (ii) For given $\varepsilon > 0$ (however small) $\lim[m\{E(|f_n - f| \geq \varepsilon)\}] = 0$, i.e., for each $\varepsilon > 0 \; \exists \; n_0(\delta) > 0$ such that for all $n \geq n_0(\delta)$ we have $m[E(|f_n - f| \geq \varepsilon)] < \delta$

7.4.1 EQUIVALENT DEFINITION

A sequence $<f_n>$ of measurable functions is said to convergence in measure to a measurable function f on a measurable set E if

$$\lim_{n \to \infty} m[\{x \in E : |f_n(x) - f(x)| \geq \varepsilon\}] = 0 \quad \text{for each } \varepsilon > 0.$$

It is denoted by $f_n \xrightarrow{m} f$

☛ REMRAK

- The concept of $f_n \xrightarrow{m} f$ on a measurable set E means that for all sufficiently large values of n, the function f_n in the sequence $<f_n>$ differ from the limit function f by a small quantity (less than ε) with the exception of a set of points whose measure is arbitrary small (less than δ).

7.4.2 SOME RESULTS

If $<f_n>$ and $<g_n>$ are sequences of measurable functions and f, g are measurable functions, all defined on a common domain D. Then if $f_n \xrightarrow{m} f$ and $g_n \xrightarrow{m} g$ then

    (i) $(f_n + g_n) \xrightarrow{m} f + g$ (iv) $f_n^2 \xrightarrow{m} f^2$

    (ii) $|f_n| \xrightarrow{m} |f|$ (v) $f_n \cdot g_n \xrightarrow{m} fg$

    (iii) $(af_n + bg_n) \xrightarrow{m} af + bg$ (vi) $\dfrac{1}{f_n} \xrightarrow{m} \dfrac{1}{f} \; (f \neq 0)$

7.5 UNIFORM CONVERGENCE ALMOST EVERYWHERE

A sequence $<f_n>$ of measurable functions defined over a measurable set E is said to converge uniformly almost everywhere (a.e) if there exists a set $A \subset E$ such that

    (i) $m(A) = 0$, and

    (ii) $<f_n>$ converge uniformly to f on the set $E - A$, i.e., for arbitrarily choosen small quantity $\varepsilon > 0$, we can find a number $n_0 \in N$ (depend upon ε only, and independent of x) such that

$$|f_n(x) - f(x)| < \varepsilon \; \forall \; n \geq n_0 \text{ and } \forall \; x \in E - A$$

7.6 CONVERGENCE IN MEAN

Let $<f_n>$ be a sequence of L-integrable functions. Then $<f_n>$ is said to converge in mean to a function f if $\lim\limits_{n \to \infty} \int_E |f_n - f| dx = 0$.

7.7 FUNDAMENTAL IN MEASURE

Let $<f_n>$ be a sequence of measurable functions defined on a measurable set E then $<f_n>$ is said to be fundamental in measure if $\exists$ a positive integer $n_0 \in N$ such that

$$m[\{x \in E : |f_n(x) - f_p(x)| \geq \varepsilon\}] < \varepsilon \quad \forall n, p \geq n_0$$

7.8 RELATION BETWEEN DIFFERENT TYPE OF CONVERGENCE

'Pointwise Convergence' is more general than 'uniform convergence'. An even more general notion than that of 'pointwise convergence' is 'convergence almost everywhere'. It remains the same concept as that of pointwise convergence except that it is now on a reduced domain of definition. Further, in case of 'pointwise convergence' and 'uniform convergence' both, we get a number $n_0 \in N \ \forall \ x$, but in pointwise convergence, n_0 depends upon x also i.e., n_0 may be different for different x while in uniform convergence one number n_0 (independent of x) works for all elements x.

7.9 THEOREMS ON CONVERGENCE OF SEQUENCES OF MEASURABLE FUNCTIONS

THEOREM 1.

Let $<f_n>$ be a sequence of integrable functions which converges in mean to a function $f(x)$ then $f_n \to f$ in measure.

PROOF. Let $<f_n>$ be a sequence of integrable functions defined on a measurable set E.

Define $\qquad E_n = E(|f_n - f| \geq \delta)$, where $\delta > 0$

Now, since $|f_n(x) - f(x)| \geq \delta \ \forall \ x \in E_n$, therefore

$$\int_{E_n} |f_n(x) - f(x)| \, dx \geq \delta \cdot m(E_n) \qquad \qquad \ldots(1)$$

Further, since $f_n \to f$ in mean (given) therefore, by definition

$$\lim_{n \to \infty} \int_E |f_n(x) - f(x)| \, dx = 0 \qquad \qquad \ldots(2)$$

From (1) we have

$$\delta \cdot m(E_n) \leq \int_E |f_n(x) - f(x)| \, dx$$

Using (2) we get

$$\lim_{n \to \infty} \delta \cdot m(E_n) \leq \lim_{n \to \infty} \int_E |f_n(x) - f(x)| \, dx = 0$$

$$\Rightarrow \qquad \lim_{n \to \infty} \delta \cdot m(E_n) \leq 0$$

But since $\delta > 0$ and $m(E_n) \geq 0$, therefore,

$$\lim_{n \to \infty} \delta m(E_n) = 0$$

$$\Rightarrow \qquad \lim_{n \to \infty} m(E_n) = 0$$

Hence, $f_n \to f$ is measure.

THEOREM 2.

Let $<f_n>$ be a sequence of measurable functions on a measurable set E and if $\lim_{n \to \infty} f_n(x) = f(x)$ a.e. on E. Then f is measurable over E.

PROOF. Let $<f_n>$ be a sequence of measurable functions defined on a measurable set E and if $\lim_{n \to \infty} f_n(x) = f(x)$ a.e. on E.

We have to prove that f is measurable over E.

Define a set $A = \{x \in E : \lim f_n(x) \neq f(x)\}$

Since, $f_n \to f$ a.e. therefore $m(A) = 0$

Further, define $g_n(x) = \begin{cases} f_n(x) & \text{if } x \notin A \\ 0 & \text{if } x \in A \end{cases}$

and $\qquad\qquad g(x) = \begin{cases} f(x) & \text{if } x \notin A \\ 0 & \text{if } x \in A \end{cases}$

Clearly, g_n is a measurable function for all $n \in N$.

Also, for $x \in A$, $\lim\limits_{n \to \infty} g_n(x) = 0 = g(x)$

and for $x \notin A$, $\lim\limits_{n \to \infty} g_n(x) = \lim\limits_{n \to \infty} f_n(x) = f(x) = g(x)$

$\Rightarrow$ The sequence $<g_n(x)>$ converges pointwise to g on E.

Further, since each g_n is measurable, therefore limit function g is also measurable.

Hence, f is measurable over E.

THEOREM 3. (F. Riesz Theorem)

Let $<f_n>$ be a sequence of measurable functions which converges in measure to the function f then $\exists$ a subsequence $< f_{n_k} >$ of $<f_n>$ which is also converges to f almost everywhere.

[MEERUT–2001, 10, 12, 15, 16, 18; ROHTAK–2000, 01; NAGPUR–2006; HPU–2009]

PROOF.   Define a monotonic decreasing sequence $<g_n>$ of positive terms such that $\lim g_n = 0$. It is given that the sequence $<f_n>$ converges in measure to f, therefore, we can write

$$\lim\limits_{n \to \infty} m[E(|f_n - f| \geq g_k)] = 0$$

which implies that corresponding to each g_k we can find a number $n_k \in N$ such that for all $n \geq n_0$.

$$|m[E(|f_n - f| \geq g_k)] - 0| < g_k$$

In particular, for $n = n_k$, we get

$$m[E(|f_{n_k} - f| \geq g_n)] < g_k \qquad\qquad\qquad\qquad ...(1)$$

$\Rightarrow$ Corresponding to the sequence $<g_n>$, we can construct a sequence $<g_k>$ satisfies (1).

We have to prove that $\lim\limits_{k \to \infty} f_{n_k}(x) = f(x)$ a.e. on E.

Define $E_i = \bigcup\limits_{k=1}^{\infty} [E(|f_{n_k} - f| \geq g_k)]$ and $B = \bigcap\limits_{i=1}^{\infty} E_i$

It is clear that $<E_i>$ is a monotonic decreasing sequence of measurable sets, so

$$\lim\limits_{n \to \infty} m(E_n) = m(B)$$

From (1) $m(E_n) < \sum\limits_{k=n}^{\infty} g_k$ or $|m(E_n) - 0| < \sum\limits_{k=n}^{\infty} g_k$

which implies $\lim\limits_{n \to \infty} m(E_n) = 0$

$$m(B) = 0$$

Further, let $y \in E - B$ be arbitrary, then $y \notin B$ implies there exist at least one $n_0 \in N$ such that $y \notin E_{n_0}$.

So, $y \notin E(|f_{n_k} - f| \geq g_k)$ $\forall k \geq n_0$

$\Rightarrow \qquad |f_{n_k}(y) - f(y)| < g_k \ \forall k \geq n_0$

Therefore, $\lim_{k \to \infty} f_{n_k}(y) = f(y) \ \forall y \in E - B$

Hence, $\lim_{k \to \infty} f_{n_k} = f$ a.e. on E.

THEOREM 4. (D.F. Egoroff's Theorem)

If a sequence of almost everywhere finite valued measurable functions is convergent almost everywhere on a measurable set E of finite measure, then for $\varepsilon > 0$ there exists a measurable set $A \subset E$ such that

(i) $m(A) < \varepsilon$

(ii) *the sequence is uniformly convergent on $(E - A)$.*

[MEERUT–2003, 05, 09, 11, 14, 16, 17; GARHWAL–2001, 12; AMRITSAR–2008; ROHTAK–2001, 03]

PROOF.   Let $<f_n>$ be a sequence of finite valued measurable function defined on the measurable set E such that $<f_n>$ converges a.e. on E to a finite measurable function f.

Suppose that B is that set on which $\lim_{n \to \infty} f_n(x) = f(x)$

Then clearly, $m(E - B) = 0$

$\Rightarrow \quad f$ is measurable on $(E - B)$

$(\because$ Every function is measurable on a set of measure zero)

$\Rightarrow \quad f$ is measurable on E.

Further define $E_n^p = \bigcap_{i=n}^{\infty} \left[E\left(|f_i - f| < \dfrac{1}{p}\right)\right]$, for any positive integer p.

By definition of E_n^p, we observe that

$$E_1^p \subset E_2^p \subset \ldots \subset E$$

So, $E - E_n^p = E - \bigcap_{i=n}^{\infty}\left[E\left(|f_i - f| < \dfrac{1}{p}\right)\right]$

$\qquad\qquad = \bigcup_{i=n}^{\infty}\left[E - E\left(|f_i - f| < \dfrac{1}{p}\right)\right] \qquad$ (By Demorgan's law)

$\qquad\qquad = \bigcup_{i=n}^{\infty} E\left(|f_i - f| \geq \dfrac{1}{p}\right) \qquad\qquad\qquad$ ...(2)

Further, since f and f_i both are measurable over E, therefore $E\left(|f_i - f| \geq \dfrac{1}{p}\right)$ is

measurable and hence being the enumerable union of measurable sets, $E - E_n^p$ is measurable.

Which implies that $< E - E_n^p >$ is a non-increasing sequence of measurable sets

and $\bigcap_{n=1}^{\infty} [E - E_n^p] \subseteq B \ \Rightarrow \ m\left(\bigcap_{n=1}^{\infty} [E - E_n^n]\right) \leq m(B) \qquad$ ...(3)

So, $\displaystyle\lim_{n\to\infty} m[E - E_n^p] = m\left(\bigcap_{n=1}^{\infty}(E - E_n^p)\right) \le m(B) = 0$ (Using (3))

$\Rightarrow \qquad \displaystyle\lim_{n\to\infty} m[E - E_n^p] = 0$

$\Rightarrow \qquad$ For given $\varepsilon > 0 \,\exists\, n_0 \in N$ such that $\forall n \ge n_0, |m(E - E_n^p - 0| < \dfrac{\varepsilon}{2^p}$

or $\qquad\qquad m(E - E_n^p) < \dfrac{\varepsilon}{2^p}$ $(\because\ m(E - E_n^p) \ge 0)$

In particular, let us take $n = n_0$, we get

$$m[E - E_{n_0}^p] < \frac{\varepsilon}{2^p} \qquad\qquad\qquad \text{...(4)}$$

Now, define $A = \displaystyle\bigcup_{p=1}^{\infty}[E - E_{n_0}^p] \,\Rightarrow\, A \subseteq E$

Here, A is measurable. $(\because$ enumerable union of measurable sets is measurable)

Then $\qquad\qquad m(A) = m\left[\displaystyle\bigcup_{p=1}^{\infty}[E - E_{n_0}^p]\right] \le \sum_{p=1}^{\infty} m[E - E_{n_0}^p]$

$$\le \sum_{p=1}^{\infty} \frac{\varepsilon}{2^p} < \varepsilon \qquad\qquad \left(\because\ \sum_{p=1}^{\infty}\frac{1}{2^p} = 1 \text{ sum of infinite G.P.}\right)$$

$\Rightarrow \qquad\qquad m(A) < \varepsilon \qquad\qquad\qquad\qquad\qquad\qquad$ ...(3)

Further $\qquad\qquad E - A = E - \displaystyle\bigcup_{p=1}^{\infty}(E - E_{n_0}^p) = E \cap \left[\bigcup_{p=1}^{\infty}\left(E - E_{n_0}^p\right)\right]' \quad [\because\ A - B = A \cap B']$

Therefore, for all $n \ge n_0$ and $x \in E - A \Rightarrow x \in E_{n_0}^p$

$\Rightarrow \qquad\qquad\qquad x \in \displaystyle\bigcap_{i=n_0}^{\infty}\left[E \,|\, f_i - f| < \frac{1}{p}\right]$

$\Rightarrow \qquad |f_n(x) - f(x)| < \dfrac{1}{p} \quad \forall n \ge n_0$

Hence, $\langle f_n \rangle$ converges unifomly on $E - A$.

THEOREM 5. (E-Borel Theorem)

Let f be a measurable function defined on a closed interval [a, b] which is finite almost everywhere on [a, b] then for all δ, $\varepsilon \ge 0$ there exists a continuous function g on [a, b] such that

$$m[E\,|f - g| \ge \delta] < \varepsilon \qquad\qquad \text{[MEERUT–1991, 2001; GARHWAL–2006]}$$

PROOF. $\qquad$ Let f be a measurable function defined on a closed interval $[a, b]$ which is finite almost everywhere on $[a, b]$.

Case I. If f is bounded.

Since f is bounded, therefore by definition $\exists$ a number $k > 0$ such that

$\qquad\qquad f(x) < k\ \forall\ x \in [a, b]$ ...(1)

Let m be a positive integer such that $\dfrac{k}{m} < \delta$

Define, $\qquad E_r = E\left[\dfrac{r-1}{m}k \le f(x) \le \dfrac{r}{m}\cdot k\right]; r = 1 - m, 2 - m, \ldots, m$

and $\qquad E_m = E\left[\dfrac{m-1}{m}k \le f(x) \le k\right]$

Clearly, $E_r \cap E_m = \phi$ for $r \ne m$, $r, j = 1 - m, 2 - m, \ldots, m$

and $\qquad \displaystyle\bigcup_{r=1}^{m} E_r = [a, b]$

Further, suppose that F_r be a closed interval contained in E_r such that

$$m(E_r) < m(F_r) + \frac{\varepsilon}{2m}$$

Take $\qquad F = \displaystyle\bigcup_{r=1-m}^{m} F_r$

Then $m([a, b]) - m(F) < \varepsilon$ ...(2)

Now, define a function h on F such that

$$h(x) = r \cdot \frac{k}{m} \quad \forall x \in H_r, r = 1 - m, 2 - m, \ldots m.$$

We observe that h is constant on F_r and $B_r \cap B_s = \phi$ from $r \ne s$.

Then h is continuous on F.

Further $|h(x)| = \left|r\dfrac{k}{m}\right| = \dfrac{rk}{m} \le k$

So, $|f(x) - h(x)| = \left|k - \dfrac{rk}{m}\right| = \dfrac{k}{m}|m - r| \le \dfrac{k}{m} < \delta$

$\Rightarrow \quad |f(x) - h(x)| < \delta \ \forall \ x \in H$

Thus we conclude that H is closed set contained in $[a, b]$ and if the function h is defined and continuous of F then there exists a function g on $[a, b]$ such that

(i) g is continuous

(ii) $g(x) = h(x) \ \forall \ x \in F$

(iii) $\max|g(x)| = \max|h(x)|$

Therefore, $E(|f(x) - g(x)| \ge \delta) < [a, b] - F$

$\Rightarrow \qquad m[E(|f(x) - g(x)| \ge \delta)] \le m([a, b]) - m(F)$

$$< \varepsilon$$

Hence $m[E(|f(x) - g(x)| \ge \delta)] < \varepsilon$

Case II. If f is unbounded

Since, f is unbounded, therefore, we can find a bounded (dominated) function ϕ such that

$$m[E(f(x) \ne \phi(x))] < \varepsilon/2 \qquad \ldots(3)$$

Now, since ϕ is bounded, then by case-I, we can find a continuous function g such that

$$m[E(|\phi(x) - g(x)| \ge \delta)] < \varepsilon/2 \qquad \ldots(4)$$

Therefore, $m[E(|f(x) - g(x)| \ge \delta)] \le m[E(f(x) \ne g(x))] + m[E(|\phi(x) - g(x)|)] \ge \delta$

$$< \varepsilon/2 + \varepsilon/2 \qquad \text{[By (3) and (4)]}$$

Hence, $m[E(|f(x) - g(x)| \ge \delta)] < \varepsilon$

THEOREM 6. (Lebesgue Bounded Convergence Theorem)

Let $<f_n>$ be a sequence of bouned measurable functions defined on a set E of finite measure. If there exists a positive real number M such that

$$|f_n(x)| \leq M \ \forall \ n \in N \ and \ \forall \ x \in E$$

and $<f_n>$ converges in measure to a measurable function f on the set E then

$$\lim_{n \to \infty} \int_E f_n(x)dx = \int_E f(x)dx \text{ [MEERUT-2001, 03, 04, 06, 09, 12, 14, 16, 18; HPU-2003;}$$

KANPUR–2001, 02; NAGPUR–2006; GARHWAL–2007, 17; ROHTAK–2004; DELHI–2012]

PROOF.   Let $<f_n>$ be a sequence of bounded measurable functions defined on a set E of finite measure.

Since f_n is bounded and measurable on E.

$\Rightarrow \quad f_n$ is integrable on E.

Since, by hypothesis $<f_n>$ converges in measure to a function f therefore, by definition

$$\lim_{n \to \infty} m[E(|f_n - f| \geq \delta)] = 0 \qquad \qquad ...(1)$$

and $\qquad\qquad |f_n(x)| \leq M \ \forall \ n \in N, x \in E$ (given)

$\Rightarrow \quad |f(x)| < M \ \forall \ x \in E \qquad\qquad\qquad\qquad\qquad\qquad ...(2)$

$\Rightarrow \quad f(x)$ is bounded and measurable function on E.

$\Rightarrow \quad f(x)$ is integrable on E.

Now, for arbitrary $\lambda > 0$, define

$$E_n = E(|f_n - f| \geq \lambda)$$

$$\Rightarrow \qquad\qquad E_n' = E(|f_n - f| < \lambda)$$

Clearly, $E = E_n \cup E_n'$ and $E_n \cap E_n' = \phi$

Since, $<f_n>$ is not convergent in E_n therefore

$$\lim_{n \to \infty} m(E_n) = 0 \qquad\qquad \text{(By definition of convergence in measure)}$$

$$...(3)$$

Now, since $E = E_n \cup E_n'$ and $E_n \cap E_n' = \phi$ then by Countable additive property of integrals, we can write

$$\int_E |f_n - f| = \int_{E_n} |f_n - f| + \int_{E_n'} |f_n - f| \qquad\qquad ...(4)$$

Since, $|f_n - f| < \lambda, \ \forall \ x \in E_n'$ therefore, by first mean value theorem

$$\int_{E_n'} |f_n - f| < \lambda \cdot m(E_n') < \lambda m(E) \qquad\qquad (\because \ E_n' \subseteq E \Rightarrow m(E_n') < m(E))$$

So, $\int_{E_n'} |f_n - f| < \lambda m(E) \qquad\qquad\qquad\qquad\qquad\qquad ...(5)$

Now for arbitrary $\varepsilon > 0$ choose λ such that

$$\lambda \cdot m(E) < \frac{\varepsilon}{2} \ \Rightarrow \ \lambda < \frac{\varepsilon}{2m(E)}$$

Then from (5) $\int_{E_n'} |f_n - f| < \varepsilon / 2 \qquad\qquad\qquad\qquad\qquad ...(6)$

Also, $|f_n - f| \leq |f_n| + |f| \leq M + M = 2M$

So, by first mean value theorem

$$\int_{E_n} |f_n - f| \leq 2M \cdot m(E_n) \qquad\qquad\qquad\qquad\qquad ...(7)$$

From (3), for arbitrary $\varepsilon > 0 \; \exists \; m_0 \in N$ such that $\forall \; n \geq m_0$

$$|m(E_n) - 0| < \frac{\varepsilon}{4M}$$

$$\Rightarrow \qquad |m(E_n)| < \frac{\varepsilon}{4M} \qquad \qquad \ldots(8)$$

Now, from (8) and (7) we get

$$\int_{E_n} |f_n - f| < \frac{\varepsilon}{2} \forall n \geq m_0 \qquad \qquad \ldots(9)$$

Finally, using (6) and (9) in (4) we get

$$\int_E |f_n - f| = \int_{E_n} |f_n - f| + \int_{E'_n} |f_n - f| \quad \forall n \geq m_0$$

$$< \frac{\varepsilon}{2} + \frac{\varepsilon}{2} = \varepsilon \; \forall n \geq m_0$$

But $\qquad \left| \int_E (f_n - f) \right| \leq \int_E |f_n - f| < \varepsilon \; \forall n \geq m_0$

$$\Rightarrow \qquad \left| \int_E (f_n - f) \right| < \varepsilon \; \forall n \geq m_0$$

$$\Rightarrow \qquad \left| \int_E (f_n - f) - 0 \right| < \varepsilon \; \forall n \geq m$$

$$\Rightarrow \qquad \lim_{n \to \infty} \int_E (f_n - f) = 0$$

$$\Rightarrow \qquad \lim_{n \to \infty} \int_E f_n(x)dx - \int_E f(x)dx = 0$$

Hence, $\lim_{n \to \infty} \int_E f_n(x)dx = \int_E f(x)dx$

☞ **REMARK**

• Lebesgue bounded convergence theorem is not true for Riemann integral.

THEOREM 7. (Lebesgue Dominated Convergence Theorem)

Let $\langle f_n \rangle$ be a sequence of measurable function defined over a measurable set E such that $|f_n(x)| < g(x) \; \forall \; x \in E, \; \forall \; n \in N$ where $g(x)$ is an integrable function (dominant function) over E. If $\langle f_n \rangle$ converges in measure to a measurable function f over E, then

$$\lim_{n \to \infty} \int_E f_n(x)dx = \int_E f(x)dx$$

[MEERUT–2000, 01, 04, 11, 14, 15; ROHTAK–2002, 03, 12; KANPUR–2007;
GARHWAL–2003, 05; PUNJAB–2002, 14; HPU–2009; NAGPUR–2007]

PROOF. Let $\langle f_n \rangle$ be a sequence of measurable functions and $g(x)$ is an integrable function such that

$$|f_n(x)| < g(x) \; \forall \; n \in N \; \forall \; x \in E$$

Since $g(x)$ is integrable $\quad \Rightarrow \quad g(x)$ is bounded

$$\Rightarrow \quad f_n(x) \text{ is bounded } \forall \; n \in N$$

Therefore, $\langle f_n \rangle$ is a sequence of bounded and measurable function over E.

$\Rightarrow \quad \langle f_n \rangle$ is Lebesgue integrable over E.

Further, it is given that $\langle f_n \rangle$ converges in measure to a measurable function f on E, therefore

$$\lim_{n \to \infty} m[E(|f_n - f| \geq p)] = 0 \; \text{ for every } p > 0$$

$\Rightarrow \langle f_n \rangle$ is a sequence of integrable function over $E \; \forall \; n \in N$ and $f_n \to f$ in measure.

$\Rightarrow f(x)$ is integrable over E.

Now, since $<f_n>$ and f both are integrable over $E \ \forall \ n \in N$.

$\Rightarrow \quad |f_n - f|$ is integrable over $E \ \forall \ n \in N$.

Let us define, for arbitrary $\delta > 0$

$$E_n = E(|f_n - f| \geq \delta)$$
$$\Rightarrow \qquad E'_n = E(|f_n - f| < \delta)$$

Obviouly, $E_n \cap E'_n = \phi$ and $E = E_n \cup E'_n$. Also, $\lim\limits_{n \to \infty} m(E_n) = 0$

$$\therefore \qquad \int_E |f_n - f| \, dx = \int_{E_n} |f_n - f| \, dx + \int_{E'_n} |f_n - f| \, dx$$

(By countable addittition property of integrals) ...(1)

Since, $|f_n - f| < \delta \ \forall x \in E'_n$, therefore by first mean value theorem

$$\int_{E'_n} |f_n - f| \, dx < \delta m(E'_n)$$

$$\leq \delta(m(E)) \qquad\qquad (\because \ E'_n \subseteq E \ \Rightarrow \ m(E'_n) \leq m(E))$$

$$\Rightarrow \qquad \int_{E'_n} |f_n - f| \, dx < \delta m(E) \qquad\qquad ...(2)$$

For $\varepsilon > 0$ (however small) choose δ such that $m(E) < \varepsilon/2\delta$

Then from (2) $\int_{E'_n} |f_n - f| \, dx < \delta \cdot \dfrac{\varepsilon}{2\delta} = \varepsilon/2$

$$\Rightarrow \qquad \int_{E'_n} |f_n - f| \, dx < \varepsilon/2 \qquad\qquad ...(3)$$

Further, consider

$$|f_n - f| \leq |f_n| + |f| < g + g = 2g$$
$$\Rightarrow \qquad |f_n - f| < 2g$$
$$\Rightarrow \qquad \int_{E_n} |f_n - f| \, dx < 2\int_{E_n} g(x) \, dx \qquad\qquad ...(4)$$

Now, since $|f_n| \leq g \ \forall \ x \in E \qquad \Rightarrow \ g(x) \geq 0 \ \forall \ x \in E$

$$\Rightarrow \ \int_{E_n} g(x) \, dx \geq 0$$

$$\Rightarrow \ \left| \int_{E_n} g(x) \, dx \right| = \int_{E_n} g(x) \, dx$$

Then from (4) we get

$$\int_{E_n} |f_n - f| \, dx < 2 \left| \int_{E_n} g(x) \, dx \right| \qquad\qquad ...(5)$$

Further, since $\lim\limits_{n \to \infty} m(E_n) = 0$ therefore, for given $\varepsilon > 0 \ \exists \ m \in N$ such that for all $n \geq m$.

$$|m(E_n) - 0| < \varepsilon$$
$$\Rightarrow \qquad m(E_n) < \varepsilon$$

By absolute continuity of the integral we have $\left| \int_{E_n} g(x) \, dx \right| < \dfrac{\varepsilon}{4}$ ...(6)

From (5) and (6) we have

$$\int_{E_n} |f_n - f| < 2 \cdot \dfrac{\varepsilon}{4} = \dfrac{\varepsilon}{2} \qquad\qquad ...(7)$$

Finally using (3) and (7) in (1) we get

$$\int_E |f_n - f| \, dx \leq \dfrac{\varepsilon}{2} + \dfrac{\varepsilon}{2} = \varepsilon$$

Letting $\varepsilon \to 0 \ \int_E |f_n - f| \, dx \leq 0$. But $\int_E |f_n - f| \, dx \geq 0$

$$\therefore \qquad \int_E (f_n - f) \, dx = 0$$
$$\Rightarrow \qquad \int_E f_n \, dx - \int_E f \, dx = 0$$

$$\Rightarrow \quad \lim_{n\to\infty}\left[\int_E f_n(x)dx - \int_E f(x)dx\right] = 0$$

$$\Rightarrow \quad \lim_{n\to\infty}\int_E f_n(x)dx = \int_E f(x)dx$$

☞ REMARK
- In Lebesgue dominated convergence theorem, the existence of dominant function g is sufficient condition, not necessary.

For; let $f_n(x) = \begin{cases} 1/x, & \text{for } n - \dfrac{1}{2} < x < n + \dfrac{1}{2} \\ 0, & \text{otherwise} \end{cases}$

Then $\lim\limits_{n\to\infty} f_n(x) = 0 \Rightarrow f(x) = 0$ so $\int_0^\infty f(x)dx = 0$

Also, $\lim\limits_{n\to\infty}\int_0^\infty f_n(x)dx = \lim\limits_{n\to\infty}\int_{(2n-1)/2}^{(2n+1)/2}\dfrac{1}{x}dx$

$$= \lim_{n\to\infty}\log\frac{(2n+1)}{(2n-1)} = 0$$

$$\Rightarrow \quad \int_0^\infty f(x)dx = \lim_{n\to\infty}\int_0^\infty f_n(x)dx$$

while if $g(x) \geq [f_n(x)]$, then $g(x) \geq \dfrac{1}{x}$ and hence, no integrable dominant function $g(x)$ exists.

THEOREM 8. (Beppo Levi's Theorem or Lebesgue Monotonic Convergence Theorem)

Let $<f_n>$ be a non-decreasing sequences of integrable function defined over a measurable set E and if

$$\lim_{n\to\infty} f_n(x) = f(x)$$

be integrable over E then $\lim\limits_{n\to\infty}\int_E f_n(x)dx = \int_E f(x)dx$.

PROOF. Let $<f_n>$ be a non-decreasing sequence of integrable function, then by definition

$$f_1 \leq f_2 \leq f_3 \leq \cdots f_n \leq \cdots$$

$$\Rightarrow \quad f_n - f_1 \geq 0 \ \forall \ n \in N$$

Let us write $f_n - f_1 = g_n$

Clearly $g_n \geq 0 \ \forall \ n \in N$

$\Rightarrow \quad <g_n>$ is a sequence of integrable function.

(∵ difference of two integrable functions is again integrable)

We have the following two cases:

Case 1. If g_n is bounded measurable function

Let g_n is bounded and measurable, then by Lebesgue bounded convergence theorem, we get

$$\lim_{n\to\infty}\int_E g_n(x)dx = \int_E \lim_{n\to\infty} g_n(x)dx \qquad \qquad \dots(1)$$

Case 2. If g_n is unbounded.

In this case we define

$$[g_n(x)]_m = \begin{cases} g_n(x); & \text{when } g_n(x) \leq m \\ m; & \text{when } g_n(x) > m \end{cases}$$

Obviously, $[g_n(x)]_m$ is bounded and measurable.

Then by Lebesgue bounded convergence theorem, we get

$$\lim_{n\to\infty} \int_E [g_n(x)]_m \, dx = \int_E \lim_{n\to\infty} [g_n(x)]_m \, dx$$

Letting $m \to \infty$ we get

$$\lim_{n\to\infty} \int_E g_n(x) dx = \int_E \lim_{n\to\infty} g_n(x) dx \qquad [\because \text{ When } m \to \infty, [g_n(x)]_m \to g_n(x)]$$

Thus in both the above cases equation (1) holds good.

i.e., $$\lim_{n\to\infty} \int_E g_n(x) dx = \int_E \lim_{n\to\infty} g_n(x) dx$$

$$\Rightarrow \quad \lim_{n\to\infty} \int_E (f_n - f_1) dx = \int_E \lim_{n\to\infty} (f_n - f_1) dx$$

$$\Rightarrow \quad \lim_{n\to\infty} \int_E f_n(x) dx - \int_E f_1(x) dx = \int_E \lim_{n\to\infty} f_n(x) dx - \int_E f_1(x) dx$$

Hence, $$\lim_{n\to\infty} \int_E f_n(x) dx = \int_E \lim_{n\to\infty} f_n(x) dx$$

$$\Rightarrow \quad \lim_{n\to\infty} \int_E f_n(x) dx = \int_E f(x) dx \qquad (\because \lim_{n\to\infty} f_n(x) dx = f(x))$$

☛ **REMARK**

- Lebesgue monotone convergence theorem may not hold good for a decreasing sequence of funcitons. For:
  Let us define a sequence $<f_n>$ of functions on R as follows.

$$f_n(x) = \begin{cases} 1 & \text{if } x \geq n \\ 0 & \text{if } x < n \end{cases}$$

$\Rightarrow <f_n>$ is a decreasing sequence of non-negative measurable functions. Also, $<f_n> \to f$ such that $f(x) = 0$.

$$\Rightarrow \qquad \int_R f(x) dx = 0.$$

While $$\int_{-\infty}^{\infty} f_n(x) dx = \int_{-\infty}^{n} f_n(x) dx + \int_{n}^{\infty} f_n(x) dx = 0 + \int_{n}^{\infty} 1 \cdot dx = \infty$$

$$\Rightarrow \qquad \lim_{n\to\infty} \int_{-\infty}^{\infty} f_n(x) dx = \infty$$

$\Rightarrow$ Lebesgue monotone convergence theorem does not hold good.

THEOREM 9. (Fatou's Lemma)

Let $<f_n>$ be a sequence of non-negative integrable functions defined over a measurable set E such that

(i) $\lim_{n\to\infty} \inf f_n = f$ a.e. on E

(ii) $\lim_{n\to\infty} \inf \int_E f_n(x) dx < \infty$

Then $\lim_{n\to\infty} \inf \int_E f_n(x) dx \geq \int_E f(x) dx$ or $\lim_{n\to\infty} \int_E f_n \geq \int_E f$

[MEERUT–2001, 08, 10, 13,14; GARHWAL–2000, 01, 04, 06, 07, 12, 16; KANPUR–2001, 02; KURUKSHETRA–1998]

PROOF. Let $<f_n>$ be a sequence of non-negative integrable functions defined over a measurable set E such that

(i) $\lim_{n\to\infty} \inf f_n = f$ a.e. on E.

(ii) $\lim_{n\to\infty} \inf \int_E f_n(x) dx < \infty$

Define $$g_r(x) = \inf. \{f_n(x); n > r\}$$

Clearly, $$g_n(x) \leq f_n(x) \; \forall \; n \in N$$

$$\Rightarrow \qquad \int_E g_n(x) dx \leq \int_E f_n(x) dx \quad \forall n \in N$$

$\Rightarrow \qquad \lim\limits_{n\to\infty} \int_E g_n(x)dx \le \lim\limits_{n\to\infty} \inf \int_E f_n(x)dx \quad \forall n \in N$ ...(1)

Evidently, $\langle g_n \rangle$ is an increasing sequence of non-negative integrable functions. Then by Lebesgue monotone convergence theorem, we get

$\lim\limits_{n\to\infty} \int_E g_n(x)dx = \int_E \lim\limits_{n\to\infty} g_n(x)dx$

$\qquad\qquad = \int_E \lim\limits_{n\to\infty} \inf f_n(x)dx = \int_E f(x)dx \quad [\because \lim\limits_{n\to\infty} \inf f_n(x) = f(x)]$

Therefore, $\lim\limits_{n\to\infty} \int_E g_n(x)dx = \int_E f(x)dx$ ...(2)

Finally, from (1) and (2) we conclude that

$\int_E f(x)dx \le \lim\limits_{n\to\infty} \inf \int_E f_n(x)dx$

DEDUCTIONS. (1) Monotone Convergence theorem can be deduce from the Fatou's lemma as follows:

Since, $\langle f_n \rangle$ is an increasing sequence of non-negative functions which converges to f almost everywhere.

Therefore, $\qquad 0 \le f_n \le f \quad \forall n \in N$

$\Rightarrow \qquad \int f_n \le \int f$

$\Rightarrow \qquad \overline{\lim\limits_{n\to\infty}} \int f_n \le \int f$ ...(1)

By Fatou's lemma

$\int f \le \underline{\lim\limits_{n\to\infty}} \int f_n$

$\Rightarrow \qquad \int f \le \underline{\lim\limits_{n\to\infty}} \int f_n \le \overline{\lim\limits_{n\to\infty}} \int f_n \le \int f$ (By (1))

Hence, $\lim\limits_{n\to\infty} \int f_n = \int f$

(2) Since, $\overline{\lim} f_n = -\underline{\lim} f_n$ therefore, by deduction (1), we can deduce that

$\int_E f = \overline{\lim} \int_E f_n$

☛ **REMARKS**

• For the result of Fatou's lemma, the non-negative condition of all function is necessary. For:
Consider the real valued function f_n defined on $E = [0, 1]$ such that

$$f_n = \begin{cases} -n, & \text{if } \dfrac{1}{n} \le x \le \dfrac{2}{n} \\ 0, & \text{otherwise} \end{cases}$$

Then $f(x) = \lim\limits_{n\to\infty} f_n = 0$ a.e. on $E \Rightarrow \int_E f(x)dx = 0$.

while $\int_E f_n(x)dx = \int_{1/n}^{2/n} -n\, dx = -1$

$\Rightarrow \quad \lim\limits_{n\to\infty} \inf \int_E f_n(x)dx = -1 \Rightarrow \lim\limits_{n\to\infty} \inf \int_E f_n \ge \int_E f(x)$

which implies that, if function f_n are not non-negative, the result of Fatou's Lemma may not hold good.

• We may have strict inequality in Fatou's lemma.
For: Consider the function $f_{2n-1} = \phi_{[0, 1]}$.

$f_{2n} = \phi_{[1, 2]}, \; n = 1, 2, \ldots$

Then $\underline{\lim} f_n(x) = 0$ for all x

But $\int f_n(x)dx = 1$

Therefore, $\int \underline{\lim} f_n(x)dx < \int f_n(x)dx$

THEOREM 10.

A measurable function can be approximated by a sequence simple functions.   [ROHTAK–2000, 02]

PROOF.   Let f be a measurable function defined over a measurable set E. We have to prove that there exists a sequence $<f_n>$ of simple functions which converges pointwise to f on E. Here, we have the following cases:

Case 1. Suppose $f \geq 0$ on E. Define

$$E_a^n = \left\{ x \in E : \frac{a-1}{2^n} \leq f(x) < \frac{a}{2^n} \right\}, a = 1, 2, 2^2, ..., 2^{2n}$$

and $E_{1+2^{2n}}^n = \{ x \in E : f(x) \geq 2^n \}$

Clearly, for all $a = 1, 2, ..., 2^{2n}$; E_a^n and $E_{1+2^{2n}}^n$ are disjoint subsets of E. Now consider the sequence $<f_n>$ of function defined by

$$f_n = \sum_{a=1}^{1+2^{2n}} \left(\frac{a-1}{2^n} \right) \chi E_a^n$$

Clearly, each f_n is a simple function. Now, since $<f_n>$ is an increasing sequence which converges to f on E.

Case 2. In general case, we construct two non-negative functions $g = f^+$ and $h = f^-$
$$\qquad\qquad\qquad\qquad\qquad\qquad\qquad ...(1)$$

Then proceed same as in Case-1, we get two sequences $<g_n>$ and $<h_n>$ of simple functions which converges to g and h respectively.

From (1) $f = f^+ - f^- = g - h$

Since, $f = g - h$, we get the sequence $<f_n>$ of simple functions such that
$$f_n = g_n - h_n$$
Clearly, $<f_n> \to f$

Hence, in both the cases, we find a sequence $<f_n>$ of simple functions which converges pointwise to f on E.

THEOREM 11. (Lusin's Theorem)

Let f be a measurable function defined on a measurable set E then for every $\varepsilon > 0$ $\exists$ a closed set $F \subset E$ such that

(i) $m(E - F) < \varepsilon$

(ii) f is continuous on F.

[ROHTAK–2000, POONA–2010]

PROOF.   We have the following two cases:

Case 1. When f is a simple function

By definition of simple function, f takes $a_1, a_2, ..., a_n$ and can be expressed

as $f = \sum_{i=1}^{n} a_i \chi_{A_i}$

where each A_i are pairwise disjoint measurable sets and χ_{A_i} is the characteristic function of A_i.

Define $A_{n+1} = E - \bigcup_{i=1}^{n} A_i$

Since each $A_1, A_2, ..., A_{n+1}$ is measurable, then for $\varepsilon' > 0$ $\left(\varepsilon' = \dfrac{\varepsilon}{n+1}\right)$ there exists closed sets $F_i \subset A_i : i = 1, 2, ..., n+1$ such that
$$m(A_i - F_i) < \varepsilon'$$

Let $\qquad F = \overset{n+1}{\underset{i=1}{\cup}} F_i$

Clearly being the countable union of closed sets, F is closed and $F \subset E$ such that
$$m(E - F) = \sum_{i=1}^{n+1} m(A_i - F_i) < (n+1) \cdot \varepsilon' < (n+1) \cdot \dfrac{\varepsilon}{n+1} < \varepsilon$$
$\Rightarrow \qquad m(E - F) < \varepsilon$

Further, since f takes constant values on each F_i, therefore f is continuous.

Case 2. General Case:

Let f be a measurable function, then by previous theorem there exist a sequence $<f_n>$ of simple functions such that
$$f_n \to f$$
So, by case-1, for given $\varepsilon > 0$ for each n there exists a closed set $E_n \subset E$ such that

(i) $m(E - E_n) < \dfrac{\varepsilon}{2^n}$

and (ii) f is continuous on E_n

Now define $A = \cap E_n$ then
$$m(E - A) = m\left[E - \underset{n}{\cap} E_n\right] = m[\cup(E - E_n)] \text{ (By Demorgan's law)}$$
$$\leq \sum_n m(E - E_n) < \sum \dfrac{\varepsilon}{2^n}$$
$$= \varepsilon \sum \dfrac{1}{2^n} = \varepsilon \qquad (\because \; \sum \dfrac{1}{2^n} = 1, \text{ sum of infinite G.P.})$$
$\Rightarrow \qquad m(E - A) < \varepsilon$

Further, since each f_n is continuous on A. Define
$$B_r = A \cap [x : r - 1 \leq |x| \leq r]$$
Clearly, B_r is a meassurable set such that $A = \underset{r}{\cup} B_r$

Then by D.F. Eqorff's theorem corresponding to each r there exists a measurable set $C_r \subset B_r$ such that

(i) $m(B_r - C_r) < \dfrac{\varepsilon}{2^r}$

(ii) $<f_n>$ converges uniformly on C_r

(iii) $\exists$ a closed set $F_r \subset B_r$ such that $m(C_r - F_r) < \dfrac{\varepsilon}{2^r}$

and (iv) $<f_n>$ converges uniformly to f on F_r

So, f is continuous on each F_r

Let $f = \cup F_r$ then being the countable union of closed set, F is closed and f is continuous on F.

Also, $\qquad m(E - F) = m(E - A + A - F) = m(E - A) + m(A - F)$

$$(\because (E - A) \text{ and } (A - F) \text{ are disjoint})$$
$$< \varepsilon + m[\cup B_r - \cup F_r] = \varepsilon + m[\cup(B_r - F_r)]$$
$$\leq \varepsilon + \Sigma m(B_r - F_r)$$
$$< \varepsilon + \Sigma \frac{\varepsilon}{2^{r-1}} = \varepsilon + 2\varepsilon = 3\varepsilon = \varepsilon'$$

$$\Rightarrow \qquad m(E - F) < \varepsilon'$$

☞ REMARK

• The above theorem can be restated as follows:

"If f is a measurable real valued function on an interval $[a, b]$ then for $\varepsilon > 0$ ∃ a continuous function f on $[a, b]$ such that
$$m[x : f(x) \neq \phi(x)] < \varepsilon$$
which is also known as "Littlewood's second principle of measurablility".

THEOREM 12.

A sequence $<f_n>$ which converges to f in measure is a Cauchy sequence in measure.

PROOF. Let $<f_n>$ be a sequence which converges to f in measure.
So, by definition

$$m\left[E\left(|f_n - f| \geq \frac{\varepsilon}{2}\right)\right] < \frac{\varepsilon}{2} \quad \forall n \geq n_0 \qquad \qquad ...(1)$$

Consider two numbers $n, p \geq n_0$ then consider

$$E(|f_n - f_p| \geq \varepsilon) \subset E\left(|f_n - f| \geq \frac{\varepsilon}{2}\right) \cup E\left(|f_p - f| \geq \frac{\varepsilon}{2}\right)$$

$$\Rightarrow m[E(|f_n - f_p| \geq \varepsilon)] \leq m[E(|f_n - f| \geq \varepsilon/2)] + m[E(|f_p - f| \geq \varepsilon/2)]$$
$$< \varepsilon/2 + \varepsilon/2 \qquad \qquad \text{(By (1))}$$
$$\Rightarrow m[E(|f_n - f_p| \geq \varepsilon] < \varepsilon \quad \forall n, p \geq n_0$$

Hence, $<f_n>$ is a Cauchy sequence in measure.

THEOREM 13.

Let $<f_n>$ be a sequence of measurable function which is fundamental (Cauchy) in measure, then there exists a subsequence $< f_{n_k} >$ which is almost uniformly.

PROOF. Since, $<f_n>$ is a sequence of measurable functions which is fundamental in measure. Then by definition of fundamental in measure.

For every $\varepsilon\left(= \frac{1}{2^k}\right)$, we get a number $n_k \in N$, such that

$$m\left[\left\{x : |f_n(x) - f_p(x)| \geq \frac{1}{2^k}\right\}\right] < \frac{1}{2^k} \quad \forall n, p \geq n_k$$

Since $n_{k+1} > n_k \quad \forall k \in N$ therefore

$< f_{n_k} >$ is a subsequence of $<f_n>$

Let us write $E_k = \left\{x : \left|f_{n_k}(x) - f_{n_{k+1}}(x)\right| \geq \frac{1}{2^k}\right\}, \quad k \leq i \leq j$

Then for each $x \notin \bigcup\limits_{i=k}^{\infty} E_i$, we get

$$\left| f_{n_i}(x) - f_{n_j}(x) \right| \le \sum\limits_{m=1}^{\infty} \left| f_{n_m}(x) - f_{n_{m+1}}(x) \right| < \frac{1}{2^{i-1}}$$

Therefore, $< f_{n_k} >$ is a uniformly Cauchy sequence in the $\left(\bigcup\limits_{i=k}^{\infty} E_k \right)$.

Also, $m\left[\bigcup\limits_{i=k}^{\infty} E_i \right] \le \sum\limits_{i=k}^{\infty} m(E_i) < \frac{1}{2^{k-1}}$

which implies that $< f_{n_k} >$ is a Cauchy sequence a.e.

Hence, $< f_{n_k} >$ is almost uniformly fundamental.

THEOREM 14.

Let $<f_n>$ be a sequence of measurable functions which is a fundamental in measure then there exists a measurable function f such that $<f_n>$ converges in measure to f.

PROOF.   Let $<f_n>$ be a sequence of measurable functions which is fundamental in measure. We have to prove that there exists a measurable function f such that $<f_n>$ converges in measure to f.

Using previous theorem we can find $< f_{n_K} >$ which is almost uniformly fundamental.

Let $\lim\limits_{n \to \infty} f_{n_K}(x) = f(x)$ $\forall x$

Then for every $\varepsilon > 0$

$$\{x : | f_n(x) - f(x)| \subset \left\{ x : \left| f_n(x) - f_{n_k}(x) \right| \ge \frac{\varepsilon}{2} \right\} \cup \left\{ x : \left| f_{n_k}(x) - f_n(x) \right| \ge \frac{\varepsilon}{2} \right\}$$

Evidently, the measure of the first term on the RHS is arbitrary small when n and n_k are sufficiently large and measure of the second term of RHS tends to 0 as $k \to \infty$.

Therefore, $<f_n>$ converges in measure to the function f.

THEOREM 15.

If a sequence $<f_n>$ converges in measure to a function f defined on a measurable set E. Then

(i) $<f_n>$ converges in measure to function g, which is equivalent to f.

(ii) limit function f is unique almost everywhere.

PROOF.   Let $<f_n>$ be a sequence converges to the function f.

(i) Let g be the function which is equivalent to f.

We have to prove that $<f_n>$ converges to g also.

Since, g is equivalent to f, therefore, by definition

$f = g$ a.e.

$\Rightarrow$ $m[E\{x : f(x) \ne g(x)\}] = 0$ ...(1)

Now for arbitrary $\varepsilon > 0$, we have

$$E\{x : | f_n(x) - g(x)| \ge \varepsilon\} \subseteq E\{x : | f_n(x) - f(x)| \ge \varepsilon\} \cup E\{x : f(x) \ne g(x)\}$$

$$\Rightarrow m[E\{x : | f_n(x) - g(x)| \ge \varepsilon\}] \le m[E\{x : | f_n(x) - f(x)| \ge \varepsilon\}] + m[E\{x : f(x) \ne g(x)\}]$$

$$\Rightarrow m[E\{x : |f_n(x) - g(x)| \geq \varepsilon\}] \leq m[E\{x : |f_n(x) - f(x)| \geq \varepsilon\}] + 0 \qquad \text{(By (1))}$$

$$\Rightarrow m[E\{x : |f_n(x) - g(x)| \geq \varepsilon\}] \leq m[E\{x : |f_n(x) - f(x)| \geq \varepsilon\}]$$

$$\Rightarrow \lim_{n \to \infty} m[E\{x : |f_n(x) - g(x)| \geq \varepsilon\}] \leq \lim_{n \to \infty} m\{E[x : |f_n(x) - f(x)| \geq \varepsilon]\} \qquad ...(2)$$

Since, $<f_n>$ converges in measure to f, therefore,

$$\lim_{n \to \infty} m\{E[x : |f_n(x) - f(x)| \geq \varepsilon]\} \leq 0 \qquad ...(3)$$

Using (3) in (2) we get

$$\lim_{n \to \infty} m[E\{x : |f_n(x) - g(x)| \geq \varepsilon]\} \leq 0$$

Hence, $<f_n>$ converges to g in measure.

(ii) We have to prove that limit function f is unique almost everywhere.

Let if possible $\exists$ another function g such that $f_n \xrightarrow{m} g$

Consider $|f - g| = |f - f_n + f_n + g|$

$$\leq |f - f_n| + |f_n - g|$$

$$\Rightarrow E\{x : |f(x) - g(x)| \geq \varepsilon\} \subseteq [E\{x : |f(x) - f_n(x)| \geq \varepsilon\}] \cup [E\{x : |f_n(x) - g(x)| \geq \varepsilon\}]$$

$$\Rightarrow m[E\{x : |f(x) - g(x)| \geq \varepsilon\}] \leq m[E\{x : |f(x) - f_n(x)| \geq \varepsilon\}]$$

$$+ m[E\{x : |f_n(x) - g(x)| \geq \varepsilon\}] \qquad ...(4)$$

Now, since, $f_n \xrightarrow{m} f$ and $f_n \xrightarrow{m} g$ therefore,

$$m[E\{x : |f(x) - f_n(x)| \geq \varepsilon\}] < \delta/2 \qquad ...(5)$$

and $m[E\{x : |f_n(x) - g(x)| \geq \varepsilon\}] < \delta/2 \qquad ...(6)$

Using (5) and (6) in (4) we get

$$m[E\{x : |f(x) - g(x)| \geq \varepsilon\}] \leq \delta/2 + \delta/2 = \delta$$

Since, δ is arbitrary therefore letting $\delta \to 0$, we get

$$m[E\{x : |f(x) - g(x)| \geq \varepsilon\}] \leq 0$$

But $m[E\{x : |f(x) - g(x)| \geq \varepsilon\}] \leq 0$

$$\Rightarrow \qquad m[E\{x : |f(x) - g(x)| \geq \varepsilon\}] = 0$$

$$\Rightarrow \qquad g = f \quad \text{a.e.}$$

Hence, the limit function f is unique.

7.10 LITTLE WOOD'S THREE PRINCIPLES

We know that the knowledge of theory of functions of real numbers is very wide. But in connection with the theory of functions knowledge required is nothing like so great as is sometimes supposed. He suggested that there are three principles are required, which are given below:

(i) Every measurable set is nearly a finite union of intervals.

(ii) Every measurable function is nearly continuous.

(iii) Every convergent sequence of measurable functions is nearly uniformly convergent.

7.10.1 ANOTHER VERSION OR INTERPRETATIONS

(i) **Second Principle:**

(1) If f is a measurable function defined on an interval [a, b] and assumes the values $\pm\infty$ only in a set of measure zero, then for arbitrary $\varepsilon > 0$, however small there exists a

step function g and a continuous function h such that
$$|f - g| < \varepsilon \text{ and } |f - h| < \varepsilon$$

(2) Lusin's theorem is also the version of second principle and is given by "If f is a measurable real valued function on an interval $[a, b]$ then for $\varepsilon > 0$ ∃ a continuous function g on $[a, b]$ such that
$$m[x : f(x) \neq g(x)] < \varepsilon$$

(3) Another version of third principle is Egiroff's theorem which states that "If a sequence of a.e. finite valued measurable function is convergent a.e. on a measurable set E of finite measure then for every $\varepsilon > 0$ ∃ a measurable set $A \subseteq E$ such that
(i) $m(A) < \varepsilon$
(ii) the sequence is uniformly convergent on $(E - A)$.

 Solved Examples

EXAMPLE 1. *Show that* $\int_{-1}^{\infty} \dfrac{dx}{x} = \infty$.

SOLUTION. Let
$$f(x) = \frac{1}{x}$$

Clearly, $\dfrac{1}{x}$ is continuous for $x > 0$, measurable and hence integrable. Therefore,
$$\int_1^{\infty} x^{-1} dx > \int_1^n x^{-1} dx$$

$\Rightarrow \qquad \int_1^{\infty} x^{-1} dx \geq \lim_{n \to \infty} \int_1^n x^{-1} dx$

We know that $[1, n] = \overset{n}{\underset{p=2}{\cup}} [p-1, p]$ and $x^{-1} > p^{-1}$ on $[p-1, p]$

Therefore, $\int_1^n \dfrac{1}{x} dx > \overset{n}{\underset{p=2}{\sum}} \int_1^p p^{-1} \phi_{[p-1,p]} dx > \overset{n}{\underset{p=2}{\sum}} p^{-1}$

which implies
$$\int_1^{\infty} x^{-1} dx = \lim_{n \to \infty} \overset{n}{\underset{p=2}{\sum}} p^{-1} \geq \frac{1}{2} + \frac{1}{3} + \frac{1}{4} + \dots$$

$$= \infty, \text{ being a divergent series.}$$

Hence, $\int_1^{\infty} \dfrac{1}{x} dx = \infty$

EXAMPLE 2. *If* $a > 1$, *show that* $\int_0^1 \dfrac{x \sin x}{1 + (nx)^a} dx = 0(n^{-1})$, *as* $n \to \infty$.

SOLUTION. Define a sequence
$$f_n(x) = \frac{nx \sin x}{1 + (nx)^{\alpha}}, n \in N$$

Since, $a > 1$ and $x \in [0, 1]$, therefore, $\left| \dfrac{nx \sin x}{1 + (nx)^a} \right| \leq 1$

If we select $g(x) = 1 \; \forall x$, then clearly, $|f_n(x)| \leq g(x) \; \forall \; x$.
Then by dominated convergence theorem, we get

$$\lim_{n \to \infty} \int_0^1 \frac{nx \sin x}{1 + (nx)^a} dx = \int_0^1 \lim_{n \to \infty} \frac{nx \sin x}{1 + (nx)^{\alpha}} dx$$

$$= \int_0^1 0 dx = 0$$

So, $\lim\limits_{n\to\infty} n\cdot\left[\int_0^1 \dfrac{x\sin x}{1+(nx)^a}dx\right]=0$

Hence, $\int_0^1 \dfrac{x\sin x}{1+(nx)^a}dx = 0[n^{-1}]$

EXAMPLE 3. *Give two examples which yield a strict inequality in Fatou's lemma.*

SOLUTION. (1) Define a function $f_n : R \to R$ such that

$$f_n(x) = \begin{cases} 2; & n \le x \le n+1 \\ 0; & \text{otherwise} \end{cases}$$

Clearly, $\lim\limits_{n\to\infty} f_n(x) = 0 \Rightarrow f(x) = 0$. So, $\int_R f = 0$.

If we take $E = [n, n+1]$ then

$$f_n(x) = \begin{cases} 2 & \text{on } E \\ 0 & \text{on } E' \end{cases}$$

So, $\int_R f_n(x)dx = \int_E f_n(x)dx + \int_{E'} f_n(x)dx$

$\qquad\qquad = \int_n^{n+1} 2dx + \int_{E'} 0dx = 2$

$\Rightarrow \qquad \lim\limits_{n\to\infty} \int_R f_n = 2 > 0 = \int_R f$

$\Rightarrow \qquad \lim\limits_{n\to\infty} \int_R f_n = \int_R f$

(2) Define $\qquad f_{2n}(x) = g(x); 0 \le x \le 1$

$\qquad\qquad\qquad f_{2n+1}(x) = g(1-x); 0 \le x \le 1$

such that $\qquad g(x) = \begin{cases} 0; & \text{if } 0 \le x < \dfrac{1}{2} \\ 1; & \text{if } \dfrac{1}{2} < x \le 1 \end{cases}$

Then $\quad \lim\limits_{n\to\infty} \inf . f_n(x) = \lim\limits_{n\to\infty k\ge n} \inf f_k(x) = \lim 0 = 0$

So, $\int_0^1 \lim\limits_{n\to\infty} \inf f(x)dx = 0$

But, $\quad \int_0^1 f_{2n}(x)dx = \int_0^{1/2} 0dx + \int_{1/2}^1 1dx = \dfrac{1}{2}$

and $\quad \int_0^1 f_{2n-1}(x)dx = \int_0^{1/2} 1dx + \int_{1/2}^1 0\cdot dx = \dfrac{1}{2}$

$\Rightarrow \qquad \lim\limits_{n\to\infty} \int_0^1 f_n(x)dx = \dfrac{1}{2}$

Hence, $\int_0^1 \lim\limits_{n\to\infty} \inf . f_n(x)dx < \lim\limits_{n\to\infty} \int_0^1 f_n(x)dx$

EXAMPLE 4. *If* $f_n(x) = \dfrac{n^{3/2}\cdot x}{1+n^2x^2}, n\in N, 0\le x \le 1$. *Then using Lebesgue dominated convergence theorem, evaluate* $\lim\limits_{n\to\infty} \int_0^1 f_n(x)dx$

[MEERUT–1996, 2007, 12]

SOLUTION. Given that $\qquad f_n(x) = \dfrac{n^{3/2}\cdot x}{1+n^2x^2} = \dfrac{1}{x}\left[\dfrac{n^{3/2}x^2}{1+n^2x^2}\right]$

$$= \frac{1}{x} \frac{\left(\frac{1}{\sqrt{n}} \cdot x^2\right)}{\frac{1}{n^2} + x^2} < \frac{1}{x} \frac{1 \cdot x^2}{0 + x^2}$$

$$\leq \frac{1}{x} = g(x) \text{ (say)}$$

$$\Rightarrow \qquad f(x) \leq g(x)$$

and $g(x) \in L[0, 1]$

Then by Lebesgue dominated convergence theorem

$$\lim_{n \to \infty} \int_0^1 f_n(x)dx = \int_0^1 \lim_{n \to \infty} f_n(x)dx$$

$$= \int_0^1 \lim_{n \to \infty} \left(\frac{n^{3/2} \cdot x}{1 + n^2 x^2}\right) dx$$

$$= \int_0^1 \lim_{n \to \infty} \left(\frac{1}{\sqrt{n}}\right) \left(\frac{x}{\frac{1}{n^2} + x^2}\right) dx = \int_0^1 0 dx = 0$$

EXAMPLE 5.   *Verify the result of bounded convergence theorem for the function*

$$f_n(x) = \frac{nx}{1 + n^2 x^2}, 0 \leq x \leq 1$$

[MEERUT–2004, 15; GARHWAL–2007; GURUKUL KANGRI–2004]

SOLUTION.   Given that $f_n(x) = \dfrac{nx}{1 + n^2 x^2} = \dfrac{1}{\dfrac{1}{nx} + nx}$

$$= \frac{1}{\left[\dfrac{1}{\sqrt{nx}} - \sqrt{nx}\right]^2 + 2} \leq \frac{1}{2}$$

So, there exist a number $\dfrac{1}{2}$ such that $|f_n(x)| \leq \dfrac{1}{2}$. Now,

$$\lim_{n \to \infty} \int_0^1 f_n(x)dx = \lim_{n \to \infty} \int_0^1 \frac{nx}{1 + n^2 x^2} dx$$

$$= \lim_{n \to \infty} \frac{1}{2n} \log(1 + n^2) \qquad\qquad (\frac{\infty}{\infty} \text{ form})$$

$$= \lim_{n \to \infty} \left[\frac{[1/(1 + n^2)]2n}{2}\right] = \lim_{n \to \infty} \frac{n}{1 + n^2} = 0 \qquad\qquad \text{...(1)}$$

and $\int_0^1 \lim_{n \to \infty} f_n(x)dx = \int_0^1 \lim_{n \to \infty} \left(\dfrac{nx}{1 + n^2 x^2}\right) dx = \int_0^1 0 \cdot dx = 0$ \qquad\qquad \text{...(2)}

which implies that (from (1) and (2))

$$\lim_{n \to \infty} \int_0^1 f_n(x)dx = \int_0^1 \lim_{n \to \infty} f_n(x)dx$$

EXAMPLE 6.   *Show that* $\lim\limits_{n\to\infty} \int_0^\infty \dfrac{dx}{\left(1+\dfrac{x}{n}\right)^n \cdot x^{1/n}} = 1, \quad n > 1, x > 0$

SOLUTION.   Consider, $\left(1+\dfrac{x}{n}\right)^n = 1 + x + \dfrac{n(n-1)}{1\cdot 2}\dfrac{x^2}{n^2} + \ldots \geq \dfrac{x^2}{4}$

Define $g(x) = \begin{cases} \dfrac{4}{x^2} & \text{for} \quad x \geq 1 \\ x^{1/2} & \text{for} \quad 0 < x < 1 \end{cases}$

Then, we have

$$\left(1+\dfrac{x}{n}\right)^{-n} \cdot x^{-1/n} < g(x)$$

Also, g(x) is integrable over]0, ∞[. Then by Lebesgue dominated convergence theorem, we have

$$\lim_{n\to\infty} \int_0^\infty \left(1+\dfrac{x}{n}\right)^{-n} \cdot x^{-1/n} dx = \int_0^\infty \lim_{n\to\infty} \left(1+\dfrac{x}{n}\right)^{-n} \cdot x^{-1/n} dx$$

$$= \int_0^\infty -e^{-x} dx = 1$$

EXAMPLE 7.   *Show that* $\lim\limits_{n\to\infty} \int_a^\infty \dfrac{n^2 x e^{-n^2 x^2}}{1+x^2} dx = 0$ *if* $a > 0$ *but not for* $a = 0$.

[DELHI–2008; GARHWAL–2005, 07]

SOLUTION.   If $a > 0$, let us put $nx = u \Rightarrow du = ndx$, we get

$$\int_0^\infty \dfrac{n^2 x e^{-n^2 x^2}}{1+x^2} dx = \int_{na}^\infty \dfrac{u e^{-u^2}}{1+u^2/n^2} du$$

$$= \int_0^\infty \phi_{(na,\infty)} \dfrac{u e^{-u^2}}{1+u^2/n^2} du$$

Also, $\left| \dfrac{u e^{-u^2}}{1+u^2/n^2} \phi_{(na,\infty)} \right| < u e^{-u^2} \in L[0,\infty]$

and $\lim\limits_{n\to\infty} \phi_{(na,\infty)} \cdot \dfrac{u e^{-u^2}}{1+u^2/n^2} = 0$ $\qquad (\because \phi_{(\infty,\infty)} = 0)$

Then by Lebesgue dominated convergence theorem we get

$$\lim_{n\to\infty} \int_a^\infty \dfrac{n^2 x e^{-n^2 x^2}}{1+x^2} dx = \lim_{n\to\infty} \int_0^\infty \phi_{(na,\infty)} \cdot \dfrac{u e^{-u^2}}{1+u^2/n^2} du$$

$$= \int_0^\infty \lim_{n\to\infty} \phi_{(na,\infty)} \cdot \dfrac{u e^{-u^2}}{1+u^2/n^2} du$$

$$= \int_0^\infty 0 \, dx = 0$$

But when $a = 0$, then

$$\int_0^\infty \frac{n^2 x e^{-n^2 x^2}}{1+x^2} dx > \int_0^1 \frac{n^2 x e^{-n^2 x^2}}{1+x^2} dx$$

$$> \frac{1}{2} \int_a^1 n^2 x e^{-n^2 x^2} dx \qquad \text{(Take 1 for } x^2)$$

$$= -\frac{1}{4} \left[e^{-n^2 x^2} \right]_0^1 > \frac{1}{4} \neq 0$$

EXAMPLE 8. Let $f(x) = \begin{cases} 0; & \text{for} \quad x = 0 \\ x^{-1/3}; & \text{for} \quad 0 < x \leq 1 \end{cases}$. *Then evaluate L-integral of f defined on* $E = [0, 1]$.

SOLUTION. Evidently, the given function is unbounded non-negative measurable function. So we can define

$$f_n(x) = \begin{cases} f(x) & \text{when } f(x) \leq n \quad i.e., x \geq \dfrac{1}{n^3} \\ n & \text{when } f(x) > n \quad i.e., x < \dfrac{1}{n^3} \end{cases}$$

Clearly, $\langle f_n \rangle$ is an increasing sequence of non-negative bounded functions such that $f_n \to f$. Then by monotone convergence theorem we get

$$\int_0^1 f = \lim_{n \to \infty} \int_0^1 f_n(x) dx = \lim_{n \to \infty} \left[\int_0^{1/n^3} n\, dx + \int_{1/n^3}^1 x^{-1/3} dx \right]$$

$$= \lim_{n \to \infty} \left[\frac{1}{n^2} + \frac{3}{2} - \frac{3}{2n^2} \right] = \frac{3}{2}$$

Hence, the given function f is integrable and its integral value is $\dfrac{3}{2}$.

EXAMPLE 9. *Verify Beppo-Levi's theorem on the following function:*

If $-1 < a < 0$ *and* $f : [0, 1] \to R$ *such that*

$$f(x) = \begin{cases} x^a; & 0 < x \leq 1 \\ 0; & x = 0 \end{cases} \qquad \text{[MEERUT–2004, 11]}$$

SOLUTION. Define the sequence $\langle f_n \rangle$ of functions as follows:

$$f_n(x) = \begin{cases} x^a & \text{for} \quad \dfrac{1}{n} \leq x \leq 1 \\ 0 & \text{for} \quad 0 \leq x < \dfrac{1}{n} \end{cases}$$

Clearly, $\langle f_n \rangle$ is an increasing sequence of non-negative measurable functions and $\lim_{n \to \infty} f_n = f$

and

$$\int_0^1 f_n(x) dx = \int_0^{1/n} 0\, dx + \int_{1/n}^1 x^a dx$$

$$= \frac{1}{a+1} \left(1 - \frac{1}{n^{a+1}} \right)$$

So,

$$\lim_{n \to \infty} \int_0^1 f_n(x) dx = \frac{1}{a+1}$$

However f is unbounded and hence it is not Riemann integrable although improper integral $\int_0^1 f(x)dx$ exists and has the value $\dfrac{1}{a+1}$.

Hence, $\quad \lim\limits_{n \to \infty} \int_0^1 f_n(x)dx = \int_0^1 f(x)dx$

$\Rightarrow \quad$ Beppo-Levi's theorem is verified.

Exercise 7.1

1. If $f : R \to R$ is Lebesgue integrable and for $n \in N$, $E_n = \{x \in R : |f(x)| > n\}$. Then show that the series $\sum\limits_{n=1}^{\infty} m(E_n)$ converges.

2. If f is finite real valued Lebesgue measurable function on $[0, 1]$ and let $En = \{x \in [0, 1] : (n - 1)\} \le f(x) \le n$, for $n = 0, \pm 1, \pm 2, \pm 3, \ldots$ Show that $\int_0^1 f d\mu < \infty$ iff $\sum\limits_{-\infty}^{\infty} |n| \mu(E_n) < \infty$.

3. For $n \in Z$, let

$$f_n(x) = \begin{cases} 2n, & if \quad \dfrac{1}{2n} \le x \le \dfrac{1}{n} \\ 0 & if \quad x \in \left]0, \dfrac{1}{2n}\right[\cup \left[\dfrac{1}{n}, 1\right[\end{cases}$$

Show that Fatou's lemma applies but that the Lebesgue dominated convergence theorem does not.

4. Given an example of a sequence which converges to zero in measure on $[0, 1]$ but does not converge for any $x \in [0, 1]$.

5. Show that $\int_0^1 \dfrac{1+nx}{(1+x)^n} dx = 0$.

6. Show that $\int_0^{\infty} \left(1+\dfrac{x}{n}\right)^{-n} \sin\dfrac{x}{n} dx = 0$.

7. Show that $\lim\limits_{n \to \infty} \int_0^n \left(1+\dfrac{x}{n}\right)^n e^{-2x} dx = 1$

8. Show that $\lim\limits_{n \to \infty} \int_0^1 f_n(x)dx = 0$ where $f_n(x) =$

   (i) $\dfrac{\log(x+n)}{n}$ (ii) $\dfrac{nx\log n}{1+n^2 x^2}$

9. Show that $\lim\limits_{n \to \infty} \int_0^1 f_n(x)dx = 0$ where $f_n(x) =$

   (i) $\dfrac{n\sqrt{x}}{1+n^2 x^2}$

   (ii) $\dfrac{n^p x^r \log x}{1+n^2 x^2}, r > 0, p < \min\{2, 1+r\}$

10. Verify Lebesgue bounded convergence theorem for the sequence of function

$$f_n(x) = \dfrac{1}{\left(1+\dfrac{x}{n}\right)^a}; 0 \le x \le 1, n \in N.$$

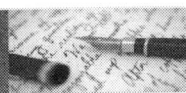
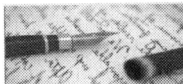

CHAPTER Summary

⮞ KEY TERMS

- **CONVERGENCE ALMOST EVERYWHERE:** Let $<f_n>$ be a sequence of measurable functions defined over a measurable set E. Then $<f_n>$ converges a.e. on E if $\exists$ a subset $A \subseteq E$ such that
  (i) $f_n(x) \to f(x) \ \forall \ x \in E - A$
  (ii) $m(A) = 0$

- **POINTWISE CONVERGENCE:** Let $<f_n>$ be a sequence of measurable set E then $<f_n>$ is said to converge pointwise in E if $\exists$ a measurable function f on E such that $f_n(x) \to f(x) \ \forall \ x \in E$.

- **CONVERGENCE IN MEASURE:** Let $<f_n>$ be a sequence of measurable defined over a measurable set E then the sequence $<f_n>$ is said to converge in measure to a function f, i.e.
  $$f_n \xrightarrow{\ m\ } f \text{ if}$$

- (i) f is measurable over E such that $f(x) < \infty$ a.e. on E.
- (ii) $\lim_{n \to \infty} m[E(|f_n - f| \geq \varepsilon)] = 0$

- **FUNDAMENTAL IN MEASURE:** The sequence $<f_n>$ of measurable function defined on the set E is said to be fundamental in measure if for arbitrary $\varepsilon > 0 \ \exists$ a $n_0 \in N$ such that
  $$m[\{x \in E : |f_n(x) - f_p(x)| \geq \varepsilon\} < \varepsilon] \ \forall n, p \geq n_0$$

- **UNIFORM CONVERGENCE A.E.:** A sequence $<f_n>$ of measurable functions defined over a measurable set E is said to converge uniformly a.e. to f if $\exists$ a set $A \subseteq E$ such that
  (i) $m(A) = 0$
  and (ii) $<f_n>$ converges uniformly to f on the set $E - A$

⮞ RESULTS

- Let $<f_n>$ be a sequence of integrable functions which converges in mean to a function $f(x)$ then $f_n \to f$ in measure.

- Let $<f_n>$ be a sequence of measurable functions on a measurable set E and if $\lim_{n \to \infty} f_n(x) = f(x)$ a.e. on E. Then f is measurable over E.

- Let $<f_n>$ be a sequence of measurable functions which converges in measure to the function f then $\exists$ a subsequence $< f_{n_K} >$ of $<f_n>$.

- If a sequence of almost everywhere finite valued measurable functions is convergent almost everywhere on a measurable set E of finite measure, then for $\varepsilon > 0$ there exists a measurable set $A \subset E$ such that
  (i) $m(A) < \varepsilon$
  (ii) the sequence is uniformly convergent on $(E - A)$.

- Let f be a measurable function defined on a closed interval $[a, b]$ which is finite almost everywhere on $[a, b]$ then for all $\delta, \varepsilon \geq 0$ there exists a continuous function g on $[a, b]$ such that $m[E|f - g| \geq \delta] < \varepsilon$.

- Let $<f_n>$ be a sequence of bouned measurable functions defined on a set E of finite measure. If there exists a positive real number M such that $|f_n(x)| \leq M \ \forall \ n \in N$ and $\forall \ x \in E$ and $<f_n>$ converges in measure to a measurable function f on the set E then
  $$\lim_{n \to \infty} \int_E f_n(x) dx = \int_E f(x) dx$$

- Let $<f_n>$ be a sequence of measurable function defined over a measurable set E such that

$|f_n(x)| < g(x) \ \forall \ x \in E, \ \forall \ n \in N$ where $g(x)$ is an integrable function (dominant function) over E. If $<f_n>$ converges in measure to a measurable function f over E, then
$$\lim_{n \to \infty} \int_E f_n(x) dx = \int_E f(x) dx$$

- Let $<f_n>$ be a non-decreasing sequences of integrable function defined over a measurable set E and if $\lim_{n \to \infty} f_n(x) = f(x)$ be integrable over E then $\lim_{n \to \infty} \int_E f_n(x) dx = \int_E f(x) dx$.

- Let $<f_n>$ be a sequence of non-negative integrable functions defined over a measurable set E such that
  (i) $\lim_{n \to \infty} \inf f_n = f$ a.e. on E
  (ii) $\lim_{n \to \infty} \inf \int_E f_n(x) dx < \infty$

  Then $\lim_{n \to \infty} \inf \int_E f_n(x) dx \geq \int_E f(x) dx$ or
  $\lim_{n \to \infty} \int_E f_n \geq \int_E f$

- A measurable function can be approximated by a sequence simple functions.

- Let f be a measurable function defined on a measurable set E then for every $\varepsilon > 0 \ \exists$ a closed set $F \subset E$ such that
  (i) $m(E - F) < \varepsilon$
  (ii) f is continuous on F.

- A sequence $<f_n>$ which converges to f in measure is a Cauchy sequence in measure.

- Let $\langle f_n \rangle$ be a sequence of measurable function which is fundamental (Cauchy) in measure, then there exists a subsequence $\langle f_{n_K} \rangle$ which is almost uniformly.
- Let $\langle f_n \rangle$ be a sequence of measurable functions which is a fundamental in measure then there exists a measurable function f such that $\langle f_n \rangle$ converges in measure to f.
- If a sequence $\langle f_n \rangle$ converges in measure to a function f defined on a measurable set E. Then
  (i) $\langle f_n \rangle$ converges in measure to function g, which is equivalent to f.
  (ii) limit function f is unique almost everywhere.

⨕ WORTHY READINGS

☞ A sequence $\langle f_n \rangle$ which converges to f in measure is a Cauchy sequence in measure.

☞ Lebesgue bounded convergence theorem is not true for Riemann integral.

☞ Fatou's lemma, Monotone Convergence, Lebesgue Convergence theorem remains valid if convergence a.e. is replaced by convergence in measure.

☞ Convergence in measure does not necessarily imply pointwise convergence.

☞ Egoroff's theorem, does not hold good for E such that $m(E) = \infty$.

☞ The "almost everywhere convergence" implies the "convergence in measure".

☞ Pointwise convergence is more general than uniform convergence.

☞ Convergence in measure is more general convergence almost everywhere.

☞ There are sequence of measurable (even continuous) functions that converge in measure but fall to converge at any point.

☞ Every subsequence of a Cauchy sequence in measure is again a Cauchy sequence in measure.

⨕ FURTHER READINGS

☞ Let $f_n \to f$ in measure where f and each f_n are measurable functions then there exists a subsequence $\langle n_k \rangle$ such that
$$f_{n_K} \to f \quad \text{a.e.}$$

☞ If $m(A) < \infty$ and $f_n \to f$ in measure than $f_n^2 \to f^2$ in measure.

☞ Uniform convergence a.e. implies almost uniform convergence.

☞ If a sequence converges to a finite valued limit function a.e. then it is fudamental a.e. and conversely, *i.e.*, corresponding to a sequence which is fundamental a.e. there always exists a finite valued limit function which is converges a.e.

☞ If $\langle f_n \rangle$ is a sequence of measurable functions which is fundamental in measure, then some sequences $\langle f_{n_K} \rangle$ is almost uniformly fundamental.

☞ If $f = 0$ a.e. then $\langle f_n^2 \rangle \xrightarrow{m} f^2$.

☞ Every subsequence of a sequence which is fundamental in measure is fundamental in measure.

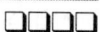

Chapter
8

Absolutely Continuous Function: Differentiation and Integration

We know that an interval may be open or closed, or right open and left closed or left open and right closed. Any function on an interval that consists only of one point is monotonic non-decreasing as well as monotonic non-increasing. Also, the constant functions are monotonic non-decreasing as well as monotonic non-increasing on every interval. In this chapter we have to characterize the functions that can be expressed as the difference of two monotonic non-decreasing functions.

8.2 FUNCTION OF A BOUNDED VARIATION

Definition 1. *A function* f *on the closed bounded interval* $[a,b]$ *is said to be of bounded variation on* $[a, b]$ *if the supremum*

$$T_{ab} = \sup \left\{ \sum_{k=1}^{n} \left| f(a_k) - f(a_{k-1}) \right| : a \le a_0 \le ... \le a_n \le b \right\}$$

which is taken over all possible finite sequences $a_0, a_1, ..., a_n$ *is finite.*

T_{ab} *is called the total variation of* f *on* (a, b). *It is denoted by* V_{ab} *or* V_a^b.

☛ REMARK
- $T_{ab} = f(b) - f(a)$, if f is monotonic non-decreasing.

Definition 2. *Let the function* f *be of bounded variation on each closed interval. Then, the monotonic non-decreasing function* T_f *defined by*

$$T_f(x) = \begin{cases} f(0) + \sup\{\Sigma \left| f(a_k) - f(a_{k-1}) \right| : 0 \le a_0 \le ... \le a_n \le x\} \text{ for } x \ge 0 \\ f(0) - \sup\{\Sigma \left| f(a_k) - f(a_{k-1}) \right| : x \le a_0 \le ... \le a_n \le 0\} \text{ for } x \le 0 \end{cases}$$

is called the total variation function of f.

If T_{ab} *denote the total variation of* f *on the bounded interval* $[a, b]$, *then*

$$T_f(x) = \begin{cases} f(0) + T_{0x} : \text{for } x \ge 0 \\ f(0) - T_{0x} : \text{for } x \le 0 \end{cases}$$

☛ REMARK
- For a monotonic non-decreasing function f
    $T_{ab} = f(b) - f(a)$. therefore $T_f = f$, if f is monotonic non decreasing.

SOME RESULTS

Let $f: [a, b] \to R$ be a function and P be any division of $[a, b]$. Then we have the following results:

(i) $\underset{a,a}{V} = \underset{a}{\overset{b}{V}} f = 0$

(ii) $|f(x) - f(a)| \le \underset{a}{\overset{x}{V}}(f), x \in [a,b]$

(iii) $P_1 \subseteq P_2 \Rightarrow \underset{a}{\overset{b}{V}}(f;P_1) \le \underset{a}{\overset{b}{V}}(f,P_2), P_1$ and P_2 are subdivisions of $[a, b]$.

(iv) $\underset{a}{\overset{b}{V}}(f) \ge 0$

(v) $a < b < c \Rightarrow \underset{a}{\overset{b}{V}}(f) < \underset{a}{\overset{c}{V}}(f)$

THEOREM 1.

For $a \le b$

$$T_f(b) - T_f(a) = T_{ab} = \sup\left\{ \sum_{k=1}^{n} \left| f(a_k) - f(a_{k-1}) \right| : a \le a_0 \le ... \le a_n \le b \right\}$$

PROOF. By definition of T_f, we have that the total variation of f on an interval $(0, x)$ is
$$T_f(x) - f(0) = T_f(x) - T_f(0) \qquad [\because T_f(0) = f(0)]$$

Similarly, the total variation of f on an interval $(x, 0)$ is $T_f(0) - T_f(x)$.

Thus, we conclude that the total variation T_{ab} of f on any closed bounded interval $[a, b]$ is $T_f(b) - T_f(a)$ if for $a \le c \le b$ implies $T_{ab} = T_{ac} + T_{cb}$.

Let us suppose $a \le c_0 \le ... \le c_s \le b$ then $c_t \le c \le c_{t+1}$ for some integer t, if we make the convention $c_{-1} = a$ and $c_{s+1} = b$, we have

$$\sum_{k=1}^{s} \left| f(c_k) - f(c_{k-1}) \right| \le \sum_{k=1}^{t} \left| f(c_k) - f(c_{k-1}) \right| + \left| f(c_{t+1}) - f(c_t) \right| + \sum_{k=t+2}^{s} \left| f(c_k) - f(c_{k-1}) \right|$$

$$\le \sum_{k=1}^{t} \left| f(c_k) - f(c_{k-1}) \right| + \left| f(c) - f(c_t) \right| + \left| f(c_{t+1}) - f(c) \right| + \sum_{k=t+2}^{s} \left| f(c_k) - f(c_{k-1}) \right|$$

$$\le T_{ac} + T_{cb}.$$

Taking its supremum an L.H.S., we get $T_{ab} \le T_{ac} + T_{cb}$.

Similarly, we can prove that if $a \le a_0 \le ... \le a_n \le c \le b_0 \le ... \le b_n \le b$ and if we let $c_0, ..., c_s$ be the sequence $a_0, ..., a_n c, b_0 ... b_m$

Then $\sum_{k=1}^{n} \left| f(a_k) - f(a_{k-1}) \right| + \sum_{k=1}^{m} \left| f(b_k) - f(b_{k-1}) \right| \le \sum_{k=1}^{s} \left| f(c_k) - f(c_{k-1}) \right| \le T_{ab}$

$$T_{ac} + T_{cb} \le T_{ab}.$$

AN IMPORTANT RESULT

Let f be a function of bounded variation on each closed bounded interval $[a, b]$. Then, the function $f_1 = \frac{1}{2}(T_f + f)$ and $f_2 = \frac{1}{2}(T_f - f)$ are both monotonic non-decreasing and

$$f = f_1 - f_2, \; T_f = f_1 + f_2, \; f(0) = f_1(0) = Tf(0), f_2(0) = 0$$

☞ **Remark**
- The functions f_1 and f_2 defined above is called its parts of positive and negative variations of f.

8.3 ABSOLUTE CONTINUOUS FUNCTION

Let $f(x)$ be a finite real valued function defined on a closed interval $[a, b]$ such that for given $\varepsilon > 0 \, \exists \, \delta > 0$ such that

$$\left| \sum_{i=1}^{n} [f(b_k) - f(a_k)] \right| < \varepsilon \text{ whenever } \sum_{k} |b_k - a_k| < \delta$$

Then the function $f(x)$ is said to be absolutely continuous function.

☞ **Remark**
- Every absolutely continuous function is continuous.

8.4 INDEFINITE INTEGRAL

Let $f(x)$ be a function which is integrable on $[a, b]$ such that

$$F(x) = \int_a^x f(t)dt + c \quad \forall x \in [a,b], c \in R$$

Then the function $F(x)$ is called the indefinite integral of $f(x)$.

8.5 VARIATION FUNCTION

Let f be a function of bounded variation on $[a, b]$ and $x \in [a, b]$. The total variation of f on $[a, x]$ denoted by $T[f, [a, x]]$ given by

$$T[f, [a, x]] = T_f(x)$$

is called variation function or total variation function. It is also denoted by $V(x)$.

☞ **Remark**
- It is also denoted by $V[f, [a, x]]$.

8.6 FUNCTION OF LOCALLY BOUNDED VARIATION

A function f is said to be of locally bounded variation if it has finite total variation on each bounded closed interval. The set of all functions of locally bounded variation is denoted by V_{loc} and the subset of monotone non-decreasing function by V_{loc}^{+}.

THEOREM 1.

Let f and g be functions of bounded variations on $[a,b]$ then $f+g, f-g, fg$ and f/g $(g(x) \neq 0 \, \forall \, x)$ are functions of bounded variation. [MEERUT–1998, 2004, 04 BP]

PROOF.   (i) Let $f + g = h$

Thus we have

$$\left| h(x_{r+1}) - h(x_r) \right| = \left| [f(x_{r+1}) + g(x_{r+1})] - [f(x_r) + g(x_r)] \right|,$$

$$\text{where } a = x_0 < x_1 ... < x_n = b$$

$$= |[f(x_{r+1}) - f(x_r)] + [g(x_{r+1}) - g(x_r)]|$$

$$\leq |f(x_{r+1}) - f(x_r)| + |g(x_{r+1}) - g(x_r)|$$

$$\Rightarrow \sum_{r=0}^{n-1} |h(x_{r+1}) - h(x_r)| \leq \sum_{r=0}^{n-1} |f(x_{r+1}) - f(x_r)| + \sum_{r=0}^{n-1} |g(x_{r+1}) - g(x_r)|$$

$$\Rightarrow \qquad T_{ab}(h) \leq T_{ab}(f) + T_{ab}(g)$$

Now, since, the function f and g are functions of bounded variation.

Therefore, $T_{ab}(f)$ and $T_{ab}(g)$ are finite.

$\Rightarrow \qquad T_{ab}(h)$ is a finite quantity.

Hence $h = f + g$ is of bounded variation in $[a, b]$.

(ii) Similarly, as above we can prove that $f - g$ is a function of bounded variation.

(iii) Now, define $h(x) = f(x) \cdot g(x)$ Then, we have

$$|h(x_{r+1}) - h(x_r)| = |f(x_{r+1}) g(x_{r+1}) - f(x_r) g(x_r)|$$
$$= |f(x_{r+1}) \cdot g(x_{r+1}) - f(x_r) g(x_{r+1}) + f(x_r) g(x_{r+1}) - f(x_r) \cdot g(x_r)|$$
$$\leq |g(x_{r+1})| |[f(x_{r+1}) - f(x_r)]| + |f(x_r)| |[g(x_{r+1}) - g(x_r)]|$$
$$\leq |g(x_{r+1})| \cdot |f(x_{r-1}) - f(x_r)| + |f(x_r)| \cdot |g(x_{r+1}) - g(x_r)|.$$

Let us define $s_1 = \sup\{|f(x)| : x \in (a, b)\}$, $s_2 = \sup\{|g(x)| : x \in (a, b)\}$

Therefore, $|h(x_{r+1}) - h(x_r)| \leq s_1 \cdot |f(x_{r+1}) - f(x_r)| + s_2 |g(x_{r+1}) - g(x_r)|$

$$\Rightarrow \quad \sum_{r=0}^{n-1} |h(x_{r+1}) - h(x_r)| \leq s_2 \sum_{r=0}^{n-1} |f(x_{r+1}) - f(x_r)| + s_1 \sum_{r=0}^{n-1} |g(x_{r+1}) - g(x_r)|$$

$\Rightarrow V_{ab}(h) \leq s_2 V_{ab}(f) + s_1 V_{ab}(g)$, which is a finite quantity.

Thus, $h(x) = f(x) \cdot g(x)$ is of bounded variation in $[a, b]$.

(iv) Here, first we shall prove that $\dfrac{1}{g}$ is of bounded variation.

Let $g(x) \geq \sigma > 0 \quad \forall x \in [a, b]$.

Since $g(x) \geq \sigma > 0 \quad \forall x \in [a, b] \Rightarrow \dfrac{1}{g(x)} \leq \dfrac{1}{\sigma} > 0 \quad \forall x \in [a, b]$.

Consider $\left| \dfrac{1}{g(x_{r+1})} - \dfrac{1}{g(x_r)} \right| = \left| \dfrac{g(x_r) - g(x_{r+1})}{g(x_r) \cdot g(x_{r+1})} \right| \leq \dfrac{1}{\sigma^2} |g(x_r) - g(x_{r+1})|$

Thus $\sum_{r=0}^{n-1} \left| \dfrac{1}{g(x_{r+1})} - \dfrac{1}{g(x_r)} \right| \leq \dfrac{1}{\sigma^2} \sum_{r=0}^{n-1} |g(x_r) - g(x_{r+1})|$

$\Rightarrow \qquad V_{ab}\left(\dfrac{1}{g}\right) \leq \dfrac{1}{\sigma^2} V_{ab}(g)$, which is a finite quantity.

$\Rightarrow \dfrac{1}{g}$ is a function of bounded variation in $[a, b]$.

Now, since f and $\dfrac{1}{g}$ are of function of bounded variation in $[a, b]$

$\Rightarrow \qquad f \cdot \dfrac{1}{g}$ is a function of bounded variation in $[a, b]$.

Hence, $\dfrac{f}{g}$ is a function of bounded variation in $[a, b]$.

THEOREM 2.

Every absolutely continuous function f defined on $[a, b]$ is of bounded variation.

[MEERUT–92, 96, 99, 2000, 03BP, 04, 05BP, 06, 07, 07BP, 10, 14; GARHWAL–94, 97, 2005, 06; ROHTAK–2001]

PROOF. As per given, we have f is absolutely continuous an $[a, b]$.

Now for $\varepsilon = 1$ there exists a $\delta > 0$ such that

$$\sum_{i=1}^{n} |f(b_i) - f(a_i)| < 1 \text{ whenever } \sum_{i=1}^{n} (b_i - a_i) < \delta$$

and $a = a_1 < b_1 \le a_2 < b_2 \le ... \le a_n < b_n = b$.

Let P be any refinement of P adjoining some additional points to P such that all the intervals can be divided into r parts each of total length less than δ.

Let the r subintervals be $[c_0, c_1], [c_1, c_2]...,[c_{r-1}, c_r]$ such that $a = c_0, c_r = b$ and $[c_{k+1} - c_k] < \delta \quad \forall k = 1, 2, ..., r$.

Clearly $\sum_i |f(x_{i+1}) - f(x_i)| < 1$ whenever $x_{i+1}, x_i \in [c_k, c_{k+1}]$

$\Rightarrow \qquad V_{c_k \cdot c_{k+1}}(f) < 1$

$\Rightarrow \qquad V_{ab}(f) = V_{c_0 c_1}(f) + V_{c_1 c_2}(f) + ... + V_{c_{r-1} \cdot c_r}(f)$

$$< 1 + 1 + 1 ... + 1$$
$$= r, \text{ a finite quantity}$$

$\Rightarrow \quad f$ is a function of bounded variation.

Hence, every absolutely continuous function f defined on $[a, b]$ is of bounded variation.

THEOREM 3. (Jordan Decomposition Theorem)

A function f is of bounded variation if and only if it can be expressed as a difference of two monotonic functions both non-decreasing. [MEERUT–2000, 01BP, 2005; ROHTAK–2000, 02, 04; HIMACHAL–2001, 03]

PROOF. Define the function $f : [a, b] \to R$.

Let us first suppose that f is a function of bounded variation on $[a, b]$.

Then, we can write

$$f = v - (v - f) \qquad ...(1)$$

so that $\qquad f(x) = v(x) - (v(x) - f(x)), \; x \in [a, b]$

If $x, y \in [a, b]$ such that $x < y$. Then, we can write

$$V_{xy}(f) = V_{ax}(f) + V_{xy}(f)$$

$\Rightarrow \qquad v(y) - v(x) = V_{xy}(f) \ge 0$

$\Rightarrow \qquad v(x) \le v(y)$

$\Rightarrow \quad v$ is a non-decreasing function on $[a, b]$.

Further, if $x < y$ on $[a, b]$, then

$$v(y) - v(x) = V_{xy}(f) \ge |f(y) - f(x)| \ge f(y) - f(x)$$

$\Rightarrow \qquad v(y) - f(y) \ge v(x) - f(x)$

$\Rightarrow \qquad (v - f)y \ge (v - f)x$

$\Rightarrow \quad (v - f)$ is a non-decreasing function on $[a, b]$.

Hence, from (1) we conclude that the function f is expressible as a difference of two monotonically non-decreasing functions.

Conversely, let $g(x)$ and $h(x)$ be increasing functions such that $f(x) = g(x) - h(x)$.

Divide the closed interval $[a, b]$ such that

$$a = x_0 < x_1 < x_2 < ... < x_n = b$$

Let $\qquad V = \sum_{r=0}^{n-1} |f(x_{r+1}) - f(x_r)|$

Consider

$$|f(x_{r+1}) - f(x_r)| = |g(x_{r+1}) - h(x_{r+1}) - (g(x_r) - h(x_r))|$$
$$= |[g(x_{r+1}) - g(x_r)] + [h(x_r) - h(x_{r+1})]|$$
$$\leq |g(x_{r+1}) - g(x_r)| + |h(x_r) - h(x_{r+1})|$$
$$\leq |g(x_{r+1}) - g(x_r)| + |h(x_{r+1}) - h(x_r)|.$$

Since, $g(x)$ and $h(x)$ are monotonically increasing function, so that

$$g(x_{r+1}) - g(x_r) \geq 0 \text{ and } h(x_{r+1}) - h(x_r) \geq 0$$

Therefore $|g(x_{r+1}) - g(x_r)| = g(x_{r+1}) - g(x_r)$

and $|h(x_{r+1}) - h(x_r)| = h(x_{r+1}) - h(x_r)$

Thus, $|f(x_{r+1}) - f(x_r)| \leq [g(x_{r+1}) - g(x_r)] + [h(x_{r+1}) - h(x_r)]$

$$\Rightarrow \sum_{r=0}^{n-1} |f(x_{r+1}) - f(x_r)| \leq \sum_{r=0}^{n-1} [g(x_{r+1}) - g(x_r)] + \sum_{r=0}^{n-1} [h(x_{r+1}) - h(x_r)]$$

$$\Rightarrow \sum_{r=0}^{n-1} [g(x_{r+1}) - g(x_r)] = [g(x_1) - g(x_0)] + [g(x_2) - g(x_1)] + \ldots + [g(x_n) - g(x_{n-1})]$$

$$= g(x_n) - g(x_0) = g(b) - g(a)$$

Similarly $\sum_{r=0}^{n-1} [h(x_{r+1}) - h(x_r)] = h(b) - h(a)$

$$\Rightarrow \sum_{r=0}^{n-1} |f(x_{r-1}) - f(x_r)| \leq g(b) - g(a) + h(b) - h(a).$$

Now, since f is finite in [a, b], therefore $g(b), g(a), h(b), h(a)$ are finite numbers

$$\Rightarrow \sum_{r=0}^{n-1} |f(x_{r+1}) - f(x_r)| < \infty$$

$$\Rightarrow V_{ab}(f) < \infty$$

Hence, f is a function of bounded variation.

☞ **REMARKS**

- A continuous function is of bounded variation if and only if it can be expressed as a deference of two continuous monotonically increasing functions.
- If f is a function of bounded variation, then $f(x)$ exists almost everywhere.
- If f is a finite valued monotonic increasing function defined on [a, b] then f is continuous on [a, b] except almost a countable number of points.
- An absolutely continuous function is differentiable almost everywhere.

THEOREM 4.

An indefinite integral is a function of bounded variation, i.e., if f is Lebesgue integrable on [a,b] and $F(x)$ is indefinite integral of f(x), i.e., $F(x) = \int_a^x f(t)dt$. Then F is a function of bounded variation on [a,b]. Also, $V_{ab}(F) \leq \int_a^x |f|$.

[MEERUT–84,89, 2000, 13; AMRITSAR–98; HIMACHAL–1999, 2000, 03; ROHTAK–1999, 2001, 02, 03]

PROOF. As per given f is Lebesgue integrable on [a, b], i.e., $f \in L[a, b]$

$$\Rightarrow |f| \in L(a, b)$$

Let $P = \{x_i : i = 0, 1, 2, \ldots, n\}$ be a subdivision of the interval $[a, b]$. Then

$$\sum_{i=1}^{n} |F(x_i) - F(x_{i-1})| = \sum_{i=1}^{n} |\int_a^{x_i} f - \int_a^{x_{i-1}} f|$$

$$= \sum_{i=1}^{n} |\int_{x_{i-1}}^{x_i} f| \le \sum_{i=1}^{n} \int_{x_{i-1}}^{x_i} |f| = \int_a^b |f| < \infty$$

$\Rightarrow$ F is of bounded variation on $[a, b]$ and $V_{ab}(F,P) \le \int_a^b |f|$.

Since this result is true for any subdivision of P on $[a, b]$, therefore, taking supremum, we get $V_{ab}(F) \le \int_a^b |f|$.

☞ **REMARK**

- If $f(x)$ and $g(x)$ are absolutely continuous function, then $f(x) \pm g(x)$ and $f(x) \cdot g(x)$ are also absolutely continuous function also if $g(x) \ne 0$, then $\dfrac{f(x)}{g(x)}$ is also absolutely continuous function.

THEOREM 5.

A necessary and sufficient condition that a function should be an indefinite integral is that it should be absolutely continuous.

[MEERUT–89, 2001, 05BP, 10, 13; GARHWAL–91, 95, 98, PUNJAB–2002; ROHTAK–2001, 04; HIMACHAL–2001, 03]

PROOF.   Let $f(x)$ be an absolutely continuous function over $[a, b]$ then by Jordan decomposition theorem f is of bounded variation and can be written as

$$f(x) = f_1(x) - f_2(x).$$

where $f_1(x)$ and $f_2(x)$ are monotonically increasing function and hence both are differentiable.

Since $f'(x)$ exists.

$\Rightarrow$ $\left|f'(x)\right| \le f_1'(x) + f_2'(x)$

$\Rightarrow$ $\int \left|f'(x)\right| \le f_1(b) + f_2(b) - f_1(a) - f_2(a) < \infty$

$\Rightarrow$ $f'(x)$ is integrable.

Let $F(x)$ be an indefinite integral of $f'(x)$.

i.e., $F(x) = F(a) + \int_a^x f'(t)dt$ $x \in [a,b]$ ...(1)

Then, using fundamental theorem of integral calculus, we have

$F'(x) = f'(x)$ a.e.

$\Rightarrow$ $F(x) = f(x) + C$ ...(2)

Using (1), we have $F(a) = f(a)$.

Then, from (2), $C = 0$.

Hence, $F(x) = f(x)$.

Thus, every absolutely continuous function $f(x)$ is an indefinite integral of its own derivative.

Conversely, let $F(x)$ be an indefinite integral of $f(x)$ defined on the closed interval $[a, b]$, so that

$$F(x) = \int_a^x f(t)dt + F(a) \quad \forall x \in [a,b]$$

and $f(x)$ is integrable over $[a, b]$.

Let for $\in > 0$ $\exists$ $\delta > 0$ such that if $m(A) < \delta$, then $\int_A |f| < \in$.

Select $2n$ real numbers such that

$$a_1 < b_1 \le a_2 < b_2 \le a_3 < ... \le a_n < b_n$$

such that $A = \bigcup_{i=1}^{n} [a_i, b_i]$ and $\sum_{i=1}^{n} (b_i - a_i) < \delta$

Then, $\sum\limits_{i=1}^{n} |F(b_i) - F(a_i)| = \sum\limits_{i=1}^{n} \left| \int_a^{b_i} f - \int_a^{a_i} f \right|$

$$= \sum_{i=1}^{n} \left| \int_{a_i}^{b_i} f \right| \le \sum_{i=1}^{n} \int_{a_i}^{b_i} |f| = \int_A |f| < \epsilon$$

$\Rightarrow$ For $\epsilon > 0$ $\exists$ a $\delta > 0$ such that $\sum\limits_{i=1}^{n} (b_i - a_i) < \delta$

$\Rightarrow$ $\sum\limits_{i=1}^{n} |F(b_i) - F(a_i)| < \epsilon$

$\Rightarrow$ F is absolutely continuous.

Hence, every indefinite integral is absolutely continuous.

THEOREM 6.

An integral is a continuous function.   [MEERUT–2005; ROHTAK–2001, 02, 03; HIMACHAL–2002, 03]

PROOF. Suppose that $F(x)$ be an indefinite integral of $f(x)$ defined over $[a, b]$, so that $f(x)$ is integrable over $[a, b]$ and

$$F(x) = \int_a^x f(t)dt + F(a) \qquad \forall x \in [a,b]$$

Let x be any element of the open interval $]a\, b[$ and $x_1, x_2 \in \,]x - \delta/2, x + \delta/2\, [$.
Define $E_k = [x_1, x_2]$, then we have $m(E_k) = m([x_1\, x_2]) < \delta$

$\Rightarrow$ $\left| \int_{E_k} f(t)dt \right| < \epsilon$ for $k > k_0$

$\Rightarrow$ $\left| \int_{x_1}^{x_2} f(t)dt \right| < \epsilon$ wherever $m([x_1, x_2]) < \delta$

or $|F(x_2) - F(x_1)| < \epsilon$ wherever $|x_2 - x_1| = m([x_1, x_2]) < \delta$

$\Rightarrow$ $|F(x_2) - F(x_1| < \epsilon$ wherever $|x_2 - x_1| = m([x_1, x_2]) < \delta$.

Hence, $F(x)$ is a continuous function.

THEOREM 7.

If a function f is absolutely continuous in an open interval $]a, b[$ and $f'(x) = 0$, a.e. in $[a, b]$, then f
is constant.   [MEERUT–84, 86, 89, 97, 2003BP, 05BP; ROHTAK–2000, 03, HIMACHAL–2001, GARHWAL– 91]

PROOF. Let c be any arbitrary point of $[a, b]$. To show $f(c) = f(a)$

Define $E = \{x \in]a, c[: f'(x) = 0\}$

For arbitrary set $E \subset]a\ c[$ $x \in E \Rightarrow f'(x) = 0$

Let $\epsilon, \eta > 0$ be arbitrary

$\therefore$ $f'(x) = 0$ for all $x \in E \Rightarrow$ There exists an arbitrary small interval $[x, x+h] \subset [a, c]$

such that $\dfrac{|f(x+h) - f(x)|}{h} < \eta \Rightarrow |f(x_1 + h) - f(x)| < \eta h$.

$\Rightarrow$ Corresponding to every $x \in E$, there exists an arbitrary small closed interval $[x, x+h]$ contained in $[a, c]$ such that

$$|f(x+h) - f(x)| < \eta h \qquad \qquad ...(1)$$

Then, by Vitali's covering lemma, we can find a finite number of non-overlapping interval I_k, where $I_k = [x_k, y_k]$ $\forall k = 1, 2...n$ such that this collection covers all of E except for a set of measure less than $\delta > 0$ where δ is pre-assigned number which corresponds to ϵ occurring in the definition of absolutely continuity of f.

Let $x_k < x_{k+1}$, then adjoining the points y_0, x_{n+1}, we have

$$a = y_0 \le x_1 < y_1 \le x_2 < y_2 \le \dots \le x_n < y_n \le x_{n+1} = c.$$

Since f is absolutely continuous, therefore for above subdivision of $[a,c]$ we have

$$\sum_{k=0}^{\dot{n}} \left| f(x_{k+1}) - f(y_k) \right| < \epsilon \text{ whenever } \sum_{k=0}^{n} \left| x_{k+1} - y_k \right| < \delta$$

Now (1) implies

$$\sum_{k=1}^{n} \left| f(y_k) - f(x_k) \right| \le \eta \sum_{k=1}^{n} (y_k - x_k) < \eta(c-a).$$

Now,
$$\left| f(c) - f(a) \right| = \left| \sum_{k=0}^{n} [f(x_{k+1}) - f(y_k)] + \sum_{k=1}^{n} [f(y_k) - f(x_k)] \right|$$

$$\le \sum_{k=0}^{n} \left| f(x_{k+1}) - f(y_k) \right| + \sum_{k=1}^{n} \left| f(y_k) - f(x_k) \right|$$

$$< \epsilon + \eta(c-a).$$

Since, ϵ, η and hence $\epsilon + \eta(c-a)$ are arbitrary small positive numbers, thus letting $\epsilon \to 0, \eta \to 0$, we get $f(c) = f(a)$.

Hence, $f(x)$ is a constant function.

☞ REMARK
- If the derivative of two absolutely continuous functions are equivalent, then the functions differ by a constant.

THEOREM 8. (Fundamental Theorem of Integral Calculus)

If f is a bounded and measurable function on $[a,b]$ and

$$F(x) = \int_a^x f(t)\, dt + F(a)$$

Then, $F'(x) = f(x)$ a.e. in $[a, b]$.   [MEERUT–90, 92, 95, 2001, 03BP, 06, 06BP, 07, 12, 15; HIMACHAL–2000, 01; PUNJAB–2003; ROHTAK–2002; GARHWAL–1997]

PROOF.   We know that every indefinite integral is a function of bounded variation, therefore, $F(x)$ is a function of bounded variation over $[a, b]$. Further, $F(x)$ can be expressed as a difference of two monotonic functions and since every monotonic function has a finite differential coefficients at every point of a set of non-zero measure, thus, $F(x)$ has a finite differential coefficients almost everywhere in $[a, b]$.

Since f is given to be bounded, therefore

$$\left| f(t) \right| \le M$$

Set
$$f_n(x) = \frac{F(x+h) - F(x)}{h}, \quad \text{where } h = \frac{1}{n}$$

Then,
$$\left| f_n(x) \right| = \left| \frac{1}{h} \int_x^{x+h} f(t)dt \right| \le \frac{1}{h} \int_x^{x+h} \left| f(t) \right| dt \le \frac{M}{h} \int_x^{x+h} dt = M$$

$$\Rightarrow \qquad \left| f_n(x) \right| \le M.$$

Now, since $f_n(x) \to F'(x)$ a.e., then by Lebesgue bounded convergence theorem

We have
$$\int_a^x F'(x)dx = \lim_{n \to \infty} \int_a^x f_n(x)dx = \lim_{h \to 0} \frac{1}{h} \int_a^x [F(x+h) - F(x)]dx$$

$$= \lim\left[\frac{1}{h}\int_x^{x+h} f(x)dx - \frac{1}{h}\int_a^{a+h} F(x)dx\right] = F(x) - F(a)$$

$$= \int_a^x F(t)dt$$

$$\Rightarrow \int_a^x (F'(t) - f(t))dt = 0 \quad \forall x$$

$$\Rightarrow \quad F'(x) - f(x) = 0 \quad a.e. \text{ in } [a, b]$$

Hence $F'(x) = f(x)$ a.e. in $[a, b]$.

THEOREM 9. (Lebesgue Differentiation Theorem)

Let $f : [a,b] \to R$ be a finite valued monotonically increasing function then f is differentiable. Also $f : [a,b] \to R$ is Lebesgue integrable and $\int_a^b f'(x)dx \le f(b) - f(a)$.

[MEERUT–2004, 07BP; GARHWAL–1997, 2001; ROHTAK–1996, 97, 2000]

PROOF. Let $< f_n >$ be a sequence of non-negative functions, where

$$f_n : (a,b) \to R$$

such that $f_n(x) = n\left[f\left(x + \frac{1}{n}\right) - f(x)\right] \forall x \in [a, b]$. ...(1)

Set $f(x) = f(b)$, $x \ge b$

By our hypothesis, $f_n : [a,b] \to R$ is an increasing function, thus $f_n : [a,b] \to R$ is also an increasing function and hence integrable in the Lebesgue sense. Using (1) we have

$$\lim_{n\to\infty} f_n(x) = \lim_{\frac{1}{n}\to 0} \frac{f\{x + (1/n)\} - f(x)}{(1/n)}, \quad \forall x \in [a,b]$$

$$= f'(x), \ a.e.$$

Using Fatau's lemma, we have

$$\int_a^b f'(x)dx \le \lim_{n\to\infty} \inf\left\{\int_a^b f_n(x)dx\right\}$$ ...(2)

Further, $\displaystyle\lim_{n\to\infty} \inf\int_a^b f_n(x)dx \le \lim_{n\to\infty} \inf n\int_a^b \left[f\left(x+\frac{1}{n}\right) - f(x)\right]dx$

$$= \lim_{n\to\infty} \inf n\left[\int_a^b\left(x+\frac{1}{n}\right)dx - \int_a^b f(x)dx\right].$$

Putting $t = x + \left(\frac{1}{n}\right)$ and using the first property of definite integral, we have

$$\int_a^b f\left(x+\frac{1}{n}\right)dx = \int_{a+\left(\frac{1}{n}\right)}^{b+\left(\frac{1}{n}\right)} f(t)dt = \int_{a+\left(\frac{1}{n}\right)}^{b+\left(\frac{1}{n}\right)} f(x)dx.$$

Thus $\displaystyle\lim_{n\to\infty} \inf\int_a^b f_n(x)dx = \lim_{n\to\infty} \inf n\left[\int_{a+\left(\frac{1}{n}\right)}^{b+\left(\frac{1}{n}\right)} f(x)dx - \int_a^b f(x)dx\right]$

$$= \lim_{n\to\infty} \inf n\left[\int_b^{b+1/n} f(x)dx - \int_a^{a+\left(\frac{1}{n}\right)} f(x)dx\right].$$ ...(3)

Extend the definition of f by assuming

$$f(x) = f(b) \quad \forall x \in \left[b, b + \frac{1}{n} \right].$$

Also, $f(a) \le f(x)$ for $x \in \left[a, a + \frac{1}{n} \right]$.

Therefore, $\int_a^{a + \left(\frac{1}{n} \right)} f(x)dx \ge \int_a^{a + \left(\frac{1}{n} \right)} f(a)dx = \frac{1}{n} f(a)$

$\Rightarrow \quad -\int_a^{a + \left(\frac{1}{n} \right)} f(x)dx \le -\frac{1}{n} f(a)$

Therefore, (3) gives

$$\lim_{n \to \infty} \inf \int_a^b f_n(x)dx = \lim_{n \to \infty} \inf . n \left[\int_b^{b + \left(\frac{1}{n} \right)} f(b)dx + \left(-\int_a^{a + \left(\frac{1}{n} \right)} f(x)dx \right) \right]$$

$$\le \lim_{n \to \infty} \inf . n \left[f(b) . \frac{1}{n} + \left(-\frac{1}{n} \right) f(a) \right] \le f(b) - f(a).$$

Therefore, using (2), we get

$$\int_a^b f'(x)dx \le f(b) - f(a).$$

Therefore, $f'(x)$ is integrable and thus finite almost everywhere. Hence, f is differentiable almost everywhere.

THEOREM 10.

If f is an absolutely continuous monotonic function on $[a, b]$ and E is a set of measure zero, then $f(E)$ has measure zero.

PROOF. Let f be a function which is monotonically increasing then, by definition of absolute continuity of f, for $\in > 0, \exists\, \delta > 0$ and non-overlapping interval $\{f_n = [a_n, b_n]\}$ such that

$$\Sigma\ (b_n - a_n) < \delta \Rightarrow \Sigma |f(b_n) - f(a_n)| < \in$$

$\Rightarrow \quad \Sigma \left(f(b_n) - f(a_n) \right) < \in$ \qquad\qquad ...(1)

Since $\qquad\qquad E \subseteq [a, b] \Rightarrow E \subseteq \cup I_n$

which implies $\qquad f(E) \subset f(\cup I_n) = \cup f(I_n)$

$\Rightarrow \qquad\qquad m\, f(E) \le \Sigma m(f(I_n)) \le \Sigma [(\overline{f}(x_n) - \underline{f}(x_n)] < \in$

when $\overline{f}(x_n)$ and $\underline{f}(x_n)$ are the maximum and minimum values of $f(x)$ in the interval $[a_n, b_n]$.

Also, we have $\quad \Sigma |\overline{x}_n - \underline{x}_n| \le \Sigma (b_n - a_n) < \delta$

$\Rightarrow \qquad\qquad m(f(E)) \le \in$

Since $\in$ is arbitrary, therefore

$$m(f(E)) = 0$$

Hence, $m(f(E)) = 0$.

THEOREM 11.

Let $G(x)$ be an indefinite integral of $g(x)$ and also $f(x)$ be an indefinite integral, then
$\int_a^b f(x)g(x)dx = [f(x).G(x)]_a^b - \int_a^b f'(x)G(x)dx$.

PROOF.
As per given, we have $G(x)$ is an indefinite integral of $g(x)$. Thus, we can write
$$G(x) = \int_a^b g(t)dt + c \text{ , where } c \text{ is a constant.} \qquad ...(1)$$
Since, f is an indefinite integral, therefore f is absolutely continuous.
Thus $f(x)$ and $G(x)$ are absolutely continuous.
$\Rightarrow \quad f(x).G(x)$ is absolutely continuous.
$(\because$ Product of two absolutely continuous function is absolutely continuous$)$
$\Rightarrow \quad f(x)$ is an indefinite integral of its own derivative $f'(x)$.
$\Rightarrow \quad f'(x)$ is Lebesgue integrable.
Since $f'(x)$ and $G(x)$ are Lebesgue integrable that $f'(x).G(x)$ is Lebesgue
integrable, so that $\int_a^b f'(x)G(x)dx$ exists.
Then, from (1), we have
$$G'(x) = g(x) \text{ a.e. on } [a,b].$$
Further, $\dfrac{d}{dx}[f(x).G(x)] = f'(x).G(x) + f(x).G'(x)$
$$= f'(x)G(x) + f(x).g(x) \qquad ...(2)$$
Also $\int_a^b \dfrac{d}{dx}[f(x).G(x)]dx = [f(x).G(x)]_a^b \qquad ...(3)$
Using (2) and (3), we get
$$\int_a^b [f'(x)G(x) + f(x)g(x)]dx = [f(x).G(x)]_a^b$$
Hence, $\int_a^b f(x)g(x)dx = [f(x).G(x)]_a^b - \int_a^b f'(x)G(x)dx$

THEOREM 12. (Generalized First Mean Value Theorem)

Let $f(x)$ is bounded and $g(x) \geq 0$ in a measurable set E and are integrable over E, then
there exists a number δ between the bounds of $f(x)$ in E, such that
$$\int_E f(x)g(x)dx = \delta \int_E g(x)dx$$

PROOF.
Since $f(x)$ is bounded in E, thus assume that α and β be the supremum and
infimum for $f(x)$ on E, i.e.,
$$\alpha \leq (f(x) \leq \beta \qquad ...(1)$$
Since $g(x)$ is non-negative, therefore from (1), we have
$$\alpha.g(x) \leq f(x).g(x) \leq \beta g(x)$$
$\Rightarrow \quad \alpha \int_E g(x)dx \leq \int_E f(x).g(x)dx \leq \beta \int_E g(x)dx$
Let $\alpha \leq \delta \leq \beta$
$$\delta \int_E g(x)dx \leq \int_E f(x)g(x)dx \leq \delta \int_E g(x)dx$$
Hence, $\int_E f(x).g(x)dx = \delta \int_E g(x)dx$.

THEOREM 13. (Second Mean Value Theorem)

Let $f(x)$ be integrable over $[a, b]$ and $g(x)$ be positive, bounded and non-decreasing, then
$\int_a^b f(x)g(x) = g(a+0)\int_a^t f(x)dx$, where $a < t < b$.

PROOF. Let us suppose that $\in > 0$ be given such that
$$\in > g(a+0) - g(b-0)$$
then there exists a point x_1 such that
$$g(a+0) - g(x) < \in \text{ for } (a < x < x_1) \ge \in \text{ for } x > x_1$$
Similarly, there exist points $x_2, x_3, ..., x_r$ such that
$$g(x_{r-1} + 0) - g(x) < \in; \text{ for } x_{r-1} < x < x_r$$
$$\ge \in; \text{ for } x > x_r$$
So long as $g(x_{r-1} + 0) - g(b-0) > \in$ otherwise take $x_n = b$.
Proceeding in this way, we get a point b after a finite number of steps.
Define $\quad \psi(x) = g(x_r + 0)$ in each interval $x_r \le x < x_{r+1}$
such that $0 \le \psi(x) - g(x) < \in$ except possible at the points
$$a = x_0, x_1, ... = b$$
and $\quad \int_a^b \psi(x) f(x) dx = \sum_{r=0}^{n-1} g(x_r + 0) \int_{x_r}^{x_{r+1}} f(x) dx$ ...(1)

Now, let k and K be the lower and upper bounds of the function $F(x)$.
Defined by $\quad F(x) = \int_a^x f(t) dt$
Then, using Abel's lemma, we get
$$k.g(a+0) \le \int_a^b \psi(x) f(x) dx = K.g(a+0)$$ ...(2)
But $\quad \left| \int_a^b \psi(x) f(x) dx - \int_a^b g(x) f(x) dx \right| \le \in \int_a^b |f(x)| dx$

$\Rightarrow \quad \lim_{\in \to 0} \left\{ \left| \int_a^b \psi(x) f(x) dx - \int_a^b g(x) f(x) dx \right| \right\} \to 0$ ...(3)

Therefore $\lim_{\in \to 0} \left| \int_a^b \psi(x) f(x) dx \right| = \lim_{\in \to 0} \left| \int_a^b g(x) f(x) dx \right|$ ...(4)

Letting $\in \to 0$ and using (4), relation (2) gives
$$k.g(a+0) \le \int_a^b g(x) f(x) dx \le K.g(a+0)$$

$\Rightarrow \quad k \le \dfrac{1}{g(a+0)} \int_a^b g(x) f(x) dx \le K$ ...(5)

Since, we know that an indefinite integrals is a continuous function, therefore $F(x)$ is a continuous function and hence $F(x)$ can assumes any value between k and K, so that
$$F(t) = \dfrac{1}{g(a+0)} \int_a^b g(x) f(x) dx$$

$\Rightarrow \quad \int_0^t f(t) dt = \dfrac{1}{g(a+0)} \int_a^b g(x) f(x) dx$

Hence, $\int_a^b g(x) f(x) dx = g(a+0) \int_a^t f(x) dx$, $a < t < b$.

THEOREM 14. (Fubini Theorem)

Let $< f_n >$ be a sequence of real valued non-decreasing functions on $[a, b]$ such that $\sum_{n=1}^{\infty} f_n(x) = f(x)$

exists for every $x \in [a, b]$. Then, f is differentiable a.e. $x \in [a, b]$ and $f'(x) = \sum_{n=1}^{\infty} f_n'(x)$.

PROOF.   Let us assume that $f_n(x) \geq 0 \; \forall n$ and $\forall x$. Since each f_n is non-decreasing, it is differentiable a.e. for x. Then obviously $f'(x) \geq 0$, if exists.

Now, define $\quad E_n = \{x \in [a, b] : f_n'(x) \text{ does not exist}\}$

and $\qquad\qquad E = \overset{\infty}{\underset{n=1}{\cup}} E_n$

Then, E is a null set and for all $x \in [a, b]$, $\left\{ \overset{n}{\underset{k=1}{\Sigma}} f_k'(x) \right\}_{n \geq 1}$ is a non-decreasing sequence.

Further $\overset{n}{\underset{k=1}{\Sigma}} \dfrac{f_k(x+h) - f_k(x)}{h} \leq \underset{n \to \infty}{\lim} \overset{n}{\underset{k=1}{\Sigma}} \dfrac{f_k(x+h) - f_k(x)}{h} = \dfrac{f(x+h) - f(x)}{h}$

Since f is also a non-decreasing function, then again $f'(x)$ exists for all $x \notin F \subset [a, b]$, where F is a null set. Therefore, for all $x \in [a, b]$, we have

$$\overset{n}{\underset{k=1}{\Sigma}} f_k'(x) = \underset{h \to 0}{\lim} \overset{n}{\underset{k=1}{\Sigma}} \dfrac{f_k(x+h) - f_k(x)}{h}$$

$$\leq \underset{h \to 0}{\lim} \dfrac{f(x+h) - f(x)}{h}$$

$$= f'(x)$$

Therefore, $\left\{ \overset{n}{\underset{k=1}{\Sigma}} f_k'(x) \right\}_{n \geq 1}$ is a non-decreasing sequence and is bounded above

by $f'(x)$, $x \in [a, b]$. So, $\overset{\infty}{\underset{k=1}{\Sigma}} f_k'(x)$ is convergent for almost everywhere x.

Now, we have to show that there is a subsequence of $\left\{ \overset{n}{\underset{k=1}{\Sigma}} f_k'(x) \right\}_{n \geq 1}$, which converges to $f'(x)$ for almost everywhere x.

For this, we shall show that there exists positive integers $n_1 < n_2 < n_3 < ... < n_k$

such that $\overset{\infty}{\underset{k=1}{\Sigma}} \left[f'(x) - \overset{n_k}{\underset{j=1}{\Sigma}} f_j'(x) \right]$ is converged a.e. $x \in [a, b]$.

We know that for every $x \in [a, b]$ and every choice of positive integers $n_1 < n_2 < ... < n_k < ...$

$$f'(x) - \overset{n_k}{\underset{j=1}{\Sigma}} f_j'(x) = \left[f(x) - \overset{n_k}{\underset{j=1}{\Sigma}} f_j(x) \right]'$$

and $\quad f(x) - \overset{n_k}{\underset{j=1}{\Sigma}} f_j(x) = \overset{\infty}{\underset{j = n_k+1}{\Sigma}} f_j(x)$

Since $f_n(x) \geq 0$ for all n and for all x, $\left\{ \overset{\infty}{\underset{j=n_k+1}{\Sigma}} f_j(x) \right\}$ is a sequence of non-decreasing

functions. So, whenever the series $\overset{\infty}{\underset{k=1}{\Sigma}} \left(\overset{\infty}{\underset{j=n_k+1}{\Sigma}} f_j \right)$ converges pointwise, then

corresponding series of derivatives will converge a.e. x. Therefore, we only have to choose $< n_k >_{k \geq 1}$ such that $\forall x \in [a, b]$

$$\sum_{k=1}^{\infty} \left(\sum_{j=n_k+1}^{\infty} f_j(x) \right) < \infty$$

Since $\displaystyle\sum_{j=n_k+1}^{\infty} f_j(x) \le \sum_{j=n_k+1}^{\infty} f_j(b)$

We only have to choose $<n_k>_{k\ge 1}$ such that $\displaystyle\sum_{k=1}^{\infty} \left[\sum_{j=n_k+1}^{\infty} f_j(b) \right] < \infty$.

But this is possible, since $f(b) = \displaystyle\sum_{j=1}^{\infty} f_j(b)$ and we can choose $<n_k>_{k\ge 1}$ with

$$\sum_{j=n_k+1}^{\infty} f_j(b) = f(b) - \sum_{j=1}^{n_k} f(b) < \frac{1}{2^k}$$

with $$\sum_{j=n_k+1}^{\infty} f_j(b) = f(b) - \sum_{j=1}^{n_k} f(b) < \frac{1}{2^k}$$

Then, $$\sum_{k=1}^{\infty} \left[\sum_{j=n_k+1}^{\infty} f_j(b) \right] \le \sum_{k=1}^{\infty} \frac{1}{2^k} < \infty$$

Hence the theorem.

8.7 SOME MORE THEOREMS

THEOREM 1.

Every function of bounded variation is bounded.   [AGRA–2002, 14; KANPUR–2000, 04, 08, 13]

PROOF.   Let $f(x)$ be a function defined on $[a, b]$. Suppose that f is of bounded variation on $[a, b]$. We have to prove that f is bounded.

Since, f is of bounded variation, so by definition

$\exists\, c \in R, c > 0$ such that $V[f, P] < c$

$\Rightarrow\quad V[f, [a, b]] \le M, \quad M > 0$ ...(1)

and $|f(x) - f(a)| \le V[f, [a, b]] \le M \ \forall\, x \in [a, b]$ [By (1)]

Now, $|f(x) - f(a)| \le M \Rightarrow\quad |f(x)| - |f(a)| \le |f(x) - f(a)| \le M$

$\Rightarrow\quad |f(x)| - |f(a)| \le M \quad \forall\, x \in [a, b]$

$\Rightarrow\quad |f(x)| \le M + |f(a)| \quad \forall\, x \in [a, b]$

$\Rightarrow\quad |f(x)| \le M_1, \quad M_1 = M + |f(a)| \Rightarrow M_1 > 0$

Hence, $f(x)$ is bounded on $[a, b]$.

THEOREM 2.

If the derivative $f'(x)$ exists and is bounded in the closed interval $[a, b]$ then function f is of bounded variation.   [KANPUR–2000, 03, 14]

PROOF.   Let f be a function defined on an interval $[a, b]$ and P a closed partition of $[a, b]$ such that

$$P = [a = x_0 < x_1 < x_2 < \ldots < x_n = b]$$

Then by definition

$$V[f; P] = \sum_{i=1}^{n} |f(x_r) - f(x_{r-1})|$$ ...(1)

and $V[f, [a, b]] = \sup\{V[f; P] : P \in P[a, b]\}$ ...(2)

It is given that $f'(x)$ exists and bounded in $[a, b]$, so $\exists\, c > 0, c \in R$ such that
$$|f'(x)| \le c \,\forall\, x \in [a, b] \qquad \ldots(3)$$

Now, by Lagrange's mean value theorem
$$\frac{f(x_r) - f(x_{r-1})}{x_r - x_{r-1}} = f'(t), \quad t \in]a, b[$$

$$\Rightarrow \quad |f(x_r) - f(x_{r-1})| = (x_r - x_{r-1}) \cdot f'(t) \qquad \ldots(4)$$

Since $x_{r-1} < x_r \quad \Rightarrow \quad x_r > x_{r-1}$
$$\Rightarrow \quad |x_r - x_{r-1}| = (x_r - x_{r-1})$$

Then from equation (3) and (4) we get
$$|f(x_r) - f(x_{r-1})| \le (x_r - x_{r-1}) \cdot c \qquad \ldots(5)$$

Then from (1) [Using (5)]
$$V[f; P] \le \sum_{r=1}^{n} (x_r - x_{r-1}) \cdot c = c(x_n - x_0) = c(b - a)$$

$$\Rightarrow \qquad V[f; P] \le c[b - a]$$

Taking supremum of both the sides, and using (2) we get
$$V[f, [a, b]] \le c(b - a)$$

$\Rightarrow \quad V[f, [a, b]]$ is finite.

Hence, the function f is of bounded variation.

THEOREM 3.

Let f be a function of bounded variation on $[a, b]$. If $c \in [a, b]$ then f is of bounded variation on $[a, c]$ and $[c, b]$. Also, $V_{ab}(f) = V_{ac}(f) + V_{cb}(f)$. [KANPUR–2004, 06]

PROOF. Let f be a function of bounded variation on $[a, b]$, i.e.,
$$f \in BV[a, b]$$

Now, $f \in BV[a, b] \quad \Rightarrow \quad V_{ab}f < \infty \qquad \ldots(1)$

Let $c \in [a, b]$ then since $[a, c] \subseteq [a, b]$

Then $\quad V_{ac}(f) < V_{ab}(f) < \infty \qquad$ [From (1)]

$\Rightarrow \qquad V_{ac}(f) < \infty$

$\Rightarrow \qquad f \in BV[a, c]$

$\Rightarrow \quad f$ is of bounded variation on $[a, c]$.

Similarly, we may prove that $f \in BV[c, b]$, i.e., f is of bounded variation on $[c, b]$.

Now, suppose that P_1 and P_2 are any subdivision of $[a, c]$ and $[c, b]$ respectively. Then clearly, $P_1 \cup P_2$ is a subdivision of $[a, b]$.

Thus, $V_{ac}(f, P_1) + V_{bc}(f, P_2) = V_{ab}(f, P) \le V_{ab}(f)$

Taking supremum on P_1 and P_2, we get
$$V_{ac}(f) + V_{cb}(f) \le V_{ab}(f) \qquad \ldots(1)$$

Now, let $P = \{a = x_0 < x_1 < \ldots < x_n = b\}$ be a subdivision of $[a, b]$ and $c \in [x_{r-1}, x_r]$

Then clearly, $P_1 = \{x_0, x_1, x_2, \ldots, x_n, c\}$ and $P_2 = \{c, x_r, x_{r+1}, \ldots, x_n\}$ are the subdivision of $[a, c]$ and $[c, b]$ respectively. Therefore,

$$V_{ab}[f, P] = \sum_{i=1}^{r-1} |f(x_i) - f(x_{i-1})| + |f(x_r) - f(x_{r-1})| + \sum_{i=r+1}^{n} |f(x_i) - f(x_{i-1})|$$

$$= \sum_{i=1}^{r-1} |f(x_i) - f(x_{i-1})| + |f(x_r) - f(c) + f(c) - f(x_{r-1})|$$

$$+ \sum_{i=r+1}^{n} |f(x_i) - f(x_{i-1})|$$

$$\leq \left[\sum_{i=1}^{n} |f(x_i) - f(x_{i-1})| + |f(c) - f(x_{r-1})| \right]$$

$$+ \left[|f(x_r) - f(c)| + \sum_{i=r+1}^{n} |f(x_i) - f(x_{i-1})| \right]$$

$$\leq V_{ac}[f; P_1] + V_{cb}[f, P_2]$$
$$\leq V_{ac}(f) + V_{cb}(f) \qquad\qquad ...(2)$$

From (1) and (2) we conclude that
$$V_{ab}(f) = V_{ac}(f) + V_{cb}(f)$$

or $$\overset{b}{\underset{a}{V}}(f) = \overset{c}{\underset{a}{V}}(f) + \overset{b}{\underset{c}{V}}(f)$$

☞ **REMARKS**

- From the above theorem, we conclude that, if $a < c_1 < c_2 < ... < c_n < b$ then
$$V_{ab}(f) = V_{ac_1}(f) + V_{c_1c_2}(f) + ... + V_{c_nb}(f)$$

- $f \in BV[a, b] \Leftrightarrow f \in BV[a, c], f \in BV[c, b]$ for all $c \in [a, b]$

THEOREM 4.

The variation function $V(x)$ of a function of bounded variation is continuous if and only if f is a continuous function. [GARHWAL–1996, 2009; MEERUT–2004]

PROOF. Let us define a function of bounded variation $f: [a, b] \to R$ and $x, c \in [a, b]$ such that $x < c$. Then by definition of variation function

$$V(x) = V[f, (a, x)] \qquad\qquad ...(1)$$
$$0 \leq |f(x) - f(c)| \leq V[f, [x, c]] \qquad\qquad ...(2)$$

and $$V[f, [x, c]] = V[f, [a, c]] - V[f, [a, x]] \qquad\qquad ...(3)$$

Equation (2) and (3) implies
$$0 \leq |f(x) - f(c)| \leq V[f, [a, c]] - V[f, [a, x]]$$
$$= V(c) - V(x)$$

i.e., $$0 \leq |f(x) - f(c)| \leq V(c) - V(x)$$

or, $$0 \leq |f(x) - f(c)| \leq V(c) - V(x) \leq |V(c) - V(x)| \qquad ...(4)$$

Let us first suppose variation function $V(x)$ is continuous on $[a, b]$. We have to prove that $f(x)$ is a continuous function.

Since, f is a function of bounded variation, therefore, $V(x), V(c) \leq \infty$. ...(5)

We claim that f is continuous at $x = c$.

Since, $V(x)$ is continuous on $[a, b]$, so by definition of continuity, for given $\varepsilon > 0 \; \exists \; \delta > 0$ such that

$$|V(x) - V(c)| < \varepsilon, \text{ whenever } |x - c| < \delta \qquad ...(6)$$

Using (6) in (4) we get

$$|f(x) - f(c)| < \varepsilon \text{ whenever } |x - c| < \delta$$

$\Rightarrow$ $f(x)$ is continuous at $x = c$.

Hence, $f(x)$ is continuous on $[a, b]$.

Conversely, let us suppose that $f(x)$ be continuous on $[a, b]$. We have to prove that $V(x)$ is continuous on $[a, b]$.

Since, $f(x)$ is continuous on $[a, b]$ then by definition, for given $\varepsilon > 0 \; \exists \; \delta > 0$ such that $|f(x) - f(c)| < \varepsilon/2$ whenever $|x - \varepsilon| < \delta \; c \in [a, b]$ ...(7)

Now, since f is the function of bounded variation, then by definition, there exists a partition P of $[c, b]$ and $P = [c = x_0, x_1, ..., x_n = b]$

such that $\displaystyle\sum_{i=1}^{n} |f(x_r) - f(x_{r-1})| > V[f, [c,b]] - \varepsilon/2$ ...(8)

Let us set, the length of first subinterval $x_1 - c$ less than δ, i.e.,
$$0 < |x_1 - c| = x_1 - c < \delta$$

Also, by (7) $|f(x_1) - f(c)| < \varepsilon/2$ ...(9)

$\Rightarrow \quad |f(x_1) - f(c)| + \displaystyle\sum_{r=2}^{n} |f(x_r) - f(x_{r-1})| > V[f, [c,b]] - \varepsilon/2$ (By (8))

$\Rightarrow \quad V[f, [c,b]] - \displaystyle\sum_{r=2}^{n} |f(x_r) - f(x_{r-1})| < |f(x_1) - f(c)| + \varepsilon/2$

$\qquad\qquad\qquad\qquad\qquad\qquad < \varepsilon/2 + \varepsilon/2$ (By (9))

$\Rightarrow \quad V[f, [c, b]] - V[f, [x, b]] < \varepsilon$

$\Rightarrow \qquad\qquad V[f, [c, x_1]] < \varepsilon$ ...(10)

But, we have
$$V[f, [a, x_1]] - V[f, [a, c]] = V[f, [c, x_1]] < \varepsilon \qquad\qquad \text{(By (10))}$$

$\Rightarrow \qquad V[f, [a, x_1]] - V[f, [a, c]] < \varepsilon$

$\Rightarrow \qquad\qquad V(x_1) - V(c) < \varepsilon$

$\Rightarrow \quad |V(x_1) - V(c)| < \varepsilon$ whenever $|x_1 - c| < \delta$

Hence, $V(x)$ is continuous at $x = c$.

THEOREM 5.

Let f be a function of bounded variation then
$$V = P + N \text{ and } P - N = f(b) - f(a)$$

where V, P, H respectively denote total, positive and negative variation on $[a, b]$.

[KANPUR–2007; MEERUT–2006, 09, 15; PUNJAB–2003; GARHWAL–2005; HPU–2001; NAGPUR–2006]

PROOF.   Let f be a function of bounded variation on $[a, b]$. Divide $[a, b]$ by mean of points $a = x_0 < x_1 < x_2 < ... < x_n = b$.

Then by definition of total variation
$$V = \sum_{r=1}^{n-1} |f(x_{r+1}) - f(x_r)|$$

Further, let us suppose that p be the sum of the difference $f(x_{r+1}) - f(x_r)$ which are positive and $-n$ that the sum of those differences which are negative. Then, we have
$$V = p + n, \; f(b) - f(a) = p - n$$

$\Rightarrow \qquad V + f(b) - f(a) = 2p \qquad \Rightarrow \qquad V = 2p + f(a) - f(b)$ ...(1)

and $\qquad V - f(b) + f(a) = 2n \qquad$ and $\quad V = 2n + f(b) - f(a)$ ...(2)

Taking supremum of (1) and (2) we get

$$V = 2P + f(a) - f(b) \qquad \qquad \ldots(3)$$

and
$$V = 2N + f(b) - f(a) \qquad \qquad \ldots(4)$$

where $V = \sup(v)$, $N = \sup(n)$, $P = \sup(p)$

Finally, by adding and subtracting (3) and (4), we get

$$V = P + N$$

and
$$f(b) - f(a) = P - N.$$

THEOREM 6.

If a function f is of bounded variation on [a, b] and if there exist k > 0 such that $|f(x)| \leq k \; \forall \; x \in [a, b]$

then $\dfrac{1}{f}(f \neq 0)$ is also of bounded variation.   [KANPUR–2002; DEKHI–2006; NAGPUR–2009; AGRA–2007]

PROOF.   Let f be a function of bounded variation on $[a, b]$. We have to prove that $\dfrac{1}{f}$ is also a function of bounded variation.

Consider, $\quad V\left[\dfrac{1}{f}, P\right] = \Sigma \left| \dfrac{1}{f(x_r)} - \dfrac{1}{f(x_{r-1})} \right| = \Sigma \left| \dfrac{f(x_{r-1}) - f(x_r)}{f(x_r) f(x_{r-1})} \right|$

$$= \Sigma \dfrac{|f(x_{r-1}) - f(x_r)|}{|f(x_r)| \cdot |f(x_{r-1})|}$$

$$\leq \dfrac{1}{k^2} \Sigma |f(x_r) - f(x_{r-1})| \qquad \qquad [\because \; |f(x)| \leq k \; (\text{given})]$$

$$= \dfrac{1}{k^2} V[f, P]$$

i.e., $\qquad V\left[\dfrac{1}{f}, P\right] \leq \dfrac{1}{k^2} V[f, P] \qquad \qquad \ldots(1)$

Also, since f is of bounded variation, therefore

$$V[f, P] < k_1, k_1 > 0$$

Using this value in (1) we get

$$V\left[\dfrac{1}{f}, P\right] < \dfrac{k_1}{k} = \text{a finite inequality}$$

$\Rightarrow \qquad V\left[\dfrac{1}{f}, P\right] < \infty$

Hence, the function $\dfrac{1}{f}$ is of bounded variation.

THEOREM 7.

If f(x) and g(x) are absolutely continuous functions then their sum, differences and product are also absolutely continuous. Also, if g(x) does not vanish for any x then $\dfrac{f(x)}{g(x)}$ is also absolutely

continuous.   [MEERUT–2010, GARHWAL–2004]

PROOF.   Let $f(x)$ and $g(x)$ be two absolutely continuous function over the closed interval $[a, b]$.

Then by definition of absolute continuity, for given $\varepsilon > 0 \; \exists \; \delta > 0$ such that

$$\sum_{r=1}^{n} |f(b_r) - f(a_r)| < \varepsilon/2 \text{ and } \sum_{r=1}^{n} |g(b_r) - g(a_r)| < \varepsilon/2 \qquad \ldots(1)$$

whenever $\sum_{r=1}^{n} (b_r - a_r) < \delta \quad \forall a_r, b_r \in [a,b]$ such that $a_1 < b_1 \le a_2 < b_2 \le \ldots \le a_n < b_n$.

(1) Firstly, we shall prove that $f(x) \pm g(x)$ is also absolutely continuous over $[a, b]$

Consider $\sum_{r=1}^{n} \left| [f(b_r) \pm g(b_r)] - [f(a_r) \pm g(b_r)] \right|$

$$\le \sum_{r=1}^{n} |f(b_r) - f(a_r)| + \sum_{r=1}^{n} |g(b_r) - g(a_r)|$$

$$< \varepsilon/2 + \varepsilon/2 = \varepsilon \qquad \text{[Using (1)]}$$

Hence, the function $f(x) \pm g(x)$ is also absolutely continuous on $[a, b]$.

(2) We have to prove that $f(x) \cdot g(x)$ is also absolutely continuous on $[a, b]$. For this, consider

$$\sum_{r-1}^{n} |f(b_r) g(b_r) - f(a_r) g(a_r)|$$

$$= \sum_{r=1}^{n} |f(b_r) g(b_r) - f(b_r) g(a_r) + f(b_r) g(a_r) - f(a_r) g(a_r)|$$

$$= \sum_{r=1}^{n} |f(b_r) [g(b_r - g(a_r)] + g(a_r) [f(b_r) - f(a_r)]|$$

$$\le \sum_{r=1}^{n} |f(b_r)| \cdot |g(b_r) - g(a_r)| + \sum_{r=1}^{n} |g(a_r)| \cdot |f(b_r) - f(a_r)| \qquad \ldots(2)$$

Since, f and g both are absolutely continuous (given)

$\Rightarrow \quad f$ and g both are continuous.

$\Rightarrow \quad f$ and g both are bounded on $[a, b]$.

$\Rightarrow \quad \exists \; m_1$ and $m_2 \;(> 0)$ such that $|f(x)| \le m_1$ and $|g(x)| \le m_2 \qquad \ldots(3)$

Now, using (1) and (3) in (2) we get

$$\sum_{r=1}^{n} |f(b_r) g(b_r) - f(a_r) g(a_r)| \le m_1 \frac{\varepsilon}{2} + m_2 \frac{\varepsilon}{2} = \left(\frac{m_1 + m_2}{2} \right) \varepsilon = \varepsilon_1 \text{ (say)}$$

$$\Rightarrow \quad \sum_{r=1}^{n} |f(b_r) g(b_r) - f(a_r) g(a_r)| < \varepsilon_1$$

Hence, $f(x) \cdot g(x)$ is absolutely continuous function.

(3) We have to prove that $\frac{f(x)}{g(x)} (g(x) \ne 0)$ is also absolutely continuous. Since,

$g(x) \ne 0$ on $[a, b]$ so there exist $k > 0$ such that $|g(x)| \ge k \; \forall \; x \in [a, b]$.

Now, consider

$$\sum_{r=1}^{n} \left| \frac{1}{g(b_r)} - \frac{1}{g(a_r)} \right| = \sum_{r=1}^{n} \left| \frac{g(a_r) - g(b_r)}{g(a_r) g(b_r)} \right|$$

$$\le \sum_{r=1}^{n} \frac{|g(b_r) - g(a_r)|}{|g(a_r)| \cdot |g(b_r)|}$$

$$< \frac{\varepsilon}{k^2} = \varepsilon_1 \text{ (say)}$$

$$\Rightarrow \quad \sum_{r=1}^{n} \left| \frac{1}{g(b_r)} - \frac{1}{g(a_r)} \right| < \varepsilon_1$$

$\Rightarrow g(x)$ is absolutely continuous.

Further, since in (2) we have already proved that product of two absolutely continuous functions is also absolutely continuous.

Therefore, $f(x) \cdot \dfrac{1}{g(x)}$ is also absolutely continuous.

$\Rightarrow \quad \dfrac{f(x)}{g(x)}$ is absolutely continuous on $[a, b]$.

THEOREM 8.

Let $f(x)$ be an absolutely continuous function on the closed interval $[a, b]$. Let a function $F(y)$ satisfy the Lipchitz condition in the segment $[A, B] \subset [a, b]$. Then the composite function $F[f(x)]$ is absolutely continuous in $[A, B]$.

PROOF.   Let $f(x)$ be an absolutely continuous function on the closed interval $[a, b]$. Then clearly $f(x)$ is absolutely continuous on $[A, B] \subset [a, b]$.

Then by definition, for given $\varepsilon > 0 \ \exists \ \delta > 0$ such that

$$\sum_{r=1}^{n} |f(b_r) - f(a_r)| < \varepsilon \qquad \qquad ...(1)$$

for all numbers $a_1, b_1, ..., a_n, b_n$ such that
$$A = a_1 < b_1 \leq a_2 < b_2 \leq ... \leq a_n < b_n = B$$

and
$$\sum_{r=1}^{n} |b_r - a_r| < \delta$$

It is also given that $F(y)$ satisfies that Lipchitz's condition in $[A, B]$ therefore, for $m > 0$ we can write

$$|F(B_r) - F(A_r)| \leq m |B_r - A_r|$$

Then $\displaystyle\sum_{r=1}^{n} |F(f(b_r)) - F(f(a_r))| \leq m \sum_{r=1}^{n} |f(b_r) - f(a_r)| < m\varepsilon$ (Using (1))

$$\Rightarrow \quad \sum_{r=1}^{n} |F[f(b_r)] - F[f(a_r)]| \leq m\varepsilon = \varepsilon_1 \text{ (say)}$$

Therefore, $\displaystyle\sum_{r=1}^{n} |F[f(b_r)] - F[f(a_r)]| < \varepsilon_1$ whenever $\displaystyle\sum_{r=1}^{n} |b_r - a_r| < \delta$

Hence, the composite function $F[f(x)]$ is absolutely continuous in $[A, B]$.

THEOREM 9.

An indefinite integral is an absolutely continuous function.

PROOF.   Let $F(x)$ be an indefinite integral of $f(x)$ defined over $[a, b]$.

Then by definition, we can write

$$F(x) = \int_a^x f(t)dt + F(a) \quad \forall x \in [a, b] \qquad \qquad ...(1)$$

where $f(x)$ is integrable over $[a, b]$.

We have to prove that $F(x)$ is absolutely continuous on $[a, b]$.

We know that, if $f(x)$ is integrable over a measurable set E and if $<E_k>$ is a sequence of subsets of E such that $\lim_{n \to \infty} m(E_k) = 0$ then $\lim_{k \to \infty} \int_{E_k} f(x)dx = 0$.

So, $\lim_{k \to \infty} \int_{E_k} f(x)dx = 0$

$\Rightarrow \qquad \left| \int_{E_k} f(x)dx \right| < \varepsilon \quad \forall k \geq k_0, m(E_k) < \delta$

Now, let $a_1, b_1, a_2, b_2, \ldots, a_n, b_n$ be $2n$ numbers such that
$$a_1 < b_1 \leq a_2 < b_2 \leq \ldots \leq a_n < b_n$$

Let $\qquad m(E_k) = \sum_{i=1}^{n} m(b_i, a_i) = \sum_{i=1}^{n} (b_i - a_i) < \delta$

Then $\left| \sum_{i=1}^{n} \int_{a_1}^{b_1} f(t)dt \right| < \varepsilon$

$\Rightarrow \left| \sum_{i=1}^{n} [F(b_i) - F(a_i)] \right| < \varepsilon$ whenever $\sum_{i=1}^{n} (b_i - a_i) < \delta$

Hence, $F(x)$ is absolutely continuous function.

THEOREM 10.

Every absolutely continuous function is an indefinite integral of its own derivative.

[HPU–2003, 12; MEERUT–2006]

PROOF. Let $f(x)$ be an absolutely continuous function in a closed interval $[a, b]$. Then $f'(x)$ and $\int_a^x f'(t)dt$ exist finitely for all $x \in [a, b]$.

Let $F(x)$ be an indefinite integral of $f'(x)$, therefore,
$$F(x) = f(a) + \int_a^x f'(t)dt \quad \forall x \in [a, b] \qquad \ldots(1)$$

We have to prove that $F(x) = f(x)$ a.e.

From (1) we have $F'(x) = f'(x)$ a.e.

$\Rightarrow \qquad \dfrac{d}{dx}[F(x) - f(x)] = 0$

$\Rightarrow \quad F(x) - f(x) = c$, a constant $\qquad \ldots(2)$

Putting $x = a$ in (1) we get
$$F(a) = f(a) + \int_a^a f'(t)dt = f(a)$$

$\Rightarrow \qquad F(a) = f(a)$

$\Rightarrow \qquad F(x) - f(x) = 0$ for $x = a$

Using this in (2), we get $c = 0$

Therefore, from (2)
$$F(x) - f(x) = 0 \text{ a.e.}$$

$\Rightarrow \qquad F(x) = f(x)$ a.e.

Hence, $f(x)$ is indefinte integral of its own derivative.

☞ REMARK

- Theorem 9 and 10 can be restated combindly as follows:

"The necessary and sufficient condition that a function should be an indefinite integral is that it should be absolutely continuous."

THEOREM 11.

Let $f(x)$ be an indefinite integral of bounded measurable function $f(x)$ then $F'(x) = f(x)$ a.e.

[MEERUT–2002, 12]

PROOF. Let $F(x)$ be an indefinite integral of bounded measurable function $f(x)$, so that $f(x)$ is integrable and

$$F(x) = \int_a^x f(t)dt + F(a) \qquad \qquad ...(1)$$

We have to prove that $F'(x) = f(x)$ a.e.

Since, $f(x)$ is bounded $\Rightarrow |f(x)| \le m$

$\Rightarrow |f(t)| \le m$

Then from (1), we find

$$\frac{F(x+h) - F(x)}{h} = \frac{1}{h}\left[\int_a^{x+h} f(t)dt + F(a) - \int_a^x f(t)dt - F(a) \right]$$

$$= \frac{1}{h}\left[\int_x^{x+h} f(t)dt \right]$$

$$\Rightarrow \quad \left| \frac{F(x+h) - F(x)}{h} \right| = \left| \frac{1}{h}\left[\int_x^{x+h} f(t)dt \right] \right|$$

$$\le \frac{1}{|h|} \int_x^{x+h} |f(t)| \, |dt|$$

$$\le \frac{m}{h} \int_x^{x+h} |dt| = \frac{m}{h}|h| = m$$

$$\Rightarrow \quad \left| \frac{F(x+h) - F(x)}{h} \right| \le m \qquad \qquad ...(2)$$

and $\dfrac{F(x+h) - F(x)}{h} \to F'(x)$ a.e. as $h \to 0$

If h takes a sequence of values tending to 0, *i.e.*, $h_n \to 0$ as $n \to \infty$. So, we can say that $\dfrac{F(x+h) - F(x)}{h}$ satisfies all the conditions of Lebesgue bounded convergence theorem, therefore,

$$\int_a^c \lim_{h \to 0}\left[\frac{F(x+h) - F(x)}{h} \right] dx = \lim_{h \to 0} \int_a^c \frac{F(x+h) - F(x)}{h} dx \qquad c \in [a,\, b]$$

$$\Rightarrow \quad \int_a^c F'(x)dx = \lim_{h \to 0}\left[\frac{1}{h}\int_a^c F(x+h)dx - \frac{1}{h}\int_a^c F(x)dx \right]$$

$$= \lim_{h \to 0}\left[\int_{a+h}^{c+h} F(t)dt - \frac{1}{h}\int_a^c F(x)dx \right]$$

(On putting $x + h = t$ in first integral)

$$= \lim_{h \to 0}\left[\frac{1}{h}\int_c^{c+h} F(t)dt - \frac{1}{h}\int_a^{a} {}_{+h} F(t)dt \right]$$

$$\left[\because \int_a^b F(x)dx = \int_a^b F(t)dt \text{ and} \right.$$

$$\left. \int_{a+h}^{c+h} + \int_a^c = \int_c^{c+h} + \int_{a+h}^a \right]$$

$$= \lim_{h \to 0} \left[\frac{1}{h} \int_c^{c+h} F(t)dt - \frac{1}{h} \int_a^{a+h} F(t)dt \right] \qquad \ldots(3)$$

Now, consider

$$\lim_{h \to 0} \frac{1}{h} \int_c^{c+h} F(t)dt = \lim_{h \to 0} \frac{1}{h} \int_c^{c+h} \frac{d}{dt}(g(t))dt = \lim_{h \to 0} \frac{1}{h} [g(x)]_c^{c+h}$$

$$= \lim_{h \to 0} \frac{g(c+h) - g(c)}{h} = g'(c) = F(c) \qquad \ldots(4)$$

Using (4) in (3) we get

$$\int_a^c F'(x)dx = F(c) - F(a) = \int_a^c f(x)dx \qquad \text{[Using (1)]}$$

$$\Rightarrow \quad \int_a^c [F'(x) - f(x)]dx = 0$$

$$\Rightarrow \qquad F'(x) - f(x) = 0 \text{ a.e.}$$

Hence, $\qquad F'(x) = f(x)$ a.e.

THEOREM 12.

If f is a finite valued monotonic increasing function defined on [a, b] then f is continuous on [a, b] except almost a countable number of points.

PROOF. Let $f(x)$ be a finite valued monotonic increasing function defined on [a, b].

Let $\delta f(x)$ be the jump function defined as follows:

$$\delta f(x) = \inf[f(x + h)] - \sup[f(x + h)], h > 0$$

Now, since f is monotonic increasing, therefore $\delta f(x) = 0$.

We know that a function f is continuous if and only if $\delta f(x) = 0$

Also, $\displaystyle\sum_{x_i \in (a,b)} \delta f(x_i) \le f(b) - f(a)$, where x_i is any sequence of points in [a, b].

Then clearly the set $E_n = \left\{ x : \delta f(x) > \dfrac{1}{n} \right\}$ contains almost $n \cdot [f(b) - f(a)]$ points.

$\Rightarrow \quad E_n$ is countable for all n.

Since, the set of points of discontinuity is $E = \displaystyle\bigcup_{n=1}^{\infty} E_n$, which is being an enumerable union of enumerable set is countable.

$\Rightarrow \quad E$ is countable.

Recapitulations

♦ If f_1 and f_2 are non-decreasing functions on [a, b] then $f_1 - f_2$ is of bounded variation on [a, b].

♦ The set of all functions of bounded variations form a linear space.

♦ An absolutely continuous function is differentiable a.e.

♦ A function of bounded variation may not be continuous.

♦ If f is monotonic function on [a, b] then $V_{ab}(f) = |f(b) - f(a)|$.

♦ If $c_1, c_2 \in R$ then $f, g \in BV[a, b]$

$\Rightarrow c_1 f + c_2 g \in BV[a, b]$.

♦ A continuous function may not be of bounded variation.

8.8 LEBESGUE POINT

A point x is said to be a Lebesgue point of the function $f(t)$ if

$$\lim_{h \to 0} \frac{1}{h} \int_x^{x+h} |f(t) - f(x)| dt = 0$$

8.9 COVERING IN THE SENSE OF VITALI

A set E is said to covered in the sense of Vitali by a family of intervals M in which none is a singleton set, if every point of the set E is contained in small intervals of M, i.e., for each $x \in E$ and $\varepsilon > 0$ there exist $I \in M$ such that $x \in I$ and $l(I) < \varepsilon$.

Here, the family M is called the Vitali cover of E.

8.10 DINI'S DERIVATIVES

Here we define four quantities called Dini's derivatives which may be defined even at the points where the functions is not differentiable.

(1) **Right Dini's Derivaties**

   (i) **Upper Right Dini's derivatie**
   $$D^+ f(x) = \overline{\lim_{h \to 0^+}} \frac{f(x+h) - f(x)}{h}$$

   (ii) **Lower Right Dini's derivative**
   $$D_+ f(x) = \underline{\lim_{h \to 0^+}} \frac{f(x+h) - f(x)}{h}$$

(2) **Left Dini's Derivatives**

   (i) **Upper Left Dini's derivative**
   $$D^- f(x) = \overline{\lim_{h \to 0^-}} \frac{f(x+h) - f(x)}{h} = \overline{\lim_{h \to 0^+}} \frac{f(x-h) - f(x)}{-h}$$

   (ii) **Lower Left Dini's derivative**
   $$D_- f(x) = \underline{\lim_{h \to 0^-}} \frac{f(x+h) - f(x)}{h} = \underline{\lim_{h \to 0^+}} \frac{f(x+h) - f(x)}{-h}$$

We observe that

(i) If $D^+f(x) = D_+f(x)$ then we say that right hand derivative of $f(x)$ exists at the point x and denoted by $f'(x^+)$.

(ii) If $D^-f(x) = D_-f(x)$ then we say that left hand derivative of $f(x)$ exists at the point x and denoted by $f'(x^-)$.

(iii) The function $f(x)$ is said to be differentiable at a point x, if all the four Dini's derivative are finite and equal, i.e.,
$$D^+ f(x) = D_+ f(x) = D^- f(x) = D_- f(x) \neq \infty.$$

8.10.1 PROPERTIES OF DINI'S DERIVATIVES

(1) If $f(x)$ is any function on an interval (a, b) then four Dini's derivatives are measurable.

(2) Dini's derivatives always exists for every function, but may have finite or infinite value.

(3) If f is a continuous function on $[a, b]$ and one of its Dini's derivative is non-negative on $]a, b[$. Then f is non-decreasing in $[a, b]$.

(4) $D^+[f + g] \leq D^+(f) + D^+(g)$
Similar results follows for other Dini's derivatives.

(5) $D_+ f(x) = -D^+[-f(x)]$ and $D_- f(x) = -D^-[-f(x)]$

(6) If f and g are continuous at a point x then
$$D^+(f \cdot g)(x) \leq f(x)D^+(g(x)) + g(x)D^+(f(x))$$

THEOREM 1. (Vitali's Covering Theorem)

If a bounded set E is covered by a family M of closed intervals in the sense of Vitali then it is possible to find a countably finite or enumerable subfamily of closed interval $<I_k>$ of M such that

$$m^*\left[E - \sum_k I_k\right] = 0, I_i \cap I_j = \phi, \text{ for } i \neq j \qquad \text{[MEERUT–2013, 17; ROHTAK–1998]}$$

PROOF. Let E be a bounded set which is covered in the sense of Vitali by a family M of closed intervals. We have to prove that $\exists$ a pointwise disjoint subfamily $<I_k>$ of M with the property $m^*\left[E - \sum_k I_k\right] = 0$. Since E is covered by M in the sense of

Vitali therefore, by definition, for $\varepsilon > 0$, $x \in E$ $\exists$ a closed interval $I_k \in M$ such that $m(I_k) < \varepsilon$ ...(1)

Select an interval $]a, b[$ such that $E \subset]a, b[$. Form a family M_0 of M such that
$$M_0 = \{I_k \in M : I_k \subset]a, b[\}$$

Evidently, $M_0 \subseteq M$ and every member of M_0 is contained in $]a, b[$ and M_0 covers E in the sense of Vitali.

Let us pick an interval $I_1 \in M_0$. If $E \subset I_1$, then theorem is proved by (1).
If not then we pick another interval $I_2 \in M_0$ such that $I_1 \cap I_2 = \phi$.

If $E \subset I_2$, then again by (1) $m^*\left[E - \sum_{k=1}^{2} I_k\right] = 0$.

In the contrary case pick an interval $I_3 \in M_0$ such that $I_m \cap I_n = \phi$, $m \neq n$, $m, n \in N$. Proceed in the same manner, repeat the process n times, we get a family of pairwise disjoint intervals $I_1, I_2, \dots I_n$.

If $E \subset \sum_{r=1}^{n} I_n$ then again from (1), proof is complete.

On the contrary case, $E \not\subset \sum_{r=1}^{n} I_n$, so that $E - \sum_{r=1}^{n} I_r \neq \phi$ ...(2)

In this situation, set $F_n = \sum_{r=1}^{n} I_r, G_n =]a, b[- F_n$

Now, we consider those intervals of M which are subsets of the open set G_n. Such interval exists by virtue of (1) and their length is less than or equal to $m(]a, b[)$. Let s_n denote the supremum of the lengths of these intervals and let I_{n+1} be one of them for which

$$m(I_{n+1}) > \frac{s_n}{2}$$

Clearly, $s_n > 0$
Therefore, $I_{r+1} \cap I_r = \phi$, for $r = 1, 2, \dots, n-1$.
If the process of constructing the interval $I_1, I_2, \dots$ ends after a finite number of steps, then theorem is proved.
But if this process does not come to an end after a finite number of steps then we are left with a sequence $<I_n>$ of pairwise disjoint intervals.
Now we shall show that this sequence also satisfies (1).
Construct a closed interval $F_k \ \forall \ k$ such that
(i) the length of F_k is five times the length of I_k, i.e., $m(F_k) = 5m(I_k)$

(ii) the middle point of F_k coincides with the middle point of I_k.

Since, every element of the sequence $<I_n>$ is contained in $]a, b[$ so that

$$m\left[\sum_{k=1}^{n} I_n\right] \leq m[\,]a,b[\,] \qquad \qquad ...(2)$$

$$\Rightarrow \qquad m\left[\sum_{i=1}^{\infty} F_k\right] = 5m\left(\sum_{k=1}^{\infty} I_k\right) \leq m[\,]a,b[\,] = \text{a finite number}$$

$$\Rightarrow \qquad m\left[\sum_{i=1}^{\infty} F_k\right] < \infty$$

Now, let $x \in E - \sum_{k=1}^{\infty} I_k$ where $x \in G_i \, \forall \, i$ \qquad ...(3)

Since, $x \in G_i$ and G_i is open therefore, there exists a closed interval $I \in M_0$ such that $x \in I \subset G$. However it is impossible that $I \subset G_n$. \qquad ...(4)

Which follows from the fact that

$$m(I) \leq s_n \leq 2m(I_{n+1}) \, \forall \, n$$

which is not possible (by virtue of (2))

Therefore, the relation (4) is not satisfied for some n and so the relation

$$I \cap I_n \neq \phi \qquad \qquad ...(5)$$

holds.

Further, let us assume that n is the least positive integer such that (5) holds. So, $n > i$, because $I \cap I_i = \phi$ and $I_1 \subset I_2 \subset I_3 \subset ...$

$\therefore$ \quad By definition of n, we have $I \cap I_{n-1} = \phi$.

which gives the following results:

(i) $I \cap I_n \neq \phi$

(ii) $I \subset G_{n-1}$ and $m(I) \leq s_{n-1} < 2m(I_n)$

From the above result (i) and (ii) we can find that

$$I \subset F_n$$

$$\Rightarrow \qquad I \subset \sum_{k=1}^{\infty} F_k$$

$$\Rightarrow \qquad x \in \sum_{k=1}^{\infty} F_k$$

Hence, the theorem.

THEOREM 2.

If x is a Lebesgue point of a function f(t) then the indefinite integral

$$F(x) = F(a) + \int_a^x f(t)dt$$

is differentiable at each point x and $F'(x) = f(x)$.

PROOF. \qquad Let x be the Lebesgue point of $f(t)$, then by definition, we have

$$\lim_{h \to 0} \frac{1}{h} \int_x^{x+h} |F(t) - f(x)| \, dt = 0 \qquad \qquad ...(1)$$

Consider $\dfrac{1}{h} \int_x^{x+h} f(x)dx = \dfrac{1}{h} f(x) \int_x^{x+h} 1 \cdot dt = \dfrac{1}{h} f(x)[t]_x^{x+h}$

$$= \frac{1}{h} f(x) \cdot h = f(x)$$

$$\Rightarrow \qquad f(x) = \frac{1}{h} \int_x^{x+h} f(x)dx \qquad \qquad \text{...(2)}$$

Now, since $\qquad F(x) = F(a) + \int_a^x f(t)dt$

$$\Rightarrow \qquad F(x+h) = F(a) + \int_a^{x+h} f(t)dt$$

$$\therefore \qquad F(x+h) - F(x) = \int_a^{x+h} f(t)dt - \int_a^x f(t)dt$$

$$= \int_a^x f(t)dt + \int_x^{x+h} f(t)dt - \int_a^x f(t)dt$$

$$= \int_x^{x+h} f(t)dt$$

$$\Rightarrow \qquad \frac{F(x+h) - F(x)}{h} = \frac{1}{h} \int_x^{x+h} f(t)dt \qquad \qquad \text{...(3)}$$

Now, from (2) and (3) we have

$$\left| \frac{F(x+h) - F(x)}{h} - f(x) \right| = \left| \frac{1}{h} \int_x^{x+h} f(t)dt - \frac{1}{h} \int_x^{x+h} f(x)dt \right|$$

$$= \left| \frac{1}{h} \int_x^{x+h} (f(t) - f(x))dt \right|$$

$$\leq \frac{1}{h} \int_x^{x+h} |f(t) - f(x)| \, dt$$

$$\Rightarrow \lim_{h \to 0} \left| \frac{F(x+h) - F(x)}{h} - f(x) \right| \leq \lim_{h \to 0} \frac{1}{h} \int_x^{x+h} |f(t) - f(x)| \, dt = 0 \qquad \text{(By (1))}$$

$$\Rightarrow \lim_{h \to 0} \left| \frac{F(x+h) - F(x)}{h} - f(x) \right| \leq 0 \qquad \qquad \text{...(4)}$$

But by definition of modulus, we have

$$\lim_{h \to 0} \left| \frac{F(x+h) - F(x)}{h} - f(x) \right| \geq 0 \qquad \qquad \text{...(5)}$$

From (4) and (5) we conclude that

$$\lim_{h \to 0} \left| \frac{F(x+h) - F(x)}{h} - f(x) \right| = 0$$

Hence, $\displaystyle \lim_{h \to 0} \left(\frac{F(x+h) - F(x)}{h} \right) = f(x)$

i.e., $\qquad F'(x) = f(x)$

THEOREM 3.

Every point of continuity of an integrable function $f(t)$ is a Lebesgue point of $f(t)$.

PROOF.   Let $f(t)$ be integrable over $[a, b]$ and continuous at the point x_0. Then by definition of continuity, we have for $x > 0$, $\exists \, \delta > 0$ s.t.

$$|f(t) - f(x_0)| < \varepsilon \quad \text{whenever} \quad |t - x_0| < \delta$$

which implies $\int_{x_0}^{x_0+h} |f(t) - f(x_0)| \, dt < \varepsilon \int_{x_0}^{x_0+h} dt + \varepsilon h \quad$ whenever $|h| < \delta$

$$\Rightarrow \quad \frac{1}{h} \int_{x_0}^{x_0+h} |f(t) - f(x_0)| \, dt < \varepsilon \qquad \qquad \text{...(1)}$$

Now, $h \to 0$ implies $\varepsilon \to 0$ then from (1), we have

$$\lim_{h \to 0} \frac{1}{h} \int_{x_0}^{x_0+h} |f(t) - f(x_0)| \, dt \le 0 \qquad \qquad \text{...(2)}$$

Also, $\left| \frac{1}{h} \int_{x_0}^{x_0+h} |f(t) - f(x_0)| \, dt \right| \le \lim_{h \to 0} \frac{1}{h} \int_{x_0}^{x_0+h} |f(t) - f(x_0)| \, dt \le 0 \qquad$ (by 2) $\qquad \text{...(3)}$

But by definition of modulus, we can write

$$\lim_{h \to 0} \left| \frac{1}{h} \int_{x_0}^{x_0+h} |f(t) - f(x_0)| \, dt \right| \ge 0 \qquad \qquad \text{...(4)}$$

Therefore, from (3) and (4) we conclude that

$$\lim_{h \to 0} \frac{1}{h} \left| \int_{x_0}^{x_0+h} |f(t) - f(x_0)| \, dt \right| = 0$$

Hence, x_0 is a Lebesgue point of f(t).

8.11 CONVEX FUNCTION

A function f defined on an interval $]a, b[$ is said to be a convex function if for all λ such that $0 \le \lambda \le 1$ and $x, y \in]a, b[$. We have

$$f(\lambda x + (1 - \lambda)y) \le \lambda f(x) + (1 - \lambda)y$$

☛ REMARKS
- Every convex function is continuous.
- If f is a convex function on $]a, b[$ and $x, y, x', y' \in]a, b[$ such that $x < x' < y'; x < y \le y'$ then
$$\frac{f(y) - f(x)}{y - x} \le \frac{f(y') - f(x')}{y' - x'}$$

8.11.1 SUPPORTING LINE

Let f be a convex function on $]a, b[$ and $\alpha \in]a, b[$ then the line $y = m(x - \alpha) + f(\alpha)$ passing through the point $(\alpha, f(x))$ is said to be a supporting line at $x = \alpha$ if it always below the graph of the function f, i.e., $m(x - \alpha) + f(a) \le f(x)$.

☛ REMARKS
- The above line will be a supporting line if and only if its slope m lies between the left and right hand derivative of f at $x = a$.
- There always exists at least one supporting line at each point of $]a, b[$.

THEOREM 1.

If f is a convex function on $]a, b[$ then f is absolutely continuous on each closed subinterval of $]a, b[$.

PROOF.   Let f be a convex function on $]a, b[$. We have to prove that f is absolutely continuous on $[c, d] \subset]a, b[$.

Since, $[c, d] \subset]a, b[$, then by above remark, we can write

For all $x, y \in [c, d]$

$$\frac{f(c) - f(a)}{c - a} \le \frac{f(y) - f(x)}{y - x} \le \frac{f(b) - f(d)}{b - d}$$

which implies that

$$|f(y) - f(x)| \le M(x - y)$$

$\Rightarrow$ $f(x)$ satisfies the Lipchitz condition and hence absolutely continuous.

☞ **REMARK**

- The right and left hand derivative of the function f discussed in the above theorem, having the following properties:
    (1)   Both exists at each point of $]a, b[$ and are equal to each other except on a countable set.
    (2)   Both are monotonically increasing functions of x.
    (3)   Left hand derivative is less than or euqal to the right hand derivative at each point of $]a, b[$.

THEOREM 2.

If one of the four Dini's derivative is non-decreasing and f is a continuous function on $]a, b[$ then f is convex.   [GWALIOR–2008; RAVISHANKAR–2003]

PROOF.   For given x, y such that $a < x < y < b$, let us define a function g on $[0, 1]$ such that
$$g(t) = f[ty + (1 - t)x] - tf(y) - (1 - t)f(x) \qquad \qquad ...(1)$$
Firstly, we shall prove that $g(t)$ is non-positive function on $[0, 1]$.
Since, f is continuous (given), therefore, g is also continuous and
$$g(0) = g(1) = 0$$
Also, $D^+g = (y - x)D^+f - f(y) + f(x)$
Now, since D^+f is non-decreasing, therefore D^+g is also non-decreasing on $[0, 1]$.
If g assumes the maximum on $[0, 1]$ at $t = a$.

Case 1 If $a = 1$
Then $g(t) \leq g(1) = 0$ on $[0, 1]$ so $g(t)$ is non-positive function on $[0, 1]$.
Thus, $f[ty + (1 - t)x] - tf(y) - (1 - t)f(x) \leq 0$
$\Rightarrow \quad f[ty + (1 - t)x] \leq tf(y) + (1 - t)f(x)$
Hence, f is convex.

Case 2 If $a \neq 1$
Then $a \in [0, 1[$. Then g has a local maxima at $t = a$ and hence $D^+g(a) \leq 0$
But D^+g is also non-decreasing therefore, $D^+g \leq 0$ on $[0, a]$.
$\Rightarrow \quad g$ is non-increasing on $[0, a]$.
$\Rightarrow \quad g(0) \geq g(a) \Rightarrow g(a) \leq 0$.
$\Rightarrow \quad g[t_1 \leq 0$ on $(0, 1)]$, i.e., $g(t)$ is non-positive on $[0, 1]$.
Hence, f is convex (as shown in case 1).

THEOREM 3. (Jenson's Inequality)

If f is a convex function on $]-\infty, \infty[$ and g is an integrable function on $[0, 1]$ then

$$\int_0^1 f(g(t))dt \geq f\left[\int_0^1 g(t)dt\right] \qquad \text{[NAGPUR–2006, 12; RAVISHANKAR–2003]}$$

PROOF.   Consider a supporting line $y = m(x - \alpha) + f(\alpha)$ at $x = \alpha$.

where $\alpha = \int_0^1 g(t)dt$ such that $\alpha \in]0, 1[$
By definition of supporting line, for every $t \in [0, 1]$
$$g(t) \geq m(g(t) - \alpha) + f(\alpha)$$
On integrating both the sides w.r.t. t over $[0, 1]$, we get
$$\int_0^1 f(g(t))dt \geq m\int_0^1[g(t) - \alpha]dt + f(\alpha)\int_0^1 dt$$
$$\geq m\left[\int_0^1 g(t)dt - \alpha\right] + f(\alpha)$$
$$\geq m[\alpha - \alpha] + f(\alpha) = f(\alpha)$$

$$\Rightarrow \quad \int_0^1 f[g(t)]dt \geq f(\alpha) = f\left[\int_0^1 g(t)dt\right]$$

Hence, $\int_0^1 f(g(t))dt \geq f\left[\int_0^1 g(t)dt\right]$

☞ **REMARK**
- If f is an exponential function, *i.e.*, $f(x) = e^x$. Then Jenson's inequality becomes
$$\int_0^1 \exp[g(t)]dt = \exp\left(\int_0^1 g(t)dt\right)$$

 Solved Examples

EXAMPLE 1. *Let f be a function defined by* $f(x) = \begin{cases} x\sin\dfrac{1}{x}, & x \neq 0 \\ 0, & x = 0 \end{cases}$. *Find $D^+f(0)$, $D_+f(0)$, $D^-f(0)$,*

$D_-f(0)$. [HPU–2004; BHOPAL–2006]

SOLUTION. By definition of Dini's derivative, we have

$$D^+f(0) = \varlimsup_{h\to0^+} \frac{f(0+h)-f(0)}{h} = \varlimsup_{h\to0}\left\{\frac{h\sin\dfrac{1}{h}-0}{h}\right\}$$

$$= \varlimsup_{h\to0} \sin\frac{1}{h} = 1 \qquad (\because \text{ Value of } \sin x \text{ always lies between 1 and } -1)$$

Now, $D_+f(0) = \varliminf_{h\to0^+} \dfrac{f(0+h)-f(0)}{h} = \varliminf_{h\to0^+} \sin\dfrac{1}{h} = -1$

$$D^-f(0) = \varlimsup_{h\to0^-} \frac{f(0-h)-f(0)}{0-h} = \varlimsup_{h\to0} \frac{(-h)\sin\left(-\dfrac{1}{h}\right)-0}{-h}$$

$$= \varlimsup_{h\to0}\left(-\sin\frac{1}{h}\right) = 1$$

and $D_-f(0) = \varliminf_{h\to0^-} \dfrac{f(0-h)-f(0)}{-h} = \varliminf_{h\to0}\left(-\sin\dfrac{1}{h}\right) = -1$

EXAMPLE 2. *Let* $f(x) = \begin{cases} ax\sin^2\dfrac{1}{x}+bx\cos^2\dfrac{1}{x}, & x > 0 \\ px\sin^2\dfrac{1}{x}+qx\cos^2\dfrac{1}{x}, & x < 0 \\ 0, & x = 0 \end{cases}$.

If $a < b$, $p < q$, evaluate all four Dini's derivatives at $x = 0$.

SOLUTION. We have

$$D^+f = \varlimsup_{h\to0^+}\left(a\sin^2\frac{1}{h}+b\cos^2\frac{1}{h}\right)$$

$$= \varlimsup_{h\to0^+} \frac{1}{2}\left[a\left(1-\cos\frac{2}{h}\right)+b\left(1+\cos\frac{2}{h}\right)\right]$$

$$= \overline{\lim_{h \to 0^+}} \frac{1}{2}\left[(a+b)+(b-a)\cos\frac{2}{h}\right]$$

$$= \frac{1}{2}[(a+b)+(b-a)] = b$$

Similarly, we may find

$$D_+f = a, D^-f = q \text{ and } D_-f = p$$

EXAMPLE 3. *If the function $f(x)$ assumes its maximum at c, show that $D^+f(c) \le 0$ and $D_-f(c) \ge 0$.*

SOLUTION. It is given that the function $f(x)$ assumes its maximum value at $x = c$. Therefore,

$$f(c+h) \le f(c) \qquad \Rightarrow \quad f(c+h) - f(c) \le 0$$

and $f(c-h) \le f(c) \qquad \Rightarrow \quad f(c-h) - f(c) \le 0$

which implies that

$$\frac{f(c+h) - f(c)}{h} \le 0 \text{ and } \frac{f(c-h) - f(c)}{-h} \ge 0$$

Hence, $D^+f(c) = \overline{\lim_{h \to 0^+}} \dfrac{f(c+h) - f(c)}{h} \le 0$

Similarly, $D_-f(c) \ge 0$.

EXAMPLE 4. *Find the four Dini's derivatives of the function $f : [0, 1] \to R$ such that $f(x) = 0$ if $x \in Q$ and $f(x) = 1$ if $x \notin Q$.*

SOLUTION. If $x \in Q$, then

$$D^+f(x) = \overline{\lim_{h \to 0}} \frac{f(x+h) - f(x)}{h} = \overline{\lim_{h \to 0}} \frac{f(x+h) - 0}{h}$$

But $f(x + h)$ will take the value 0 or 1 according as h is rational or not. Then $\dfrac{f(x+h)}{h}$ will have the value 0 or $\dfrac{1}{h}$.

Therefore,

$$D^+f(x) = \overline{\lim_{h \to 0}}\left(0 \text{ or } \frac{1}{h}\right) = \infty$$

Similarly, $D_+f(x) = 0$.

and $D^-f(x) = \overline{\lim_{h \to 0}} \dfrac{f(x+h) - f(x)}{-h} = \overline{\lim_{h \to 0}} \dfrac{f(x+h) - f(0)}{-h}$

$$= \overline{\lim_{h \to 0}}\left(0 \text{ or} - \frac{1}{h}\right) = 0$$

Similarly, $D_-f(x) = -\infty$.

Now, consider then case when $x \notin Q$, then

$$D^+f(x) = \overline{\lim_{h \to 0^+}} \frac{f(x+h) - f(x)}{h} = \overline{\lim_{h \to 0^+}}\left(\frac{f(x+h) - 1}{h}\right)$$

$$= \overline{\lim_{h \to 0^+}} \frac{(0 \text{ or } 1) - 1}{h} = \overline{\lim_{h \to 0^+}}\left(\frac{-1}{h} \text{ or } 0\right) = 0$$

Similarly, we can find

$$D_+ f(x) = \lim_{h \to 0^+} \left(-\frac{1}{h} \text{ or } 0 \right) = -\infty$$

$$D_- f(x) = \infty$$

and $D_- f(x) = 0$

EXAMPLE 5. *Show by means of an example that every bounded function is not necessarily of bounded variation.* [KANPUR–2000; RAIPUR–2012; RAJASTHAN–2006]

SOLUTION. Let us define a function

$$f(x) = \begin{cases} x \sin \dfrac{\pi}{x}, & 0 < x \le 1 \\ 0, & x = 0 \end{cases}$$

Since, $0 \le x \le 1$ and $-1 \le \sin x \le 1$, the function f is clearly bounded. Further, consider the partition of $[0, 1]$.

$$P = \left\{ 0, \frac{2}{2n+1}, \frac{2}{2n-1}, \dots, \frac{2}{7}, \frac{2}{5}, \frac{2}{3}, 1 \right\} \quad n \in N$$

Then $V_{01}(f, P) = \left| f\left(\dfrac{2}{2n+1} \right) - f(0) \right| + \dots + \left| f\left(\dfrac{2}{3} \right) - f\left(\dfrac{2}{5} \right) \right| + \left| f(1) - f\left(\dfrac{2}{3} \right) \right|$

$$= \left| \frac{2}{2n+1} (-1)^n - 0 \right| + \dots + \left| \frac{2}{3}(-1) - \frac{2}{5}(1) \right| + \left| 0 - \frac{2}{3}(-1) \right|$$

$$= \frac{2}{2n+1} + \dots + \left(\frac{2}{3} + \frac{2}{5} \right) + \frac{2}{3}$$

$$= 4 \left(\frac{1}{3} + \frac{1}{5} + \dots + \frac{1}{2n+1} \right) = 4 \sum_n \frac{1}{2n+1}$$

We know that the series $\sum_n \dfrac{1}{2n+1}$ is a divergent series. So, letting $n \to \infty$ we get

$$V_{01}(f) = \lim_{n \to \infty} \underline{V_{01}(f, P)} = \infty$$

Hence, the function f is not of bounded variation.

EXAMPLE 6. *Show that the function* $f(x) = \begin{cases} x^p \sin \dfrac{1}{x} & \text{for} \quad 0 < x \le 1 \\ 0 & \text{for} \quad x = 0 \end{cases}$, $p \ge 2$ *is of bounded variation on* $[0, 1]$.

SOLUTION. We know that if $f'(x)$ exists and bounded then f is of bounded variation.

Now, $Rf'(0) = \lim_{h \to 0} \dfrac{f(0+h) - f(0)}{h} = \lim_{h \to 0} \dfrac{(0+h)^p \sin \dfrac{1}{h} - 0}{h}$

$$= \lim_{h \to 0} h^{p-1} \cdot \sin \frac{1}{h} = 0$$

and $Lf'(0) = \lim_{h \to 0} \dfrac{f(0-h) - f(0)}{-h} = \lim_{h \to 0} \dfrac{(-h)^p \sin \left(-\dfrac{1}{h} \right) - 0}{-h} = 0$

So, $Rf'(0) = Lf'(0) = 0.$

$\Rightarrow$ $f'(0) = 0 \Rightarrow f'(x)$ exists.

and $f'(x) = x^p \cos\dfrac{1}{x}\left(-\dfrac{1}{x^2}\right) + px^{p-1} \sin\dfrac{1}{x}$

$$= x^{p-2}\left[px \sin\dfrac{1}{x} - \cos\dfrac{1}{x}\right], \text{ for } 0 < x \le 1$$

$\Rightarrow$ $f'(x)$ is bounded for $0 \le x \le 1$.

Here $f(x)$ is of bounded variation on $[0, 1]$.

EXAMPLE 7. *Let $f : [a, b] \to R$ be a function which satisfies Lipchitz's condition then show that it is absolutely continuous.*

SOLUTION. Let $f : [a, b] \to R$ be the given function which satisfies the Lipchitz's condition, *i.e.*, for any constant M.

$$|f(x) - f(y)| \le M|x - y| \ \forall \ x, y \in [a, b] \qquad \dots(1)$$

Now for given $\varepsilon > 0$, take $\delta = \dfrac{\varepsilon}{M}$ such that

$$\sum_{r=1}^{n} (b_r - a_r) < \delta = \dfrac{\varepsilon}{M}$$

where $(]a_i, b_i[) : i \in N$ is a finite non-overlapping collection of pairwise disjoint intervals. Then from (1)

$$|f(b_r) - f(a_r)| \le M(b_r - a_r) \ \forall \ r$$

$\Rightarrow$ $\displaystyle\sum_{r=1}^{n} |f(b_r) - f(a_r)| \le M\Sigma |b_r - a_r|$

$$< M\dfrac{\varepsilon}{M} = \varepsilon$$

$\Rightarrow$ $\displaystyle\sum_{r=1}^{n} |f(b_r) - f(a_r)| < \varepsilon$

Hence, f is an absolutely continuous function.

EXAMPLE 8. *If f is an absolutely continuous monotone function on $[a, b]$ and E is a set of measure zero then show that $f(E)$ has measure zero.*

SOLUTION. Without loss of any generality, we may assume that the function f is monotonically increasing. Then by definition of absolute continuity of f, for $\varepsilon > 0 \ \exists \ \delta > 0$ non-overlapping intervals $\{I_n = [a_n - b_n]\}$ such that

$$\Sigma(b_n - a_n) < \delta \qquad \Rightarrow \ \Sigma|f(b_n) - f(a_n)| < \varepsilon$$

or $\Sigma|f(b_n) - f(a_n)| < \varepsilon$ \qquad $\dots(1)$

Since, $E \subseteq [a, b] \ \Rightarrow \ E \subseteq \bigcup_n I_n$

$\Rightarrow$ $f(E) \subseteq f(\cup I_n) = \cup f(I_n)$

$\Rightarrow$ $m^*(f(E)) \le \Sigma m^*(f(I_n)) \le \Sigma[\overline{f(x_n)} - \underline{f(x_n)}] < \varepsilon$

where $\overline{f(x_n)}$ and $\underline{f(x_n)}$ are the maximum and minimum values of $f(x)$ in the interval $[a, b]$

Also, $\Sigma|\overline{x_n} - \underline{x_n}| \le \Sigma(b_n - a_n) < \delta$

Hence, $m^*(f(E)) \le \varepsilon$

Letting $\varepsilon \to 0$ we get $m^*[f(E)] \le 0$

But we know that $m^*[f(E)] \geq 0$

$\Rightarrow \qquad\qquad m^*[f(E)] = 0$

Hence, $m[f(E)] = 0$.

EXAMPLE 9. *Show that if $f'(x)$ exists and is bounded on $[a, b]$ then f is of bounded variation on $[a, b]$.*

[KANPUR–2001; MEERUT–2006]

SOLUTION. It is given that $f'(x)$ exists and bounded so $\exists\ m > 0$ such that $|f'(x)| \leq m$ on $[a, b]$.

$\Rightarrow \qquad \left| \dfrac{f(x_i) - f(x_{i-1})}{x_i - x_{i-1}} \right| \leq m$

$\Rightarrow \qquad |f(x_i) - f(x_{i-1})| \leq m(x_i - x_{i-1})$

$\Rightarrow \qquad V_{ab}(f) \leq m\Sigma(x_i - x_{i-1}) = m(b - a)$, for any partition P of $[a, b]$.

Hence, $f \in BV[a, b]$.

EXAMPLE 10. *Give an example of the function which is continuous but not absolutely continuous.*

[MEERUT–2008; ROHTAK–2000, 01]

SOLUTION. Let us consider a function $f : C \to R$ where C is the Cantor's ternary set.

Let $x \in C$. Then by definition, we can write

$$x = 0 \cdot x_1 x_2 x_3 x_4 \ldots = \sum_{k=1}^{\infty} \frac{x_k}{3^k}, \qquad x_k = 0 \text{ or } 2$$

Define $f(x) = \sum_{k=1}^{\infty} \dfrac{r_k}{2^k}$, where $r_k = \dfrac{1}{2} x_k$

$$= 0 \cdot r_1 r_2 r_3 \ldots$$

We claim that $f(x)$ is continuous but not absolutely continuous.

Clearly this function is constant on each interval contained in the complement of the Cantor's ternary set. Also, it is a decreasing function. Firstly, we shall prove that $f(x)$ is a continuous function. Let $c', c'' \in C$.

Then, $\qquad c' = 0 \cdot (2p_1)(2p_2)(2p_3)\ldots$

$\qquad\qquad c'' = 0 \cdot (2q_1)(2q_2)(2q_3)\ldots$ where each $p_i, q_i = 0$ or 1

If $|c' - c''| < \dfrac{1}{3^n}$ then $p_i = q_i$ for $1 \leq i \leq n + 1$ and therefore,

$$|f(c') - f(c'')| < \frac{1}{2^n} \qquad\qquad \ldots(1)$$

which implies that $f(c') \to f(c'')$ as $c' \to c''$ and $n \to \infty$.

So, if $c_0 \in C$ and $<C_n>$ is a sequence in C' such that $c_n \to c_0$ when $n \to \infty$ then $f(c_n) \to f(c_0)$ when $n \to \infty$.

Let $x_0 \in [0, 1]$ and let $<x_n>$ be a sequence in $[0, 1]$ such that $x_n \to x_0$ as $n \to \infty$. Now, we have the following cases:

Case 1. Let $x_0 \notin C \quad \Rightarrow \quad x_0 \in I$, say $]a, b[\subset C'$

$\qquad\qquad\qquad\qquad \Rightarrow \quad x_n \in I$ and therefore $f(x_n) = f(x_0) = f(a)$

Thus, $f(x_n) \to f(x_0)$ as $n \to \infty$.

Case 2. Let $x_0 \in C$. Then for each n such that $x_n \in C'$, set $x_n = C_n$ and hence $f(x_n) \to f(x_0)$.

If $x_n \notin C$ then $\exists$ an open interval $I \supset C'$ such that

(i) If $x_n < x_0$ then the set C_n as the upper end point of I.

(ii) If $x_0 < x_n$ then set C_n as the lower end point of I.

In both the cases, $f(x_n) \to f(x_0)$ as $n \to \infty$.

Hence, f is a continuous function.

Now, we shall show $f(x)$ is not absolutely continuous.

Since, $f'(x) = 0$ at each $x \in C'$.

Therefore, $f'(x)$ exists and zero a.e. on $[0, 1]$ and is summable on $[0, 1]$. We know that for absolute continuity.

$$f(x) = \int_0^x f'(x)dx + f(0)$$

In particular, we must have

$$f(1) - f(0) = \int_0^1 f'(x)dx$$

But $\qquad f(1) - f(0) = 1$

and $\qquad \int_0^x f'(x)dx = 0$

$\Rightarrow \qquad f'(x) = 0$ a.e.

So, $\qquad f(1) - f(0) \neq \int_0^1 f'(x)dx$

Hence, $f(x)$ is not absolutely continuous.

Exercise 8.1

1. V, P, N denote total positive and negative variations of a bounded functions f on $[a, b]$, then show that $V = P + N$ and $P - N = f(b) - f(1)$. [MEERUT–2003BP; PUNJAB–2003; HIMACHAL–2001; GARHWAL–1995]

2. If f and g be the functions of bounded variations on $[a, b]$, then show that $f + g$, $f - g$, fg and f/g, $g(x) \neq 0$ and cf are function of bounded variations, $c \in R$.

3. Let f be a function of bounded variation, then show that $f(x)$ exists a.e. [MEERUT–1986]

4. Show that an absolutely continuous function is differentiable almost everywhere. [ROHTAK–2000]

5. Give an example which is continuous but not absolutely continuous. [MEERUT–1980; ROHTAK–2000, 01]

6. Show that if $F(x) = F(a) + \int_a^x f(t)dt$, then $F'(x) = f(x)$ a.e. [AMRAVATI–1997]

7. Show that the function f defined on $[0, 1]$ by

$$f(x) = \begin{cases} x\cos\left(\dfrac{\pi x}{2}\right); & \text{for } 0 < x \leq 1 \\ 0 & \text{for } x = 0 \end{cases}$$

is continuous but not of bounded variation on $[0, 1]$ [MEERUT–1994, 2005]

8. Show that the function f defined on $[0, 1]$ by $f(x) = x\sin\dfrac{1}{x}$ when $x \neq 0$ and $f(0) = 0$ is not of bounded variation. [KANPUR–2001]

9. If f is intergrable on $[a, b]$ and $\int_a^x f(t)dt = 0$ for all $x \in [a,b]$. Show that $f(t) = 0$ a.e. in $[a, b]$. (ROHTAK–1995; HIMACHAL–2000, 02, 04)

10. Show that an absolutely continuous function satisfy a Lipschitz condition of its derivative is bounded. [AMRAVATI–1997]

11. Show that the function f defined on $[0, 1]$ as $f(x) = x\sin\dfrac{\pi}{2}$ for $x > 0$ and $f(0) = 0$ is continuous but not is of bounded variation on $[0, 1]$. [GARHWAL–2000]

12. Show that every increasing function on $[a, b]$ is of bounded variation and every function of bounded variation on $[a, b]$ is almost everywhere differentiable on $[a, b]$. [AMRITSAR–1998]

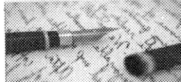

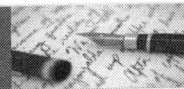

CHAPTER Summary

KEY TERMS

- **Absolutely Continuous Function:** A real valued function f defined on $[a, b]$ is said to be absolutely continuous on $[a, b]$ if for an arbitrary $\varepsilon > 0$ however small $\exists$ a $\delta > 0$ such that

  $$\sum_{r=1}^{n} |f(b_r) - f(a_r)| < \varepsilon \text{ whenever } \sum_{r=1}^{n} |b_r - a_r| < \delta$$

- **Function of Bounded Variation:** Let f be a real valued function defined on $[a, b]$ which is divided by means of point $a = x_0 < x_1 < x_2 < \dots < x_n = b$.

  If $V_{ab}[f, P] = \sum_{r=0}^{n-1} |f(x_{r+1}) - f(x_r)| < \infty$ then f is called the function of bounded variation for the partition P of $[a, b]$.

- **Lebesgue Point:** A point x is said to be a Lebesgue point of the function $f(t)$ if

  $$\lim_{h \to 0} \frac{1}{h} \int_x^{x+h} |f(t) - f(x)| \, dt = 0$$

- **Vitali's Cover of a Set:** A set E is said to covered in the sense of Vitali by a family of intervals M in which none is a singleton set, if every point of the set E is contained in small intervals of M.

- **Indefinite Integral:** Let $f(x)$ be L-integrable over $[a, b]$ then the function $F(x)$ defined by

  $$F(x) = \int_a^x f(t)dt + c \quad \forall x \in [a, b]$$

  is called indefinite integral of $f(x)$.

- **Convex Function:** A function f defined on an open interval $]a, b[$ is said to be a convex function if for all λ s.t. $0 \le \lambda \le 1$ and $x, y \in]a, b[$, i.e., $0 \le a < x < y < \infty$, we have

  $$f(\lambda x + (1 - \lambda)y) \le \lambda f(x) + (1 - \lambda)f(y)$$

RESULTS

- Every absolutely continuous function is continuous.
- A function f defined on $[a, b]$ is said to satisfy Lipschitz condition if there exists a function $M > 0$ such that $|f(x) - f(y)| \le M|x - y|$, $\forall x, y \in [a, b]$.
- A point x is said to be Lebesgue point of the function $f(t)$ if $\lim_{h \to 0} \frac{1}{h} \int_x^{x+h} |f(t) - f(x)| dt = 0$
- A monotonic function is of bounded variation.
- Every absolutely continuous function f defined on $[a, b]$ is of bounded variation.
- A function f is of bounded variation if and only if it can be expressed as a difference of two monotonic function both non-decreasing.
- Every absolutely continuous function is differentiable a.e.
- If f is a finite valued monotonic increasing function defined on $[a, b]$, then f is continuous

- on $[a, b]$ except almost a countable number of points.
- Every absolutely continuous functions $f(x)$ is an indefinite integral of its own derivative.
- If a function f is absolutely continuous in an interval $[a, b]$, and if $f'(x) = 0$, a.e. in $[a, b]$, then f is constant.
- If the derivative of two absolutely continuous function are equivalent then the functions differ by a constant.
- Every point of continuity of an integrable function $f(t)$ is a Lebesgue point of $f(t)$.
- A continuous function may not be of bounded variation.
- A function of bounded variation may not be continuous.
- Integration by parts in the Lebesgue integration is the same as in ordinary integration.

WORTHY READINGS

☞ Fundamental theorem of integral calculus states that integration and differentiation are reverse process of each other.

☞ Monotone function are always regarded as finite valued functions.

☞ The continuity of a function is not necessary for its property of bounded variation, since a monotone function need not be continuous. Also, continuity of a function is

also not sufficient in its property of bounded variation function.

☞ Since, a monotone function has atmost a countable set of discontinuities all of the first kind, it is true as well as function of bounded variation.

☞ A function of bounded variation is R-integrable but the converse is not true.

☞ If f is absolutely continuous then $f'(x)$ exists a.e.

☞ Every monotonic function is differentiable a.e.

☞ If $f(x)$ is absolutely continuous in an interval and $f(x) = 0$ a.e. then $f(x)$ is constant.

☞ If f is an absolutely continuous monotone function on $[a, b]$ and E is a set of measure zero then $f(E)$ has measure zero.

☞ If function f is Lipschitzian, then it is absolutely continuous.

☞ If $f'(x)$ exists and bounded on $[a, b]$ then $f \in BV[a, b]$.

☞ Monotone function can have only countable number of discontinuities and if f is continuous function on $]a, b[$ then f is a Convex function.

☞ Each Dini's derivative are monotonic and the two derivatives will be equal if one of them is continuous.

☞ A bounded function need not be of bounded variation.

☞ An absolutely continuous function satisfies Lipschitz condition if its derivative is bounded.

⮛ FURTHER READINGS

☞ If f is a differentiable function on an interval I then f' is measurable on I.

☞ If f is a function of bounded variation on $[a, b]$ then f' exists a.e. on $[a, b]$.

☞ If f is a function of bounded variation then it is measurable.

☞ A step function defined on $[a, b]$ is of bounded variation on $[a, b]$.

☞ The set of points of discontinuity of a function of bounded variation is countable.

☞ Every absolutely continuous function is uniformly continuous but converse is not necessarily true. For ex. the Cantor's function is uniformly continuous in $[0, 1]$ but not absolutely continuous.

☞ Any monotonic increasing function is the sum of an absolutely continuous function and a singular function.

☞ The class of absolutely continuous function over $[a, b]$ is identical with the class of functions obtained by integrating Lebesgue integrable functions over $[a, b]$, except that the corresponding functions in two classes differ at the most by a constant.

☞ $BV[a, b]$ is a vector space over the set of real numbers.

☞ If f is a non-negative integrable functions then its indefinite integral is a finite measure on the class of all measurable sets.

☐☐☐

Chapter

9 The Lebesgue L^P-spaces

9.1 INTRODUCTION

The L^p-spaces have many important and remarkable properties which are widely used in Analysis. The concept of L^p-spaces based on the norm. In this chapter we shall discuss the L^p-spaces followed by many important inequalities.

9.2 CONCEPT OF NORMS

Let L be a linear space over the field of reals or complex. Then a real valued function $\|\cdot\| : L \to L$ is said to be norm, if following conditions are satisfied:

(1) $\|x\| \geq 0 \; \forall \; x \in L$

and $\|x\| = 0$ if and only if $x = 0 \; \forall \; x \in L$

(2) $\|x + y\| \leq \|x\| + \|y\| \; \forall \; x, y \in L$

(3) $\|\alpha x\| = |\alpha| \cdot \|x\| \; \forall \; x \in L, \alpha \in R$ or C

9.3 L^P-SPACE

Let $f(x)$ be a function. Then the class of all measurable functions $f(x)$ is defined as L^p-space over $[a, b]$ if f is Lebesgue integrable over $[a, b]$ for each p, $0 < p < \infty$, i.e.,

$$\int_a^b |f|^p \, dx < \infty \quad (p > 0)$$

It is denoted by $L^p[a, b]$.

ALTERNATIVE DEFINITION

By $L^p[a, b]$ we mean a class of function $f(x)$ such that

(i) $f(x)$ is measurable over $[a, b]$.

(ii) $|f|^p$ is L-integrable over $[a, b]$ for $p > 0$

i.e., $\int_a^b |f|^p \, dx < \infty$, for $p > 0$.

☞ REMARKS

• Sometimes, we denote the class of such functions by the symbol L^p when mention of interval is not necessary.

• L or L^1 denote the class of measurable of measurable function $f(x)$ which are also L-integrable.

9.3.1 SOME RELATED DEFINITIONS

(1) **Conjugate Numbers:** Two non-negative extended real numbers p and q are said to be conjugate to each other if $\dfrac{1}{p} + \dfrac{1}{q} = 1$.

☞ REMARKS
- $p \geq 1, q \geq 1$
- 2 is a self conjugate number.
- If $p \neq 2$ then $q \neq 2$
- 1 and ∞ are conjugate numbers.

(2) **Norm of an Element of L^P-space:** Let $f(x) \in L^p[a, b]$ be arbitrary. Then norm of $f(x)$, denoted by $\|f\|_p$ is defined as follows:

$$\|f\|_p = \left(\int_a^b |f|^p \ dx\right)^{1/p}$$

In particular, if $p = 1$ then $\|f\|_1 = \|f\| = \int_a^b |f| \ dx$

(3) **Metric or Distance Function:** Let $f(x), g(x) \in L^p[a, b]$. Then metric or distance function $d(f, g)$ is defined as follows:

$$d[f, g] = \|f - g\|_p$$

Here, $d(f, g)$ denote the distance between the functions f and g.

(4) **Convergent sequence:** Let $<f_n>$ be a sequence of function in $L^p[a, b]$. Then $<f_n>$ is said to converge in mean with index p, if for given $\varepsilon > 0 \ \exists \ n_0 \in N$ such that

$$\|f_n(x) - f(x)\|_p < \varepsilon \ \forall \ n \geq n_0$$

or $\qquad \int_a^b |f_n(x) - f(x)|^p \ dx \to 0 \text{ as } n \to \infty.$

(5) **Cauchy Sequence:** Let $<f_n>$ be a sequence of functions belonging to $L^p[a, b]$. Then $<f_n>$ is said to be fundamental sequence or Cauchy sequence if for given $\varepsilon > 0 \ \exists \ n_0 \in N$ such that $m, n \geq n_0$.

$$\|f_m - fn\|_p < \varepsilon$$

☞ REMARKS
- Every convergent sequence is Cauchy.
- An L^P-space is said to be complete if every Cauchy's sequence is convergent.
- A complete normed linear space is called Banach space.

THEOREM 1.

If $f \in L^P[a, b]$ and $g \leq f$ then $g \in L^P[a, b]$.

PROOF. Let $f \in L^P[a, b]$. Then by definition, f is measurable and $\int |f|^p < \infty$.

Let a be any poitive real number. Then

$$\{x \in [a,b] : g(x) > \alpha\} = \{x \in [a,b] : \alpha < g(x) \leq f(x)\} \qquad [\because g \leq f]$$
$$= \{x \in [a,b] : f(x) > \alpha\}$$

Also, $f \in L^P[a, b]$
⇒ f is measurable over $[a, b]$.
⇒ $\{x \in [a, b] : f(x) \leq \alpha\}$ is a measurable set.
⇒ $\{x \in [a, b] : g(x) \leq \alpha\}$ is a measurable set. $\qquad [\because g \leq f]$
⇒ g is a measurable function on $[a, b]$.
Also, since $g(x) \leq f(x) \ \forall \ x \in [a, b]$

⇒ $\int_a^b |g|^p \ dx \leq \int_a^b |f|^p \ dx < \infty \qquad [\because \int_a^b |f|^p \ dx \in L^P[a,b]]$

⇒ $\int_a^b |g|^p \ dx < \infty$

Therefore, we conclude that g is measurable function over $[a, b]$ such that
$$|g|^P \in L[a, b]$$
Hence, $g \in L^P[a, b]$.

THEOREM 2.

If $f \in L^P[a, b]$, $p > 1$ then $f \in L[a, b]$.

PROOF.   It is given that $f \in L^P[a, b]$, $p > 1$

We shall prove that $f \in L[a, b]$. Here, it is sufficient to prove that

(i) f is measurable over $[a, b]$

(ii) $|f|$ is integrable over $[a, b]$

Since, $f \in L^P[a, b]$, therefore f is measurable and $|f|^P$ is integrable over $[a, b]$.

Let $E = [a, b]$.

Define two sets A and B such that

$$A = \{x \in [a, b] : |f(x)| \geq 1\}$$

and $\qquad B = \{x \in [a, b] : |f(x)| < 1\}$

Then $E = A \cup B$ and $A \cap B = \phi$.

Then by countable additive property of integrals, we can write

$$\int_a^b |f| \, dx = \int_A |f| \, dx + \int_B |f| \, dx \qquad \qquad ...(1)$$

Since, $f(x) \geq 1 \ \forall \ x \in A$ therefore $|f| \leq |f|^P$ on A.

Further, since $p > 1$, therefore, $\int_A |f| \, dx \leq \int_A |f| \, dx < \infty$ $\qquad ...(2)$

Now, $\qquad \qquad f(x) < 1 \ \forall \ x \in B$

Then by first mean value theorem we can write

$$\int_B |f| \, dx < m(B) = \text{a finite quantity} < \infty \qquad \qquad ...(3)$$

Now, from (1), (2) and (3) we conclude that

$$\int_a^b |f| \, dx < \infty$$

Therefore, f is measurable over [a, b] and $\int_a^b |f| \, dx < \infty$.

Hence, $f \in L[a, b]$.

THEOREM 3.

If $f, g \in L^P[a, b]$ then $(f + g) \in L^P[a, b]$.

[MEERUT–2004, 06, 07, 08, 10, 16, 17; GARHWAL–2007, 11; KANPUR–2006]

PROOF.   Let $f \in L^P[a, b]$ and $g \in L^P[a, b]$. We have to prove that $f + g \in L^P[a, b]$.

Since, $f, g \in L^P[a, b]$, so by definition,

$\qquad \qquad f$ and g both are measurable over $[a, b]$

$\Rightarrow \qquad \qquad (f + g)$ is measurable over $[a, b]$.

$\qquad \qquad \qquad$ [$\because$ Sum of two measurable functions is again measurable]

Now, it remains to prove that

$$\int_a^b |f + g|^P \, dx < \infty$$

Define two sets A and B such that

$$A = \{x \in [a, b] : |f(x)| \geq |g(x)|\}$$

and $\qquad \qquad B = \{x \in [a, b] : |f(x)| < |g(x)|\}$

Then clearly $A \cup B = [a, b]$ and $A \cap B = \phi$

Then by countable additive property of integrals, we have

$$\int_a^b |f + g|^P \, dx = \int_A |f + g|^P \, dx + \int_B |f + g|^P \, dx \qquad ...(1)$$

Now, $\qquad \qquad |f + g|^P \leq (|f| + |g|)^P$

$$\leq [|g| + |g|]^P \text{ on } B \text{ and } \leq (|f| + |f|)^P \text{ on } A$$

$$\leq 2^p |g|^p \text{ on } B \text{ and } \leq 2^p |f|^p \text{ on } A.$$

Therefore, $\int_A |f+g|^p \, dx \leq 2^p \int_A |f|^p$ ...(2)

and $\qquad \int_B |f+g|^p \, dx \leq 2^p \int_B |g|^p$ ...(3)

Now, since $f, g \in L^p[a, b]$, therefore, by definition

$$\int_A |f|^p \, dx < \infty \text{ and } \int_B |g|^p \, dx < \infty$$

$$2^p \int_A |f|^p \, dx < \infty \text{ and } 2^p \int_B |g|^p \, dx < \infty$$

Using these results in (2) and (3), we get

$$\int_A |f+g|^p \, dx < \infty \text{ and } \int_B |f+g|^p \, dx < \infty \qquad \text{...(4)}$$

Finally using (4) in (1) we get

$$\int_a^b |f+g|^p \, dx < \infty$$

Hence, $(f+g) \in L^p[a,b]$.

AN IMPORTANT LEMMA

Let A and B are any two non-negative real numbers and $0 < \lambda < 1$ then $A^\lambda B^{1-\lambda} \leq \lambda A + (1-\lambda)B$ with equally when $A = B$.

PROOF. In case of $A = 0$ or $B = 0$, result is trivially true. So, assume that $A > 0$ and $B > 0$. Let us define a function

$$g(x) = x^\lambda - \lambda x, \; 0 \leq x < \infty \text{ and } 0 < \lambda < 1$$

which implies

$$\frac{dg}{dx} = \lambda x^{\lambda-1} \text{ and } \frac{d^2 g}{dx^2} = \lambda(\lambda-1)x^{\lambda-2}$$

Now, $\dfrac{dg}{dx} = 0 \Rightarrow x = 1$

At $x = 1, \dfrac{d^2 g}{dx^2} < 0$ as $0 < \lambda < 1$

Therefore, by the principle of maxima and minima, we can say that
$g(x)$ is maximum at $x = 1 \Rightarrow g(1)$ is maximum.

$\Rightarrow \qquad\qquad g(x) \leq g(1)$

$\Rightarrow \qquad\qquad x^\lambda - \lambda x \leq 1^\lambda - \lambda = 1 - \lambda$ ...(1)

Let us put $x = \dfrac{A}{B}$ in (1) we get

$$\left(\frac{A}{B}\right)^\lambda - \lambda\left(\frac{A}{B}\right) \leq 1 - \lambda$$

$\Rightarrow \qquad A^\lambda B^{-\lambda} - \lambda\left(\dfrac{A}{B}\right) \leq 1 - \lambda$

$\Rightarrow \qquad A^\lambda B^{1-\lambda} - \lambda A \leq (1-\lambda)B$

Hence, $\qquad A^\lambda B^{1-\lambda} \leq \lambda A + (1-\lambda)B$

DEDUCTION. **(Young's Inequality)**

If $\lambda = \dfrac{1}{p}$ then $1 - \lambda = \dfrac{1}{q}$

So, we get $A^{1/p} \cdot B^{1/q} \leq \dfrac{a^p}{p} + \dfrac{b^q}{q}$

Setting $A^{1/p} = a$, $B^{1/q} = b$ then

We get $\qquad ab \leq \dfrac{a^p}{p} + \dfrac{b^q}{q}$

THEOREM 4. (Riesz-Holder's Inequality)

Let p and q be non-negative extended real numbers such that $\dfrac{1}{p} + \dfrac{1}{q} = 1$. If $f \in L^P[a, b]$ and $g \in L^q[a, b]$.

then

(i) $f \cdot g \in L[a, b]$

(ii) $\|fg\| \leq \|f\|_p \cdot \|g\|_q$, i.e., $\int |f + g| \leq (\int |f|^p)^{1/p} (\int |g|^q)^{1/q}$

equality holds if and only if for some non-zero constants α and β we have

$$\alpha |f|^p = \beta |g|^q \ a.e.$$

[MEERUT–2009, 10, 11, 14, 16, 17; KANPUR–2003, 04, 07, 08 ,09; AVADH–2008; GARHWAL–2007]

PROOF. Let p and q be non-negative extended real numbers such that $\dfrac{1}{p} + \dfrac{1}{q} = 1$. If $p = 1$

then $q = \infty$. In this case, result is obvious.

So, let us assume that $1 < p < \infty$ and $1 < q < \infty$.

Set $\lambda = \dfrac{1}{p}, p > 1$ implies $\lambda > 1$.

$\Rightarrow \qquad \dfrac{1}{q} = 1 - \lambda \qquad\qquad (\because p$ and q are conjugate nos., i.e., $\dfrac{1}{p} + \dfrac{1}{q} = 1)$

Using previous lemma, we can write

$$A^{1/p} B^{1/q} \leq \dfrac{A}{p} + \dfrac{B}{q} \qquad\qquad ...(1)$$

If one of the function $f(x)$ and $g(x)$ is zero almost everywhere, then result is trivially true. Further, assume that $f \neq 0$, $g \neq 0$ a.e.

$\therefore \qquad \int_a^b |f|^p \, dx > 0$ and $\int_a^b |g|^q \, dx > 0$

$\Rightarrow \qquad \|f\|_p > 0$ and $\|g\|_p > 0$

Write $\qquad F(x) = \dfrac{f(x)}{\|f\|_p}, \ G(x) = \dfrac{g(x)}{\|g\|_q} \qquad\qquad ...(2)$

and $\qquad A^{1/p} = |F(x)|, B^{1/q} = |G(x)|$

Putting all these values in (1) we get

$$|F(x) \cdot G(x)| \leq \dfrac{|F(x)|^p}{p} + \dfrac{|G(x)|^q}{q}$$

$$\Rightarrow \quad \int_a^b |F(x) \cdot G(x)| \, dx \le \frac{1}{p} \int_a^b |F(x)|^p \, dx + \frac{1}{q} \int_a^b |G(x)|^q \, dx$$

$$= \frac{1}{p} \int_a^b \frac{|f(x)|^p}{\int_a^b |f|^p \, dx} \, dx + \int_a^b \frac{|g(x)|^q}{\int_a^b |g|^q \, dx} \, dx$$

$$= \frac{1}{p} \frac{\int_a^b |f|^p \, dx}{\int_a^b |f|^p \, dx} + \frac{1}{q} \frac{\int_a^b |g|^q \, dx}{\int_a^b |g|^q \, dx}$$

$$= \frac{1}{p} + \frac{1}{q} = 1 \qquad \qquad (\because p \text{ and } q \text{ are conjugate numbers})$$

$$\Rightarrow \quad \int_a^b |F(x) \cdot G(x)| \, dx \le 1 \qquad \qquad \dots(3)$$

Now, using (2) in (3) we get

$$\frac{\int_a^b |f(x)g(x)| \, dx}{\|f\|_p \cdot \|g\|_q} \le 1$$

$$\Rightarrow \quad \int_a^b |f(x)g(x)| \, dx \le \|f\|_p \cdot \|g\|_q$$

$$\Rightarrow \quad \|fg\| \le \|f\|_p \cdot \|g\|_q \qquad \qquad \dots(4)$$

Further $f \in L^p[a, b]$, $g \in L^q[a, b] \Rightarrow f$ and g both are integrable.

$$\Rightarrow \quad \int_a^b |f|^p \, dx < \infty \text{ and } \int_a^b |g|^q \, dx < \infty$$

$$\Rightarrow \quad \|f\|_p < \infty \text{ and } \|g\|_q < \infty$$

Using these results in (4) we get

$$\|fg\| < \infty$$

Hence $fg \in L[a, b]$.

CASE OF EQUALITY :

The equality holds when $A = B$, *i.e.*, if $\qquad |F(x)|^p = |G(x)|^q$ a.e.

i.e., if $\qquad \dfrac{|f|^p}{\|f\|_p^p} = \dfrac{|g|^q}{\|g\|_q^q}$ a.e.

i.e., if $\qquad \|g\|_q^q \, |f|^p = \|f\|_p^p \, |g|^q$ a.e.

i.e., if we have found some non-zero constants α, β such that
$$\alpha |f|^p = \beta |g|^q$$

THEOREM 5. (Cauchy-Schwarz's Inequality)

If f and g are square integrable functions then $fg \in L[a, b]$ and

$$\|fg\| \le \|f\|_2 \|g\|_2 \qquad \qquad \text{[MEERUT–2001, 09, 12; GARHWAL–2003, 07]}$$

PROOF.   Let f and g be square integrable function, *i.e.*, $f, g \in L^2[a, b]$.

We have to prove that $fg \in L[a, b]$ and $\|fg\| \le \|f\|_2 \cdot \|g\|_2$

Let $x \in [a, b]$ be arbitrary, then by definition

$$[f(x) - g(x)]^2 \geq 0$$

$$\Rightarrow \quad 2|f(x)| \cdot |g(x)| \leq |f(x)|^2 + |g(x)|^2$$

$$\Rightarrow \quad 2\int_a^b |f(x)| \cdot |g(x)| \, dx \leq \int_a^b |f(x)|^2 \, dx + \int_a^b |g(x)|^2 \, dx \qquad \ldots(1)$$

Since $f, g \in L^2[a, b]$

$$\Rightarrow \quad f \text{ and } g \text{ are measurable and integrable over } [a, b].$$

$$\Rightarrow \quad \int_a^b |f(x)|^2 \, dx < \infty \text{ and } \int_a^b |g(x)|^2 \, dx < \infty \qquad \ldots(2)$$

Using (2) in (1) we get

$$\int_a^b |f(x) \cdot g(x)| \, dx < \infty$$

Also, f, g are measurable $\Rightarrow$ $f \cdot g$ is also measurable.

$$\Rightarrow \quad fg \in L[a, b]$$

Further, let $\alpha \in R$, then

$$(\alpha|f| + |g|)^2 \geq 0$$

$$\Rightarrow \quad \int_a^b (\alpha|f| + |g|)^2 \geq 0$$

$$\Rightarrow \quad \alpha^2 \int_a^b |f|^2 \, dx + 2\alpha \int_a^b |fg| \, dx + \int_a^b |g|^2 \, dx \geq 0 \qquad \ldots(3)$$

For the sake of convenience, let us write

$$A = \int_a^b |f|^2 \, dx, B = \int_a^b |fg| \, dx \text{ and } C = \int_a^b |g|^2 \, dx$$

Then (3) reduces to

$$(\alpha^2 \cdot A) + \alpha B + C = 0 \qquad \ldots(4)$$

If $A = 0$, then $f(x) = 0$ a.e. and therefore, $B = 0$. Then required inequality is trivally true.

Now, let $A \neq 0$, write $\alpha = -\dfrac{B}{2A}$

Then from (4)

$$A\left(-\frac{B}{2A}\right)^2 + B\left(-\frac{B}{2A}\right) + C \geq 0$$

$$\Rightarrow \quad 4AC - B^2 \geq 0$$

$$\Rightarrow \quad B^2 \leq 4AC$$

Finally, putting the values of A, B and C in the above equation, we get

$$4\left[\int_a^b |fg| \, dx\right]^2 \leq 4\left[\int_a^b |f|^2\right]\left[\int_a^b |g|^2\right]$$

$$\Rightarrow \quad \int_a^b |f(x)g(x)| \, dx \leq \left(\int_a^b |f(x)|^2\right)^{1/2} + \left(\int_a^b |g(x)|^2\right)^{1/2}$$

$$\Rightarrow \quad \|fg\| \leq \|f\|_2 \cdot \|g\|_2$$

DEDUCTION. From above inequality we can easily deduce that

$$\left|\int_a^b fg\right| \leq \left(\int_a^b f^2 dx\right)^{1/2} \left(\int_a^b g^2 dx\right)^{1/2}$$

THEOREM 6. (Riesz-Minkowski's Inequality)

Let $f, g \in L^P[a, b]$, $1 \leq p \leq \infty$ then $(f + g) \in L^P[a, b]$ and

$$\|f + g\|_p \leq \|f\|_p + \|g\|_p.$$

[MEERUT–2005, 06, 10, 11, 12, 15, 17; GARHWAL–2001, 02, 03, 15,16, 18; NAGPUR–2006, 08; POONA–2010; HPU–2000, 01, 03, 04, 16]

PROOF. **Case 1.** If $p = 1$, then result is obvious.

Case 2. If $p = \infty$ then

$$|f| \leq \|f\|_\infty \text{ a.e. and } |g| \leq \|g\|_\infty \text{ a.e.}$$

$$\Rightarrow \quad |f + g| \leq |f| + |g| \leq \|f\|_\infty + \|g\|_\infty$$

$$\Rightarrow \quad \text{Result holds for } f = \infty.$$

Case 3. If $f = 0$ or $g = 0$ then result is obvious.

Case 4. If $1 < p < \infty$ and $f \neq 0, g \neq 0$

We have already proved that $f, g \in L^p[a, b] \Rightarrow f + g \in L^p[a, b]$

Now, since $\dfrac{1}{p} + \dfrac{1}{q} = 1 \Rightarrow (p-1)q = p$

$\therefore \quad \int (|f + g|^{p-1})^q = \int |f + g|^p$

$\Rightarrow \quad |f + g|^{p-1} \in L^q[a, b] \qquad\qquad (\because f + g \in L^p[a, b])$

$\Rightarrow \quad (f + g)^{p/q} \in L^q[a, b]$

Now apply Holder's inequality for f and $(f + g)^{p/q}$, we get

$$\int_a^b |f| \cdot |f + g|^{p/q}\, dx \leq \left(\int_a^b |f|^p\, dx \right)^{1/p} \left(\int_a^b |f + g|^{\left(\frac{p}{q}\right) \cdot q}\, dx \right)^{1/q} \qquad \ldots(1)$$

On interchanging f and g in (1) we get

$$\int_a^b |g| \cdot |f + g|^{p/q}\, dx \leq \left(\int_a^b |g|^p\, dx \right)^{1/p} \left(\int_a^b |f + g|^p\, dx \right)^{1/q} \qquad \ldots(2)$$

Adding (1) and (2) we get

$$\int_a^b |f| \cdot |f + g|^{p/q}\, dx + \int_a^b |g| \cdot |f + g|^{p/q}\, dx$$

$$\leq \left[\int_a^b |f|^p\, dx + \int_a^b |g|^p\, dx \right] \left[\int_a^b |f + g|^p\, dx \right]^{1/q} \qquad \ldots(3)$$

But since p and q are conjugate numbers, therefore

$$\dfrac{1}{p} + \dfrac{1}{q} = 1 \Rightarrow 1 + \dfrac{p}{q} = p$$

Therefore, $|f + g|^p = |f + g| \cdot |f + g|^{p/q} \leq (|f| + |g|) \cdot |f + g|^{p/q}$

$\Rightarrow \quad |f + g|^p \leq |f| \cdot |f + g|^{p/q} + |g| \cdot |f + g|^{p/q}$

On integrating we get

$$\int_a^b |f + g|^p\, dx \leq \int_a^b |f| \cdot |f + g|^{p/q}\, dx + \int_a^b |g| \cdot |f + g|^{p/q}\, dx \qquad \ldots(4)$$

Using (3) in (4) we get

$$\int_a^b |f + g|^p\, dx \leq \left[\left(\int_a^b |f|^p\, dx \right)^{1/p} + \left(\int_a^b |g|^p\, dx \right)^{1/p} \right] \left[\int_a^b |f + g|^p\, dx \right]^{1/q}$$

$$\Rightarrow \left(\int_a^b |f + g|^p\, dx \right)^{1 - \frac{1}{q}} \leq \left(\int_a^b |f|^p\, dx \right)^{1/p} + \left(\int_a^b |g|^p\, dx \right)^{1/p}$$

$$\Rightarrow \left(\int_a^b |f + g|^p\, dx \right)^{1/p} \leq \left(\int_a^b |f|^p\, dx \right)^{1/p} + \left(\int_a^b |g|^p\, dx \right)^{1/p} \qquad \ldots(6)$$

$$\left(\because \dfrac{1}{p} + \dfrac{1}{q} = 1 \Rightarrow 1 - \dfrac{1}{q} = \dfrac{1}{p} \right)$$

Hence, $\|f + g\|_p \leq \|f\|_p + \|g\|_p$

THEOREM 7.

If f and g are square integrable in the Lebesgue sense, then $f + g$ is also square integrable in the Lebesgue sense and $\left\| f + g \right\|_2 \leq \left\| f \right\|_2 + \left\| g \right\|_2$ [MEERUT–2004, 09]

PROOF. Let f and g be Lebesgue square integrable functions. Firstly we shall prove that $(f + g)$ is also Lebesgue square integrable.

Now $f, g \in L^2[a, b]$ $\Rightarrow$ f, g are measurable over $[a, b]$.

$\Rightarrow$ $f + g$ are measurable over $[a, b]$.

Also $f, g \in L^2[a, b]$ $\Rightarrow$ f, g are square integrable over $[a, b]$.

$\Rightarrow$ $f + g$ is square integrable over $[a, b]$.

Therefore, $(f + g) \in L^2[a, b]$

Now, it remains to prove that $\left\| f + g \right\|_2 \leq \left\| f \right\|_2 + \left\| g \right\|_2$

Consider $|f + g|^2 \leq [\, |f| + |g|\,]^2 = |f|^2 + |g|^2 + 2|f| \cdot |g|$

$$= |f|^2 + |g|^2 + 2|fg|$$

Therefore, $\int_a^b |f + g|^2 \leq \int_a^b |f|^2 + \int_a^b |g|^2 + 2\int_a^b |fg|$

Using Schwarz's inequality, we have

$$\int_a^b |f + g|^2 \leq \int_a^b |f|^2 + \int_a^b |g|^2 + 2\left[\int_a^b |f|^2\right]^{1/2}\left[\int_a^b |g|^2\right]^{1/2}$$

$$= \left[\left(\int_a^b |f|^2\right)^{1/2} + \left(\int_a^b |g|^2\right)^{1/2}\right]^2$$

On taking positive square root, we get

$$\left[\int_a^b |f + g|^2\right]^{1/2} = \left[\int_a^b |f|^2\right]^{1/2} + \left[\int_a^b |g|^2\right]^{1/2}$$

Hence, $\left\| f + g \right\|_2 \leq \left\| f \right\|_2 + \left\| g \right\|_2$

THEOREM 8.

If $1 < p < \infty$ then equality of Minkowski's inequality can be true iff there are non-negative constants α and β such that

$$\beta f = \alpha g$$ [HPU–2003, 07; DELHI–2011]

PROOF. Minkowski's inequality is given by

$$\left\| f + g \right\|_p \leq \left\| f \right\|_p + \left\| g \right\|_p$$

Let us first suppose $\beta f = \alpha g$, i.e., $g = \left(\dfrac{\beta}{\alpha}\right) f$

$$\text{LHS} = \left\| f + g \right\|_p = \left(\int_a^b \left| f + \frac{\beta}{\alpha} f \right|^p\right)^{1/p}$$

$$= \left[\left(1 + \frac{\beta}{\alpha}\right)^p\right]^{1/p} \left[\int_a^b |f|^p\right]^{1/p} = \left(1 + \frac{\beta}{\alpha}\right)\left\| f \right\|_p$$

$$\text{RHS} = \left(\int_a^b |f|^p\right)^{1/p} + \left(\int_a^b \left|\frac{\beta}{\alpha} f\right|^p\right)^{1/p} = \left(1 + \frac{\beta}{\alpha}\right)\left(\int_a^b |f|^p\right)^{1/p}$$

$$= \left(1 + \frac{\beta}{\alpha}\right)\left\| f \right\|_p = \text{LHS}$$

Hence, in this case

$$\|f+g\|_p = \|f\|_p + \|g\|_p$$

Conversely, suppose that equality holds.

Clearly the equality holds in inequality

$$\left(\int_a^b |f+g|^p \, dx\right)^{1/p} \le \left(\int_a^b |f|^p \, dx\right)^{1/p} + \left(\int_a^b |g|^p \, dx\right)^{1/p}$$

only if there exists numbers, α, β, γ such that

$$\alpha |f|^p = \gamma |f+g|^p = \beta |g|^p \text{ a.e.}$$

$\Rightarrow$ only if there exists non-negative constants α, $\beta \ge 0$ such that $\beta f = \alpha g$.

☞ **REMARK**

• If $p = 1$, the equality will hold iff $fg = 0$ a.e.

THEOREM 9. (Riesz-Holder's Inequality for $0 < p < 1$)

If $0 < p < 1$ and p and q are conjugate numbers. If $f \in L^P$ and $g \in L^q$ then

$$\int |fg| \ge \|f\|_p \cdot \|g\|_q , \text{ provided } \int |g|^q \ne 0.$$

PROOF. Let p and q are conjugate numbers. Therefore, $\dfrac{1}{p}+\dfrac{1}{q}=1$

$\Rightarrow$
$$\frac{1}{q}=1-\frac{1}{p}$$

$\Rightarrow$
$$\frac{-p}{q}=1-p, i.e., p+\left(-\frac{p}{q}\right)=1$$

Let us write $p=\dfrac{1}{P}$ and $\dfrac{-p}{q}=\dfrac{1}{Q}$ then $\dfrac{1}{P}+\dfrac{1}{Q}=1$

Also, since $0 < p < 1$

$\Rightarrow \quad 0<\dfrac{1}{P}<1 \qquad \Rightarrow \quad P>1, \text{ i.e., } 1<P<\infty$

and $\dfrac{1}{Q}=\dfrac{-p}{q}=1-p \quad \Rightarrow \quad 0<\dfrac{1}{Q}<1 \text{ becomes } 0<p<1$

$$\Rightarrow \quad Q>1$$

Thus, we can say that P and Q are conjugate numbers such that $1 < P < \infty$.

Let us take $|fg| = F^p$ and $|g|^q = G^Q$

Then $FG = |fg|^{1/p}, |g|^{q/Q} = |f|^p \cdot |g|^{\frac{1}{P}+\left(\frac{q}{Q}\right)\left(\frac{-p}{q}\right)}= |f|^p$ $\qquad \left[\because \dfrac{-p}{q}=\dfrac{1}{Q}\right]$

which shows that F and G are non-negative measurable functions such that $F \in L^P$ and $G \in L^q$

Then by Holder's inequality for P, Q to the functions F and G, we get

$$\int |FG| \le \|F\|_P \cdot \|G\|_Q$$

Therefore, $\qquad \int |f|^p \le \left(\int |F|^P\right)^{1/p} \left(\int |G|^Q\right)^{1/Q}$ $\qquad (\because |FG| = FG = |f|^p)$

$\Rightarrow \qquad \int |f|^p \le \left(\int |fg|^p\right)\left(\int |g|^q\right)^{-p/q}$

$$\Rightarrow \qquad \left(\int |f|^p\right)^{1/p} \le \left(\int |fg|\right)\left(\int |g|^q\right)^{-1/q}$$

$$\Rightarrow \qquad \left(\int |f|^p\right)^{1/p} \le \frac{\int |fg|}{\left(\int |g|^q\right)^{1/q}}, \text{ provided } \int |g|^q \ne 0$$

Hence, $\qquad \int |f+g| \ge \left(\int |f|^p\right)^{1/p}\left(|g|^q\right)^{1/q} \ge \|f\|_p \cdot \|g\|_q$

$$\Rightarrow \qquad \int |f+g| \ge \|f\|_p \cdot \|g\|_q$$

☞ **REMARK**

• The above inequality (for $0 < p < 1$) is reversed than that of the case for $1 \le p < \infty$.

THEOREM 10. (Minkowski Inequality for $0 < p < 1$)

If $0 < p < 1$ and f, g are non-negative functions in L^p, then

$$\|f+g\|_p \ge \|f\|_p + \|g\|_p$$

PROOF. Let f and g be two non-negative functions in L^P then proceed as in main Minkowski inequality, we have

$$f \in L^P, (f+q)^{p/q} \in L^q$$

Now, apply the Holder's inequality for $0 < p < 1$ for the function $f \in L^P$ and $[f+g]^{p/q} \in L^q$, we get

$$\int |f| \cdot |f+g|^{p/q} \ge \left(\int |f|^p\right)^{1/p} \cdot \left(\int |f+g|^p\right)^{1/q} \qquad \qquad ...(1)$$

Similarly, for the function $g \in L^P$ and $(f+g)^{p/q} \in L^q$, apply Holder's inequality we get

$$\int |g| \cdot |f+g|^{p/q} \ge \left(\int |g|^p \, dx\right)^{1/P}\left(|f+g|^p\right)^{1/q} \qquad \qquad ...(2)$$

On adding (1) and (2) we get

$$\int |f+g|^{p/q}(|f|+|g|) \ge [\{\int |f|^p\}^{1/p} + \{\int |g|^p\}^{1/p}] \times [\int |f+g|^p]^{1/q} \qquad ...(3)$$

Since $\dfrac{1}{p}+\dfrac{1}{q} = 1 \Rightarrow 1+\dfrac{p}{q} = p$

Therefore, $\qquad |f+g|^p = |f+g|^{1+\frac{p}{q}} = |f+g| |f+g|^{\frac{p}{q}}$

$$= (|f|+|g|) \cdot |f+g|^{p/q} \qquad \qquad (\because f \ge 0, g \ge 0)$$

So, $\qquad \int |f+g|^p \ge [\{\int |f|^p\}^{1/p} + \{\int |g|^p\}^{1/p}](\int |f+g|^p)^{1/q}$

Dividing both sides by $(\int |f+g|^p)^{1/q}$, we get

$$(\int |f+g|^p)^{1-\frac{1}{q}} \ge [\|f\|_p + \|g\|_p]$$

$$\Rightarrow \qquad (\int |f+g|^p)^{1/p} \ge \|f\|_p + \|g\|_p$$

Hence, $\qquad \|f+g\|_p \ge \|f\|_p + \|g\|_p$

☛ **REMARK**
* The above inequality (for $0 < p < 1$) is reversed than that of the case for $p > 1$.

9.4 L^P-SPACE FOR $p = \infty$

Before defining the L^∞-space, let us introduce the following definitions:

(i) **Essential Bound:** A non-negative real number m is said to be essential bound for the real valued measurable function f defined on $E = [a, b]$ such that $m(E) > 0$ if
$$|f(x)| \le m \text{ a.e. on } E.$$

(ii) **Essentially Bounded Function:** A function f is said to be essentially bounded if there exists an essential bound for it, *i.e.*, function f is bounded on E a.e. (f is bounded on E except on a set of measure zero).

(iii) **Essential Supremum:** Let f be a function then greatest lower bound (g.l.b.) of the function f on E is called essential supremum of f on E and is denoted by ess. sup $|f(x)|$. Therefore, ess. $\sup|f(x)| = \inf.\{M : |f(x)| \le M \text{ a.e. on } E\}$
$$= \inf. \{M : m[x \in E : |f(x)| > M] = 0\}$$
$$= \sup.\{M : m[x \in E : (f(x) \ge M \ne 0)]\}$$

☛ **REMARK**
* $|f(x)| \le$ ess. $\sup|f(x)|$

(iv) **$L^\infty(E)$ space:** The class of all the essential bounded measurable functions defined on E is defined as $L^\infty(E)$ space. Therefore, $L^\infty(E) = \{f : \text{ess. sup } |f| < \infty\}$.

9.4.1 SOME OBSERVATIONS

(1) ess. $\sup|af + bg| \le |a|$ ess. $\sup(f) + |b|$ ess. $\sup|g|$
(2) Every bounded function on E is $L^\infty(t)$.
(3) The space $L^\infty(E)$ is a linear space.

9.4.2 SOME DEFINITIONS RELATED TO NORM ON $L^P[a, b]$

(1) **Distance function:** Let $f, g \in L^P[a, b]$ then the distance function d on $L^P[a, b]$ is defined by
$$d[f, g] = \|f - g\|_p$$

(2) **Convergent Sequence:** A sequence $<x_n>$ in a normed linear space X with norm $\|\cdot\|$ is said to converge to an element $x \in X$ if for arbitrary $\varepsilon > 0$ (however small) $\exists n_0 \in N$ such that
$$\|x_n - x\| < \varepsilon \ \forall n \ge n_0$$
The number x is called the limit of x_n and can be written as
$$\lim_{n \to \infty} x_n = x$$

(3) **Cauchy Sequence:** A sequence $<x_n>$ in a normed linear space X with norm $\|\cdot\|$ is said to be Cauchy if for arbitrary $\varepsilon > 0$ (however small) $\exists n_0 \in N$ such that
$$\|x_n - x_m\| < \varepsilon \ \forall \ n, m \ge n_0$$

(4) **Complete Space:** A normed linear space $(X, \|\cdot\|)$ is said to be complete if every cauchy sequence $<x_n>$ in X converges to an element $x \in X$.

(5) **Banach Space:** A complete normed linear space is called Banach space.

Illustrations

✦ The spaces R and C with norm given by $\|x\| = |x|$ are Banach spaces.

✦ The spaces $R^n = \{x = (x_1, x_2, ..., x_n) : x_i \in R\}$ and C^n are Banach spaces with the norm defined by $\|x\| = \left(\sum\limits_{i=1}^{n} x_i^2 \right)^{1/2}$

(6) **Summable Sequence:** A sequence $<x_n>$ in a normed linear space X with norm $\|\cdot\|$ is said to be summable if the sequence $<s_n>$ of partial sum [i.e., $s_n = x_1 + x_2 + ... + x_n$] converses to its sum s, i.e.,

$$\|s_n - s\| = \left\| \sum_{r=1}^{n} x_r - s \right\| \to 0 \text{ as } n \to \infty$$

i.e., for $\varepsilon > 0 \; \exists \; n_0 \in N$ such that $\|s_n - s\| < \varepsilon \; \forall \; n \geq n_0$ and then $s = \sum\limits_{r=1}^{\infty} x_r$.

(7) **Absolutely Summable Sequence:** The sequence $<x_n>$ is said to be absolutely summable if $\sum\limits_{n=1}^{\infty} \|x_n\| < \infty$.

THEOREM 1.

The space (L^P, d) is a metric space. [GARHWAL–2007, 12]

PROOF. Let $(f_m, f_n) \in L^P$ be a arbitrary then we define

$$d(f_n, f_m) = \|f_n - f_m\|_p = \left(\int_a^b |f_n - f_m|^p \, dx \right)^{1/p}$$

We shall prove that (L_p, d) is a metric space.

(i) Since, $|f_n(x) - f_m(x)| \geq 0$ which implies $\left(\int_a^b |f_n - f_m|^p \, dx \right)^{1/p} \geq 0$.

$$\Rightarrow \quad \|f_n - f_m\|_p \geq 0$$
$$\Rightarrow \quad d(f_n, f_m) \geq 0$$

(ii) Consider $d(f_n, f_m) = 0$ iff $\|f_n - f_m\| = 0$

$$\Leftrightarrow \quad \int_a^b |f_n - f_m|^p \, dx = 0$$
$$\Leftrightarrow \quad |f_n - f_m|^p = 0 \text{ a.e.}$$
$$\Leftrightarrow \quad |f_n - f_m| = 0 \text{ a.e.}$$
$$\Leftrightarrow \quad f_n = f_m = 0 \text{ a.e.}$$

(iii) Consider $d(f_n, f_m) = \|f_n - f_m\|$

$$= \|f_m - f_n\|$$
$$= d(f_m, f_n)$$

(iv) Consider $\|f_n - f_m\| = \|f_n - h_p + h_p - f_m\|, \quad f_n, f_m, h_p \in L^P$

$$= \|(f_n - h_p) + (h_p - f_m)\|$$
$$\leq \|f_n - h_p\| + \|h_p - f_m\| \qquad \text{(By Minkowski's inequality)}$$
$$= d(f_n, h_p) + d(h_p, f_m)$$
$$\Rightarrow \quad d(f_n, f_m) \leq d(f_n, h_p) + d(h_p, h_m)$$

Finally from (i), (ii), (iii) and (iv), we conclude that $[L^P, d]$ is a metric space.

THEOREM 2.

An L^p-space is a linear space.

PROOF.   Let $f, g \in L^P[a, b]$. We have to prove that L^P is a linear space. Here it is sufficient to prove that $f, g \in L^P[a, b], c \in R$.

$\Rightarrow \quad f + g \in L^P$ and $cf \in L^P[a, b]$.

We have already proved that

$$f, g \in L^P[a, b] \quad \Rightarrow \quad f + g \in L^P[a, b]$$

Now, let $f \in L^P[a, b], c \in R$

$\therefore \quad f \in L^P[a, b] \quad \Rightarrow \quad f$ is measurable and $\int_a^b |f|^P \, dx < \infty$ ...(1)

We know that f is measurable then for any $c \in R$, cf is also measurable. Further, consider

$$\int_a^b |cf|^P \, dx = c^P \int_a^b |f|^P \, dx$$
$$< c^P \cdot \infty \qquad\qquad\qquad \text{(Using (1))}$$

$\Rightarrow \qquad\qquad \int_a^b |cf|^P \, dx < \infty$

which shows that $cf \in L^P[a, b]$.

Hence, $L^P[a, b]$ is a linear space.

THEOREM 3.

An L^P-space is a normed linear space.

[MEERUT–2005, 06, 09, 12, 15, 17; GARHWAL–2003, 07; ALLAHABAD–2010; ASSAM–2008]

PROOF.   In previous theorem, we have proved that L^P-space is a linear space; so, here it is sufficient to prove that conditions of norms are also satisfies.

(i)   Since, $|f| \geq 0 \qquad \Rightarrow \qquad \left(\int_a^b |f|^P\right)^{1/p} \geq 0$

$\Rightarrow \quad \|f\|_p \geq 0$

Also, $f = 0 \qquad \Leftrightarrow \quad \|f\|_p = 0$

(ii) $\|cf\|_p = \left(\int_a^b |cf|^P \, dx\right)^{1/p} = |c| \left(\int_a^b |f|^P \, dx\right)^{1/p} = |c| \cdot \|f\|$

(iv)   From Minkowski's inequality, it is clear that

$$\|f + g\|_p \leq \|f\|_p + \|g\|_p$$

Hence, we conclude that L^P-space is a normed linear space.

THEOREM 4. (Riesz-Fischer Theorem)

An L^P-space is a complete space $(p \geq 1)$.

[MEERUT–2003, 04, 05, 12, 14, 15; GARHWAL–2003, 04, 06, 07; HPU–2000, 01, 02, 04]

PROOF.   Let $\langle f_n \rangle$ be a sequence of functions belonging to $L^P[a, b]$. We have to prove that L^P is a complete space.

By definition of complete space, we can say that a space in which every Cauchy sequence is convergent is said to be complete space. Here it is sufficient to prove that every Cauchy sequence in it is converges to some point in it.

Suppose $\langle f_n \rangle$ is a cauchy sequence in $L^P[a, b]$. By definition of Cauchy sequence we can write for given $\varepsilon > 0, \exists \, n_0 \in N$ such that $\|f_m - f_n\| < \varepsilon \; \forall \; m, n \geq n_0$ ...(1)

We have to prove that $\langle f_n \rangle$ converges in mean to a function $f \in L^P[a, b]$.

Let us take $\varepsilon = \dfrac{1}{2^k}$ and $n_0 = n_k$ in (1) we get

$$\|f_m - f_n\| < \frac{1}{2^k} \quad \forall m, n \geq n_k$$

or $\qquad \|f_m - f_{n_k}\| < \varepsilon \quad \forall m > n_k$ ...(2)

Let $g_k = f_{n_k}$. Then

$$\sum_{k=1}^{\infty} \|g_{k+1} - g_k\|_p < \sum_{k=1}^{\infty} \frac{1}{2^k} = 1 \qquad \text{(Being an infinite G.P.)}$$

$$\Rightarrow \quad \sum_{k=1}^{\infty} \|g_{k+1} - g_k\|_p < 1 \qquad \qquad ...(3)$$

$$\Rightarrow \quad \sum_{k} \|g_{k+1} - g_k\|_p \text{ is convergent.}$$

Further define $g(x) = |g_1(x)| + \sum_{k=1}^{\infty} |g_{k+1} - g_k|$ ...(4)

With the property that $g(x) = \infty$ if RHS of the above series is divergent.

Frorm (3),

$$\left(\int_a^b |g|^p \, dx \right)^{1/p} = \left\{ \int_a^b \left[|g_1| + \sum_{k=1}^{\infty} |g_{k+1} - g_k| \right]^p \right\}^{1/p}$$

$$\Rightarrow \qquad \|g\|_p \leq \left[\|g_1\| + \sum_{k=1}^{\infty} \|g_{k+1} - g_k\|_p \right] \qquad \text{(By Minkowski's inequality)}$$

$$< \|g_1\|_p + 1, \text{ a finite quantity} \qquad \text{(From (3))}$$

$$\Rightarrow \qquad g \in L^P[a, b]$$

Now suppose that E is the set of those points x for which $g(x) = \infty$.

Define $f(x) = 0 \; \forall \; x \in E$ and $f(x) = g_1 + \sum_{k=1}^{\infty} (g_{k+1} - g_k), x \notin E, x \in]a,b[$

If $x \notin E$, then $f(x) = \lim_{m \to \infty} \left[g_1 + \sum_{k=1}^{m-1} (g_{k+1} - g_k) \right]$

$$= \lim_{m \to \infty} g_m(x)$$

Also, $f(x) = 0$, $x \in E$ such that $x \in [a, b]$.

$$\Rightarrow \qquad f(x) = \lim_{m \to \infty} g_m(x) \text{ a.e. on } [a, b] \qquad ...(5)$$

$$\Rightarrow \quad \lim_{m \to \infty} |f - g_m| = 0 \text{ a.e. in } [a, b] \qquad ...(6)$$

Clearly, $\qquad g_m(x) = g_1 + \sum_{k=1}^{m-1} (g_{k+1} - g_k)$

$$\Rightarrow \qquad |g_m| \leq |g_1| + \sum_{k=1}^{m-1} |g_{k+1} - g_k|$$

$$\leq |g| + \sum_{k=1}^{\infty} |g_{k+1} - g_k| = g \qquad \text{(By (4))}$$

$$\Rightarrow \qquad |g_m| \leq |g| \; \forall \; m$$

Letting $m \to \infty$ and using (5) we can write

$$|f| \leq g$$

Also, $\qquad |f - g_m| \leq |f| + |g_m| \leq g + g = 2g$

$$\Rightarrow \qquad |f - g_m| \leq 2g \qquad \qquad ...(7)$$

Clearly (6) and (7) are the conditions of Lebesgue's dominated convergence theorem. Hence by Lebesgue's dominated convergence theorem, we get

$$\lim_{n \to \infty} \int_a^b |f - g_m|^p \, dx = \int_a^b \lim_{m \to \infty} |f - g_m|^p \, dx = \int_a^b 0 \, dx = 0$$

$$\Rightarrow \quad \lim_{m \to \infty} \left[\int_a^b |f - g_m|^p \, dx \right]^{1/p} = 0$$

$$\Rightarrow \quad \lim_{m \to \infty} \|f - g_m\|_p = 0$$

$$\Rightarrow \quad \lim_{m \to \infty} \|f - f_{n_m}\|_p = 0 \qquad\qquad (\because \; g_m(x) = f_{n_m}(x))$$

$$\Rightarrow \quad \lim_{m \to \infty} \|f - f_m\|_p = 0 \qquad\qquad \text{(By (2))}$$

$\Rightarrow \quad <f_n>$ is convergent in mean to a function $f \in L^P[a, b]$.

Hence, an L^P-space is complete.

☞ REMARK

- The above theorem can be restated as follows:

  Every Cauchy sequence $<f_n>$ in L_p-space converges to a limit function $f \in L^P$-space.

THEOREM 5.

An L^P-space is a Banach space.

PROOF. We know that a normed linear space which is complete is called Banach space. Since, we know that an L^P-space is a normed linear space (Theorem 3). Also, by previous theorem-4, we have proved that every normed linear space is complete.

Hence, an L^P-space is Banach.

THEOREM 6.

A sequence of function belonging to an L^P-space is Cauchy sequence has its limit in the space.

[MEERUT–2000, 07, 10]

PROOF. Let $<f_n>$ be a convergent sequence in $L^P[a, b]$ such that it converges to a function $f \in L^P$-space. In other words, we can say $\exists f \in L^P[a, b]$ such that $\lim_{n \to \infty} f_n = f$ a.e.

We have to prove that $<f_n>$ is a Cauchy sequence.

Since, $\lim_{n \to \infty} f_n = f$ a.e. then by definition, for given $\varepsilon > 0 \; \exists \; n_0 \in N$ such that

$$\|f_n - f\|_p < \varepsilon/2 \; \forall \; m, n \geq n_0$$

Now, $\|f_n - f_m\|_p = \|f_n - f + f - f_m\|_p$

$$\leq \|f_n - f\|_p + \|f - f_m\|_p \qquad\qquad \text{(By Minkowski's inequality)}$$

$$< \frac{\varepsilon}{2} + \frac{\varepsilon}{2}$$

$\Rightarrow \quad \|f_n - f_m\| < \varepsilon \; \forall \; n, m \geq n_0$

Hence, $<f_n>$ is a Cauchy sequence.

THEOREM 7.

A sequence $<f_n>$ of functions belonging of an L^P-space has atmost one limit.

PROOF. Let if possible $\exists$ two limit functions f and g such that $f_n \to f, f_n \to g$

Consider $\|f - g\| = \|f - f_n + f_n - g\|$

$$\leq \|f - f_n\| + \|f_n - g\| \qquad \text{(By Minkowski's inequality)}$$
$$\qquad \ldots(1)$$

Since, $\qquad f_n \to f \qquad \Rightarrow \qquad \|f - f_n\| \to 0$ as $n \to \infty$

and $\qquad f_n \to g \qquad \Rightarrow \qquad \|f_n - g\| \to 0$ as $n \to \infty$

Then from (1)

$$\|f - g\| \leq 0 \text{ as } n \to 0 \qquad \ldots(2)$$

But by definition of norm, $\|f - g\| \geq 0$ $\qquad \ldots(3)$

From (2) and (3) we conclude that

$$\|f - g\| = 0$$

$\Rightarrow \qquad f - g = 0$ a.e. $\qquad\qquad (\because \|x\| = 0 \Leftrightarrow x = 0)$

$\Rightarrow \qquad f = g$ a.e.

Hence, the sequence $\langle f_n \rangle$ has atmost one limit.

THEOREM 8.

Let f be a bounded measurable function on [a, b] then for a given $\varepsilon > 0$ $\exists$ a continuous function g on [a, b] such that $\|f - g\|_2 < \varepsilon$ [KANPUR–2006; DELHI–2006]

PROOF. Let f be a bounded measurable functions defined on $[a, b]$.

Let us define $F(x) = \int_a^x f(t)dt, x \in [a, b]$

Clearly $F'(x) = f(x)$ a.e. $x \in [a, b]$

Now, $\qquad \left| F(x+h) - F(x) \right| = \left| \int_a^{x+h} f(t)dt - \int_a^x f(t)dt \right|$

$$= \left| \int_x^{x+h} f(t)dt \right| \leq \int_x^{x+h} |f(t)| \, dt \qquad \ldots(1)$$

$$\leq mh, \qquad\qquad (\because |f(x)| \leq m \ \forall \ x \in [a, b])$$

Set $h < \delta$ and $mh < \varepsilon_1$ we get $|x + h - x| < \delta \Rightarrow |F(x + h) - F(x)| < \varepsilon_1$

$\Rightarrow \quad F(x)$ is continuous on $[a, b]$

Further let $G_n(x) = n\int_x^{x+h} f(t)dt, x \in [a, b], n \in N$

Then $\qquad G_n(x) = n\left[F\left(x + \dfrac{1}{n}\right) - F(x) \right]$ $\qquad$ [From (1)]

$$\Rightarrow \quad \lim_{n \to \infty} G_n(x) = \lim_{n \to \infty} \frac{F\left(x + \dfrac{1}{n}\right) - F(x)}{1/n} = \lim_{h \to 0} \frac{F(x+h) - F(x)}{h} \ , \left(h = \frac{1}{n} \right)$$

$$= F'(x) = f(x) \text{ a.e. on } [a, b]$$

$$\Rightarrow \quad \lim_{n \to \infty} [G_n(x) - f(x)]^2 = 0$$

Also, $\qquad |G_n(x)| = \left| \int_x^{x+1/n} f(t)dt \right| \leq n\int_x^{x+1/n} |f(t)| \, dt = m$ [$\because f$ is bounded so $|f(t)| \leq m$]

$\Rightarrow \qquad |G_n(x)| \leq m \ \forall \ n \in N, \ \forall \ x \in [a, b]$

Therefore, $\quad [G_n(x) - f(x)]^2 \leq [m + m]^2 = 4m^2, x \in [a, b]$

Then by Lebesgue bounded convergence theorem, we get

$$\lim_{n \to \infty} \int_a^b (G_n - f)^2 = \int_a^b \lim_{n \to \infty} (G_n - f)^2 = 0$$

$$\Rightarrow \qquad \lim_{n \to \infty} [G_n - f]_2^2 = 0$$

$$\Rightarrow \qquad \lim_{n\to\infty} \left\| G_n - f \right\|_2 = 0$$

$$\Rightarrow \qquad \lim_{n\to\infty} \left\| f - G_n \right\|_2 = 0$$

Therefore, we can say that for given $\varepsilon > 0$ $\exists\, n_0 \in N$ such that $\left\| f - G_n \right\|_2 < \varepsilon \; \forall\, n \geq n_0$
In particular for $n = n_0$

$$\left\| f - G_{n_0} \right\|_2 < \varepsilon$$

$$\Rightarrow \qquad \left\| f - g \right\|_2 < \varepsilon \qquad\qquad \text{(Taking } G_{n_0} = g)$$

THEOREM 9.

The necessary and sufficient condition for a sequence $\langle f_n \rangle$ of functions in $L^p[a, b]$ to converge in mean to a function $f \in L^P[a, b]$ is that $\left\| f_m - f_n \right\|_p \to 0$ as $m, n \to \infty$.   [MEERUT–2001; GARHWAL–1996]

PROOF.   Let us first suppose $\langle f_n \rangle \to f$ in mean and $f \in L^P[a, b]$.
Then by definition for arbitrary $\varepsilon > 0$ $\exists\, n_0 \in N$ such that for all $m \geq n_0$

$$\left\| f - f_m \right\| < \varepsilon/2 \qquad\qquad\qquad\qquad ...(1)$$

and
$$\left\| f_n - f_m \right\|_p = \left\| f_n - f + f - f_m \right\|_p \leq \left\| f_n - f \right\|_p + \left\| f - f_m \right\|_p \qquad ...(2)$$
$$\text{(By Minkowski's Inequality)}$$
$$< \varepsilon/2 + \varepsilon/2 \qquad\qquad \text{(Using (1))}$$

$$\Rightarrow \qquad \left\| f_n - f_m \right\| < \varepsilon \quad \forall n, m \geq n_0$$

which implies that $\left\| f_n - f_m \right\|_p \to 0$ as $m, n \to \infty$
Conversely, if $\left\| f_m - f_n \right\| \to 0$ then by Riesz's theorem, the Cauchy sequence $\langle f_n \rangle$ definitely converge to some $f \in L^P[a, b]$.

THEOREM 10.

A normed linear space is complete if and only if every absolutely summable sequence is summable.
            [MEERUT–2008, 14; HPU–2000, 01, 04, 09, 12, 15; NAGPUR–2006]

PROOF.   Let us first suppose X be a complete normed linear space and $\langle f_n \rangle$ be an absolutely summable sequence of elements of X.

So,
$$\sum_{n=1}^{\infty} \left\| f_n \right\| = m < \infty$$

Therefore, for given $\varepsilon > 0$ $\exists\, n_0 \in N$ such that $\displaystyle\sum_{n=n_0}^{\infty} \left\| f_n \right\| < \varepsilon \qquad\qquad ...(1)$

Let $S_n = \displaystyle\sum_{i=1}^{n} f_i$

Then $\left\| S_n - S_m \right\|_p = \left\| \displaystyle\sum_{i=m+1}^{n} f_i \right\| \leq \displaystyle\sum_{i=m+1}^{n} \left\| f_i \right\| \leq \displaystyle\sum_{i=n_0}^{\infty} \left\| f_i \right\| < \varepsilon \; \forall n, m \geq n_0$

$\Rightarrow$ Sequence of partial sum of $\langle S_n \rangle$ is Cauchy.
$\Rightarrow$ Sequence $\langle f_n \rangle$ is summable to some elements S in X.
$\Rightarrow$ $\langle S_n \rangle$ converges to S in X.   ($\because X$ is complete)
Conversely let us suppose that every absolutely summable sequence in X is summable. We have to prove that X is complete.
Let $\langle f_n \rangle$ be a Cauchy sequence in X. Then by definition

$$\left\| f_n - f_m \right\| < \frac{1}{2^k} \quad \forall\, n, m \geq n_k \qquad\qquad ...(2)$$

$\Rightarrow\quad <f_{n_k}>$ is subsequence of $<f_n>$.

Let us set $g_1 = f_{n_1}, g_k = f_{n_k} - f_{n_{k-1}}\qquad (k > 1)$

Then we get a sequence $<g_k>$ such that its partial sum

$$S_k = g_1 + g_2 + \ldots + g_k = f_{n_1} - (f_{n_2} - f_{n_1}) + \ldots + (f_{n_k} - f_{n_{k-1}}) = f_{n_k}$$

$$\therefore \ \|g_k\| = \left\|f_{n_k} - f_{n_{k-1}}\right\| < \frac{1}{2^{k-1}}, \quad k > 1 \qquad\qquad \text{(From (2))}$$

$$\Rightarrow\ \sum_{k=1}^{\infty} \|g_k\| \le \|g_1\| + \sum_{k=2}^{\infty} \frac{1}{2^{k-1}} = \|g_1\| + 1 \qquad \left[\because \sum_{k=2}^{\infty} \frac{1}{2^{k-1}} = 1\right]$$

$\Rightarrow\quad <g_k>$ is absolutely summable.

$\Rightarrow\quad <g_k>$ is summable. $\qquad$ (By hypothesis)

$\Rightarrow\quad$ The sequence of partial sums of this sequence converges to some $S \in X$

$\Rightarrow\quad <S_k>$ converges and hence $< f_{n_k} >$ converges to f in X.

Now, it remains to prove that limit $f_n = f$

Since, $<f_n>$ is a Cauchy sequence then

$$\|f_n - f_m\| < \varepsilon/2 \qquad\qquad \ldots(3)$$

Further, since $f_{n_k} \to f\ \exists\ n' \in N$ such that for all $k > n'$

$$\left\|f_{n_k} - f\right\| < \varepsilon/2 \qquad\qquad \ldots(4)$$

Now, $\qquad \left\|f_n - f\right\| \le \left\|f_n - f_{n_k}\right\| + \left\|f_{n_k} - f\right\|$

$$< \varepsilon/2 + \varepsilon/2 = \varepsilon \qquad\qquad \text{(Using (3) and (4))}$$

$\Rightarrow\qquad\qquad f_n \to f \in X$

Hence, X is complete.

THEOREM 11.

$\|f + g\|_\infty \le \|f\|_\infty + \|g\|_\infty$ $\hfill$ [HPU–2001, 02]

PROOF. $\quad$ Let us define $\qquad E_n = \{x : f(x) > \dfrac{1}{n} + \text{ess. sup } f\}$

Then clearly, $E_n \subseteq E_{n+1}$, i.e., $<E_n>$ is monotonically non-decreasing sequence and if $E_n = \cup E_n$ then

$$E = \{x : f(x) > \text{ess. sup } f\}$$

Since, $<E_n>$ is monotonically non-decreasing sequence of measurable sets, therefore,

$$m(E) = \lim_{n \to \infty} m(E_n)$$

If $m(E) > 0$ then $m(E_n) > 0$ for some n, which contradict the definition of ess. sup f.

$\Rightarrow\quad$ none of the $m(E_n) > 0$

which implies $m(E) = 0 \qquad \Rightarrow \quad f \le \text{ess. sup } f$ a.e.

In a similar manner, $g \le \text{ess. sup. } g$ a.e.

Thus, we conclude that

$$f + g \le \text{ess. sup } f + \text{ess. sup } g \text{ a.e.}$$

But $\quad$ ess. sup $[f + g] = \inf.\{\alpha : f + g \le \alpha \text{ a.e.}\}$

$\Rightarrow\quad$ ess. sup. $(f + g) \le$ ess. sup $f +$ ess. sup g

Hence, $\qquad \|f + g\|_\alpha \le \|f\|_\alpha + \|g\|_\alpha$

Solved Examples

EXAMPLE 1. *Prove that* $\|f+g\|_1 \le \|f\|_1 + \|g\|_1$ [HPU–2002, 10]

SOLUTION. We know that $|f+g| \le |f| + |g|$

On integrating both the sides we get

$$\int |f+g|\, dx \le \int |f|\, dx + \int |g|\, dx$$

which shows that

$$\|f+g\|_1 \le \|f\|_1 + \|g\|_1$$

EXAMPLE 2. *If* $f \in L^2[0, 1]$, *show that* $\left| \int_0^1 f(x)dx \right| \le \left[\int_0^1 |f(x)|^2\, dx \right]^{1/2}$. [MEERUT–2002, 03, 04, 08]

SOLUTION. Using Schwarz's inequality for $f, g \in L^2[0, 1]$, we can write

$$\|fg\| \le \|f\|_2 + \|g\|_2$$

$$\Rightarrow \qquad \int_0^1 |fg|\, dx \le \left[\int_0^1 |f|^2\, dx \right]^{1/2} \left[\int_0^1 |g|^2\, dx \right]^{1/2}$$

If we take $g(x) = 1$, for all x, then we get

$$\int_0^1 |f|\, dx \le \left[\int_0^1 |f|^2\, dx \right]^{1/2}$$

$$\Rightarrow \qquad \left| \int_0^1 f dx \right| \le \int_0^1 |f|\, dx \le \left[\int_0^1 |f|^2\, dx \right]^{1/2}$$

Hence, $\left| \int_0^1 f dx \right| \le \left[\int_0^1 |f|^2\, dx \right]^{1/2}$

EXAMPLE 3. *Let* $f(x)$ *be a real valued function defined on* $[a, b]$ *such that*

$$f(x) = \begin{cases} 1, & \text{if } x \text{ is rational} \\ \infty, & \text{if } x \text{ is irrational} \end{cases} \quad \forall\, x \in [a, b]$$

Show that $f \in L^\infty[a, b]$.

SOLUTION. Since, we know that

$$m\{x \in [a, b] : |f(x)| > M, M \ge 1\} = m\{\text{set of all rationals in } [a, b]\}$$
$$= 0$$

Therefore, for all $M \ge 1$, $|f(x)| \le M$ a.e. on $[a, b]$

$\Rightarrow$ ess. sup $|f(x)| = \inf.\{M : |f(x)| \le M \text{ a.e. on } E\}$
$$= \inf.\{M, m \ge 1\} = 1$$

$\Rightarrow$ ess. sup. $|f(x)| < \infty$

Hence, $f \in L^\infty[a, b]$.

EXAMPLE 4. *Show that the inequalities* $\int_0^\pi [f(x) - \sin x]^2\, dx \le \frac{4}{9}$ *and* $\int_0^\pi [f(x) - \cos x]^2\, dx \le \frac{1}{9}$, $f \in L^2[0, \pi]$ *are not consistent.*

SOLUTION. Consider,

$$\|\sin x - \cos x\|_2 = \|(f - \cos x) + (\sin x - f)\|_2$$

$$\le \|f - \cos x\|_2 + \|\sin x - f\|_2$$

$$\le \left(\int_0^\pi (f - \cos x)^2\, dx \right)^{1/2} + \left(\int_0^\pi (f - \sin x)^2\, dx \right)^{1/2}$$

$$\leq \left(\frac{4}{9}\right)^{1/2} + \left(\frac{1}{9}\right)^{1/2} = \frac{2}{3} + \frac{1}{3} = 1 \qquad\qquad\qquad ...(1)$$

But

$$\|\sin x - \cos x\|_2 = \left[\int_0^\pi (\sin x - \cos x)^2 \, dx\right]^{1/2}$$

$$= \left[\int_0^\pi (1 - \sin 2x) dx\right]^{1/2}$$

$$= \sqrt{\pi} < 1$$

which contradict the inequality (1). Hence, the given inequalities are not consistent.

EXAMPLE 5. *Show that space* $L^\infty[0, 1]$ *is complete.*   [HPU–2001, 04, 06]

SOLUTION. We know that a space in which every Cauchy sequence is convergent, so consider a Cauchy sequence $\langle f_n \rangle$ in $L^\infty[0, 1]$.
Since, $\langle f_n \rangle$ is Cauchy, so by definition
$$\|f_n - f_m\|_\infty \to 0, \text{ as } n, m \to \infty \qquad\qquad\qquad ...(1)$$
Let us denote
$$A_n = \{x : |f_n(x)| > \|f_n\|_\infty\}$$
and $\qquad B_{m,n} = \{x : |f_n(x) - f_m(x)| > \|f_n - f_m\|_p\}$
Clearly, we have $m(A) = 0$ and $m[B_{m,n}] = 0$

which implies if $E = \overset{\infty}{\underset{n=1}{\cup}} A_n$ and $\underset{n \neq m}{\cup} B_{m,n}$ then $m(E) = 0$

$\Rightarrow \quad |f_n(x)| \leq \|f_n\|_\infty$ on $F = [0, 1] - E$

$\Rightarrow \quad |f_n(x) - f_m(x)| \leq \|f_n - f_m\|_\infty \to 0$ as n, m, ∞ \qquad\qquad (By (1))

$\Rightarrow \quad \langle f_n(x) \rangle$ is Cauchy on F.

$\Rightarrow \quad \langle f_n(x) \rangle$ converges to some f on F

So, define $f : [0, 1] \to R$ such that

$$f = \begin{cases} \lim_{n\to\infty} f_n(x) & \text{if} \quad x \in F \\ 0 & \text{if} \quad x \in E \end{cases}$$

Then clearly $f \in L^\infty$ such that $|f - f_n(x)| \to 0$ as $m \to \infty \Rightarrow \langle f_n \rangle$ is convergent.
Hence, L^∞ is complete.

EXAMPLE 6. *Let* $f \in L^1[0, 1]$ *and* $g \in L^\infty[0, 1]$, *show that* $fg \in L^1[0, 1]$ *and* $\int_0^1 |fg| \leq \|f\|_1 \cdot \|g\|_\infty$

[HPU–2002, 10, 14]

SOLUTION. By definition, we have
$$|g| \leq \text{ess. sup } |g| \text{ a.e.}$$
$\Rightarrow \qquad |fg| \leq |f| \cdot |g| \leq |f| \cdot \|g\| \text{ a.e.} \qquad\qquad (\because \|g\|_\infty = \text{ess. sup} |g|)$
On integrating both the sides from $[0, 1]$ we get
$$\int_0^1 |fg| \leq \|f\|_1 \|g\|_\infty$$

EXAMPLE 7. *If* $\langle f_n \rangle$ *is a sequence of function belonging to* $L^2[a, b]$ *and also* $f \in L^2[a, b]$ *and also* $f \in L^2[a, b]$ *and* $\lim \|f_n - f\|_2 = 0$ *then prove that*
$$\int_a^b f^2 dx = \lim \int_a^b f_n^2 dx$$

SOLUTION. Using Minkowski's inequality, we can write

$$\left| \|f_n\|_2 - \|f\|_2 \right| \le \|f_n - f\|_2$$

$$\Rightarrow \quad \lim \left| \|f_n\|_2 - \|f\|_2 \right| \le \lim \|f_n - f\| = 0$$

$$\Rightarrow \quad \lim \left| \|f_n\|_2 - \|f\|_2 \right| = 0$$

$$\Rightarrow \quad \lim \|f_n\| = | \|f\| |_2$$

Hence, $\lim \left(\int_a^b (f_n)^2 \, dx \right)^{1/2} = \left(\int_a^b f^2 \, dx \right)^{1/2}$

$$\Rightarrow \quad \lim \int_a^b f_n^2 \, dx = \int_a^b f^2 \, dx$$

Exercise 9.1

1. Let $f, g \in L(]-\infty, \infty[)$. Define

   $$h(x) = \int_{-\infty}^{\infty} f(x-y)g(y)dy, \quad -\infty < x < \infty.$$

   Prove that $h \in L^1(]-\infty, \infty[)$.

2. Show that the space $L^2[a, b]$ is a complete metric space.

3. Let $f_n : R \to R$ be a function such that

   $$f_n(x) = \begin{cases} 2^n; & x \in [2^n, 2^{-n+1}] \\ 0; & \text{otherwise} \end{cases} \quad \text{for all } n$$

   If $f(x) = \lim f_n(x)$, show that $\int f \ne \lim \int f_k$

4. If $f, g \in L^p$, show that $fg \in L^{p/2}$.

5. If $f_1, f_2, \dots \in L^p$, prove that the necessary and sufficient condition that $\|f_n - f\|_p \to 0$ as $n \to \infty$ is that $\|f_n - f_m\| \to 0$ as $m \to \infty, n \to \infty$.

6. Illustrate that L^1 consists precisely of the Lebesgue integrable function on [0, 1].

7. Prove the inequality $\left| \int_0^{\pi} x^{-1/4} \sin x dx \right| \le \pi^{3/4}$.

8. If $0 < q < p < \infty$ and $f \in L^p \cap L^q$ then show that $f \in L^2$ for all r such that $q < r < p$.

9. If $1 \le p < \infty$ and E is a measurable set such that $m(E) < \infty$ then show that $L^{\infty}(E) \subset L^p(E)$, for each p. Also, show that

   $$\lim_{p \to \infty} \|f\|_p = \|f\|_{\infty} \quad \forall f \in L^{\infty}(E)$$

10. Let f be a bounded function on [0, 1], show that

    $$\lim_{p \to \infty} \|f\|_p = \|f\|_{\infty}$$

11. If $0 < q < p < \infty$, then prove that $L^p \subset L^q$ and there exists a positive constant in such that

    $$\|f\|_q \le M \|f\|_p \quad \forall f \in L^p$$

12. Let $f \ge 0$ be such that $f \in L^p$, $p > 0$ and let $f_n = \min[f, n]$. Show that $f_n \in L^p$ and

    $$\lim_{n \to \infty} \|f - f_n\|_p = 0.$$

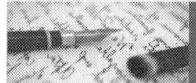
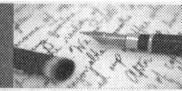
CHAPTER Summary

📖 KEY TERMS

- **CONJUGATE NUMBERS:** Let p and q be two positive numbers such that $p > 1$ and $\dfrac{1}{p} + \dfrac{1}{q} = 1$ then q is called conjugate to p.

- **L^P-SPACE:** By $L^p[a, b]$ we mean a class of function $f(x)$ such that
    - (i) $f(x)$ is measurable over $[a, b]$.
    and (ii) $|f|^p$ is L-integrable over $[a, b]$, for $p > 0$

- **NORM:** The norm of $f(x)$ denoted by $\|f\|_p$ is defined by $\|f\|_p = \left(\int_a^b |f|^p\, dx\right)^{1/p}$.

- **CAUCHY SEQUENCE:** A sequence $<f_n> \in L^p[a, b]$ is said to be Cauchy or fundemental sequence if for given $\varepsilon > 0$ $\exists\ n_0 \in N$ such that $\|f_m - f_n\|_p < \varepsilon$ $\forall\ m, n \geq n_0$.

- **BANACH SPACE:** A complete normed linear space is called Banach space.

- **COMPLETE SPACE:** An L^P-space is said to be complete if evey Cauchy sequence in the space is convergent at some point in the space.

- **DISTANCE FUNCTION:** Let $f(x), g(x) \in L^P[a, b]$ then $d(f, g) = \|f - g\|_p$ is called the distance function or metric on $L^P[a, b]$.

📖 RESULTS

- If $f \in L^P[a, b]$, $p > 1$ then $f \in L[a, b]$.

- If $f \in L^P[a, b]$, $g \in L^P[a, b]$ then $f + g \in L^P[a, b]$.

- **Holder's Inequality:** $\|fg\| \leq \|f\|_p \cdot \|g\|_p$

- **Schwarz's Inequality:** $\|fg\| \leq \|f\|_2 \cdot \|g\|_2$

- **Minkowski's Inenquality:** $\|f+g\|_p \leq \|f\|_p + \|g\|_p$

- If f is a bounded measurable fucntions defined on $[a, b]$ then for given $\varepsilon > 0$ $\exists$ a continuous function g on $[a, b]$ such that $\|f - g\|_2 < \varepsilon$.

- **Riesz-Fisher Theorem:** The normed L^P-space is complete for $p \geq 1$.

- A normed linear space is complete if and only if every absolutely summable sequence is summable.

- A sequence of function in an L^P-space has atmost one limit.

- If f and g are square L-integrable then
$$\|f + g\|_2 \leq \|f\|_2 + \|g\|_2$$

- L^P-space is a normed linear space.

- (L^P, d) is a metric space.

- In case of $0 < p < 1$, the Riesz-Holder inequality and Minkowski's inequality are reversed than that of the case for $1 \leq p < \infty$.

📖 WORTHY READINGS

☞ Every bounded function on E is in $L^\infty(E)$.

☞ Riesz-Minkowski equality holds if and only if one of the functions f and g is a multiple of other.

☞ Covergence in the mean neither implies nor is implied by the pointwise convergence or convergence almost everywhere.

☞ If we replace the interval $[a, b]$ by an infinite interval or more generally by any measurable set E with $m(E) = \infty$, then a function $f \in L^P$ may not be approximated by a continuous function.

☞ No family of continuous function is dense in L^∞.

☞ The family of step function is dense in L^∞.

☞ Let $<f_n>$ be a sequence of integrable fuctions which converges in mean to a function f, then sequence converges in measure to f.

☞ If $f(x) \in L^p[a, b]$ and $f(x) \in L^q[a, b]$, then $f(x) \in L^r[a, b]$ if $p < r < q$.

☞ Every bounded functions belongs to $L^p[a, b]$ for all p where $[a, b]$ is finite.

☞ Every convergent sequence is a Cauchy sequence.

☞ If $<f_n>$ is a Cauchy sequence in $L^P[a, b]$, then it has a limit.

☛ FURTHER READINGS

☞ A sequence $\langle f_n \rangle$ in L^P is said to converge weakly to f in L^P if for every fucntion $g \in L^q$ (where p and q are conjugate numbers), we have

$$\lim_{n \to \infty} \int g f_n = \int g f$$

☞ Let f be a real valued function on $[a, b]$, $1 \le p \le \infty$ and p and q are conjugate to each other then

$$\|f\|_p = \sup \int_a^b fg$$

☞ (Arithmetic-Geometric Mean Inequality). If $a^i > 0$, $i \in N$, then

$$\left(\prod_{i=1}^n a_i \right)^{1/n} \le \frac{1}{n} \sum_{i=1}^n a_i$$

with equality if and only if all $a_i's$ are equal.

☞ The sets of measurable simple function, step functions and of continuous functions are each dense in the metric space $L^P[a, b]$, $p > 1$, when a and b are functions.

☞ A continuous function $f : R \to R$ is said to have **compact support** if there is a compact set $K \subset R$ such that $f(x) = 0$ whenever $x \notin K$.

☞ Let $\langle f_n \rangle$ be a sequence of functions in L^∞. Then $\langle f_n \rangle$ converges to f in L^∞ if and only if there is a set E of measure zero such that $\langle f_n \rangle$ converges to f uniformly on $[a, b] - E$.

Chapter

10 Signed Measure

10.1 INTRODUCTION

We know that a measure is a non-negative function. In this chapter, we consider some of the possibilities which may arise if a measure is allowed to take on both positive and negative values. Suppose that μ_1 and μ_2 are two measures on a σ-ring of subsets of X. If we define for every set E

$$\mu(E) = \mu_1(E) + \mu_2(E)$$

Then, clearly μ is a measure which extends immediately to any finite sum. Another way of manufacturing new measures is to multiply a given measure by an arbitrary non-negative constant. Combining above two methods, we observe that if $\{\mu_1, \mu_2, \ldots, \mu_n\}$ is a finite set of measure and $\{\alpha_1, \alpha_2, \ldots, \alpha_n\}$ is a finite set of non-negative real numbers, then the set function μ is defined over E is given by

$$\mu(E) = \sum_{i=1}^{n} \alpha_i \, \mu_i(E)$$

is a measure.

On the other hand, if we define μ by $\mu(E) = \mu_1(E) - \mu_2(E)$, then there are following two possibilities :

(i) μ may be negative on some sets.

(ii) $\mu_1(E) = \mu_2(E) = \infty$

To avoid the difficulty of above indeterminate form, we subtract two measures only if at least one of them is finite. Therefore, if f is a measurable function such that $\int f \, d\mu$ is defined, then the set function ν, defined by

$\nu(E) = \int_E f \, d\mu$, is the difference of two functions.

☞ REMARK

- $\int f \, d\mu$ is defined for a measurable function f if and only if at least one of the two functions f^+ and f^- is integrable.

10.2 SIGNED MEASURE

[MEERUT–2006 BP, 07BP, 09, 09 BP,12]

To deal with set functions, the concept of measure is extended to a signed measure – a σ-additive set function which need not be non-negative and it is shown that this can be equated to the difference of two non-negative measures.

Definition. *Let A be a σ-algebra of subsets of X. An extended real valued set function*
$$\mu : A \to [-\infty, \infty]$$
is called a signed measure on a measurable space (X, A) if it satisfies the following conditions :

(i) μ *takes atmost one of the values* $-\infty$ *or* ∞.

(ii) $\mu(\phi) = 0$

(iii) μ *is countably additive, i.e.*

$$\mu\left(\bigcup_{i=1}^{\infty} A_i \right) = \sum_{i=1}^{\infty} \mu(A_i)$$

for any sequence $< A_i >$ of disjoint measurable sets.

We observe that implicit in the requirement of countable additivity is the requirement that if $< A_n >$ is a disjoint sequence of measurable sets, then the series $\sum_{n=1}^{\infty} \mu(A_n)$ is either convergent or definitely divergent to $+\infty$ or $-\infty$.

☞ **REMARK**

• Measure is a special case of a signed measure, but a signed measure is not in general a measure.

10.2.1 POSITIVE SET

A subset E of X is said to be positive relative to a signed measure μ defined on a measurable space (X, A) if

(i) E is measurable.

(ii) For all $A \subset E$ such that A is measurable implies $\mu(A) \geq 0$.   [MEERUT–2008]

10.2.2 NEGATIVE SET

A subset E of X is said to be negative relative to a signed measure μ defined on a measurable space (X, A) if

(i) E is measurable.

(ii) For all $A \subset E$ such that A is measurable implies $\mu(A) \leq 0$.

10.2.3 NULL SET

A set $E \subset X$ is said to be a null set relative to a signed measure μ if E is both negative and positive.

10.2.4 TOTALLY FINITE SIGNED MEASURE

A signed measure μ is said to be totally finite if E is measurable and $|\mu(E)| < \infty$.

10.2.5 HAHN DECOMPOSITION OF A SET

A Hahn decomposition of X with respect to signed measure signed μ is a decomposition $X = P \cup Q$ of X into disjoint subsets $P > 0$ and $Q < 0$.   [MEERUT–2006 BP]

10.2.6 JORDAN DECOMPOSITION OF A SET

A Jordan decomposition of measure μ is a representation $\mu(E) = \mu^+(E) - \mu^-(E)$ where μ^+ and μ^- are measures, which are non-negative σ-additive set functions.

10.2.7 COMPLEX MEASURE

A complex measure on the class of all measurable sets of a measurable space is a set function μ such that for every measurable set such that $\mu(E) = \mu_1(E) + i\,\mu_2(E)$, where μ_1 and μ_2 are signed measures and $i = \sqrt{-1}$.

☞ REMARKS
- We know that a measurable set E is a set of measure zero if and only if every measurable subset of it has μ measure zero.
- The measure of every null set is zero.
- A set of measure zero may be a union of two measurable sets whose measures are not zero but are negative of each other.
- A signed measure is finitely additive and subtractive.

THEOREM 1.

Let E and F are measurable sets and μ is a signed measure such that

$$E \subset F \quad and \quad |\mu(F)| < \infty$$

Then, $|\mu(E)| < \infty$

PROOF. If E and F are measurable sets such that $E \subset F$. Then, we can write

$$\mu(F) = \mu(F - E) + \mu(E)$$

If exactly one of the summands is infinite then clearly $\mu(F)$ is infinite. If they are both infinite, then, since μ assumes at most one of the values $+\infty$ and $-\infty$, they are equal and again $\mu(F)$ is infinite. Only one possibility remains, namely that both summands are finite and this prove that every measurable subset of a set of finite signed measure has finite signed measure. Hence

$$E \subset F \text{ and } |\mu(F)| < \infty \ \Rightarrow \ |\mu(E)| < \infty$$

THEOREM 2.

Let μ be a signed measure and $< E_n >$ be a disjoint sequence of measurable sets such that

$$\left|\mu\left(\bigcup_{n=1}^{\infty} E_n\right)\right| < \infty, \text{ then the series } \sum_{n=1}^{\infty} \mu(E_n) \text{ is absolutely convergent.}$$

PROOF. Define

$$E_n^+ = \begin{cases} E_n, & \text{if } \mu(E_n) \geq 0 \\ 0, & \text{if } \mu(E_n) < 0 \end{cases}$$

and

$$E_n^- = \begin{cases} E_n, & \text{if } \mu(E_n) \leq 0 \\ 0, & \text{if } \mu(E_n) > 0 \end{cases}$$

Then, clearly, we have

$$\mu\left(\bigcup_{n=1}^{\infty} E_n^+\right) = \sum_{n=1}^{\infty} \mu(E_n^+)$$

and

$$\mu\left(\bigcup_{n=1}^{\infty} E_n^-\right) = \sum_{n=1}^{\infty} \mu(E_n^-).$$

Now, since the terms of both the above series are of constant sign and since μ takes on at most one of the values $+\infty$ and $-\infty$ it follows that at least one of these series is convergent. Also, since the sum of two series is the convergent series $\sum_{n=1}^{\infty} \mu(E_n)$, therefore, they both converge and since the convergence of the series of positive terms and the series of negative terms is equivalent to absolute convergence. Hence, the series $\sum_{n=1}^{\infty} \mu(E_n)$ is absolutely convergent.

THEOREM 3.

A union of any countable collection of positive subsets of X is positive.

PROOF. Let $< E_n >$ be a sequence of positive sets in X.

Also, let $A = \bigcup_{i=1}^{\infty} E_i$ and B be any subset of A. To show A is positive.

Let us write

$$B_n = B \cap E_n' \cap E_{n-1}' \cap \ldots\ldots \cap E_1' \qquad \forall\, n \in N \qquad \ldots(1)$$

where $\qquad E_i' = X - E_i$

Since, the complement of a measurable set is again measurable. Further, the countable intersection of measurable sets is measurable. Therefore, B_n is a measurable subset of the positive set E_n.

Thus, $\mu(B_n) \geq 0$.

It is also clear from (1) that sets B_n are disjoint.

Also, $\quad B = \bigcup_{n=1}^{\infty} B_n \quad \Rightarrow \quad \mu(B) = \bigcup_{n=1}^{\infty} \mu(B_n) \geq 0$

Thus, we conclude that

(1) A is a measurable set

For E_n is a positive set $\Rightarrow E_n$ is a measurable set.

$\Rightarrow \qquad \bigcup_{n=1}^{\infty} E_n$ is measurable.

$\Rightarrow \qquad A$ is measurable.

(2) For all $B \subset A$ such that B is a measurable set

$\Rightarrow \qquad \mu(B) \geq 0$

which implies $A\left(= \bigcup_{i=1}^{\infty} E_i \right)$ is positive.

Hence, countable union of positive subsets of X is positive.

☞ **REMARK**

• Every subset of a negative set is negative and countable union of negative sets is negative.

THEOREM 4.

If E is a measurable set with finite negative measure, i.e., if $-\infty < \mu(E) < 0$, then E contains a negative set A with the property $\mu(A) < 0$.

PROOF. If E itself is a negative set, then we can easily prove the theorem by assuming $A = E$.

Now, consider E itself is not a negative set. Then, E must contain a subset of positive measure.

i.e., there exists $E_1 \subset E$ such that

$$\mu(E_1) > \frac{1}{n_1} \text{ for smallest positive integer } n_1.$$

Now, $\qquad E = (E - E_1) \cup E_1 \quad \text{and} \quad (E - E_1) \cap E_1 = \phi$

$\Rightarrow \qquad \mu(E) = \mu(E - E_1) + \mu(E_1)$ ...(1)

$\Rightarrow \qquad \mu(E - E_1) = \mu(E) - \mu(E_1)$ ...(2)

Since, $\mu(E)$ is finite then clearly $\mu(E_1)$ and $\mu(E - E_1)$ both must be finite.

Since $\mu(E) < 0 \Rightarrow \mu(E)$ is a negative finite number.

Then, using (2), we have

$$\mu(E - E_1) < 0$$

Now, let $E - E_1$ is a negative set. Then take $A = E - E_1$ otherwise $E - E_1$ contains subsets of positive measure. Therefore for any positive integer n_2, there is a measurable set $E_2 \subset E - E_1$ such that

$$\mu(E_2) > \frac{1}{n_2}$$

Since $\qquad E = (E - E_1 \cup E_2) \cup (E_1 \cup E_2) \text{ and } (E - E_1 \cup E_2) \cap (E_1 \cup E_2) = \phi$

$\therefore \qquad \mu(E) = \mu(E - E_1 \cup E_2) + \mu(E_1 \cup E_2)$

$\qquad\qquad = \mu(E - E_1 \cup E_2) + \mu(E_1) + \mu(E_2)$

$\qquad \mu(E - E_1 \cup E_2) = \mu(E) - \mu(E_1) - \mu(E_2) < 0$

Now for $\mu(E) < 0$, $\mu(E_r) > 0$ for $r = 1, 2$, we have $\mu(E - E_1 \cup E_2) < 0 \Rightarrow E - E_1 \cup E_2$ is a set of negative measures. If $E - E_1 \cup E_2$ is a negative set, then, we take $A = E - E_1 \cup E_2$. Continuing the process, we shall get either a negative subset A of E, such that $\mu(A) < 0$ or a sequence $< n_k : k \in N >$ of positive integers and a sequence $< E_k >$ of disjoint measurable sets such that $\frac{1}{n_k} < \mu(E_k) < \infty$.

Suppose that $\qquad A = \left(E - \bigcup_{i=1}^{\infty} E_i \right)$ ...(3)

Proceeding as usual, we get

$$\mu(E) = \mu(A) + \mu\left(\bigcup_{i=1}^{\infty} E_i \right)$$

$$= \mu(A) + \sum_{k=1}^{\infty} \mu(E_k)$$

$$> \mu(A) + \sum_{k=1}^{\infty} \frac{1}{n_k}$$

$\Rightarrow \qquad \mu(E) > \mu(A) + \sum_{k=1}^{\infty} \frac{1}{n_k}.$ ...(4)

By definition of signed measure, we know that μ assumes atmost one of the values $-\infty$ or $+\infty$ and $\mu(E)$ is finite, thus from (4), we conclude that $\mu(A)$ is finite and the series $\sum_{k=1}^{\infty} \frac{1}{n_k}$ is convergent.

Using (4), we get

$$\mu(A) < \mu(E) - \sum_{k=1}^{\infty} \frac{1}{n_k}$$

= a finite negative number (difference of two finite negative number)

$$\Rightarrow \quad \mu(A) < 0$$

Now, since arbitrary union of measurable sets is measurable. Also difference of two measurable sets is measurable. Then, using (3), we have A is a measurable set.

Let $B \subset A$ be any arbitrary measurable set.

$$B \subset A = E - \bigcup_{k=1}^{\infty} E_k \subset E - \bigcup_{k=1}^{i-1} E_k$$

$$\Rightarrow \qquad B \subset E - \bigcup_{k=1}^{i-1} E_k \ .$$

By choosing a suitable positive integer, we can show that

$$\mu(B) \ge \frac{1}{n_i - 1} \quad \forall\, i \in \mathbf{N} \qquad \qquad ...(5)$$

Letting $n \to \infty$, we get $\mu(B) \le 0$.

Thus, we conclude that A is a measurable set such that $\mu(A) < 0$ and for all $B \subset A$ such that B is a measurable set implies $\mu(B) \le 0$.

Hence, A is a negative set with $\mu(A) < 0$.

THEOREM 5.

Let E be a measurable set of finite measure, i.e., $0 < \mu(E) < \infty$, then E contains a positive set A with $\mu(A) > 0$.

[MEERUT–2007 BP]

PROOF.   If E itself is a positive set, then we can easily prove the theorem by assuming $A = E$.

Now, let E itself is not a positive set. Then E must contain subsets of negative measures.

Therefore, there exists a measurable set $E_1 \subset E$ and a smallest positive integer n_1 such that

$$\mu(E_1) < -\frac{1}{n_1}$$

We have

$$E = (E - E_1) \cup E_1 \text{ such that } (E - E_1) \cap E_1 = \phi$$

$$\Rightarrow \qquad \mu(E) = \mu(E - E_1) + \mu(E_1) \qquad \qquad ...(1)$$

$$\Rightarrow \quad \mu(E - E_1) = \mu(E) - \mu(E_1) \qquad \qquad ...(2)$$

Since $\mu(E)$ is finite, then (2) gives that $\mu(E - E_1)$ and $\mu(E_1)$ both are finite.

By our assumption, we have $\mu(E_1)$ is negative.

Then, (2) gives $\mu(E - E_1)$ is finite.

If $E - E_1$ is a positive set, then take $A = E - E_1$. Otherwise $E - E_1$ contains subset of negative measure. Let n_2 be a small positive integer such that there exists a measurable set $E_2 \subset E - E_1$ and with $\mu(E_2) < -\frac{1}{n_2}$.

Since, $(E - E_1 \cup E_2) \cap (E_1 \cup E_2) = \phi$

and $E = (E - E_1 \cup E_2) \cup (E_1 \cup E_2)$.

Therefore, $\mu(E) = \mu(E - E_1 \cup E_2) + \mu(E_1 \cup E_2)$

$\Rightarrow \quad \mu(E) - \mu(E_1) - \mu(E_2) = \mu(E - E_1 \cup E_2)$

$\Rightarrow \quad \mu(E - E_1 \cup E_2) > 0$

For $\mu(E) > 0$ and $\mu(E_r) < 0$, we have

$$-\mu(E_r) > 0 \text{ for } r = 1, 2.$$

Thus, $E - E_1 \cup E_2$ is a set of positive measure. If $E - E_1 \cup E_2$ is a positive set, then we take $A = E - E_1 \cup E_2$. Otherwise, we repeat above process.

Continuing this process, we shall get either a positive subset A of E such that $\mu(A) > 0$ or a sequence $< n_k : k \in \mathbf{N} >$ of positive integers and a sequence $< E_k >$ of disjoint measurable sets such that $-\infty < \mu(E_k) < -\dfrac{1}{n_k}$.

In the later case, suppose that

$$A = E - \overset{\infty}{\underset{k=1}{\cup}} E_k \qquad \qquad ...(3)$$

Then proceeding as usual, we get

$$\mu(E) = \mu(A) - \sum_{k=1}^{\infty} \mu(E_k) < \mu(A) - \sum_{k=1}^{\infty} \frac{1}{n_k}$$

$$\Rightarrow \qquad \mu(E) < \mu(A) - \sum_{k=1}^{\infty} \frac{1}{n_k} \qquad \qquad ...(4)$$

By definition of signed measure, we can say that μ assumes atmost one of values $-\infty$ and ∞ and $\mu(E)$ is finite. Then, from (4), we conclude that $\mu(A)$ is finite and the series $\overset{\infty}{\underset{k=1}{\sum}} \dfrac{1}{n_k}$ is convergent.

Using (4)

$$\mu(A) > \mu(E) + \sum_{k=1}^{\infty} \frac{1}{n_k}$$

$\qquad \qquad$ = a positive number (sum of two positive numbers)

$\Rightarrow \qquad \qquad \mu(A) > 0$

Now, since we know that enumerable union of measurable sets is measurable. Also, difference of two measurable sets is measurable. Therefore, from (3), A is a measurable set.

Now, to show A is a positive set.

Let $B \subset A$ be arbitrary measurable set.

Then, $\quad B \subset A = E - \overset{\infty}{\underset{k=1}{\cup}} E_k \subset E - \overset{i-1}{\underset{k=1}{\cup}} E_k$

$$\Rightarrow \qquad B \subset E - \bigcup_{k=1}^{i-1} E_k .$$

By choosing a suitable positive integer, we can show that

$$\mu(B) \geq \frac{1}{n_{i-1}} \quad \forall \, i \in \mathbf{N}$$

Letting $n \to \infty$, we get $\mu(B) \geq 0$.

Thus, we conclude that A is a measurable set such that $\mu(A) > 0$ and for all $B \subset A$ such that B is measurable, $\mu(A) \geq 0$.

Hence, A is a positive set with $\mu(A) > 0$.

THEOREM 6. (Hahn Decomposition Theorem)

Let μ be a signed measure on a measurable space $(X, \, \mathcal{A})$. Then there exists a positive set P and a negative set Q such that $P \cap Q = \phi$, $X = P \cup Q$. [MEERUT–2006, 08, 09, 09 BP, 14, DELHI–2012]

PROOF. Let $\mathcal{A}$ be a σ-algebra of subsets of X. Also, let μ be a signed measure on a measurable space $(X, \, \mathcal{A})$. By definition of signed measure μ assumes at most one of the values ∞ or $-\infty$.

Assume that μ does not take $-\infty$.

Let B be a family of all negative subsets of X.

Define $\qquad \lambda = \inf \left\{ \, \mu(E) : E \in B \, \right\}$ ...(1)

Then, there exists a sequence $< E_n >$ in B such that $\lim_{n \to \infty} \mu(E_n) = \lambda$.

Since B is a family of negative sets, therefore $< E_n >$ is a sequence of negative sets.

$$\Rightarrow \quad \bigcup_{i=1}^{\infty} E_i \text{ is a negative set.}$$

$$\Rightarrow \quad Q = \bigcup_{i=1}^{\infty} E_i \text{ is a negative set.}$$

Therefore, Q is a negative subset of X. Then, using (1), $\mu(Q) \geq \lambda$. ...(2)

Now, consider the subset $Q - E_n$.

Clearly, $Q - E_n \subset Q$.

$$\Rightarrow \qquad Q = (Q - E_n) \cup E_n$$

$$\Rightarrow \qquad \mu(Q) = \mu(Q - E_n) + \mu(E_n) \leq \mu(E_n)$$

$$\Rightarrow \qquad \mu(Q) \leq \mu(E_n) \quad \forall \, n \in \mathbf{N} \text{ and } E_n \in B.$$

Then, using (1), we conclude that

$$\mu(Q) \leq \lambda \qquad \qquad \qquad \text{...(3)}$$

Then, from (2) and (3), we conclude that

$$\mu(Q) = \lambda \quad \Rightarrow \quad \lambda > -\infty.$$

Now, it remains to prove that $P = X - Q$ is a positive subset of X. Let, if possible, P is not positive, *i.e.*, P is negative. Then, by definition, for every measurable set $E \subset P$, $\mu(E) < 0$. Since E is a measurable subset of X with negative measure, then E contains a set A with $\mu(A) < 0$, we get a negative set $A \subset E$ such that

$\mu(A) < 0$. Now, since A and Q both are disjoint negative subsets of X and their union $A \cup Q$ is also negative.

Now, using (1) $\mu(A \cup Q) \geq \lambda$.

But $\lambda \leq \mu(A \cup Q) = \mu(A) + \mu(Q) = \mu(A) + \lambda$

$\Rightarrow$ $\qquad\qquad \lambda \leq \mu(A) + \lambda$

$\Rightarrow$ $\qquad\qquad \mu(A) \geq 0$

which is a contradiction, because $\mu(A) < 0$.

Hence, P is a positive subset of X.

Thus, $P = X - Q$ is positive and Q is negative.

Therefore, $X = P \cup Q, \ P \cap Q = \phi$.

☞ REMARKS

- The Hahn decomposition is not unique.
- If $\{P, Q\}$ is a Hahn decomposition for μ, then we may define two signed measure μ^+ and μ^- such that $\mu = \mu^+ - \mu^-$ by setting

$$\mu^+(E) = \mu(E \cap P)$$
$$\mu^-(E) = -\mu(E \cap Q)$$

- The two set functions μ^+ and μ^- on the class of all measurable sets called respectively the upper variation and the lower variation of μ.
- The set function $|\mu|$ defined for every measurable set E by $|\mu|(E) = \mu^+(E) + \mu^-(E)$ is the total variation of μ.

THEOREM 7.

The upper, lower and total variations of a signed measure μ are measures and $\mu(E) = \mu^+(E) - \mu^-(E)$ for every measurable set E. If μ is totally finite or σ-finite, then so also are μ^+ and μ^- at least one of the measures μ^+ and μ^- is always finite.

PROOF.   Since the variations of μ are clearly non-negative. If every measurable set is a countable union of measurable sets for which μ is finite. Then by Theorem 1, the same is true for μ^+ and μ^-. By definition of μ^+ and μ^-, we get $\mu = \mu^+ - \mu^-$.

Since μ takes on at most one of the values $+\infty$ and $-\infty$. Therefore, at least one of the set functions μ^+ and μ^- is always finite.

☞ REMARKS

- Every signed measure is the difference of two measures (of which at least one is finite) the representation of μ as the difference of its upper and lower variations is called the Jordan decomposition of μ.
- If μ is a signed measure and if E is a measurable set, then
$$\mu^+(E) = \sup\{\mu(F) : E \supset F\} \quad \text{and} \quad \mu^-(E) = -\inf\{\mu(F) : E \supset F\}.$$
- If μ is a finite signed measure and if $<E_n>$ is a sequence of measurable sets such that $\lim_{n \to \infty} E_n$ exists *(i.e., $\overline{\lim} E_n = \underline{\lim} E_n$)* then $\mu(\lim_{n \to \infty} E_n) = \lim_{n \to \infty} \mu(E_n)$.
- If μ is a signed measure and f is a measurable function such that f is integrable with respect to $|\mu|$, then $\int f \, d\mu = \int f \, d\mu^+ - \int f \, d\mu^-$.

THEOREM 8. (Jordan Decomposition Theorem)

Let μ be a signed measure, μ^+ and μ^- on (X, S) with the following properties :

(i) $\mu = \mu^+ - \mu^-$ and at least one of the measure μ^+ and μ^- is finite.

(ii) $\mu^+ \perp \mu^-$, i.e., there exist disjoint sets $A, B \in S$ such that $\mu^+(B) = \mu^-(A) = 0$ and $A \cup B = X$.

(iii) If $\mu = \nu - \eta$, where ν and η are measures with at least one of them being finite and $\nu \perp \eta$, then $\mu^+ = \nu$ or η and μ^- equals the other.

(iv) In other words, the decomposition of μ as a difference of two singular measures is unique.

PROOF. Let $X = A \cup B$ be a Hahn decomposition of X with respect to μ, where A is a positive set for μ and B is a negative set for μ. Define μ^+ and μ^- on S as follows:

$$\mu^+(E) = \mu(A \cap E) \quad \text{and} \quad \mu^{-1}(E) = \mu(B \cap E), \ E \in S$$

Clearly, μ^+ and μ^- are measures on S with $\mu = \mu^+ - \mu^-$ and at least one of μ^+ and μ^- is finite, since μ takes at most one of the values $+\infty$ or $-\infty$. That $\mu^+ \perp \mu^-$ is obvious. Finally, let $\mu = \nu - \eta$, where ν and η are measures with $\nu \perp \eta$, and say ν is finite. Then μ never takes the value $+\infty$ and hence μ^+ is also finite. Let $C, D \in S$ be such that $\nu(C) = \eta(D) = 0$ with $C \cap D = \phi$ and $C \cup D = X$. Clearly, C is a positive set for μ and D is a negative set for μ. Thus, $C \cdot D$ is also a Hahn decomposition of X with respect to μ. Hence, we have $\forall E \in S$.

$$\mu^+(E) = \mu(E \cap A) = \mu(E \cap C) = \nu(E)$$

and
$$\mu^-(E) = \mu(E \cap B) = \mu(E \cap D) = \eta(E)$$

10.3 ABSOLUTE CONTINUITY OF SET FUNCTIONS

Definition 1. A finite signed measure together with its variations is said to be of bounded variation.

Definition 2. Two measure μ and ν are said to be mutually singular $(\mu \perp \nu)$ if there exists a measurable set $A \subset X$ such that

$$\mu(A) = 0 = \nu(X - A)$$

[MEERUT–2007 BP]

☞ REMARK
- The measures μ^+ and μ^- defined above are mutually singular.

Definition 3. Let μ be a signed measure on a measurable space $(X, \mathcal{A})$. Then measure μ is said to be absolutely continuous w.r.t. ν if and only if

$$\nu(A) = 0 \quad \forall A \in \mathcal{A} \implies \mu(A) = 0$$

It is denoted by $\mu \ll \nu$.

[MEERUT–2007 BP]

☞ REMARK
- If ν is σ-finite then μ is also σ-finite.

THEOREM 1.

Let μ and ν are signed measures, then following conditions are equivalent

(i) $\nu \ll \mu$

(ii) $\nu^+ \ll \mu$ and $\nu^- \ll \mu$

(iii) $|\nu| \ll |\mu|$

PROOF. Let (i) be valid.

Then $v(E) = 0$ whenever $|\mu|(E) = 0$.

If $X = A \cup B$ is a Hahn decomposition with respect to v, then we have whenever $|\mu|(E) = 0$.

$$0 \le |\mu|(E \cap A) \le |\mu|(E) = 0$$

and
$$0 \le |\mu|(E \cap B) \le |\mu|(E) = 0$$

Thus
$$v^+(E) = v(E \cap A) = 0$$

and $\quad v^-(E) = v(E \cap B) = 0$.

Hence, $v^+ \ll \mu$ and $v^- \ll \mu$.

This proves the validity of (ii).

Now using the relations

$$|v|(E) = v^+(E) + v^-(E)$$

and
$$0 \le |v(E)| \le |v|(E)$$

We can prove that (ii) implies (iii) and (iii) implies (i).

THEOREM 2.

If v is a finite signed measure and if μ is a signed measure such that $v \ll \mu$ corresponding to every positive number ϵ there is a positive number δ such that $|v|(E) < \epsilon$ for every measurable set E for which $|\mu|(E) < \delta$.

PROOF. Let us suppose that it is possible, for some $\epsilon > 0$, to find a sequence $< E_n >$ of measurable sets such that $|\mu|(E_n) < \dfrac{1}{2^n}$.

and $\quad |v|(E_n) \ge \epsilon, \quad n \in \mathbf{N}$

If $\quad\quad E = \lim E_n$

Then, $\quad |\mu|(E_n) \le \sum\limits_{i=n}^{\infty} |\mu|(E_i) < \dfrac{1}{2^{n-1}}, \quad n \in \mathbf{N}$

and therefore, $|\mu|(E) = 0$.

Also, since v is finite,
$$|v|(E) = \lim_{n \to \infty} |v|(E_n \cup E_{n+1} \cup \ldots\ldots)$$
$$\ge \lim |v|(E_n)$$
$$\ge \epsilon$$

which is a contradiction (because $v \ll \mu$)

Hence, corresponding to every positive number ϵ, there is a positive number δ such that $|v|(E) < \epsilon$ for every measurable set E for which $|\mu|(E) < \delta$.

☞ **REMARKS**
- The relation $\ll$ is reflexive and transitive.
- Two signed measures μ and v for which both $v \ll \mu$ and $\mu \ll v$ are called equivalent. It is written as $\mu \equiv v$.

THEOREM 3.

If μ and v are totally finite measures such that $v \ll \mu$ and v is not identically zero, then there exists a positive number $\epsilon > 0$ and a measurable set A such that $\mu(A) > 0$ and such that A is positive set for the signed measure $v - \epsilon \mu$.

PROOF. Let us suppose $X = A_n \cup B_n$ be a Hahn decomposition with respect to the signed measure $v - \frac{1}{n}\mu$, $n = 1, 2, \ldots$

We can write

$$A_0 = \bigcup_{n=1}^{\infty} A_n, \quad B_0 = \bigcap_{n=1}^{\infty} B_n$$

Since $B_0 \subset B_n$, we have

$$0 \le v(B_0) \le \frac{1}{n} \cdot \mu(B_0), \quad n = 1, 2, \ldots$$

and therefore, $v(B_0) = 0$.

It follows that $v(A_0) > 0$ and therefore, by absolute continuity, $\mu(A_0) > 0$. Hence, we must have $\mu(A_n) > 0$ for at least one value of n. Let us write $A_n = A$ and $\frac{1}{n} = \in$. Then, we can say that for a positive number ε and a measurable set A such that $\mu(A) > 0$ and such that A is a positive set for signed measure $v - \in \mu$.

SOME IMPORTANT RESULTS

(1) If μ is a signed measure and f is a function integrable with respect to $|\mu|$ and if v is defined for every measurable set E by $v(E) = \int_E f \, d\mu$, then $v \ll \mu$.

(2) For every signed measure μ, the variations μ^+ and μ^- are mutually singular and they are each absolutely continuous with respect to μ.

(3) For every signed measure μ, $|\mu| \equiv \mu$.

(4) If μ is a signed measure and E is a measurable set, then $|\mu|(E) = 0$ if and only if $\mu(F) = 0$ for every measurable subset F of E.

(5) If μ and v are any two measures on a σ-ring, then $v \ll \mu + v$.

(6) Let f_1 and f_2 be integrable functions on a totally finite measure space and let μ_i be the indefinite integral of $f_i : i = 1, 2, \ldots$. If $\mu(\{x_i, f_1(x) = 0\} \Delta \{x : f_2(x) = 0\}) = 0$, then $\mu_1 \equiv \mu_2$.

(7) If μ and v are signed measures such that v is both absolutely continuous and singular with respect to μ, then $v = 0$.

(8) If v_1, v_2 and μ are finite signed measures such that both v_1 and v_2 are singular with respect to μ, then $v = v_1 + v_2$ is also singular with respect to μ.

(9) If μ and v are measures on a σ-algebra such that μ is finite and $v \ll \mu$ then there exists a measurable set E such that $X - E$ is of σ-finite measure with respect to v and such that for every measurable subset F of E, $v(F)$ is either 0 or ∞.

10.4 RADON NIKODYM THEOREM

STATEMENT. Let $(X, \mathcal{A}, \mu)$ be a σ-finite measure space. Let v be a measure defined on $\mathcal{A}$ such that v is absolutely continuous with respect to μ. Then there exists a non-negative measurable function f such that

$$v(E) = \int_E f \, d\mu \quad \forall E \in \mathcal{A}$$

The function f is unique in the sense that if g is any measurable function with this property, then g(x) = f(x) almost everywhere in X with respect to μ.

[MEERUT–2007, 09; BURDWAN–1990]

PROOF.

Let us suppose that μ is finite.

If μ is finite then $v - \alpha\mu$ is a signed measure on $\mathcal{A}$ for each rational number α. Let us assume that T denotes the set of all non-negative rational numbers. Then for every $t \in T$, let (P_i, Q_i) be a Hahn decomposition for the signed measure $v - t\mu$. If $\alpha \geq t$, then Q_t is negative for $v - \alpha\mu$.

Further, if E is a measurable subset of Q_t, then

$$v(E) - \alpha\mu(E) \leq v(E) - t$$
$$\Rightarrow \quad v(E) - \alpha\mu(E) \leq v(E) - t\mu(E) \leq 0$$
$$\Rightarrow \quad v(E) - \alpha\mu(E) \leq 0$$
$$\Rightarrow \quad (v - \alpha\mu)(E) \leq 0$$

Similarly, P_t is positive for each signed measure $v - \alpha\mu$ if $\alpha \leq t$. Let

$$P = \cap(P_t : t \in T)$$

Since each P_t is measurable and we know that countable collection of measurable sets is measurable, therefore P is measurable.

Let E be any measurable subset of P.

Then, $\quad E \subset P = \cap P_t \Rightarrow E \subset \cap P_t \subset P \quad \forall t \in T$

$$\Rightarrow E \subset P_t \quad \forall t \in T$$
$$\Rightarrow (v - t\mu) \, E \geq 0 \qquad\qquad [\because P_t \text{ is positive }]$$
$$\Rightarrow v(E) - t\mu(E) \geq 0$$
$$\Rightarrow v(E) \geq t\mu(E) \Rightarrow t\mu(E) \leq v(E) \quad \forall \, t \in T$$
$$\Rightarrow \mu(E) = 0 \quad \text{or} \quad v(E) = \infty$$

Next, define a non-negative function.

$$f : X \to (-\infty, \infty)$$

such that $\quad f(x) = \inf\{t \in T : x \in Q_t\} \quad \forall x \in X$

We know that the infimum of any empty collection of real numbers is 0.

$\therefore \qquad\qquad f(x) = 0 \quad \forall x \in P$

Now, let $r \in R$ and $q \in Q$ be arbitrary.

Let us write $\quad S_q = \cup\{Q_t : \forall \, t < q\}$

$\qquad\qquad\qquad = $ Measurable $\qquad (\because$ union of measurable sets is measurable)

Now, we define f such that

$$\{x \in X : f(x) \leq r\} = \cap[S_q : q \in Q \text{ such that } q > r]$$

$\qquad\qquad\qquad = $ Measurable $\qquad$ (Being the intersection of measurable sets)

Therefore, $\{x \in X : f(x) \leq r\}$ is measurable.

$\Rightarrow$ f is measurable.

Next, we want to show that

$$v(E) = \int_E f \, d\mu \quad \forall E \in \mathcal{A}$$

Let $\quad \mu(E \cap P) = 0$

If $\mu(E \cap P) > 0$, then $v(E \cap P) = 0$

and $\quad \int_E f \, d\mu \geq \int_{E \cap P} d\mu = \infty$

Because $f(x) = 0$, $\forall\, x \in P$, therefore $f : E \to (-\infty, \infty)$ is not integrable.

$$\int_E f\, d\mu = \infty$$

Thus, $\quad \nu(E) = \int_E f\, d\mu$

which implies that result is true in case of $\mu\, (E \cap P) > 0$.

Since $\nu\, (E \cap P) = 0$ for absolute continuity of ν with respect to μ.

Choose a positive integer n such that

$$E_k = \left\{ x \in E : \frac{k-1}{n} < f(x) \le \frac{k}{n} \right\}$$

$\Rightarrow\; E_k \subset \{ x \in X : f(x) \le n \} \subset S_q = \cup [Q_t : \forall\, t < q]$ for each rational number $q < \dfrac{k}{n}$.

Since Q_t is a negative set for the signed measure $\nu - q\mu$ and E_k is a subset of Q_t.

Thus, E_k is a negative set.

$\therefore \quad (\nu - q\mu)\, (E_k) \le 0$

$\Rightarrow \qquad \nu\, (E_k) \le\, q\, \mu(E_k)$

$\Rightarrow \qquad \nu(E_k) \le \dfrac{k}{n}\, \mu\, (E_k)$ \hfill ...(1)

Also, since $\quad E_k \subset \left\{ x \in X : f(x) > \dfrac{k-1}{n} \right\} \subset P_{(k-1)/n}$

$\Rightarrow \left(\nu - \dfrac{k-1}{n}\, \mu \right) (E_k) \ge 0$, for $P_{(k-1)/n}$ is positive.

$\Rightarrow \qquad \nu\, (E_k) \ge \left(\dfrac{k-1}{n} \right) \mu\, (E_k)$. \hfill ...(2)

Using (1) and (2), we conclude that

$$\left(\frac{k-1}{n} \right) \mu(E_k) \le \nu(E_k) \le \frac{k}{n}\, \mu\, (E_k). \hspace{2cm} ...(3)$$

Now, since E is a disjoint union of sets $E \cap P$ and E_k

$\Rightarrow \qquad \mu\, (E \cap P) = 0\; =\; \nu\, (E \cap P)$

By countable additive property of integrals, we get

$$\int_E f\, d\mu\; =\; \sum_{k=0}^{\infty} \int_{E_k} f\, d\mu \;\text{ and } \nu(E) = \sum_{k=0}^{\infty} \nu\, (E_k)$$

Now, by definition of E_k

$$\frac{k-1}{n} \le f(x) \le \frac{k}{n} \text{ on } E_k.$$

Applying first mean value theorem, we get

$$\frac{k-1}{n}\, \mu\, (E_k) \le \int_{E_k} f\, d\mu \le \frac{k}{n}\, \mu\, (E_k). \hspace{2cm} ...(4)$$

Using (3) and (4), we conclude that

$$\frac{k-1}{n}\, \mu\, (E_k) \le \int_{E_k} f\, d\mu - \nu(E_k) \le \frac{k}{n}\, \mu\, (E_k)$$

Summing this result over k, we get

$$-\frac{1}{n}\, \mu\, (E) \le \int_E f\, (x)\, d\mu - \nu(E) \le \frac{1}{n}\, \mu\, (E)$$

Letting $n \to \infty$, we get

$$0 \le \int_E f(x)\, d\mu - v(E) \le 0$$

$$\Rightarrow \quad \int_E f(x)\, d\mu = v(E) \qquad\qquad \dots(5)$$

Now, it remains to prove the almost uniqueness of the function $f : X \to [-\infty, \infty]$. Let, if possible, there exists a function

$$g : X \to [-\infty, \infty]$$

which is measurable and satisfying the condition

$$v(E) = \int_E g\, d\mu \qquad \forall\, E \in \mathcal{A}$$

Define $\quad A_n = \{ x \in X : f(x) - g(x) \ge \dfrac{1}{n} \} \in \mathcal{A}$

and $\quad B_n = \{ x \in X : g(x) - f(x) \ge \dfrac{1}{n} \} \in \mathcal{A}$

Then, clearly $\quad f(x) - g(x) \ge \dfrac{1}{n}$ on A_n.

Then, applying first mean value theorem, we get

$$\int_{A_n} (f - g)\, d\mu \ge \frac{1}{n}\mu(A_n)$$

$$\Rightarrow \quad \int_{A_n} f\, d\mu - \int_{A_n} g\, d\mu \ge \frac{1}{n}\mu(A_n).$$

Using (5) in the above equation, we get

$$v(A_n) - v(A_n) \ge \frac{1}{n}\mu(A_n)$$

$$\Rightarrow \qquad \mu(A_n) \le 0$$

But $\qquad \mu(A_n) \ge 0$

$\therefore \qquad \mu(A_n) = 0.$

Similarly, we can assume that $\mu(B_n) = 0$.

Define $\quad C = \{ x \in X : f(x) \ne g(x) \} = \bigcup_{n=1}^{\infty} (A_n \cup B_n)$

Then, $\qquad \mu(C) = \sum_n \mu(A_n) + \sum \mu(B_n)$

$$= \Sigma.0 + \Sigma.0 = 0$$

$$\Rightarrow \qquad \mu(C) = 0$$

Therefore, $f = g$ almost everywhere on X w.r.t. μ.

☞ REMARKS

• The function $f : X \to [-\infty, \infty]$ defined in the above theorem is known as Radon Nikodym derivative of the measure v w.r.t. μ. It is denoted by $f = \dfrac{dv}{d\mu}$.

• The Radon-Nikodym theorem is not necessarily true if μ is not totally σ-finite even if v remains finite.

• The Radon-Nikodym theorem remains true even if μ is only a signed measure.

• The Radon-Nikodym theorem remains true even if v is not σ-finite but in this case the integral f is not necessarily finite valued.

THEOREM.

Let μ, ν be a σ-finite signed measures on (X, S) such that $\nu \ll \mu$. Then there is a real valued measurable function f on X such that $\forall E \in S$

$$r(E) = \int_E f \, d\mu$$

Further, f is unique in the sense that if g is any other real measurable function on X such that

$$r(E) = \int_E g \, d\mu, \quad \forall E \in S$$

then $f(x) = g(x)$ for a.e. $x(|\mu|)$.

PROOF. Let A, B be a Hahn decomposition of X with respect to μ.

Then, $\forall E \in S$

$$\mu^+(E) = \mu(A \cap E) \text{ and } \mu^-(E) = -\mu(B \cap E)$$

For $E \subseteq A$, $\mu(E) = \mu^+(E) + \mu^-(E) = |\mu|(E)$.

Thus $\mu^+(E) = 0 = |\mu|(E) = 0$ implies that $r(E) = 0$.

Hence, $r \ll \mu^+$ on $(A, S \cap A)$. Since both ν and μ^+ are σ-finite, which gives a measurable function f_A on A such that $\forall E \in A \cap S$

$$\nu(E) = \int_E f_A \, d\mu^+$$

Similarly, we will have a measurable function f_B on B such that $\forall E \in B \cap S$,

$$\nu(E) = \int_E f_B \, d\mu^-$$

Define $f_A = 0$ on B and $f_B = 0$ on A. Then $f := f_A + f_B$ is a measurable function on X and $\forall E \in S$,

$$r(A) = \nu(E \cap A) + \nu(E \cap B)$$

$$= \int_{E \cap A} f_A \, d\mu^+ + \int_{E \cap B} f_B \, d\mu^-$$

$$= \int_E f d\mu^+ + \int_E f d\mu^- = \int_E f d\mu$$

The unique of f follows from the fact that $f_A(x)$ is unique for a.e. $x(\mu^+)$ and the fact that $f_B(x)$ is unique for a.e. $x(\mu^-)$ and the fact that $\mu^+ \ll |\mu|$, $\mu^- \ll |\mu|$.

SOME IMPORTANT OBSERVATIONS

(1) There is a condition of measure spaces, which is more general than total σ-finiteness and more restrictive than σ-finiteness, in the presence of which the Radon-Nikodym theorem is still true. The condition is that the space be the union of a disjoint class D of measurable sets of finite measure with the property that every measurable set may be covered by countably many sets of D and a set of measure zero. For example, let X be the Euclidean plane, and let S be the class of all those sets which may be covered by countably many horizontal lines and which are Lebesgue measurable on each such line. If E is a Lebesgue measurable subset of a horizontal line, define $\mu(E)$ to be the Lebesgue measure of E for the general E in S, μ is thereby uniquely determined by the requirement of countable additivity.

(2) If $(X, \mathcal{A})$ is a measurable space and μ and ν are σ-finite measures on $\mathcal{A}$ such that $\nu \ll \mu$, then the Radon-Nikodym theorem may be applied to each measurable set separately. It must be noted that there is no need to define the function once for all on the whole space X so as to serve as a suitable integrand simultaneously for every measurable set.

10.5 DERIVATIVES OF SIGNED MEASURES

If μ is a totally σ-finite measure and

$$v(E) = \int_E f \, d\mu \text{ for every measurable set } E.$$

Then, we can write $f = \dfrac{dv}{d\mu}$ or $dv = f \, d\mu$.

This derivative is known as Radon-Nikodym derivatives.

☞ REMARK

- The Radon-Nikodym derivative $\dfrac{dv}{d\mu}$ is unique almost everywhere with respect to μ.

AN IMPORTANT NOTATION

If, for each point x of a measurable space $(X, \mathcal{A})$, $\pi(x)$ is a projection concerning x and if μ is a signed measure on $\mathcal{A}$, then the symbol

$$\pi(x)[\mu] \text{ or } \pi[\mu]$$

shall mean that $\pi(x)$ is true for almost everywhere x with respect to the measure $[\mu]$. For example, if f and g are two functions on X, we shall write $f = g \, [\mu]$ for the statement that $\{x : g(x) \neq g(x)\}$ is a measurable set of measure zero with respect to $|\mu|$. The symbol $|\mu|$ may be read as "modulo μ".

THEOREM I.

If λ and μ are totally σ-finite measures such that $\mu \ll \lambda$, and if v is a totally σ-finite measures such that $v \ll \mu$, then

$$\frac{dv}{d\lambda} = \frac{dv}{d\mu} \cdot \frac{d\mu}{d\lambda} [\lambda].$$

PROOF. Let us write $\dfrac{dv}{d\mu} = f$ and $\dfrac{d\mu}{d\lambda} = g$

Since v is non-negative, then, we have

$$f \geq 0 [\mu]$$

and therefore, without loss of any generality, we assume that f is everywhere non-negative.

Let $< f_n >$ be an increasing sequence of non-negative simple function which converging at every point to f.

Then, $\displaystyle\lim_{n \to \infty} \int_E f_n \, d\mu = \int_E f \, d\mu$

and $\displaystyle\lim_{n \to \infty} \int_E f_n \, g \, d\lambda = \int_E f \, g \, d\lambda$, for every measurable set E.

Now, since for every measurable set F

$$\int X_F \, d\mu = \mu(E \cap F) = \int_{E \cap F} g \, d\lambda = \int_E X_F \, g \, d\lambda.$$

Therefore, $\int_E f_n \, d\mu = \int_E f_n \, g \, d\lambda, \; n = 1, 2, \ldots$

Hence, $v(E) = \int_E f \, d\mu = \int_E f \, g \, d\lambda$.

Finally, using the usual notations, we can write $\dfrac{dv}{d\lambda} = \dfrac{dv}{d\mu} \cdot \dfrac{d\mu}{d\lambda} [\lambda].$

THEOREM 2.

If λ *and* μ *are totally* σ*-finite measures such that* $\mu \ll \lambda$ *and f is a finite valued measurable function for which* $\int f \, d\mu$ *is defined, then*

$$\int f \, d\mu = \int f \frac{d\mu}{d\lambda} . d\lambda .$$

PROOF.   Let E be any measurable set. Then, by Radon-Nikodym theorem, we have

$$v(E) = \int_E f \, d\mu .$$

Now, using previous theorem, we can write

$$v(E) = \int_E f \frac{d\mu}{d\lambda} . d\lambda , \text{ for every measurable set } E.$$

Generalising this result, we get

$$v(E) = \int_X f \frac{d\mu}{d\lambda} . d\lambda$$

10.6 LEBESGUE DECOMPOSITION

Now, we have to study concerning the relations among signed measures treats the Lebesgue decomposition of a totally σ-finite signed measure into an absolutely continuous part and a singular part with respect to another totally σ-finite signed measure.

THEOREM 1. (Lebesgue Decomposition Theorem)

Let $(X, \mathcal{A}, \mu)$ *be a* σ*-finite measurable space and* v *a* σ*-finite measure defined on* $\mathcal{A}$*. Then, there exist two uniquely determined measures* v_0 *and* v_1 *such that*

$$v = v_0 + v_1, \quad v_0 \perp \mu, \quad v_1 \ll \mu \qquad \text{[MEERUT–2005 BP, 07BP; KANPUR–2005]}$$

PROOF.   Let us write $\lambda = \mu + v$.

Since μ and v are σ-finite, therefore, λ is σ-finite. Clearly $\mu \ll \lambda$ and $v \ll \lambda$, where $\mu \ll \lambda$ means 'μ is absolutely continuous w.r.t. λ'.

Using Radon-Nikodym theorem, we can find non-negative functions f and g from X to $[-\infty, \infty]$, such that

$$\mu(E) = \int_E f \, d\lambda, \quad v(E) = \int_E g \, d\lambda, \quad \forall E \in \mathcal{A}$$

Write $A = \{ x \in X : f(x) > 0 \}, \quad B = \{ x \in X : f(x) = 0 \}$

Then, clearly $X = A \cup B, \quad A \cap B = \phi$

Also, $\mu(B) = \int_B f \, d\lambda = 0$

Next, define two functions v_0 and v_1, *i.e.,*

$$v_0, v_1 : \mathcal{A} \to [-\infty, \infty]$$

such that $v_0(E) = v(E \cap B)$

$$v_1(E) = v(E \cap A), \quad \forall E \in \mathcal{A}.$$

Then, v_0 and v_1 are measures on $\mathcal{A}$ with the condition

$$v = v_0 + v_1$$

$$v_0(A) = v(A \cap B) = v(\phi) = 0 \quad \text{or} \quad v_0(A) = 0 .$$

Therefore, $\mu(B) = 0 = v_0(A) = v_0(X - B)$

$\Rightarrow$ $\mu(B) = 0 = v_0(X - B)$

which implies that v_0 is mutually singular to μ

$\Rightarrow \qquad\qquad v_0 \perp \mu$

Now, to show that $v_1 \ll \mu$

Let $E \in \mathcal{A}$ be arbitrary such that $\mu(E) = 0$

Then, $\quad \int_E f \, d\lambda = \mu(E) = 0$

$\Rightarrow \qquad \int_E f \, d\lambda = 0.$

Also, $\qquad f(x) \geq 0 \quad \forall \, x \in E$

Therefore, $f = 0$ almost everywhere on E relative to λ.

Since $f > 0$ on $A \cap E$ and therefore

$$v_1(E) = v(E \cap A) \qquad \text{(By definition of } v_1)$$
$$\leq \lambda(E \cap A) = 0$$

$\Rightarrow \qquad v_1(E) \leq 0$

But, $\qquad v_1(E) \geq 0 \quad \Rightarrow \quad v_1(E) = 0.$

Thus, we conclude that $v_1(E) = 0$ for $\mu(E) = 0$

Hence, $v_1 \ll \mu$.

It remains to prove the uniqueness of v_0 and v_1.

Let if possible there exist two measures v_0' and v_1' such that $v = v_0' + v_1'$ and with the same property as that of the measures v_0 and v_1, respectively.

Then, $v = v_0 + v_1$ and $v = v_0' + v_1'$.

Therefore, $v = v_0 + v_1$ and $v = v_0' + v_1'$ are two Lebesgue decompositions of v.

We have $v_0 - v_0' = v_1' - v_1$

Further, $v_1' - v_1$ is absolutely continuous and $v_0 - v_0'$ is singular relative to v.

Thus, $v_0 = v_0'$ and $v_1 = v_1'$.

Hence, v_0 and v_1 are unique.

THEOREM 2.

Let A and B be two measurable sets and v be a signed measures such that $A \subset B$ and $|v(B)| < \infty$. Then, $|v(A)| < \infty$.

PROOF. Since $A \subset B$, then we can write

$$B = (B - A) + A, \quad (B - A) \cap A = \phi.$$

$\Rightarrow \qquad v(B) = v(B - A) + v(A)$

If $v(B - A)$ and $v(A)$ both are ∞, then $v(B)$ is ∞. If $v(B - A)$ or $v(A)$ is ∞, then $v(B)$ is ∞.

It is given that $|v(B)| < \infty$, *i.e.*, $v(B)$ is finite.

Hence, $v(B)$ will be finite if both $v(B - A)$ and $v(A)$ are finite. Therefore, $|v(A)| < \infty$.

10.7 RIESZ REPRESENTATION THEOREM

Riesz representation theorem is an application of Radon-Nikodym theorem. Here, we shall present theorems concerning the representation of bounded linear functional on the space L_p, $1 \leq p < \infty$.

(1) **Linear Functional :** A linear functional on L_p $(X, \mathcal{A}, \mu)$ is a mapping T of L_p into R such that

$$T(af + bg) = aT(f) + bT(g), \qquad \forall\, a, b \in R$$
$$f, g \in L_p$$

(2) **Bounded Linear Functional :** The linear functional T is bounded if there exists a constant M such that

$$|T(f)| \leq M \left\| f \right\|_p, \qquad \forall\, f \in L_p$$

In this case, the bound or the norm of T is defined by

$$\left\| T \right\| = \sup \{\, |T(f)| : f \in L_p, \; \left\| f \right\|_p \leq 1 \}$$

☞ **REMARKS**

- If $g \in L_q$ (where $q = \infty$, when $p = 1$ and $q = p(p-1)$, otherwise) and if we define T on L_p by $T(f) = \int fg\, d\mu$.

  Then T is a linear functional with norm at most equal to $\left\| g \right\|_q$.

- Any bounded linear functional on L_p can be written as the difference of two positive linear functional.

THEOREM 3.

Let T be a bounded linear functional on L_p. Then there exist two positive bounded linear functional T^+, T^- such that

$$T(f) = T^+(f) - T^-(f) \;\; \text{for all } f \in L_p.$$

PROOF. Let $f \geq 0$

Define $T^+(f) = \sup\{\, T(g) : g \in L_p, \; 0 \leq g \leq f \}$.

Clearly, $T^+(cf) = cT^+(f)$ for $c \geq 0$ and $f \geq 0$

If $0 \leq g_j \leq f_j$, then

$$T(g_1) + T(g_2) = T(g_1 + g_2) \leq T^+(f_1 + f_2)$$

Taking the supremum over all g_j in L_p, we get

$$T^+(f_1) + T^+(f_2) \leq T^+(f_1 + f_2). \qquad \ldots(1)$$

Conversely, if $0 \leq h \leq f_1 + f_2$

Define $\qquad g_1 = \sup(h - f_2, 0)$

and $\qquad g_2 = \inf(h, f_2)$

$\therefore \qquad g_1 + g_2 = h$ and $0 \leq g_j \leq f_j$

Thus, $\qquad T(h) = T(g_1) + T(g_2)$

$$\leq T^+(f_1) + T^+(f_2). \qquad \ldots(2)$$

Since the above inequality holds for all such $h \in L_p$, we get

$$T^+(f_1 + f_2) = T^+(f_1) + T^+(f_2), \text{ for all } f_j \text{ in } L_p, \; f_j \geq 0.$$

If f is an arbitrary element of L_p, define

$$T^+(f) = T^+(f^+) - T^+(f^-)$$

Then, we can easily show that T^+ is a bounded linear functional on L_p.

Next, define T^{-1} for $f \in L_p$ by

$$T^-(f) = T^+(f) - T(f)$$

so that T^{-1} is clearly a bounded linear functional on L_p. From the definition of T^+, it is seen that T^{-1} is a positive linear functional and obviously, we have

$$T = T^+ - T^-$$

THEOREM 4. (Riesz Representation Theorem)

For $p = 1$, Let $(X, \mathcal{A}, \mu)$ be a σ-finite measurable space and T is a bounded linear functional on $L_1(X, \mathcal{A}, \mu)$, then there exists a $g \in L_\infty(X, \mathcal{A}, \mu)$ such that equation

$$T(f) = \int f\, g\, d\mu$$

holds for all f. Moreover $\|T\| = \|g\|_\infty$ and $g \geq 0$ if T is a positive linear functional.

[MEERUT-2006, 07, 13]

PROOF. Let us suppose that $\mu(X) < \infty$ and that T is positive. Define λ on $\mathcal{A}$ to R by $\lambda(E) = T_{\chi_E}$.

Clearly, $\lambda(\phi) = 0$.

If $< E_n >$ is an increasing sequence in X and $E = \bigcup E_n$

Then, $< \chi_{E_n} >$ converges pointwise to χ_E.

Since $\mu(X) < \infty$, then the sequence converges in L_1 to χ_E.

Since
$$0 \leq \lambda(E) - \lambda(E_n) = T(\chi_E) - T(\chi_{E_n})$$

$$= T(\chi_E - \chi_{E_n})$$

$$\leq \|T\| \, \|\chi_E - \chi_{E_n}\|_1$$

Therefore, λ is a measure.

Also, if $M \in \mathcal{A}$ and $\mu(M) = 0$, then $\lambda(M) = 0$, so that $\lambda << \mu$.

Applying Radon-Nikodym theorem, we obtain a non-negative measurable function on X to R such that

$$T(\chi_E) = \lambda(E) = \int \chi_E\, g\, d\mu, \quad \forall\, E \in \mathcal{A}$$

Then, by linearity, we have

$$T(\psi) = \int \psi\, g\, d\mu, \text{ for all } \mathcal{A}\text{-measurable simple function } \psi.$$

If f is a non-negative function in L_1, let $< \psi_n >$ be a monotonic increasing sequence of simple functions converging almost everywhere and in L_1 to f. Using the boundedness of T, it is seen that

$$T(f) = \lim T(\psi_n)$$

Also, by Monotone convergence theorem, we have

$$T(f) = \lim_{n \to \infty} \int \psi_n \, g \, d\mu = \int f \, g \, d\mu$$

If $X = \bigcup F_n$, where $< F_n >$ is an increasing sequence of sets in $\mathcal{A}$ with finite measure, therefore,

$$T(f \chi_{F_n}) = \int f \chi_{F_n} \, g_n \, d\mu, \qquad \forall f \in L_p$$

If $m \le n$, it is easily seen that

$$g_m(x) = g_n(x) \text{ for almost all } x \text{ in } F_m.$$

Therefore, we get a function g which represent T.

If T is an arbitrary bounded linear functional on L_1, then using previous theorem, we can write $T = T^+ - T^-$.

where T^+ and T^- are bounded positive linear functionals. Next, we get non-negative functions g^+ and g^- which represents T^+, T^-. If we get $g = g^+ - g^-$.

We get $\quad T(f) = \int fg \, d\mu \qquad \forall f \in L_1$.

☞ **REMARK**

- The general Riesz-representation theorem can be stated as follows : "If $(X, \mathcal{A}, \mu)$ is an arbitrary measure space and T is a bounded linear functional on $L_p(X, \mathcal{A}, \mu), 1 < p < \infty$, then there exists a g in $L_q(X, \mathcal{A}, \mu)$, where $q = \dfrac{p}{p-1}$ s.t. $T(f) = \int f g \, d\mu$ holds for all f in L_p. Moreover, $\|T\| = \|g\|_q$.

10.8 CARATHEODORY EXTENSION

Definition. *A subset E of X is said to μ^*-measurable (μ^* = outer measure of μ) if*

$$\mu^*(A) = \mu^*(A \cap E) + \mu^*(A \mid E),$$

where $\qquad A \mid E = A' = E - A$ *for all subset A of X.*

The collection of all μ^*-measurable sets is denoted by A^*.

THEOREM. (Caratheodory Extension Theorem)

The collection A^* of all μ^*-measurable sets is σ-algebra containing A. Also if $< E_n >$ is a disjoint sequence in A^*, then

$$\mu^*\left(\bigcup_{n=1}^{\infty} E_n \right) = \sum_{n=1}^{\infty} \mu^*(E_n)' \qquad \text{[MEERUT–2007, 07BP, 09, 15; DELHI–2012]}$$

PROOF. By definition, we have

ϕ and X are μ^*-measurable, *i.e.*, outer measurable. Also, if $E \in A^*$, then E' is also outer measurable, therefore

$$E' \in A^*$$

Now, we shall prove that A^* is closed under intersections.

Let us suppose that E and F are μ^*-measurable. Then, for any $A \subset X$ and $E \in A^*$, we have

$$\mu^*(A \cap F) = \mu^*(A \cap F \cap E) + \mu^*((A \cap F) \mid E) \qquad \ldots(1)$$

Since $F \in A^*$, then

$$\mu^*(A) = \mu^*(A \cap F) + \mu^*(A \mid F). \qquad \ldots(2)$$

Let us write $B = A \mid (E \cap F)$.

Then, it is easily seen that

$$B \cap F = (A \cap F) \mid E$$

and $\qquad B \mid F = A \mid F.$

Since $F \in A^*$, it follows that

$$\mu^*(A \mid (E \cap F) = \mu^*((A \cap F) \mid E) + \mu^*(A \mid F) \qquad \ldots(3)$$

Combining (1), (2) and (3), we get

$$\mu^*(A) = \mu^*(A \cap E \cap F) + \mu^*(A \mid (E \cap F))$$

Therefore, $E \cap F$ belongs to A^*.

Since A^* is closed under intersection and complementation, therefore A^* is an algebra.

Now, suppose that Λ^* is a σ-algebra and μ^* is countably additive on A^*.

Let $< E_k >$ be a disjoint sequence in A^* and let $E = \bigcup E_k$.

We know that $F_n = \bigcup\limits_{k=1}^{n} E_k$ belongs to A^*.

and that if A is any subset of X, then

$$\mu^*(A) = \mu^*(A \cap F_n) + \mu^*(A \mid F_n)$$

$$= \sum_{k=1}^{n} \mu^*(A \cap E_k) + \mu^*(A \mid F_n) \qquad \ldots(4)$$

Since $F_n \subset E$, then $A \mid E \subseteq A \mid F_n$ and letting $n \to \infty$, (4) gives

$$\sum_{k=1}^{\infty} \mu^*(A \cap E_k) + \mu^*(A \mid E) \le \mu^*(A) \qquad \ldots(5)$$

But, we know that

$$\mu^*(A \cap E) \le \sum_{k=1}^{\infty} \mu^*(A \cap E_k) \qquad \ldots(6)$$

$$\mu^*(A) \le \mu^*(A \cap E) + \mu^*(A \mid E) \qquad \ldots(7)$$

On combining (5), (6) and (7), we get

$$\mu^*(A) = \mu^*(A \cap E) + \mu^*(A \mid E)$$

$$= \sum_{k=1}^{\infty} \mu^*(A \cap E_k) + \mu^*(A \mid E).$$

In particular, this shows that $E = \bigcup\limits_{k=1}^{\infty} E_k$ is μ^*-measurable.

Then taking $A = E$, then by definition of measure, we have

$$\mu^*\left(\bigcup_{n=1}^{\infty} E_n\right) = \sum_{n=1}^{\infty} \mu^*(E_n).$$

Finally, it remains to prove that $A \subset A^*$. We know that if $E \in \mathcal{A}$, then

$$\mu^*(E) = \mu(E).$$

But we need to show that E is μ^*-measurable.

Let A be any arbitrary subset of X, then

$$\mu^*(A) \le \mu^*(A \cap E) + \mu^*(A | E).$$

Let $\epsilon > 0$ be arbitrary and let $< F_n >$ be a sequence in $\mathcal{A}$ such that $A \subset \bigcup F_n$ and

$$\sum_{n=1}^{\infty} \mu(F_n) \le \mu^*(A) + \epsilon.$$

Since $A \cap E \subseteq \bigcup(F_n \cap E)$ and $A | E \subseteq \bigcup(F_n | E)$, therefore

$$\mu^*(A \cap E) \le \sum_{n=1}^{\infty} \mu(F_n \cap E), \qquad \mu^*(A | E) \le \sum_{n=1}^{\infty} \mu(F_n | E).$$

Hence, we have

$$\mu^*(A \cap E) + \mu^*(A | E) \le \sum_{n=1}^{\infty} \left\{\mu(F_n \cap E) + \mu(F_n | E)\right\}$$

$$= \sum_{n=1}^{\infty} \mu(F_n) \le \mu^*(A) + \epsilon.$$

Since ϵ is arbitrary. Hence, the desired inequality is established.

☛ **REMARKS**
- The above theorem shows that a measure μ on an algebra $\mathcal{A}$ can always be extended to a measure μ^* on a σ-algebra $\mathcal{A}^*$ containing $\mathcal{A}$.
- The σ-algebra $\mathcal{A}^*$ obtained (Remark 1) is automatically complete in the sense that if $E \in \mathcal{A}^*$ with $\mu^*(E) = 0$ and if $B \subset E$, then $B \in \mathcal{A}^*$ and $\mu^*(B) = 0$.

10.9 HAHN EXTENSION THEOREM

STATEMENT :

Let μ be a σ-finite measure on an algebra $\mathcal{A}$, then there exists a unique extension of μ to a measure on $\mathcal{A}^*$.

PROOF.   In the above theorem, we have already proved that μ^* gives a measure on $\mathcal{A}^*$. To establish the uniqueness, let ν be a measure on $\mathcal{A}^*$ which agrees with μ on $\mathcal{A}$. Firstly, suppose that μ and therefore μ^* and ν are finite measures. Let E be any set in $\mathcal{A}^*$ and let $< E_n >$ be a sequence in $\mathcal{A}$ such that $E \subset \bigcup E_n$. Since ν is a measure and agrees with μ on $\mathcal{A}$, we have

$$\nu(E) \le \nu\left(\bigcup_{n=1}^{\infty} E_n\right) \le \sum_{n=1}^{\infty} \nu(E_n) = \sum_{n=1}^{\infty} \mu(E_n)$$

Thus, $\nu(E) \le \mu^*(E)$ for any $E \in \mathcal{A}^*$.

Since μ^* and v are additive, therefore,

$$\mu^*(E) + \mu^*(X \mid E) = v(E) + v(X \mid E).$$

The terms on RHS are finite and not greater than the corresponding terms on the left side, we get

$$\mu^*(E) = v(E) \text{ for all } E \in \mathcal{A}^*.$$

which gives the uniqueness, when μ is a finite measure.

Now, suppose that μ is σ-finite and let $< F_n >$ be an increasing sequence of sets in $\mathcal{A}$, with $\mu(F_n) < +\infty$ and $X = \bigcup F_n$. Therefore, we conclude that

$$\mu^*(E \cap F_n) = v(E \cap F_n), \text{ for each } E \text{ in } \mathcal{A}^*.$$

Thus, $\mu^*(E) = \lim \mu^*(E \cap F_n) = \lim v(E \cap F_n) = v(E)$

Hence, μ^* and v agree on $\mathcal{A}^*$.

Exercise 10.1

1. If μ and v are totally σ-finite signed measures such that $\mu \equiv v$, then show that

$$\frac{d\mu}{dv} \equiv \frac{1}{(dv/d\mu)}.$$

2. If $< E_n >$ is a sequence of measurable sets such that $\bar{\mu}_n(E_n) = 0, n = 1, 2, \dots$, then show that $\mu (\limsup_n E_n) = 0$.

3. If v and μ are totally σ-finite signed measures such that $v \ll \mu$, then show that

$$v\left(\left\{x : \frac{dv}{d\mu}(x) = 0\right\}\right) = 0.$$

4. Prove that the set of absolutely continuous function is a linear space.

5. Prove that the product of two absolutely continuous function is again absolutely continuous.

6. Suppose f is differentiable at every point. If f' is bounded on every bounded interval, then f is absolutely continuous and hence

$$f(t) = \int_0^t f' \, dx + f(0).$$

7. Prove that the function f defined by

$$f(x) = \begin{cases} x^2 \left| \sin\dfrac{1}{x} \right| & \text{for } x \neq 0 \\ 0 & \text{for } x = 0 \end{cases}$$

is absolutely continuous (and non-negative) but $\sqrt{f}$ is not absolutely continuous.

8. If μ is a complex measure, show that $\mu = \mu_{real} + i\,\mu_{imag}$, where μ_{real} and μ_{imag} are signed measures.

9. If λ is a signed measure on a σ-ring, show that $|\lambda|(E) = \sup \sum_j |\lambda(E_j)|$, where the summation is taken over all finite partitions $E = \bigcup_{j=1}^{n} E_j$ of E into disjoint sets in $\mathcal{A}$.

10. For the measure v defined by

$$v(E) = \int_E x^2 \, dx$$

$m(E) = 0 \Rightarrow v(E) = 0$ (where m is the Lebesgue measure on R) but v is not absolutely continuous on R. Discuss.

11. Show that the Hahn decomposition is unique except for null sets.

12. Show that there is only one pair of mutually singular measures v^+ and v^- such that

$$v = v^+ - v^-.$$

13. Show that if v_1 and v_2 are any two finite signed measures, then so is $\alpha v_1 + \beta v_2$, where α, β are real numbers. Show that

$$|\alpha v| = |\alpha| |v|$$

and $|v_1 + v_2| \leq |v_1| + |v_2|$

where $v \leq \mu$ means $v(E) \leq \mu(E)$ for all measurable sets E.

14. Show that the Radon-Nikodym theorem for a finite measure μ implies the theorem for σ-finite measure μ.

15. Show that the Radon-Nikodym derivatives $\left[\dfrac{dv}{d\mu}\right]$ has the following properties.

   (i) If $v \ll \mu$ and f is a non-negative measurable function then

   $$\int f\, dv = \int f\left[\frac{dv}{d\mu}\right] d\mu$$

   (ii) $\left[\dfrac{d(v_1 + v_2)}{d\mu}\right] = \left[\dfrac{dv_1}{d\mu}\right] + \left[\dfrac{dv_2}{d\mu}\right]$

   (iii) If $v \ll \mu \ll \lambda$, then $\left[\dfrac{dv}{d\lambda}\right] = \left[\dfrac{dv}{d\mu}\right]\left[\dfrac{d\mu}{d\lambda}\right]$

   (iv) If $v \ll \mu$ and $\mu \ll \lambda$, then

   $$\left[\frac{dv}{d\mu}\right] = \left[\frac{d\mu}{dv}\right]^{-1}$$

16. Show that if v is a signed measure such that $v \perp \mu$ and $v \ll \mu$, then $v = 0$.

17. Show that if v_1 and v_2 are singular with respect to μ, then $c_1 v_1 + c_2 v_2$ is singular.

18. Show that if v_1 and v_2 are absolutely continuous with respect to μ, then $c_1 v_1 + c_2 v_2$ is absolutely continuous.

19. Show the uniqueness of the function f in the Radon-Nikodym theorem.

20. Extend the Radon-Nikodym theorem to the case of signed measures.

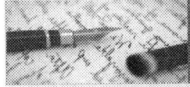

 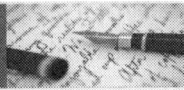

CHAPTER Summary

⬡ KEY TERMS

- **POSITIVE SET:** A subset E of X is said to be positive relative to a signed measure μ defined on a measurable space $(X, \mathcal{A})$ if
  (i) E is measurable.
  (ii) For all $A \subset E$ such that A is measurable implies $\mu(A) \geq 0$.

- **NEGATIVE SET:** A subset E of X is said to be negative relative to a signed measure μ defined on a measurable space (X, A) if
  (i) E is measurable.
  (ii) For all $A \subset E$ such that A is measurable implies $\mu(A) \leq 0$.

- **NULL SET:** A set $E \subset X$ is said to be a null set relative to a signed measure μ if E is both negative and positive.

- **TOTALLY FINITE SIGNED MEASURE:** A signed measure μ is said to be totally finite if E is measurable and $|\mu(E)| < \infty$.

- **HAHN DECOMPOSITION OF A SET:** A Hahn decomposition of X with respect to signed measure signed μ is a decomposition $X = P \cup Q$ of X into disjoint subsets $P > 0$ and $Q < 0$.

- **JORDAN DECOMPOSITION OF A SET:** A

- Jordan decomposition of measure μ is a representation $\mu(E) = \mu^{+}(E) - \mu^{-}(E)$.
  where μ^{+} and μ^{-} are measures, which are non-negative σ-additive set functions.

- **COMPLEX MEASURE:** A complex measure on the class of all measurable sets of a measurable space is a set function μ such that for every measurable set such that $\mu(E) = \mu_1(E) + i\,\mu_2(E)$, where μ_1 and μ_2 are signed measures and $i = \sqrt{-1}$.

- **BOUNDED VARIATION:** A finite signed measure together with its variations is said to be of bounded variation.

- **SINGULAR MEASURE:** Two measure μ and ν are said to be mutually singular if there exists a measurable set $A \subset X$ such that $\mu(A) = \mu(X - A)$.

- **ABSOLUTE CONTINUOUS MEASURE:** A signed measure μ on a measurable space $(X, \mathcal{A})$ is said to be absolutely continuous w.r.t. ν if and only if $\nu(A) = 0 \ \forall \, A \in \mathcal{A} \implies \mu(A) = 0$.

⬡ RESULTS

- Let $\mathcal{A}$ be a σ-algebra of subset of X. An extended real valued set function
  $$\mu : \mathcal{A} \to [-\infty, \infty]\,]$$
  is called a signed measure on $(X, \mathcal{A})$ if
  (i) μ takes atmost one of the values $-\infty$ or ∞.
  (ii) $\mu(\phi) = 0$.
  (iii) μ is countably additive.

- Measure is a special case of signed measure.

- A signed measure μ is said to be totally finite if E is measurable and $|\mu(E)| < \infty$.

- A Hahn decomposition of X with respect to signed measure μ is a decomposition $X = P \cup Q$ of X into disjoint subsets $P > 0$ and $Q < 0$.

- A signed measure is finitely additive and subtractive.

- If E be a measurable set of finite measure then E contains a positive set A with $\mu(A) < \infty$.

- Let μ be a signed measure on a measurable space $(X, \mathcal{A})$, then there exists a positive set P and a negative set Q such that

- $P \cap Q = \phi$, $X = P \cup Q$ [Hahn decomposition theorem].

- Every signed measure is the difference of two measures (of which at least one is finite), the representation of μ as the difference of its upper and lower variation is called the Jordan decomposition of μ.

- A finite signed measure together with its variations is bounded is said to be of bounded variation.

- If μ and ν are any two measures on a σ-ring then $\nu \ll \mu + \nu$.

- If μ and ν are signed measures such that ν is both absolutely continuous and singular with respect to μ, then $\nu = 0$.

- The Radon-Nikodym theorem is not measurably true if μ is not totally σ-finite even if ν remains finite.

- The Radon-Nikodym derivative $\dfrac{d\nu}{d\mu}$ is unique almost everywhere with respect to μ.

☞ WORTHY READINGS

- A measure is a particular case of signed measure, i.e., every measure of a σ-algebra $\mathcal{A}$ is also a signed measure. But signed measure is not a measure in general.
- Every measurable subset of a positive set is a positive set.
- The measure of every null set is zero.
- A set of measure zero may be a union of two measurable sets whose measure are not zero but are negative of each other.
- The null set is a positive set.
- A countable union of negative sets or null sets, respectively, a negative or a null set.
- Hahn decomposition is not unique.
- If ν is a signed measure such that $|\nu(E)| < \infty$ and $F \subseteq E$ then $|\nu(E)| < \infty$.
- The condition μ σ-finite is necessary in the Radon-Nikodym theorem.

☞ FUTHER READINGS

- A signed measure is defined as an extended real valued, countably additive set function ν on the class of all measurable sets of a measurable space such that $\nu(0) = 0$ and such that ν assumes atmost one of the values $+\infty$ and $-\infty$.
- A signed measure is finitely additive and subtractive.
- A complex measure on the class of all measurable sets functions μ such that for every measurable set $\mu(E) = \mu_1(E) + i\mu_2(E)$ where μ_1 and μ_2 are the signed measure.
- For every signed measure $\mu, \mu = |\mu|$.
- If μ is a signed measure and E is a measurable set then $|\mu|(E) = 0$ if and only if $\mu(F) = 0$ for every measurable subset F of E.
- If μ and ν are signed measure such that ν is both absolutely continuous and singular with respect to ν then $\nu = 0$.
- If ν_1, ν_2 and μ are finite signed measure such that both ν_1 and ν_2 are singular w.r.t. μ then $\nu = \nu_1 + \nu_2$ is also singular w.r.t. μ.
- The Radon-Nikodym theorem remains true even if μ is only a signed measure.
- The Radon-Nikodym theorem remains true even if ν is not σ-finite but in this case, the integrand f is not necessarily finite valued.
- The Radon-Nikodym theorem is not necessarily true if μ is not totally ν-finite, even if ν remains finite.
- If $(X, \mathcal{A})$ is a measurable space and μ and ν are σ-finite measure on $\mathcal{A}$ such that $\nu \ll \mu$ then Radon-Nikodym theorem may be applied to each measurable set separately.

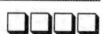

Chapter

11 Product Measures

11.1 INTRODUCTION

Let X and Y be two sets, then the Cartesian Product of X and Y denoted by $X \times Y$ is the set of all ordered pairs (x, y) where $x \in X$ and $y \in Y$. In this chapter we shall discuss that the cartesian product of two measurable space can be made into a measurable space. Next, we shall discuss that if measures are given on each of the factor spaces, we can define a measure on the product space.

(1) **Rectangle:** If $A \subset X$ and $B \subset Y$ then the set $E = A \times B$ (a subset of $X \times Y$) is called rectangle. The component sets A and B are known as its sides.

☞ **REMARK**
  • The rectangle defined above, is also called measurable rectangle.

(2) **Z-Measurable Set:** Let $(X, \mathcal{A}_2)$ and $(Y, \mathcal{A}_1)$ be two measurable spaces, then $Z = \mathcal{A}_1 \times \mathcal{A}_2$ denote the σ-algebra of subsets of $Z = X \times Y$ generated by rectangles $A \times B$ with $A \in \mathcal{A}_1$ and $B \in \mathcal{A}_2$. We shall refer to a set in Z as a Z-measurable set or as a measurable subset of Z.

THEOREM 1.

A rectangle is empty if and only if one of its sides is empty.

PROOF.   Let $\qquad A \times B \neq 0$

If $(x, y) \in A \times B$, then $x \in A$ and $y \in B$

$\Rightarrow \quad A \neq 0$ and $B \neq 0$

On the other hand, neither A nor B is empty, then there exists a point (x, y) such that $(x, y) \in A \times B$. Hence, $A \times B \neq 0$.

THEOREM 2.

If $E_1 = A_1 \times B_1$ and $E_2 = A_2 \times B_2$ are non-empty rectangle, then $E_1 \subset E_2$ if and only if $A_1 \subset A_2$ and $B_1 \subset B_2$.

PROOF.   The 'if' part of this theorem is quite obvious. To prove the converse part, let (x, y) be any arbitrary part of $A_1 \times B_1$. Also, suppose that there exists a part x_1 in A_1 such that $x_1 \notin A_2$.

Then $\qquad (x, y) \in A_1 \times B_1$ and $(x, y) \notin A_2 \times B_2$

$\Rightarrow$ There is no such point x_1 can exist and therefore $A_1 \subset A_2$.

Similarly, we can prove that $B_1 \subset B_2$.

☞ **REMARK**

- If $A_1 \times B_1 = A_2 \times B_2$ is a non-empty rectangle, then $A_1 = A_2$ and $B_1 = B_2$.

THEOREM 3.

If $E = A \times B$, $E_1 = A_1 \times B_1$ and $E_2 = A_2 \times B_2$ are non-empty rectangles, then a necessary and sufficient condition that E be the disjoint union of E_1 and E_2 is that either A is the disjoint union of A_1 and A_2 and $B = B_1 = B_2$ or else B is the disjoint union of B_1 and B_2 and $A = A_1 = A_2$.

PROOF.   **Necessary condition:** Since it is given that $E = E_1 \cup E_2$

Therefore, either $E_1 \subset E$ and $E_2 \subset E$.

Using Theorem 2, we conclude that $A_1 \subset A$ and $A_2 \subset A$ and thus we have $A_1 \cup A_2 \subset A$.

Similarly $B_1 \cup B_2 \subset B$

Now, Since $E_1 \cup E_2 \subset (A_1 \cup A_2) \times (B_1 \cup B_2)$

Therefore, $A \subset A_1 \cup A_2$ and $B \subset B_1 \cup B_2$

$\Rightarrow \quad A = A_1 \cup A_2$ and $B = B_1 \cup B_2$

Similarly, we can prove that

$$0 = E_1 \cap E_2 \supset (A_1 \cap A_2) \times (B_1 \cap B_2)$$

Using Theorem 1 it follows that at least one of the two sets $A_1 \cap A_2$ and $B_1 \cap B_2$ is empty. Let us suppose that $A_1 \cap A_2 = 0$, we have to show that $B = B_1 = B_2$.

Let if possible, there exists a point y in $B - B_1$. Then if x is any point in A_1, we have $(x, y) \in E$ but (Since $y \notin B_1$) $(x, y) \notin E_1$ and since $x \notin A_2$, $(x, y) \notin E_2$, which contradict the assumption $E = E_1 \cup E_2$. It follows that $B - B_1 = 0$.

Similarly we can prove that $B - B_2 = 0$.

Sufficient condition : Let A be the disjoint union of A_1 and A_2 and $B = B_1 = B_2$

Then $\quad\quad A_1 \subset A, A_2 \subset A, B_1 \subset B, B \subset B_2$

Therefore $E_1 \cup E_2 \subset E$

Also if $\quad (x, y) \in E$, then $(x, y) \in E_1$ or $(x, y) \in E_2$.

Hence, E is the disjoint union of E_1 and E_2.

THEOREM 4.

If A_1 and A_2 are rings of subsets of X and Y respectively, then the class $\mathbf{R}$ of all finite disjoint union of rectangles of the form $A \times B$ where $A \in A_1$ and $B \in A_2$, is a ring.

PROOF.   We know that the intersection of the two sets of the form $A \times B$ is another set of that form. If either of the given sets or their intersection is empty, then result is trivial.

Now if $\quad E_1 = A_1 \times B_1, E_2 = A_2 \times B_2$ and $(x, y) \in E_1 \cap E_2$.

Then $\quad x \in A_1 \cap A_2$ and $y \in B_1 \cap B_2$

So that $\quad E_1 \cap E_2 \subset (A_1 \cap A_2) \times (B_1 \cap B_2)$

Also, using theorem (2)

$$(A_1 \cap A_2) \times (B_1 \cap B_2) \subset E_1$$

and $\quad\quad (A_1 \cap A_2) \times (B_1 \cap B_2) \subset E_2$

which implies that

$$(A_1 \cap A_2) \times (B_1 \cap B_2) \subset E_1 \cap E_2$$

So that $E_1 \cap E_2 = (A_1 \cap A_2) \times (B_1 \cap B_2)$.

Since $\mathcal{A}_1$ and $\mathcal{A}_2$ are rings therefore $A_1 \cap A_2 \in \mathcal{A}_1$ and $B_1 \cap B_2 \in \mathcal{A}_2$ which implies that the class R is closed under the finite intersection.

Now, since $(A_1 \times B_1) - (A_2 \times B_2) = [(A_1 \cap A_2) \times (B_1 - B_2)] \cup [(A_1 - A_2) \times B_1]$.

We observe that the difference of two sets of the given form is a disjoint union of two other sets of that form.

Now since $\bigcup\limits_{i=1}^{n} E_i - \bigcup\limits_{j=1}^{m} F_j = \bigcup\limits_{i=1}^{n} \bigcap\limits_{j=1}^{m} (E_i - F_j)$.

Therefore, using above result, the class R is closed under the formation of differences.

Hence, the class R is a ring.

SOME IMPORTANT FACTS

(1) It $(X, \mathcal{A}_1)$ and $(Y, \mathcal{A}_2)$ are measurable spaces, then $(X \times Y, \mathcal{A}_1 \times \mathcal{A}_2)$ is again a measurable space.

(2) The class of measurable sets in the cartesian product of two measurable spaces is the σ-ring generated by the class of all measurable rectangles.

(3) The intersection of any countable class of measurable rectangles is a measurable rectangle.

(4) A necessary and sufficient condition that $\mathcal{A}_1 \times \mathcal{A}_2$ be a σ-algebra is that both $\mathcal{A}_1$ and $\mathcal{A}_2$ be σ-algebra.

11.2 SECTION

Definition 1. *Let $(X, \mathcal{A}_1)$ and $(Y, \mathcal{A}_2)$ be measurable spaces and let $(X \times Y, \mathcal{A}_1 \times \mathcal{A}_2)$ be their cartesian product. If E is any subset of $X \times Y$ and $x \in X$, then the set*

$$E_x = \{y : (x, y) \in E\}$$

is called the section of E or section of E determined by x.

Definition 2. *Let f be any function defined on a subset E of the product space $X \times Y$ and x is any point an X. Then, the function f_x defined on the section E_x by*

$$f_x(y) = f(x, y)$$

is called a section of f or X-section of f.

Similarly, we can define the concept of Y-section.

THEOREM 1.

Every section of a measurable set is measurable set.

PROOF.   Let X and Y be two non-empty sets. Let E be the class of all those subsets of $X \times Y$ which have the property that each of their sections is measurable. If $E = A \times B$ is a measurable rectangle, then every section of E is either empty or else equal to one of the sides A or B according as the section is a Y-section or an X-section. Thus, $E \in E$ we can easily verify that E is a σ-ring. Hence $\mathcal{A}_1 \times \mathcal{A}_2 \subset E$.

☞ **REMARKS**
- Every section of a measurable function is a measurable function.
- If χ is the characteristic function of subset E of $X \times Y$ then χ_x and χ_y are the characteristic functions of a rectangle $A \times B$. Then $\chi_{(x,y)} = \chi_A(x)\chi_B(y)$.
- Every section of a simple function is simple.
- A non-empty rectangle is a measurable set if and only if it is a measurable rectangle.

11.3 PRODUCT MEASURES

[MEERUT–2006 BP]

If (X, A_1, μ) and (Y, A_2, v) are measure spaces, then we can define a measure π on the subset $A = A_1 \times A_2$ which is the product of μ and v in the sense that

$$\pi(A \times B) = \mu(A)v(B) \qquad A \in A_1, \ B \in A_2$$

Any such measure, defined as above will be called a product measure of μ and v.

THEOREM I. (Product Measure Theorem)

If (X, A_1, μ) and (Y, A_2, v) are measure spaces. Then there exists a measure π defined an $A = A_1 \times A_2$ such that

$$\pi(A \times B) = \mu(A) \, v(B) \qquad \qquad \dots(1)$$

for all $A \in A_1$ and $B \in A_2$. If these measure spaces are $\sigma-$finite then there is a unique measure π with property (1).

PROOF. Let us suppose that the rectangles $A \times B$ is the disjoint union of a sequence $(A_j \times B_j)$ of rectangles. Therefore,

$$\chi_{A \times B}(x, y) = \chi_A(x) \, \chi_B(y) = \sum_{i=1}^{\infty} \chi_{A_i}(x) \, \chi_{B_i}(y), \quad \forall x \in X, \ y \in Y.$$

Keeping x fixed, integrate with respect to v and apply the monotone convergence theorem, we have

$$\chi_A(x) \, v(B) = \sum_{i=1}^{\infty} \chi_{A_i}(x) \, v(B_i).$$

Again applying the monotone convergence theorem, we get

$$\mu(A) \, v(B) = \sum_{i=1}^{\infty} \mu(A_i) \, v(B_i).$$

Without loss of any generality, we may assume that

$$E = \bigcup_{i=1}^{n} (A_i \times B_i)$$

Where the sets $A_i \times B_i$ are mutually disjoint rectangles

If we define $\pi_0(E)$ by $\pi_0(E) = \sum_{i=1}^{n} \mu(A_i) v(B_i)$.

Then clearly π_o is well defined and countably additive. Hence, we can say that there is an extension of π_o to a measure π on the $\sigma-$algebra.

Since π is an extension of π_o.

Hence, $\qquad \pi(A \times B) = \mu(A) \, v(B)$.

☞ REMARKS
- If μ and v are both σ–finite, then they have a unique product.
- The Cartesian product of two σ–finite and complete measure spaces need not be complete.

11.4 FUBINI'S THEOREM

[KANPUR–2007]

11.4.1 DOUBLE INTEGRAL

If f is Lebesgue integrable over a measurable set E, then $\int_E \int f(x,y)dx\,dy$ is called iterated

integral and $\int f(x,y)d\pi$ is called double integral.

If A is a measurable subset of E, then we define

$$\int_E \int f(x,y)dx\,dy = \int_E \int f(x,y)\chi_A(x,y)dx\,dy.$$

THEOREM 1.

A necessary and sufficient condition that a measurable subset E of $X \times Y$ have measure zero is that almost every X-section (or almost every Y-section) have measure zero.

PROOF. By definition of product measure, we have

$$\pi(E) = \begin{cases} \int v(E_x)d\mu(x) \\ \int \mu(E^y)dv(y) \end{cases}$$

If $\pi(E) = 0$, then the integrals on RHS are in particular finite and hence, their non-negative integrands must vanish almost every where. If on the other hand, either of the integrands vanishes almost everywhere, then $\pi(E) = 0$.

THEOREM 2.

Let (x, A_1, μ) and (y, A_2, v) be σ–finite measure spaces. If $E \in A = A_1 \times A_2$, then the function defined by

$$f(x) = v(E_x), \quad g(y) = \mu(E^y)$$

are measurable and

$$\int_x f d\mu = \pi(E) = \int_y g dv.$$

PROOF. Firstly, we suppose that the measure spaces are finite and let M be the collection of all $E \in A$ for which the above as section is true.

We claim that $M = A$

If $E = A \times B$ with $A \in A_1$ and $B \in A_2$, then

$$f(x) = \chi_A(x)\, v(B)$$
$$g(y) = \chi_B(y)\, \mu(A)$$
$$\int_x f d\mu = \mu(A)\, v(B) = \int_y g dv.$$

Since an arbitrary element of Z_0 (Collection of all finite unions of rectangles) can be written as a finite disjoint union of rectangles,

Therefore $Z_0 \subseteq M$.

Now, suppose that $\mathcal{M}$ is a monotone class. Let $< E_n >$ be a monotonic increasing sequence in $\mathcal{M}$ with union E, thus,

$$f_n(x) = v((E_n)_x)$$
$$g_n(y) = \mu((E_n)_y)$$

are measurable and

$$\int_x f_n d\mu = \pi(E_n) = \int_y g_n dv.$$

Clearly, the monotonic increasing sequence $< f_n >$ and $< g_n >$ converges to the functions f and g defined by

$$f(x) = v(E_x) \quad g(y) = \mu(E^y).$$

Apply the monotone convergence theorem for measure π, we get

$$\int_x f d\mu = \pi(E) = \int_y g dv$$

$$\Rightarrow \qquad E \in \mathcal{M}.$$

Since π is finite measure, it can be proved in the same way that if $< f_n >$ is a monotonic decreasing sequence in $\mathcal{M}$, then $F = \cap F_n \in \mathcal{M}$.

Therefore, $\mathcal{M}$ is a monotonic class, thus we conclude that $\mathcal{M} = \mathcal{A}$.

THEOREM 3. (Tonelli's Theorem)

Let $(X, \mathcal{A}_1, \mu)$ and $(Y, \mathcal{A}_2, v)$ be σ-finite measure spaces and let F be a non-negative measurable function on $Z = X \times Y$ to R.

Then, the function defined on X and Y by

$$f(x) = \int_y F_x dv, \quad g(y) = \int_x F^y d\mu$$

are measurable and

$$\int_x f d\mu = \int_z F d\pi = \int_y g dv.$$

In other symbols

$$\int_x \left(\int_y F dv \right) d\mu = \int_z F d\pi = \int_y \left(\int_x F d\mu \right) dv. \qquad \text{[MEERUT–2006, 06BP, 07]}$$

PROOF.   Let F be an arbitrary non-negative measurable functions an Z to R. Then there exists a sequence $< \phi_n >$ of non-negative measurable simple functions which converges in a monotonic increasing fashion.

If t_n and P_n are defined by

$$t_n(x) = \int_y (\phi_n)_x dv, \quad P_n(y) = \int_x (\phi_n)^y d\mu$$

Then, t_n and P_n are measurable and monotonic in n. Then by monotone convergence theorem, $< t_n >$ converges on X to f and $< P_n >$ converges on Y to g. Further, on applying the monotone convergence theorem, we have

$$\int_x f d\mu = \lim \int_x t_n d\mu = \lim \int_z \phi_n d\pi$$
$$= \lim \int_y P_n dv = \int_y g dv$$

Using the similar arguments, we can prove that

$$\int_z F d\pi = \lim \int_z \phi_n d\pi.$$

Hence, $$\int_x f d\mu = \int_z F d\pi = \int_y g dv.$$

☞ REMARK
- Tonellis theorem may fail if we drop the hypothesis that F is non-negative or if we drop the hypothesis that the measures μ and ν are σ–finite.

THEOREM 4. (Fubini's Theorem) (For product measure)

Let $(X, \mathcal{A}_1, \mu)$ and $(Y, \mathcal{A}_2, \nu)$ be σ–finite spaces and let the measure π on $\mathcal{A} = \mathcal{A}_1 \times \mathcal{A}_2$ be the product of μ and ν. If the function F and $Z = X \times Y$ to $\mathbf{R}$ is integrable with respect to π then, the extended real valued function defined almost everywhere by

$$f(x) = \int_y F_x d\nu, \quad g(y) = \int_x F^y d\mu$$

have finite integrals and

$$\int_X f d\mu = \int_z F d\pi = \int_y g d\nu .$$

In other symbols

$$\int_x \left(\int_y F d\nu \right) d\mu = \int_z F d\pi = \int_y \left(\int_x F d\mu \right) d\nu \quad \text{[MEERUT-2005, 05 (BP), 06, 07, 08, 10; KANPUR-2007]}$$

PROOF. As per given, the function F is integrable with respect to π therefore, its positive and negative parts F^+ and F^- are integrable.

Apply Tonelli's theorem to F^+ and F^- to deduce that the corresponding F^+ and F^- have finite integrals with respect to μ.

Therefore, F^+ and F^- are finite valued μ-almost everywhere, so their difference f is defined μ-almost everywhere. Hence

$$\int_X f d\mu = \int_z F d\pi$$

Similarly we can prove the other part.

ALTERNATIVE FORM OF FUBINI'S THEOREM

Let us suppose $E = (a,b) \times (c,d)$. Also, suppose that f is Lebesgue integrable over E. Then

$$\int_E \int f(x,y) dx\, dy = \int_a^b \left[\int_c^d f(x,y) dy \right] dx$$

$$\int_E \int f(x,y) dx\, dy = \int_c^d \left[\int_a^b f(x,y) dx \right] dy$$

☞ REMARKS
- Fubini's theorem may fail if the hypothesis that f is integrable is dropped.
- In order to apply the Fubini's theorem, one must first verify that f is integrable with respect to $\mu \times \nu$, i.e., one must show that f is a measurable function on $X \times Y$ and that $\int |f| d(\mu \times \nu) < \infty$.
- When μ and ν are σ–finite, the integrability of f can be determined by iterated integration using Tonelli's Theorem.

Solved Examples

EXAMPLE 1. *Using Fubini's theorem, verify*

$$\int_0^1 \left\{ \int_0^1 \frac{x^2 - y^2}{(x^2 + y^2)^2} \, dx \right\} dy \neq \int_0^1 \left\{ \int_0^1 \frac{x^2 - y^2}{(x^2 + y^2)^2} \, dy \right\} dx$$

[MEERUT–2005 BP, 06, 06 BP, 08; GWALIOR–2009; BANARAS–1967; KANPUR–2005]

SOLUTION. We have

$$\int_{x=0}^1 \frac{x^2 - y^2}{(x^2 + y^2)^2} \, dx = \int_{x=0}^1 \frac{\partial}{\partial x}\left(\frac{-x}{x^2 + y^2} \right) dx$$

$$= \left(\frac{-x}{x^2 + y^2} \right)_0^1 = \left\{ \frac{-1}{1 + y^2} + 0 \right\}$$

$$\Rightarrow \quad \int_{x=0}^1 \frac{x^2 - y^2}{(x^2 + y^2)^2} dx = \frac{-1}{1 + y^2}$$

Thus $\int_0^1 \left\{ \int_0^1 \frac{x^2 - y^2}{(x^2 + y^2)^2} \, dx \right\} dy = \int_0^1 \left(\frac{-1}{1 + y^2} \right) dy$

$$= -(\tan^{-1} y)_0^1 = -\tan^{-1} 1 + \tan^{-1} 0$$

$$\Rightarrow \quad \int_0^1 \left\{ \int_0^1 \frac{x^2 - y^2}{(x^2 + y^2)^2} \, dx \right\} dy = -\frac{\pi}{4} \qquad \qquad \ldots(1)$$

Again $\int_0^1 \frac{x^2 - y^2}{(x^2 + y^2)^2} \, dy = \int_0^1 \frac{\partial}{\partial x}\left(\frac{y}{x^2 + y^2} \right) dy$

$$= \left(\frac{y}{x^2 + y^2} \right)_0^1 = \left\{ \frac{1}{x^2 + 1} - 0 \right\}$$

$$\Rightarrow \quad \int_0^1 \frac{x^2 - y^2}{(x^2 + y^2)^2} \, dy = \frac{1}{1 + x^2}$$

Thus $\int_0^1 \left\{ \int_0^1 \frac{x^2 - y^2}{(x^2 + y^2)^2} \, dy \right\} dx = \int_0^1 \left(\frac{1}{x^2 + 1} \right) dx$

$$= (\tan^{-1} x)_0^1 = \tan^{-1} 1 - \tan^{-1} 0$$

$$\Rightarrow \quad \int_0^1 \left\{ \int_0^1 \frac{x^2 - y^2}{(x^2 + y^2)^2} \, dy \right\} dx = \frac{\pi}{4} \qquad \qquad \ldots(2)$$

From eq. (1) and eq. (2), we have

$$\int_0^1 \left\{ \int_0^1 \frac{x^2 - y^2}{(x^2 + y^2)^2} \, dx \right\} dy \neq \int_0^1 \left\{ \int_0^1 \frac{x^2 - y^2}{(x^2 + y^2)^2} \, dy \right\} dx$$

EXAMPLE 2. *Show that* $\int_0^1 dx \int_0^1 \dfrac{x^2 - y^2}{x^2 + y^2} dy = \int_0^1 dy \int_0^1 \dfrac{x^2 - y^2}{x^2 + y^2} dx$

[MEERUT–2006, 06 BP]

SOLUTION.   We have $\int_0^1 \dfrac{x^2 - y^2}{x^2 + y^2} dy = \int_0^1 \left(\dfrac{2x^2}{x^2 + y^2} - \dfrac{x^2 + y^2}{x^2 + y^2} \right) dy$

$$= \int_0^1 \left(\dfrac{2x^2}{x^2 + y^2} - 1 \right) dy$$

$$= 2x^2 \cdot \dfrac{1}{x} \left(\tan^{-1} \dfrac{y}{x} \right)_0^1 - (y)_0^1$$

$$= 2x \left\{ \tan^{-1} \dfrac{1}{x} - \tan^{-1} 0 \right\} - 1$$

$\Rightarrow \qquad \int_0^1 \dfrac{x^2 - y^2}{x^2 + y^2} dy = 2x \tan^{-1} \dfrac{1}{x} - 1$

Thus, $\int_0^1 dx \int_0^1 \dfrac{x^2 - y^2}{x^2 + y^2} dy = \int_0^1 \left(2x \tan^{-1} \dfrac{1}{x} - 1 \right) dx$

$$= \left[x^2 \tan^{-1} \dfrac{1}{x} \right]_0^1 - \int_0^1 x^2 \dfrac{1}{1 + \dfrac{1}{x^2}} \left(-\dfrac{1}{x^2} \right) dx - (x)_0^1$$

$$= \left[\tan^{-1} 1 - (\tan^{-1} \infty) . 0 \right] + \int_0^1 \dfrac{x^2 + 1 - 1}{1 + x^2} dx - 1$$

$$= \dfrac{\pi}{4} + \int_0^1 \left(\dfrac{x^2 + 1}{1 + x^2} - \dfrac{1}{1 + x^2} \right) dx - 1$$

$$= \dfrac{\pi}{4} + (x)_0^1 - (\tan^{-1} x)_0^1 - 1$$

$\Rightarrow \quad \int_0^1 dx . \int_0^1 \dfrac{x^2 - y^2}{x^2 + y^2} dy = \dfrac{\pi}{4} + 1 - \dfrac{\pi}{4} - 1 = 0$ \qquad\qquad ...(1)

Again $\int_0^1 \dfrac{x^2 - y^2}{x^2 + y^2} dx = \int_0^1 \left(\dfrac{x^2 + y^2}{x^2 + y^2} - \dfrac{2y^2}{x^2 + y^2} \right) dx$

$$= \int_0^1 \left(1 - \dfrac{2y^2}{x^2 + y^2} \right) dx$$

$$= (x)_0^1 - 2y^2 \cdot \dfrac{1}{y} \left(\tan^{-1} \dfrac{x}{y} \right)_0^1$$

$$= 1 - 2y \left\{ \tan^{-1} \dfrac{1}{y} - \tan^{-1} 0 \right\}$$

$$\Rightarrow \quad \int_0^1 \left(\frac{x^2 - y^2}{x^2 + y^2}\right) dx = 1 - 2y \tan^{-1}\left(\frac{1}{y}\right)$$

Thus, $\int_0^1 dy \int_0^1 \frac{x^2 - y^2}{x^2 + y^2} dx = \int_0^1 \left[1 - 2y \tan^{-1}(1/y)\right] dy$

$$= (y)_0^1 - \left[y^2 . \tan\frac{1}{y}\right]_0^1 + \int_0^1 y^2 . \frac{1}{1 + \frac{1}{y^2}} . \left(-\frac{1}{y^2}\right) dy$$

$$= 1 - \left[\tan^{-1} 1 - 0. \tan^{-1} \infty\right] - \int_0^1 \frac{y^2 + 1 - 1}{1 + y^2} dy$$

$$= 1 - \tan^{-1} 1 - \int_0^1 \left(\frac{1 + y^2}{1 + y^2} - \frac{1}{1 + y^2}\right) dy$$

$$= 1 - \frac{\pi}{4} - (y)_0^1 + (\tan^{-1} y)_0^1$$

$$\Rightarrow \quad \int_0^1 dy \int_0^1 \frac{x^2 - y^2}{x^2 + y^2} dx = 1 - \frac{\pi}{4} - 1 + \frac{\pi}{4} = 0 \qquad \qquad \ldots(2)$$

From (1) and (2), we conclude that

$$\int_0^1 dx \int_0^1 \frac{x^2 - y^2}{x^2 + y^2} dy = \int_0^1 dy \int_0^1 \frac{x^2 - y^2}{x^2 + y^2} dx$$

EXAMPLE 3. *Show that* $\int_0^1 \left\{ \int_0^1 \frac{x - y}{(x + y)^3} dx \right\} dy \neq \int_0^1 \left\{ \int_0^1 \frac{x - y}{(x + y)^3} dy \right\} dx$ [MEERUT–2006 BP, 07]

SOLUTION. We have $\int_0^1 \frac{x - y}{(x + y)^3} dx = \int_0^1 \left\{ \frac{x + y}{(x + y)^3} - \frac{2y}{(x + y)^3} \right\} dx$

$$= \int_0^1 \left\{ \frac{1}{(x + y)^2} - \frac{2y}{(x + y)^3} \right\} dx$$

$$= \int_0^1 \frac{dx}{(x + y)^2} - 2y \int_0^1 \frac{dx}{(x + y)^3}$$

$$= \left(\frac{(x + y)^{-1}}{-1}\right)_0^1 - 2y \left\{\frac{(x + y)^{-2}}{-2}\right\}_0^1$$

$$= \left(\frac{-1}{x + y}\right)_0^1 + 2y \left\{\frac{1}{2(x + y)^2}\right\}_0^1$$

$$= \left\{\frac{-1}{1 + y} + \frac{1}{y}\right\} + y \left\{\frac{1}{(1 + y)^2} - \frac{1}{y^2}\right\}$$

$$= \left(\frac{-1}{1+y}\right) + \frac{1}{y} + \frac{y}{(1+y)^2} - \frac{1}{y}$$

$$\Rightarrow \quad \int_0^1 \frac{x-y}{(x+y)^3} dx = \frac{-(1+y)+y}{(1+y)^2} = \frac{-1}{(1+y)^2}$$

Thus,

$$\int_0^1 \left\{ \int_0^1 \frac{x-y}{(x+y)^3} dx \right\} dy = \int_0^1 \frac{-dy}{(1+y)^2}$$

$$= -\left\{ \frac{(1+y)^{-1}}{-1} \right\}_0^1$$

$$\Rightarrow \quad \int_0^1 \left\{ \int_0^1 \frac{x-y}{(x+y)^3} dx \right\} dy = \left(\frac{1}{1+y} \right)_0^1 = \frac{1}{2} - 1 = -\frac{1}{2} \qquad \ldots(1)$$

Again, $\quad \int_0^1 \frac{x-y}{(x+y)^3} dy = \int_0^1 \left(-\frac{x+y}{(x+y)^3} + \frac{2x}{(x+y)^3} \right) dy$

$$= \int_0^1 \left(\frac{2x}{(x+y)^3} - \frac{1}{(x+y)^2} \right) dy$$

$$= 2x \int_0^1 \frac{dy}{(x+y)^3} - \int_0^1 \frac{dy}{(x+y)^2}$$

$$= 2x \left\{ \frac{(x+y)^{-2}}{-2} \right\}_0^1 - \left(\frac{(x+y)^{-1}}{-1} \right)_0^1$$

$$= -x \left\{ \frac{1}{(x+y)^2} \right\}_0^1 + \left(\frac{1}{x+y} \right)_0^1$$

$$= -x \left\{ \frac{1}{(1+x)^2} - \frac{1}{x^2} \right\} + \left(\frac{1}{1+x} - \frac{1}{x} \right)$$

$$= -\frac{x}{(1+x)^2} + \frac{1}{x} + \frac{1}{1+x} - \frac{1}{x}$$

$$\Rightarrow \quad \int_0^1 \frac{x-y}{(x+y)^3} dy = \frac{-x+1+x}{(1+x)^2} = \frac{1}{(1+x)^2}$$

Thus,

$$\int_0^1 \left\{ \int_0^1 \frac{x-y}{(x+y)^3} dy \right\} dx = \int_0^1 \frac{dx}{(1+x)^2}$$

$$= \left\{ \frac{(1+x)^{-1}}{-1} \right\}_0^1 = \left(\frac{-1}{1+x} \right)_0^1 = -\frac{1}{2} + 1$$

$$\int_0^1 \left\{ \int_0^1 \frac{x-y}{(x+y)^3} dy \right\} dx = +\frac{1}{2} \qquad \qquad \ldots(2)$$

From eq. (1) and eq. (2), we conclude that

$$\int_0^1 \left\{ \int_0^1 \frac{x-y}{(x+y)^3} dx \right\} dy \neq \int_0^1 \left\{ \int_0^1 \frac{x-y}{(x+y)^3} dy \right\} dx$$

11.5 PRODUCT OF FINITELY MANY MEASURES

For $n \geq 2$, let (X_i, A_i, μ_i), $i = 1, 2, \ldots, n$, be σ-finite measure space. Suppose we have defined the product measure space $(X_1 \times X_2 \times \ldots \times X_{n-1}, A_1 \otimes \ldots \otimes A_{n-1}, \mu_1 \times \mu_2 \ldots \times \mu_{n-1})$, which we write as

$$\left(\prod_{i=1}^{n-1} X_i, \, \bigotimes_{i=1}^{n-1} A_i, \, \prod_{i=1}^{n-1} \mu_i \right)$$

We can define the product measure space

$$\left(\left(\prod_{i=1}^{n-1} X_i \right) \times X_n, \left(\bigotimes_{i=1}^{n-1} A_i \right) \otimes A_n, \left(\prod_{i=1}^{n-1} \mu_i \right) \times \mu_n \right).$$

The sets $\left(\prod_{i=1}^{n-1} X_i \right) \times X_n$ and $\prod_{i=1}^{n} X_i = X_1 \times \ldots \times X_{n-1} \times X_n$ can be identified via the bijection

$$((x_1, \ldots, x_{n-1}), x_n) \mapsto (x_1, \ldots, x_n), \, x_i \in X_i, \, 1 \leq i \leq n.$$

Let $R_n := \{ A_1 \times A_2 \times \ldots \times A_n \mid A_i \in A_i \}$. It is easy to verify that R_n is a semi-algebra of subsets of $\prod_{i=1}^{n} X_i$. Let $\bigotimes_{i=1}^{n-1} A_i$ denote the σ-algebra of subsets of $\prod_{i=1}^{n} X_i$ generated by R_n. It is easy to check that

$$\left(\bigotimes_{i=1}^{n-1} A_i \right) \otimes A_n = \bigotimes_{i=1}^{n} A_i$$

Keeping in mind the identification $\left(\prod_{i=1}^{n-1} X_i \right) \times X_n = \prod_{i=1}^{n} X_i$.

Next, it is easy to see that the measure $\left(\prod_{i=1}^{n-1} \mu_i \right) \times \mu_n$ on $\bigotimes_{i=1}^{n} A_i$ has the property that $\forall A_i \in A_i$, $i = 1, 2, \ldots, n$.

$$\left[\left(\prod_{i=1}^{n-1} \mu_i \right) \times \mu_n \right] (A_1 \times \ldots \times A_n) = \prod_{i=1}^{n} \mu_i(A_i).$$

Moreover, that this is only measure with this property follows from the uniqueness theorem. We denote the measure $\left(\prod_{i=1}^{n-1} \mu_i \right) \times \mu_n$ by $\prod_{i=1}^{n} \mu_i$ and call it the product measure. The measure space

$$\left(\prod_{i=1}^{n} X_i, \, \bigotimes_{i=1}^{n} A_i, \, \prod_{i=1}^{n} \mu_i \right)$$

is called the product of the measure space (X_i, A_i, μ_i), $i = 1, 2, ..., n$ and is usually denoted by $\prod\limits_{i=1}^{n} (X_i, A_i, \mu_i)$.

Exercise 11.1

1. Discuses the applicability of Fubini's theorem to the function $f(x,y) = \dfrac{x^2 - y^2}{(x^2 + y^2)^2}$, $x^2 + y^2 \neq 0$ $x \in (0,1)$; $y \in [0, 1]$.

2. Develop the concept of product measure to the state needed to prove Fubini's theorem.

3. Let f and g be real valued functions on X and Y respectively. Suppose that f is X-measurable and that g is Y-measurable. If h is defined by (x, y) in $X \times Y$ by $h(x \times y) = f(x)g(y)$, show that $X \times Y$ is measurable.

4. Let $A_j \subset x$ and $B_j \subset y$, $j = 1, 2$. If $A_1 \times B_1 = A_2 \times B_2$ then show that $A_1 = A_2$ and $B_1 = B_2$.

5. Let (X, A_1) and (Y, A_2) be measurable spaces. If $A_j \in A$ and $B_j \in A_2$ for $j = 1,...m$, then show that the set $\bigcup\limits_{j=1}^{n} (A_j \times B_j)$ can be written as disjoint union of a finite number of rectangles.

6. Let (X, A_1, μ) be the measure space an the natural numbers $X = N$. With the counting measure defined on all subsets of $X = N$. Let (Y, A_2, v) be an arbitrary measure space. Since that a set E in $Z = X \times Y$ belongs to $Z = A_1 \times A_2$ if and only if each section E_n of E belongs to A_2. In this case there is a unique product measure π and $\pi(E) = \sum\limits_{n=1}^{\infty} v(E_n)$.

7. Let f be integrable on (X, A_1, μ) let g be integrable an (Y, A_2, v) and define h on Z by $h(x,y) = f(x)g(y)$. If π is the product of μ and v, show that h is π-integrable and $\int_z h d\pi = [\int_x f d\mu][\int_y g dv]$.

8. Suppose that (X, A_1, μ) and (Y, A_2, v) are σ-finite. Let E, F belong to $A_1 \times A_2$. If $v(E_x) = v(F_x)$ for all $x \in X$ then, show that $\pi(E) = \pi(F)$.

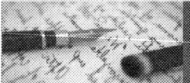
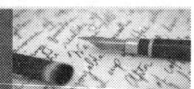

CHAPTER Summary

❧ KEY TERMS

- **RECTANGLE:** If $A \subset X$ and $B \subset Y$ then the set $E = A \times B$ (a subset of $X \times Y$) is called rectangle.

- **SECTION:** Let $(X, \mathcal{A}_1)$ and $(Y, \mathcal{A}_2)$ be two measurable spaces and let $(X \times Y, \mathcal{A}_1 \times \mathcal{A}_2)$ be the cartesian product. If E is any subset of $X \times Y$ and $x \in X$, then the set

$$E_x = \{y : (x, y) \in E\}$$

  is called the section of E determined by x.

- **PRODUCT MEASURE:** If $(X, \mathcal{A}_1, \mu)$ and $(Y, \mathcal{A}_2, \nu)$ are two measure spaces, then we can define a measure π on the subset $A = \mathcal{A}_1 \times \mathcal{A}_2$ which is the product of μ and ν in the sense that

$$\pi(A \times B) = \mu(A)\nu(B) \quad A \in \mathcal{A}_1, \ B \in \mathcal{A}_2$$

  such type of measure is called a product measure.

- **ITERATED INTEGRAL:** If f is Lebesgue integrable over a measurable set E, then $\int\limits_{E} \int f(x, y)dx\,dy$ is called iterated integral and $\int f(x, y)d\pi$ is called double integral.

❧ RESULTS

- Let X and Y be two sets, then the cartesian product $Z = X \times Y$ is the set of all ordered pairs (x, y) such that $x \in X$ and $y \in Y$.

- Cartesian product of two measurable spaces can be made into a measurable space.

- If measures are given each of the factor spaces, we can define a measure on the product space.

- If $(X, \mathcal{A}_1)$ and $(Y, \mathcal{A}_2)$ are measurable spaces, then a set of the form $A \times B$ with $A \in \mathcal{A}_1$ and $B \in \mathcal{A}_2$ is called a measurable rectangle or simply a rectangle in $Z = X \times Y$.

- The collection of all finite unions of rectangles is an algebra of subsets of Z.

- A necessary and sufficient condition that a measurable subset E of $X \times Y$ have measure zero is that almost every X-section (or almost every Y-section) have measure zero.

❧ WORTHY READINGS

☞ The cartesian product of two σ-finite and complete measure spaces need not be complete.

☞ The necessary and sufficient condition that a measurable subset E of $X \times Y$ have measure zero is that almost every X-section (or almost every Y-section) have measure zero.

☞ If f and g are integrable functions on X and Y respectively, then the function h defined by $h(x, y) = f(x)g(y)$ is an integrable function on $X \times Y$ and $\int hd(\mu \times \nu) = \int fd\mu \cdot \int gd\nu$.

❧ FUTHER READINGS

☞ If A and B are arbitrary (not necessarily measurable) subset of X and Y respectively, then $\lambda^*(A \times B) = \mu^*(A) \cdot \nu^*(B)$

☞ If X_i is the real line, S_i is the class of all Borel sets and μ_i is Lebesgue measure, $i \in N$, then

$$(X, S, \mu) = \underset{i=1}{\overset{n}{X}}[X, S_i, \mu_i]$$

☞ Sets of all σ-ring S, are called the Borel sets of n-dimensional Euclidean space. The class of all Borel sets coincides with σ-ring generated by the class of all open sets.

☞ We can easily generalise the theory of product space to uncountably many factors.

☞ If $X = \underset{i=1}{\overset{\infty}{X}}X_i$ is a product space and for each i, E_i is a measurable set in X_i then $E = \underset{i=1}{\overset{\infty}{X}}E_i$ is measurable on X and

$$\mu(E) = \prod_{i=1}^{\infty}\mu(E_i) = \lim_{n \to \infty}\prod_{i=1}^{n}\mu_i(E_i)$$

12

Lebesgue-Stieltjes Integrals : Bair Sets and Bair Functions

12.1 INTRODUCTION

Let us denote the linear space of function of locally bounded variation by V_{loc}. This space contains as a subset the set V_{loc}^{+} of monotonic non-decreasing function. For composition product, we have

$$\alpha, \beta \in V_{loc}^{+}$$

$$\Rightarrow \qquad \alpha \circ \beta \in V_{loc}^{+} \text{ if } \alpha, \beta \in V_{loc}^{+}$$

where $\qquad (\alpha \circ \beta)(x) = \alpha(\beta(x))$

The identity function $i \in V_{loc}^{+}$ defined by

$$i(x) = x$$

for all real numbers x serves as an identity for the composition operation

$$i \circ \alpha = \alpha \circ \sigma = \alpha \text{ for } \alpha \in V_{loc}^{+}$$

The inverse of α, i.e., α^{-1} satisfying

$$\alpha o \alpha^{-1} = \alpha^{-1} o \alpha = i$$

Definition 1. *Let* $\alpha \in V_{loc}^{+}$, *then* J_{α} *will denote the smallest interval containing all the values of* α, *i.e., the interval with end points*

$$\alpha(-\infty) = \lim_{x \to -\infty} \alpha(x)$$

$$\alpha(\infty) = \lim_{x \to \infty} \alpha(x)$$

where the first end point is included in the interval if and only if there is a real number y *such that* $\alpha(y) = \alpha(-\infty)$ *and correspondingly for the second part.*

Definition 2. *If* $\alpha \in V_{loc}^{+}$ *then any function* α_1 *defined an* J_{α} *and satisfying*

$$\text{Sup. } \{y : \alpha(y) < x\} \le \alpha_1(x) \le \inf\{y : x < \alpha(y)\}, \quad x \in J_{\alpha}$$

is called an inverse of α.

☛ REMARKS

- In the above definition the sup. is to be interpreted as $-\infty$ if no y with $\alpha(y) < x$ exists; this is the case when x is the left end point of J_{α}. Similarly, the inf. is to be interpreted as $+\infty$ if no y with $\alpha(y) > x$ exists; which is the case when x is the right end point of J_{α}.
- The function α can have more than one inverse only if there is a point $c \in J_{\alpha}$ with Sup. $\{y : \alpha(y) < c\} < \inf .\{y : c > \alpha(y)\}$
  i.e., if for same $c \in J_{\alpha}$, α *assumes the value c at more than one point.*

12.2 LEBESGUE-STIELTJES INTEGRAL

Definition. *Let L be a linear space and ϕ be a step function. The Lebesgue-Stieltjes integral $\int \phi d\alpha$ of a step function $\phi \in L$ with respect to a function $\alpha \in V_{loc}^+$ is defined by*

$$\int \phi d\alpha = \int_{J_\alpha} \phi \circ \alpha_1 dx \text{ , where } \alpha_1 \text{ is the inverse of } \alpha .$$

[MEERUT–2006 BP, 08]

 Recapitulations

✦ If α_1 is an inverse of a function $\alpha \in V_{loc}^+$, then α_1 is monotonic non-decreasing on J_α and for any $\in > 0$.

$\alpha_1(\alpha(a-0)-\in) < a$ if $(\alpha(a-0)-\in) \in J_\alpha$,
$\alpha_1(\alpha(a-0)+\in) \geq a$ if $(\alpha(a-0)+\in) \in J_\alpha$,
$\alpha_1(\alpha(a+0)-\in) \leq a$ if $(\alpha(a+0)-\in) \in J_\alpha$,
$\alpha_1(\alpha(a+0)+\in) > a$ if $(\alpha(a+0)+\in) \in J_\alpha$.

✦ If χ is the characteristic function of the closed bounded interval $[a, b]$ then $\chi \circ \alpha_1$ is the characteristic function defined on J_α , of a bounded interval with end points $\alpha(a - 0)$ and $\alpha(b + 0)$ so that

$$\int_{J_\alpha} \chi \circ \alpha_1 dx = \alpha(b+0) - \alpha(a-0) .$$

12.3 PROPERTIES OF LEBESGUE-STIELTJES INTEGRAL

THEOREM 1.

If f is a $d\alpha$ – integrable function on the real line and α_1 is any inverse to α , then $f \circ \alpha_1$ is $d\alpha$ – integrable on J_α and $\int f d\alpha = \int_{J_\alpha} f \circ \alpha_1 dx$. Conversely, if f is a function on the real line such that $f \circ \alpha_1$ is $d\alpha$ -integrable, on J_α for same inverse α_1 of α , then f is $d\alpha$ -integrable.

PROOF. Let us suppose that f be a $d\alpha$ -integrable function on the real line then there is a series $\sum \phi_n$ of step function satisfying

$$\sum_{n=1}^{\infty} \int |\phi_n| dx < \infty \text{ and } f(x) = \sum_{n=1}^{\infty} \phi_n(x)$$

where the series of $f(x)$ converges absolutely. Then $\sum \phi_n \circ \alpha_1$ is a series of step function on J_α that satisfies

$$\sum_{n=1}^{\infty} \int_{J_\alpha} |\phi_n \circ \alpha_1| dx = \sum_{n=1}^{\infty} \int |\phi_n| d\alpha < \infty$$

$$f(\alpha_1(y)) = \sum_{n=1}^{\infty} \phi_n(\alpha_1(y))$$

for all $y \in J_\alpha$ for which the last series converges absolutely. Therefore we have $f \circ \alpha_1$ is $d\alpha$ -integrable on J_α and $\int_{J_\alpha} f \circ \alpha_1 dx = \sum_{n=1}^{\infty} \int_{J_\alpha} \phi_n \circ \alpha_1 dx = \sum_{n=1}^{\infty} \int \phi_n d\alpha = \int f d\alpha$

Conversely, let if $\alpha(x-0) < \alpha(x+0)$ for some x , then $\alpha(x-0) < \alpha(x) < \alpha(x+0)$ and if sup $\{y : \alpha(y) < x\} < \inf \{y : \alpha(y) > x\}$ then

sup $\{y : \alpha(y) < x\} < \alpha_1(x) < \inf \{y : \alpha(y) > x\}$.

Now suppose that $f \circ \alpha_1$ is $d\alpha$ -integrable and that $\sum \phi_n$ of series of step function, not zero for any point of J_α and satisfying

$$\sum_{n=1}^{\infty} \int |\phi_n| dx < \infty, \ f(\alpha_1(x)) = \sum_{n=1}^{\infty} \phi_n(x)$$

for all $x \in J_\alpha$ for which the series of f converges absolutely, let $\{J_k\}$ be an enumeration of the intervals of constancy of α_1 , if ϕ_n is not constant on J_k , then we replace ϕ_n on J_k by its mean value

$|J_k|^{-1} \int_{J_k} \phi_n dx$, where $|J_k| = \int_{J_k} dx$.

Therefore, the relation

$$f(\alpha_1(x)) = \sum_{n=1}^{\infty} \phi_n(x)$$

will hold for $x \in J_k$, since both sides equal their mean values over J_k.

Thus, we may suppose that all ϕ_n are constant on each J_k further, consider the function $\alpha_0 \alpha_1$ on J_α. By condition of α, it maps each interval of constancy of α_1 into itself whereas by the condition on α_1 it equals the identity on the range of values $\alpha(R)$ of α. Since, this range of values and the intervals of constancy of α_1 together cover J_α, it follows that

$$\phi_n \circ \alpha \circ \alpha_1 = \phi_n \text{ on } J_\alpha \forall n.$$

Now putting $\psi_n = \phi_n \circ \alpha$, we have

$$\sum_{n=1}^{\infty} \int |\psi_n| d\alpha = \sum_{n=1}^{\infty} \int_{J_\alpha} |\phi_n \circ \alpha \circ \alpha_1| dx$$

$$= \sum_{n=1}^{\infty} \int |\phi_n| dx < \infty$$

$$f(x) = \sum_{n=1}^{\infty} \psi_n(x) \quad \forall x$$

in the range of values $\alpha_1(J_\alpha)$ of α_1 for which the last series converges absolutely, i.e., ϕ_α a.e. on $\alpha_1(J_\alpha)$. But $R - \alpha_1(J_\alpha)$ is a $d\alpha$-null set, since it is covered by the d_α-null intervals I_k on which α is constant. Namely, suppose I_k has end points $a_k < b_k$, say for instance $I_k =]a_k \, b_k]$. Then

$$\alpha(b_k) = \alpha(b_k - 0)$$

so that α must be continuous at b_k by our assumption on α.

Therefore, $\alpha(b_k + 0) = \alpha(b_k - 0)$

Thus, $d\alpha$-measure of I_k is

$$\alpha(b_k + 0) - \alpha(a_k + 0) = \alpha(b_k - 0) - \alpha(a_k + 0) = 0$$

$$\Rightarrow \qquad f = \sum_{n=1}^{\infty} \psi_n d\alpha \text{ a.e.}$$

Hence, f is $d\alpha$-integrable.

THEOREM 2.

If $\int \phi d\alpha = \int \phi d\beta$ for all $\phi \in L$, then the two functions $\alpha, \beta \in V_{loc}^+$ differ by a fixed constant at all their points of continuity.

PROOF.   Let α, β be two continuous functions. The set of points in R where α and β are continuous is the compliment of a denumerable set.

Let t be such a point and let x be any other point of continuity for both α and β. Suppose that $x < t$.

Define the characteristic function χ in $[x, t]$ then

$$\int \chi d\alpha = \alpha(t) - \alpha(x) = \int \chi d\beta = \beta(t) - \beta(x).$$

Therefore, $\alpha(x) - \beta(x) = \alpha(t) - \beta(t)$.   ...(1)

Same result can be obtained in the case $x > t$.

Since $\alpha(t) - \beta(t)$ is a fixed constant.

Hence, we conclude that α, β differ by a fixed constant at all their points of continuity.

THEOREM 3.

If $\int \phi d\alpha = \int \phi d\beta$ for all $\phi \in L$, then α, β have the same discontinuities.

PROOF.   Let a be a point of discontinuity for α. Since the set of points where both α and β are continuous is a dense set, therefore, we may select a sequence $< x_n >$, $x_n > a$ of such points which tends to a then

$$\alpha(a+0) - \beta(a+0) = \lim_{n + \infty}(\alpha(x_n) - \beta(x_n)) = \alpha(t) - \beta(t)$$

Similarly, we can prove that

$$\alpha(a-0) - \beta(a-0) = \alpha(t) - \beta(t).$$

Therefore, $\alpha(a+0) - \alpha(a-0) = \beta(a+0) - \beta(a-0)$.

Hence, β is discontinuous at all points of discontinuity of α. Similarly we can show that α is discontinuous at all points of discontinuity of β.

THEOREM 4. (Riesz Representation Theorem For L-S-integral)

Every integral $\int \phi d\mu$ on the linear space L of step functions on the real line can be written as the Stieltjes integral with respect to some function $\mu \in V_{loc}^+$.

PROOF.   Let us define the step function ψ_x, x is real such that

$$\psi_x = \begin{cases} \chi_{]0,x]} & ; \text{ if } x > 0 \\ 0 & ; \text{ if } x = 0 \\ -\chi_{]x,0]} & ; \text{ if } x < 0 \end{cases}$$

Define the function μ by $\mu(x) = \int \psi_x d\mu$

we know that the function μ is monotonic non-decreasing. It is also right continuous, therefore,

$$\mu(x+0) = \lim_{\substack{y_n \to x \\ y_n > x}} \int \psi_{y_n} d\mu = \int \psi_x d\mu = \mu(x)$$

(By monotone convergence theorem)

Let x and b be two real numbers such that $x < b$.

Then $\psi_b - \psi_x$ is simply the characteristic function of the half closed interval $]x,b]$. Let ψ be the characteristic function of a closed bounded interval $[a,b]$, then $\chi = \psi_b - \lim_{\substack{x \to a \\ x < a}} \psi_x$ everywhere, so that

$$\int \chi d\mu = \int \psi_b d\mu - \lim_{\substack{x \to a \\ x < a}} \int \psi_x d\mu$$

$$= \mu(b) - \mu(a-0) = \mu(b+0) - \mu(a-0)$$

$\Rightarrow$ $\int \psi d\mu$ is the Stieltjes integral of χ with respect to μ.

Since, every function in L is a linear combination of characteristic functions of closed bounded intervals, it follows that the integral $\int \phi d\mu$ an linear space L is really the Stieltjes integral with respect to the function μ.

12.4 BAIR SETS AND BOREL SETS

[MEERUT–2006 BP, 08]

Let X be a locally compact Housedorff space we shall denote by C, the class of all compact subsets of X, by S, the σ– ring generated by C and by U, the class of all open sets belonging to S. The set S is called the Borel set of X. Therefore, U may be described as the class of all open Borel sets.

Definition 1. *A real valued function on X is said to be Borel measurable or Borel function, if it is measurable with respect to the σ– ring S.*

Definition 2. *The class of Bair sets is defined to be the smallest σ– algebra B of subsets of X such that each function in $C(X)$ is measurable with respect to B. Thus, B is the σ– algebra generated by the sets $\{x : f(x) \geq \alpha\}$ with $f \in (X)$.* [MEERUT–2005 BP]

Definition 3. *A set E is said to be of the type F_σ if it is expressible as a union of an enumerable number of closed sets F_k, i.e., $E = \bigcup\limits_{k=1}^{\infty} F_k$.* [MEERUT–2006 BP, 08]

Definition 4. *A set E is said to be of the type G_δ if it is expressible as an intersection of an enumerable number of open sets G_k, i.e., $E = \bigcap\limits_{k=1}^{\infty} G_k$.* [MEERUT–2006 BP, 08]

Definition 5. *A set E is called a Borel set if it can be obtained from closed and open sets by using a finite or an enumerable number of union and intersection operations.*

Definition 6. *A set is called σ– compact if it is the union of a countable collection of compact sets. A set which is contained in a compact set is called bounded and one which is contained in a σ– compact set is called σ– bounded.*

☞ REMARKS
- The sets of F_σ and G_δ type are compliment of each other.
- The sets of the types F_σ and G_δ are Borel sets.

THEOREM I.

A Borel measurable set is Lebesgue measurable. [MEERUT–1992, 99]

PROOF. Let E be a Borel measurable set. Then by definition of Borel set, E is bounded. To show E is Lebesgue measurable.

Let
$$E = (\cup G_k) \cap (\cap F_k)$$

Since, E is bounded therefore all G_k and F_k are bounded such that G_k is open and F_k is closed.

$\Rightarrow$ G_k and F_k both are Lebegue measurable sets.

$\Rightarrow$ $\bigcup\limits_k G_k, \cap F_k$ are Lebesgue measurable sets.

[∵ Countable union or intersection of measurable sets is measurable]

$\Rightarrow$ $(\cup G_k) \cap (\cap F_k)$ is Lebesgue measurable.

Hence, E is Lebesgue measurable.

☞ **REMARK**

- If X is any topological space, the smallest σ–algebra containing the closed sets is called the Borel sets. Therefore, if X is locally compact, every Bair set is a Borel set. The converse is true when X is a locally compact metric space, but there are compact spaces where the class of Borel sets is larger than the class of Bair sets. The reader should be careful that not everyone uses the same definitions for Bair and Borel sets, when X is compact, everyone agrees that the Bair sets are the smallest σ–algebra such that each f in C is measurable and that the Borel sets are smallest σ–algebra containing the closed sets but definition differ when X is allowed to be locally compact.

THEOREM 2.

Every Borel set is σ − *bounded if and only if every* σ − *bounded open set is a Borel set.*

PROOF.   We know that every compact set is trivially bounded and therefore σ − bounded. Further, the class of all σ − bounded sets is a σ − ring, since this is a σ − ring includes C, it contains every set of the σ − ring generated by C.

Conversely, suppose that U is open and $<C_n>$ is a sequence of compact sets such that

$$U \subset \overset{\infty}{\underset{n=1}{\cup}} C_n = K$$

Since, for $n = 1, 2, ..., C_n - U$ is compact, it follows that

$$D = \overset{\infty}{\underset{n=1}{\cup}} (C_n - U) \in S$$

Since $D = K - U$, therefore, $U = K - (K - U) \in S$.

12.5 BAIR FUNCTION

Definition. *A smallest linear space of functions on the real line which contains all continuous function and is closed under point wise everywhere limit is called the space of Bair functions* β.

☞ **REMARK**

- The family of all vector spaces that have this property and contain all continuous function is not empty, since the space of all real valued function of one real variable is one such space. The space of Bair functions is the intersection of all the vector spaces in this family. The space of Lebesgue measurable function is also a vector space of functions containing the continuous function and closed under points wise everywhere limits; Since β is the smallest such space, every Bair function is measurable with respect to Lebesgue measure.

NOTATIONS

C_0: The class of all those compact subsets of X which are G_δ type.

S_0: The σ − ring generated by C_0.

U_0: The class of all open sets belonging to S_0. It may be described as the class of all open Bair sets.

THEOREM 1.

If B is a subbase and if S is a σ − *ring containing B then* $S \supset S_0$.

PROOF.   Let C be a compact set and U be open set containing C then, there exists a set E which is a finite union of finite intersections of sets of B, and which therefore belongs to S such that $C \subset E \subset U$. Therefore, if

$$C = \overset{\infty}{\underset{n=1}{\cap}} U_n, \text{ where each } U_n \text{ is open.}$$

Then, for every $n \in N$, these exists a set E_n in S such that $C \subset E_n \subset U_n$. Therefore,

$$C = \bigcap_{n=1}^{\infty} E_n \in S$$

$$\Rightarrow \qquad C_0 \subset S.$$

Hence, by using the definition of S_0, we conclude that $S_0 \subset S$.

THEOREM 2.

Every compact Bair set is G_δ type.

PROOF.   Let C be a compact set in S_0. Then, there exists a sequence $<C_n>$ of set in C_0 such that C belongs to the σ–ring $S(<C_n>)$. Then for every $n = 1, 2, \ldots$, there exists a function f_n such that

$$C_n = \{x : f_n(x) = 0\}$$

If for each pair, x and y of points in X, we can write

$$d(x,y) = \sum_{n=1}^{\infty} \frac{1}{2^n} |f_n(x) - f_n(y)|.$$

Then, by the property of metric space, we have

$$d(x,x) = 0, d(x,y) = d(y,x)$$

and $\qquad 0 \le d(x,y) \le d(x,z) + d(x,y).$

Thus, if we write $x \equiv y$ whenever $d(x,y) = 0$. Then, the relation $\equiv$ is reflexive, symmetric and transitive and hence it is an equivalence relation let us write $t = T(x)$ for every $x \in X$ and unequally determined equivalence class which contains x.

Now, if $\qquad T(x_1) = T(y_1)$

and $\qquad T(x_2) = T(y_2),$ i.e.

If $\qquad x_1 \equiv y_1$ and $x_2 \equiv y_2,$

then $\qquad d(x_1, x_2) \le d(x_1, y_1) + d(y_1, y_2) + d(y_2, x_2) = d(y_1, y_2)$

$\Rightarrow \qquad d(x_1, x_2) \le d(y_1, y_2)$

Similarly, by symmetry, we have

$$d(y_1, y_2) \le d(x_1, x_2)$$

Thus $\qquad d(x_1, x_2) = d(y_1, y_2)$

which implies that if $t_1 = T(x_1)$ and $t_2 = T(x_2)$ be two elements of set of equivalence class. Let δ be a metric on the set of equivalence class. Then, the equation $\delta(t_1, t_2) = d(x_1, x_2)$

Since $\qquad \delta(t_1, t_2) = 0 \Rightarrow t_1 = t_2$

If $t_0 = T(x_0)$ is any point of the metric on the set of equivalence classes if $r_0 > 0$ and $E = \{t : \delta(t_0, t) < r_0\}$

$\Rightarrow \qquad T^{-1}(E) = \{x : d(x_0, x) < r_0\}$

Since $d(x_0, x)$ depends continuous on x, then T is a continuous transformation from X onto the set of equivalence classes.

We know that a subset of X is the inverse image (under T) of a subset set of equivalence classes if and only if it has the property that if contains, along with any of its points, all points equivalent to that one. Since, each C_n has this property, therefore there exist a subset P of set of equivalence classes with $T^{-1}(P) = C$.

Also $T(T^{-1}(P)) = P$

Since, T is continuous and C is compact, therefore P is compact also, every closed compact subset of a metric space is G_δ type therefore, there exists a sequence $< \Delta_n >$ of open subsets of set of equivalence classes with

$$P = \bigcap_{n=1}^{\infty} \Delta_n$$

Write $U_n = T^{-1}(\Delta_n), \; n \in \mathbf{N}$

Then $C = \bigcap_{n=1}^{\infty} U_n$; Since, by the continuity of T, U_n is open.

Hence, $C \in C_o$.

THEOREM 3.

If X and Y are locally compact T_2-space and if A_0, B_0 and S_0 are the σ-rings of Bair sets in X, Y and $X \times Y$ respectively Then, $S_0 = A_0 \times B_0$.

PROOF.

Let X and Y be two locally compact T_2-spaces. Suppose A and B are compact Bair sets in X and Y respectively. Clearly $A \times B$ is a compact set of G_δ type and hence a compact Bair set in $X \times Y$. Since A_0 and B_0 are the σ-ring therefore $A_0 \times B_0$ is the σ-ring generated by the class of all sets of the form $A \times B$. Thus, $A_0 \times B_0 \subset S_0$.

Let U and V are open Bair sets in X and Y respectively.

Then $U \times V \in A_0 \times B_0$.

Further, since the less of all sets of the form $U \times V$ is a base $X \times Y$.

Therefore, using theorem (1), we have $S_0 \subset A_0 \times B_0$.

Hence, we conclude that $S_0 = A_0 \times B_0$.

SOME IMPORTANT FACTS

1. The entire space X is a Borel set if and only if it is σ-compact.
2. The σ-ring generated by the class of all bounded open sets or equivalently the σ-ring generated by U considers with S.
3. The term 'Bair set' is suggested by the term 'Bair function' if B is the smallest class of functions which contains all continuous functions and contains the limit of every point wise (not necessarily uniformly) convergent sequence of function in it, then the function of B are called the Bair function on X.
4. A necessary and sufficient condition that a set be a Bair set is that it be a Borel set and that its characteristic function be a Bair function.
5. The σ-ring generated by the class of all bounded open Bair sets or equivalently the σ-ring generated by U_0 coincides with S_0.
6. Every Boolean σ-algebra is isomorphic to the class of all Bair sets, modulo Bair sets of the first category, in a totally disconnected, compact T_2-space.

12.6 REGULAR MEASURES

Definition I. *A Borel measure is a measure μ defined on the class S of all Borel sets and such that $\mu(c) < \infty$ for every $c \in C$.*

A Bair measure is a measure μ_0 defined on the class S_0 of all Bair sets and such that $\mu_o(C_o) < \infty$ for every $C_0 \in C_0$.

Notation : In this section, we shall use $\hat{C}$, $\hat{U}$ and $\hat{S}$ to stand either for C, U and S or else for C_0, U_0 and S_0 respectively. Also, we shall study a measure $\hat{\mu}$ which is a Borel measure if $\hat{S} = S$ and a Bair measure if $\hat{S} = S_0$.

Definition 2. *A set* E *in* $\hat{S}$ *is said to be outer regular, with respect to the measure* $\hat{\mu}$ *if*
$$\hat{\mu}(E) = \inf.\{\hat{\mu}(U) : E \subset U \in \hat{U}].$$

Definition 3. *A set* E *in* $\hat{S}$ *is said to be inner regular, with respect to* μ *if*
$$\hat{\mu}(E) = \sup.\{\hat{\mu} \subset (C) : E \supset C \in \hat{C}].$$

Definition 4. *A set* E *in* $\hat{S}$ *is said to be regular if it is both inner regular and outer regular.*

Definition 5. *A measure* $\hat{\mu}$ *is said to be regular if every set* E *in* $\hat{S}$ *is regular.*

☞ **REMARKS**

- If $E \in \hat{S}$ and $\hat{\mu}(E) = \infty$ or if $E \in \hat{U}$ or if E is the intersection of a sequence of sets finite measure in $\hat{U}$, then E is other regular.
- If $E \in \hat{S}$ and $\hat{\mu}(E) = 0$ or if $E \in \hat{C}$ or if E is the union of a sequence of sets in $\hat{C}$, then E is inner regular.

THEOREM I.

If every set in $\hat{C}$ *is outer regular, then every proper difference of two sets of* $\hat{C}$ *is outer regular. If every bounded set in* $\hat{U}$ *is inner regular, then every proper difference of two sets in* $\hat{C}$ *is inner regular.*

PROOF.   Let C and D be two sets in $\hat{C}$ such that $C \supset D$. Firstly, we shall prove that $C - D$ is outer regular.

If C is outer regular, then for every $\epsilon > 0$, the exists a set $U \in \hat{U}$ such that $C \subset U$ and
$$\hat{\mu}(U) \leq \hat{\mu}(C) + \epsilon \qquad \qquad \dots(1)$$
Now, since
$$C - D \subset U - D \in \hat{U}$$
Therefore
$$\hat{\mu}(U - D) - \hat{\mu}(C - D) = \hat{\mu}[(U - D) - (C - D)]$$
$$= \hat{\mu}(U - C)$$
$$= \hat{\mu}(U) - \hat{\mu}(C)$$
$$< \epsilon \qquad \qquad \text{[Using (1)]}$$
$\Rightarrow$ $C - D$ is outer regular.

Next, let U be a bounded set in $\hat{U}$ such that $C \subset U$.

If the bounded set $U - D$ is inner regular, then for every $\epsilon > 0$, there is a set E in $\hat{C}$ such that
$$E \subset U - D \text{ and } \hat{\mu}(U - D) \leq \hat{\mu}(E) + \epsilon \qquad \qquad \dots(2)$$
We can write
$$C - D = C \cap (U - D) \supset C \cap E \in \hat{C}$$

Therefore

$$\hat{\mu}(C-D)-\hat{\mu}(C\cap E)=\hat{\mu}[(C-D)-(C\cap E)]$$
$$=\hat{\mu}[(C-D)-E]$$
$$\le\hat{\mu}[(U-D)-E]$$
$$=\hat{\mu}(U-D)-\hat{\mu}(E)\le\epsilon$$

Hence, $C-D$ is inner regular.

THEOREM 2.

A finite disjoint union of inner regular sets of finite measure is inner regular.

PROOF. Let $<E_n>$ be a finite disjoint class of inner regular sets of finite measure. Then for every $\epsilon>0$ and for every $i\in\mathbf{N}$ there exists a set $C_i\in\hat{C}$ such that

$$C_i\subset E_i \text{ and } \hat{\mu}(E_i)\le\hat{\mu}(C_i)+\epsilon/n$$

If $C=\bigcup_{i=1}^{n}C_i$ and $E=\bigcup_{i=1}^{n}E_i$, then $E\supset C\in\hat{C}$

Thus, $\quad \hat{\mu}(E)=\sum_{L=1}^{n}\hat{\mu}(E_i)\le\sum_{L=1}^{n}\hat{\mu}(C_i)+\epsilon=\hat{\mu}(c)+\epsilon$

Hence, E is inner regular.

THEOREM 3.

The intersection of a sequence of inner regular sets of finite measure is inner regular. Also, the intersection of a decreasing sequence of outer regular sets of finite measure is outer regular.

PROOF. Let $<E_i>$ be a sequence of inner regular sets of finite measure then for every $i\in\mathbf{N}$, then exists a set $C_i\in\hat{C}$
such that

$$C_i\subset E_i \text{ and } \hat{\mu}(E_i)\le\hat{\mu}(C_i)+\frac{\epsilon}{\alpha^i}$$

Let us write $C=\bigcap_{i=1}^{\infty}C_i$

If $E=\bigcap_{i=1}^{\infty}E_i$, then $E\supset C\in\hat{C}$

Also, $\quad\hat{\mu}(E)-\hat{\mu}(C)=\hat{\mu}(E-C)$

$$\le\hat{\mu}\left(\bigcup_{i=1}^{\infty}(E_i-C_i)\right)$$

$$\le\sum_{i=1}^{\infty}\hat{\mu}(E_i-C_i)$$

$$=\sum_{i=1}^{\infty}(\hat{\mu}(E_i)-\hat{\mu}(C_i))$$

$$\le\epsilon.$$

If $<E_i>$ is a decreasing sequence of outer regular sets of finite measure and

$$E=\bigcap_{i=1}^{\infty}E_i.$$

Then, we use the following relation
$$\hat{\mu}(E) = \lim_{i} \hat{\mu}(E_i).$$

To show that for every real number C with $C > \hat{\mu}(E)$ there exists a set $U \in \hat{U}$ such that $E \subset U$ and $C > \hat{\mu}(U)$. For this we select a value i so that $C > \hat{\mu}(E_i)$ and then using the outer regularity of E_i, we can find a set $U \in \hat{U}$ such that
$$E_i \subset U \text{ and } \hat{\mu}(U) < C.$$

THEOREM 4.

The union of sequence of outer regular sets is outer regular. Also, the union of an increasing sequence of inner regular sets is inner regular.

PROOF. Consider a sequence $< E_i >$ of outer regular sets then, for every $\epsilon > 0$ and for every $i \in \mathbf{N}$, there exists a set $U_i \in \hat{U}$.
such that
$$E_i \subset U_i \text{ and } \hat{\mu}(U_i) \leq \hat{\mu}(E_i) + \frac{\epsilon}{\alpha^i}$$

Let us write $\qquad U = \overset{\infty}{\underset{i=1}{\bigcup}} \, U_i$

If $E = \overset{\infty}{\underset{i=1}{\bigcup}} E_i$ and $\hat{\mu}(E) = \infty$, then trivially, E is outer regular if $\hat{\mu}(E) < \infty$, then

$$\begin{aligned}
\hat{\mu}(U) - \hat{\mu}(E) &= \hat{\mu}(U - E) \\
&\leq \hat{\mu}\left(\overset{\infty}{\underset{i=1}{\bigcup}} \, (U_i - E_i) \right) \\
&\leq \overset{\infty}{\underset{i=1}{\sum}} \, \hat{\mu}(U_i - E_i) \\
&= \overset{\infty}{\underset{i=1}{\sum}} \, [\hat{\mu}(U_i) - \hat{\mu}(E_i)] \\
&< \epsilon
\end{aligned}$$

If $< E_i >$ is an increasing sequence of inner regular sets and $E = \overset{\infty}{\underset{i=1}{\bigcup}} E_i$, we use the relation
$$\hat{\mu}(E) = \lim_{i} \hat{\mu}(E_i)$$

Now, to show that, for every real number c with $c < \hat{\mu} \subset E$, there exists a set E in $\hat{C}$ such that $\hat{C} \subset E$ and $c < \mu(\hat{C})$. For this, we need only select a value of i so that $c < \hat{\mu}(E_i)$ and then using the inner regularity if E_i, find a set $c \in \hat{C}$ such that $\hat{C} \subset E_i$ and $c < \hat{\mu}(C)$.

THEOREM 5.

A necessary and sufficient condition that every set in $\hat{C}$ be outer regular is that every bounded set in $\hat{U}$ be inner regular.

PROOF. Let us suppose that every set in $\hat{C}$ is outer regular and U be a set in $\hat{U}$, which is bounded. Let $\epsilon > 0$. Also, let C be a set in $\hat{C}$ such that $U \subset C$.

Since $C-U$ is compact and belongs to $\hat{S}$.

Therefore, $\qquad C-U \in \hat{C}$

Thus, there exists a set $V \in \hat{U}$ such that
$$C-U \subset V$$

and $\qquad \hat{\mu}(V) \leq \hat{\mu}(C-U) + \in$

Since, $U = C - (C-U) \supset C - V \in \hat{C}$, therefore the relations
$$\hat{\mu}(U) - \hat{\mu}(C-V) = \hat{\mu}[U - (C-V)]$$
$$= \hat{\mu}(U \cap V)$$
$$\leq \hat{\mu}(V - (C - (U))$$
$$= \hat{\mu}(V) - \hat{\mu}(C - U)$$
$$\leq \in$$

Hence, U is inner regular.

Further, suppose that every bounded set in $\hat{U}$ is inner regular, let $C \in \hat{C}$ be any set and let $\in > 0$. Let U be bounded set in $\hat{U}$ such that $C \subset U$.

Since, $U - C$ is a bounded set in $\hat{U}$, there exists a set D in $\hat{C}$ such that
$$D \subset U - C \text{ and } \hat{\mu}(U - C) \leq \hat{\mu}(D) + \in$$

Since $C = U - (U - C) \subset U - D \in \hat{U}$, then the relations
$$\hat{\mu}(U - D) - \hat{\mu}(C) = \hat{\mu}((U - D) - C)$$
$$= \hat{\mu}((U - C) - D)$$
$$= \hat{\mu}(U - C) - \hat{\mu}(D)$$
$$< \in$$

Hence, C is outer regular.

THEOREM 6.

Every Bair measure v is regular if $C \in C$, then
$$v^*(C) = \inf (v(U_0) : C \subset U_0 \in \mathbf{U}_0]$$

PROOF. We know that every set in C_0 may be written as the intersection of a decreasing sequence of sets of finite measure in $\mathbf{U}_0$.

By definition of outer measure, we have
$$v^*(C) = \inf \{v(E_0) : C \subset E_0 \in S_0\}$$
$$\leq \inf .\{v(U_0) : C \subset U_0 \in \mathbf{U}_0\}$$

Further, for every $\in > 0$, there exists a set $E_0 \in S_0$ such that $C \subset E_0$ and
$$v(E_0) \leq v^*(C) + {}^{\in}\!/_2$$

By the outer regularity of E_0, these exists a set U_0 in $\mathbf{U}_0$ such that
$$E_0 \subset U_0 \text{ and } v(U_0) \leq v(E_0) + {}^{\in}\!/_2$$

which implies
$$C \subset U_0 \text{ and } v(U_0) \leq v^*(C) + \in$$

Hence, we conclude that
$$v^*(C) = \inf .\{v(U_0) : C \subset U_0 \in \mathbf{U}_0\}$$

SOME IMPORTANT FACTS

(1) If μ is a Borel measure and if there exists a countable set Y such that $\mu(E) = \mu(E \cap Y)$, for every Borel set E, then μ is Regular.

(2) Every Borel measure is σ − finite.

(3) If μ_1, μ_2 and μ are Borel measure such that $\mu = \mu_1 + \mu_2$ then, the regularity of any two of them implies that of the third.

(4) The Borel measure μ is not regular.

(5) If, for every Borel set E in $\bar{X}$, $\mu(E) = 1$ or 0 according as E does or does not contain an unbounded closed subset of X, then μ is a Borel measure.

(6) If μ and ν are Borel measure such that μ is regular and $\nu \ll \mu$ then ν is regular.

(7) If μ is regular Borel measure, then for every σ − bounded set E

$$\mu^{*}(E) = \inf.\{\mu(U) : E \subset U \subset \mathbf{U}\}$$
$$\mu_{*}(E) = \sup.\{\mu(C) : E \supset C \in \mathbf{C}\}$$

12.7 GENERALISATION OF BOREL MEASURES

Definition 1. *A 'Content' is a set function* λ *on C which is such that*

(1) $0 \le \lambda(C) < \infty \ \forall C \in \mathbf{C}$

(2) If C and D are compact sets for which $C \subset D$ then, $\lambda(C) \le \lambda(D)$

(3) If C and D are disjoint compact sets, then $\lambda(C \cup D) = \lambda(C) + \lambda(D)$

(4) If C and D are any two compact sets, then $\lambda(C \cup D) \le \lambda(C) + \lambda(D)$

☛ REMARKS

- A 'Content' is a non-negative, finite, monotonic, additive and sub additive set function on the class C of all compact set.

- Since $\lambda(0) + \lambda(0) = \lambda(0 \cup 0) = \lambda(0) < \infty$, therefore, a content must always vanish on the empty set.

Definition 2. *The inner content* λ_*, *induced by a content* λ *is the set function defined for every* U *in* **U** *such that*

$$\lambda_*(U) = \sup.\{\lambda(C) : U \supset C \in \mathbf{C}\}$$

Definition 3. *Let* λ *us a content and* λ_* *is the inner content induced by* λ, *then a set function* μ^{*} *defined on* σ − *ring of all* σ − *bounded set by*

$$\mu^{*}(E) = \inf.\{\lambda_*(U) : E \subset U \in \mathbf{U}\}$$

is called the outer measure induced by λ.

THEOREM I.

The inner contents λ_* *induced by a content* λ *vanishes at* 0 *and is monotonic, countably sub additive, and countably additive.*

PROOF.   By definition of inner content, we have

$$\lambda_*(0) = 0$$

Let U and V be any two sets in U such that $U \subset V$.

If C is a compact set contained in U, then $C \subset V$.

Now $C \subset V \Rightarrow \lambda(C) \le \lambda_*(V)$

$\Rightarrow$ $\lambda_*(U) = \sup \lambda(C) \le \lambda_*(V)$

If U and V are in $\mathbf{U}$ and if C is a compact set such that $C \subset U \cup V$, then there exist compact sets $D \subset U$, $E \subset V$ and $C = D \cup E$.

Since $\lambda(C) \le \lambda(D) + \lambda(E) \le \lambda_*(U) + \lambda_*(V)$.

Therefore, $\lambda_*(U \cup V) = \sup \lambda(C) \le \lambda_*(U) + \lambda_*(V)$. Thus, λ_* is sub additive. Similarly by using mathematical induction, we can prove that λ_* is finitely sub additive.

Further, let $<U_i>$ be a sequence of sets in U and if C is a compact set such that

$$C \subset \bigcup_{i=1}^{\infty} U_i$$

Then, since C is compact, therefore, there is a positive integer n such that

$C \subset \bigcup_{i=1}^{n} U_i$. Therefore,

$$\lambda(C) \le \lambda_*\left(\bigcup_{i=1}^{n} U_i \right) \le \sum_{i=1}^{n} \lambda_*(U_i) \le \sum_{i=1}^{\infty} \lambda_*(U_i)$$

$$\Rightarrow \quad \lambda_*\left(\bigcup_{i=1}^{\infty} U_i \right) = \sup \lambda(C) \le \sum_{i=1}^{\infty} \lambda_*(U_i)$$

Thus, λ_* is countably sub additive.

Next, suppose that U and V are any two disjoint sets in U. Also, let C and D be compact sets such that $C \subset U$ and $D \subset V$. Since C and D are disjoint and since $C \cup D \subset U \cup V$.

Therefore, we have

$$\lambda(C) + \lambda(D) = \lambda(C \cup D) \le \lambda_*(U \cup V)$$

$$\Rightarrow \quad \lambda_*(U) + \lambda_*(V) = \sup.\lambda(C) + \sup.\lambda(D) \le \lambda_*(U \cup V)$$

Also, λ_* is sub addition hence, λ_* is finitely additive.

Now, if $<V_i>$ is a disjoint sequence of sets in U, then

$$\lambda_*\left(\bigcup_{i=1}^{\infty} U_i \right) \ge \lambda_*\left(\bigcup_{i=1}^{n} U_i \right) = \sum_{i=1}^{n} \lambda_*(U_i)$$

Letting $n \to \infty$, we get

$$\lambda_*\left(\bigcup_{i=1}^{\infty} U_i \right) \ge \sum_{i=1}^{\infty} \lambda_*(U_i)$$

Hence, λ_* is countably additive.

THEOREM 2.

The outer measure μ^* *induced by a content* λ *is an outer measure.*

PROOF. Since $O \subset O \in U$ and $\lambda_*(0) = 0$ therefore, clearly we have $\mu^*(0) = 0$. Now, let E and F are two σ-bounded sets such that $E \subset F$ and if U is a set in U such that $F \subset U$, then $E \subset U$.

Thus, $\mu^*(E) \le \lambda_*(U)$

$\Rightarrow \qquad \mu^*(E) \le \inf.\lambda_*(U) = \mu^*(F)$

$\Rightarrow \quad \mu^*$ is monotonic.

Further, let $<E_i>$ be a sequence of σ-bounded sets, then for every $\in > 0$ and for every $i \in \mathbf{N}$, Hence, there exists set $U_i \in \mathbf{U}$ such that

$$E_i \subset U_i \text{ and } \lambda*(U_i) \le \mu^*(E_i) + \frac{\epsilon}{2^i}$$

$$\Rightarrow \quad \mu^* \left(\bigcup_{i=1}^{\infty} E_i \right) \le \lambda* \left(\bigcup_{i=1}^{\infty} U_i \right) \le \sum_{i=1}^{\infty} \lambda*(U_i) \le \sum_{i=1}^{\infty} \mu^*(E_i) + \epsilon$$

Since ϵ is arbitrary, letting $\epsilon \to 0$, therefore

$$\mu^* \left(\bigcup_{i=1}^{\infty} E_i \right) \le \sum_{i=1}^{\infty} \mu^*(E_i)$$

$\Rightarrow \quad \mu^*$ is countably sub additive.

Hence, μ^* is and outer measure.

THEOREM 3.

If $\lambda*$ is the inner content and μ^* is the outer measure induced by a content λ, then $\mu^*(U) = \lambda*(U)$ for every $U \in \mathbf{U}$ and $\mu^*(C^0) \le \lambda(C) \le \mu^*(C)$ for every C in $\mathbf{C}$. Here C^0 is the interior of C.

PROOF.   Since $U \subset U \in \mathbf{U}$

$$\mu^*(U) \le \lambda*(U)$$

If $V \in \mathbf{U}$ and $U \subset V$, then $\lambda*(U) \le \lambda*(V)$

Therefore, $\lambda*(U) \le \inf . \lambda*(V) = \mu^*(U)$.

Now, if $C \in \mathbf{C}$, $U \in \mathbf{U}$ and $C \subset U$

Then $\lambda(C) \le \lambda*(U)$

$\Rightarrow$ $\lambda(C) \le \inf . \lambda*(U) = \mu^*(C)$

If $C \in \mathbf{C}$, $D \in \mathbf{C}$ and $D \subset C^0 \subset C$, then $\lambda(D) \le \lambda(C)$

Thus, $\mu^*(C^0) = \lambda*(C^0) = \sup \lambda(D) \le (C)$.

THEOREM 4.

Let μ^* be the outer measure induced by a content λ, then a $\sigma-$ bounded set E is μ^* -measurable if and only if

$$\mu^*(U) \ge \mu^*(U \cap E) + \mu^*(U \cap E')$$

For every U in U.

PROOF.   Let $\lambda*$ be the inner content induced by λ. Also, let A be an arbitrary $\sigma-$ bounded set and $U \in \mathbf{U}$ such that $A \subset U$

Then, since

$$\lambda*(U) = \mu^*(U) \ge \mu^*(U \cap E) + \mu^*(U \cap E')$$

$$\ge \mu^*(A \cap E) + \mu^*(A \cap E')$$

Therefore,

$$\mu^*(A) = \inf . \lambda*(U) \ge \mu^*(A \cap E) + \mu^*(A \cap E') \qquad \dots(1)$$

Next using the sub additively of μ^*, we have

$$\mu^*(A) \le \mu^*(A \cap E) + \mu^*(A \cap E') \qquad \dots(2)$$

From (1) and (2), we conclude that

$$\mu^*(A) = \mu^*(A \cap E) + \mu^*(A \cap E')$$

Hence, E is measurable.

Converse part of the theorem follows from the sub additively and definition of μ^*-measurability.

THEOREM 5.

If μ^* is the outer measure induced by a content λ, then the set function μ, defined for every Borel set E by $\mu(E) = \mu^*(E)$ is a regular Borel measure.

PROOF.   Firstly, we shall prove that every compact set C is μ^*-measurable using Theorem-4 , it is sufficient to prove that

$$\mu^*(U) \geq \mu^*(U \cap C) + \mu^*(U \cap C')$$

Let D be a compact subset of $U \cap C'$ and let E be a compact subset of $U \cap D'$.

Clearly $U \cap C'$ and $U \cap D'$ belongs to U.

Now, since $D \cap E = 0$ and $D \cup E \subset V$

Thus $\mu^*(U) = \lambda_*(U) \geq \lambda(D \cup E) = \lambda(D) + \lambda(E)$

$\Rightarrow$ $\mu^*(U) \geq \mu^*(U \cap C) + \sup . \lambda(D)$

$$= \mu^*(U \cap C) + \lambda_*(U \cap C^1)$$

$$= \mu^*(U \cap C) + \mu^*(U \cap C^1).$$

Further, to show that $\mu(C) < \infty$. There exists a compact set F such that $C \subset F^o$, therefore

$$\mu(C) = \mu^*(C) \leq \mu^*(F) \leq \lambda(F) < \infty$$

Now, since

$$\mu(C) = \mu^*(C) = \inf .(\lambda_*(U) : C \subset U \in \mathbf{U}\}$$

$$= \inf .\{\mu^*(U) : C \subset U \in \mathbf{U}\}$$

$$= \{\mu(U) : C \subset U \in \mathbf{U}\} .$$

12.8 REGULARITY OF MEASURES ON LOCALLY COMPACT SPACES

Definition. *A content λ is regular if, for every C in $\mathbf{C}$*

$$\lambda(C) = \inf .\{\lambda(D) : C \subset D^o \subset D \in \mathbf{C}\}.$$

THEOREM I.

If μ is the Borel measure induced by a regular content λ, then $\mu(C) = \lambda(C)$ for every C in $\mathbf{C}$.

PROOF.   Let $C \in \mathbf{C}$ then, by definition of regularly of λ, for every $\epsilon > 0 \;\exists\; D$ in $\mathbf{C}$ such that

$$C \subset D^o$$

and $\lambda(D) \leq \lambda(C) + \epsilon$

Therefore $\lambda(C) \leq \mu(C) \leq \mu(D^0) \leq \lambda(D) \leq \lambda(C) + \epsilon$

Since $\in$ is arbitrary, letting $\in \to 0$, we get
$$\lambda(C) \le \mu(C) \le \lambda(C)$$

Hence, $\mu(C) = \lambda(C)$ for every C in $\mathbf{C}$.

THEOREM 2.

Let μ be a regular measure and if for every C in $\mathbf{C}$, $\lambda(C) = \mu(C)$, then λ is a regular content and the Borel measure induced by λ coincides with μ.

PROOF.   Clearly, λ is a content. Since μ is given to be regular, therefore, by definition for every C in C and for every $\in > 0$ there exists a set U in $\mathbf{U}$ such that
$$C \subset U \text{ and } \mu(U) \le \mu(C) + \in$$
If D is a set in C such that
$$C \subset D^o \subset D \subset U$$
Then $\lambda(D) = \mu(D) \le \mu(U) \le \mu(C) + \in$
$$= \lambda(C) + \in$$
Thus, λ is regular.

If μ^* is the Borel measure induced by λ, then by previous theorem
$$\hat{\mu}(C) = \lambda(C) = \mu(C) \text{ for every } C \text{ in } \mathbf{C}.$$
Hence, $\hat{\mu} = \mu$.

THEOREM 3.

If μ_0 is a Bair measure and if, for every C in $\mathbf{C}$
$$\lambda(C) = \inf .\{\mu_0(U_0) : C \subset U_0 \in \mathbf{U}_0]$$
Then, λ is a regular content.

PROOF.   If can be easily verify that λ is non-negative, finite and monotonic.

Let C and D be the sets in C and U_0 and V_0 are sets in $\mathbf{U}_0$ such that
$$C \subset U_0 \text{ and } D \subset V_0$$
Then $C \cup D \subset U_0 \cup V_0 \in V_0$

$\Rightarrow$ $\lambda(C \cup D) \le \mu_0(U_0 \cup V_0) \le \mu_0(U_0) + \mu_0(V_0)$

Thus, $\lambda(C \cup D) \le \inf .\mu_0(U_0) + \inf .\mu_0(V_0)$
$$= \lambda(C) + \lambda(D)$$
$\Rightarrow$ λ is sub additive.

Further, if C and D are disjoint sets in C.

Then, there exists disjoint sets U_0 and V_0 in $\mathbf{U}_0$ such that $C \subset U_0$ and $D \subset V_0$.

If $C \cup D \subset W_0 \in \mathbf{U}_0$, then
$$\lambda(C) + \lambda(D) \le \mu_0(U_0 \cap W_0) + \mu_0(V_0 \cap W_0) \le \mu_0(W_0)$$
$\Rightarrow$ $\lambda(C) + \lambda(D) \le \inf .\mu_0(W_0) = \lambda(C \cup D)$

Also λ is sub additive

Hence, λ is additive.

Now, it remains to prove that λ is regular.

Let C be any compact set and let $\epsilon > 0$

Then, by definition of λ, there exists a set U_0 such that

$$C \subset U_0 \text{ and } \mu_0(U_0) \le \lambda(C) + \epsilon$$

If D is a compact set such that $C \subset D^0 \subset D \subset U_0$, then

$$\lambda(D) \le \mu_0(U_0) \le \lambda(C) + \epsilon.$$

Hence, λ is regular.

THEOREM 4.

If μ_0 is a Bair measure then there exists a unique, regular Borel measure μ such that $\mu(E) = \mu_0(E)$ for every Bair set E.

PROOF. Using previous Theorem-3 we can say that for every C in $\mathbf{C}$

$$\lambda(C) = \inf\{\mu_0(U_0) : C \subset U_0 \in U_0\}.$$

Then λ is regular contact.

If μ is the regular Borel measure induced by λ, there by Theorem-1 $\mu(C) = \lambda(C)$ for every C in $\mathbf{C}$.

Since, every Bair measure is regular, we have

$$\lambda(C) = \mu_0(C)$$

$\Rightarrow \quad \mu(C) = \mu_0(C)$ for every C in $\mathbf{C}_0$.

$\Rightarrow \quad \mu$ is unique.

SOME IMPORTANT FACTS

1. If μ is a Borel measure and if, for every C in $\mathbf{C}$, $\lambda(C) = \sup\{\mu(C_0) : C \supset C_0 \in \mathbf{C}\}$ then μ is completion regular if and only if λ is a regular content.

2. A content λ is inner regular if for every C in $\mathbf{C}$, $\lambda(C) = \sup\{\lambda(D) : C^0 \supset D \in \mathbf{C}\}$ then, following are true:

   (a) If μ is the Borel measure induced by an inner regular content λ, then $\mu(C^0) = \lambda(C)$ for every C in $\mathbf{C}$.

   (b) If μ is a regular Borel measure and if for every C in $\mathbf{C}$, $\lambda(C) = \mu(C^0)$, then λ is an inner regular content and the Borel measure induced by λ coincides with μ.

12.9 INTEGRATION OF CONTINUOUS FUNCTIONS

Let X be a locally compact T_2 space and J denote the class of all those real valued continuous function an X which vanish outside a complete set, *i.e.*, J is the class of all those continuous functions f an X for which the set $N(F) = \{x : f(x) \ne 0)$ is bounded.

Definition. *Let X is not compact and if X^* be the one point campatification of X by x^*, then x^* is called point at infinity.*

☞ **REMARK**

• Using the above definition, we conclude that J is the class of all those continuous functions which vanish in a neighborhood of infinity.

THEOREM 1.

Let C be a compact Bair set, then there exists a decreasing sequence $< f_n >$ of functions in J_+ such that $\lim_{n \to \infty} f_n(x) = \chi_c(x)$, for every x in X, where J_+ is the class of all non-negative functions in J.

PROOF.   Let $C = \bigcap_{n=1}^{\infty} U_n$, where each U_n is bounded open set then for every positive integer n, there exists a function g_n in J such that

$$g_n(x) = \begin{cases} 1, & \text{if } x \in C \\ 2, & \text{if } x \notin U_n \end{cases}$$

If $f_n = g_1 \cap \ldots \cap g_n$, then $< f_n >$ is a decreasing sequence of non-negative continuous function such that $\lim_{n \to \infty} f_n(x) = \chi_c(x)$ for all $x \in X$.

Since, U_n is bounded, therefore, $f_n \in J_+$.

☛ **REMARK**

• Let μ_0 be a Bair measure in x and if $f \in J$ and if $\{x : f(x) \neq 0\} \subset C \in C_0$ then $\mu_0(C) < \infty$, f is bounded and Bair measure imply that f is integrable with respect to μ_0 and $\int f d\mu_0 = \int_c f d\mu_0$.

THEOREM 2.

Let μ be a Bair measure such that the measure of every non-empty Bair open set is positive and if $f \in J_+$ then a necessary and sufficient condition that $\int f d\mu = 0$ is that $f(x) = 0$ $\forall x \in X$.

PROOF.   **Condition is Necessary:** Let us suppose that

$$\int f d\mu = 0$$

And U be a bounded open Bair set such that $\{x : f(x) \neq 0\} \subset U$ further, if $E = \{x : f(x) = 0\}$.

Then, since

$$0 = \int f d\mu \geq \int_{U-E} f d\mu$$

And f is non-negative, therefore $\mu(U - E) = 0$.

Since $U - E$ is an open Bair set, we must have either $U - E = 0$, *i.e.,* $U = E$ or $U \subset E$.

Condition is sufficient : The sufficiency of the condition is trivial.

THEOREM 3.

If μ_0 is a Bair measure and $\in > 0$ then, corresponding to every integrable simple Bair function f there exists an integrable simple function g,

$$g = \sum_{i=1}^{n} \alpha_i \chi_{C_i}$$

such that C_i is a compact Bair set, $i \in \mathbf{N}$, and $\int |f - g| d\mu_0 \leq \in$

PROOF.   Let us write $f = \sum_{i=1}^{n} \alpha_i \chi_{E_i}$

If C be a positive number such that $|f(x)| \leq C$ for every $x \in X$, *i.e.,* such that $|\alpha_i| \leq C$ for $i \in \mathbf{N}$.

Since, μ_o is regular, therefore, by definition, for each $i \in N$, there exists a compact Bair set C_i such that $C_i \subset E_i$ and $\mu_o(E_i) \leq \mu_o(C_i) + \dfrac{\epsilon}{n.c}$.

Thus if $g = \sum\limits_{i=1}^{n} \alpha_i \chi_{C_i}$, then $\int |f - g| d\mu_o = \sum\limits_{i=1}^{n} |\alpha_i| \mu_o(E_i - C_i) \leq \epsilon$.

THEOREM 4.

If μ_o is a Bair measure if $\epsilon > 0$ and if $g = \sum\limits_{i=1}^{n} \alpha_i \chi_{C_i}$ is a simple function such that C_i is a compact Bair set, $i \in N$ then there exists a function h in J such that $\int |g - h| d\mu_o \leq \epsilon$.

PROOF.   Let $\{C_1, C_2, ..., C_n\}$ be a finite disjoint class of compact sets then there exists, a finite disjoint class $\{U_1, ..., U_n\}$ of open bounded open Bair sets such that $C_i \subset U_i, i \in N$.

Since, μ_o is regular, therefore without loss of any generality, we may assume that $\mu_o(U_i) \leq \mu_o(C_i) + \dfrac{\epsilon}{nc}$; $i \in N$.

where C is a positive number such that $|g(x)| \leq C$ for every $x \in X$.

Now, for each $i \in N$, there exists a function h_i in J such that $h_i(x) = 1$ for x in C_i and $h_i(x) = 0$ for x in $\chi - U_i$; we can write $h = \sum\limits_{i=1}^{n} \alpha_i h_i$.

Further, since $h_i \in J_+, i \in N$, therefore clearly, $h \in J$ and disjointness of U_i implies that $|h(x)| \leq C$ for all x in X Hence, we have

$$\int |g - h| d\mu_o = \sum\limits_{i=1}^{n} \int_{U_i - C_i} |h| d\mu_o \leq \sum\limits_{i=1}^{n} C\mu_o(U_i - C_i) \leq \epsilon$$

$$\Rightarrow \quad \int |g - h| d\mu_o \leq \epsilon$$

SOME IMPORTANT FACTS

1. If μ is a regular Borel measure, then the class of all finite linear combinations of characteristic functions of compact sets is dense in $J_p(\mu)$, $1 \leq p < \infty$.

2. If μ is a regular Borel measure, then J is dense in $J_p(\mu)$, $1 \leq p < \infty$.

3. If μ is a regular Borel measure, E is a Borel set of finite measure and f is a Borel measurable function on E then, for every $\epsilon > 0$, there exists a compact set C in E such that $\mu(E - C) \leq \epsilon$ and such that f is continuous on C.

Exercise 12.1

1. Show that the collection of compact G_δ 's is closed with respect to finite union and inter sections.

2. Let μ and μ^* restricted to the Bair sets. If f is a non-negative function in $C(x)$ and $f \geq 1$ an a Bair set E, then $\mu(E) \leq I(f)$. If $f \leq 1$ and the support of f is contained in a compact Bair set K, then $\mu(K) \geq I(f)$.

3. Let X be a locally compact T_2-space, K a compact subset, U an open subset and $K \subset U$, then show that exists an open subset V with compact closure $\overline{V}$ such that $K \subset V \subset \overline{V} \subset U$.

4. Let X be a locally compact T_2-space and K be a compact subset of X. Then show that the necessary and sufficient condition for the existence of a continuous function

$\psi : X \rightarrow [0,1]$ of compact support with $K = \{x \in X : \psi(x) = 1\}$ is that K should by a G_δ type.

5. Let X be locally compact T_2-space. Then show that the σ–algebra of Bair sets in X is generated by the compact G_f type.

6. If μ_o is a Bair measure, then show that there exists a unique, regular Borel measure μ such that $\mu(E) = \mu_o(E)$ for every Bair set E.

7. Suppose that T is a homeomorphism of X onto itself and that λ is a contact. If, for every C in $\mathbf{C}$, $\lambda(C) = \hat{\lambda}(T(C))$ and if μ and μ are the Borel measure induced by λ and λ respectively, then show that $\hat{\mu}(E) = \mu(T(E))$ for every Borel set E.

8. Show that the Borel measure μ is not regular.

9. If, for every Borel set E in $\overline{X}$, $\mu(E) = 1$ or 0 according as E does or does not contain an unbounded closed subset of X, then show that μ is a Borel measure.

10. If μ and ν are Borel measure such that μ is regular and $\nu \ll \mu$ then show that ν is regular.

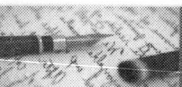 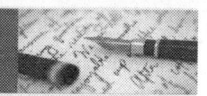

CHAPTER Summary

KEY TERMS

- **L-S Integral:** Let L be a linear space and ϕ be a step function. The Lebesgue-Stieltjes integral $\int \phi d\alpha$ of a step function $\phi \in L$ with respect to a function $\alpha \in V_{loc}^+$ is defined by $\int \phi d\alpha = \int_{J_\alpha} \phi \circ \alpha_1 dx$, where α_1 is the inverse of α.

- **Borel Measurable Function:** A real valued function on X is Borel measurable, if it is measurable with respect to the σ-ring.

- **Baire's Set:** The class of Baire sets is defined to be the smallest σ-algebra B of subsets of X such that each function in $C(X)$ is measurable w.r.t. B.

- **σ-Compact:** A set is called σ-compact if it is the union of a countable collection of compact sets.

- **Baire Function:** A smallest linear space of functions on the real line which contains all continuous function and is closed under point wise everywhere limit is called the space of Baire functions.

- **Baire Measure:** A measure μ_0 defined on the class of all Baire sets is called Baire measure if $\mu_0(C_o) < \infty$.

RESULTS

- A real valued function an X is Borel measurable or simply a Borel function if it is measurable with respect to the $\sigma-$ring S.

- A real valued function on X is Bair measurable or simply a Bair function if it is measurable with respect to the $\sigma-$ring S_0 where S_0 denote the ring generated by C_o.

- Every compact Bair set Y is G_δ.

- A necessary and sufficient condition that a set be a Bair set is that it be a Borel set and that its

characteristic function be a Bair function.

- A Borel measure is a measure μ defined on the class S all Borel sets and such that $\mu(C) < \infty$ for every C in $\mathbf{C}$ and a Bair measure is a measure μ_o defined on the class S_o of all Bair sets and such that $\mu(C_o) < \infty$ for every C_o in $\mathbf{C}$.

- A finite, disjoint union of inner regular sets of finite measure is inner regular.

- Every Borel measure is $\sigma-$finite.

WORTHY READINGS

☞ The entire space X is a Borel set if and only if it is σ-compact.

☞ Let X be a product space then the class of Baire's sets coincides with the class of measurable sets.

☞ A necessary and sufficient condition that a set be a Bair set is that it be a Borel set and that its characteristic function be a Bair function.

☞ The regularity of certain sets implies the regularity of many others.

☞ Every Borel measure is σ-finite.

☞ If X is the Euclidean plane and if μ is Lebesgue measure on the class of all Borel sets then μ is regular measure.

☞ If μ and ν are Borel measure such that μ is regular and $\nu << \mu$ then ν is regular.

FURTHER READINGS

☞ A necessary and sufficient condition that a set be a Bair set is that it be a Borel set and that its characteristic function be a Bair function.

☞ Every Boolean σ-algebra is isomorphic to the class of all Baire sets, modulo Baire set of the first category, in a totally disconnected, compact T_2-space.

☞ The class of all bounded closed subsets of X is closed under the formation of countable intersection.

☞ The Borel measure μ is not regular.

☞ If X is a discrete space consisting of a finite number of points, then $\lambda(C) = 1$ for every compact set C.

Chapter
13 More Theorems on Convergence and Integrations

INTRODUCTION

In this chapter we shall discuss some miscellaneous topics such as integration by parts, mean value theorems, Weirstrass' approximation theorem and semicontinuous functions etc.

13.2 INTEGRATION BY PARTS

In ordinary integral calculus, we have the following formula of integration by parts.

$$\int_a^b f(x)g(x)dx = \left\{[\int f(x)dx]g(x)\right\}_a^b - \int_a^b \left[\frac{dg}{dx}\int fdx\right]dx$$

This formula of integration by parts is same in Lebesgue theory, which is discussed in the following theorems.

THEOREM I.

Let f(x) be an indefinite integral and if G(x) is an indefinite integral of g(x) then

$$\int_a^b f(x)g(x)dx = \left[f(x)\cdot G(x)\right]_a^b - \int_a^b f'(x)G(x)dx$$

PROOF.   By definition of indefinite integral, we can write

$$G(x) = \int_a^x g(t)dt + C, \qquad\qquad ...(1)$$

Since, f is an indefinite integral therefore f is absolutely continuous. Now from (1), we can say that $G(x)$ is an absolutely continuous on $[a, b]$ and $g(x)$ is Lebesgue integrable in $[a, b]$.

$\Rightarrow$ $f(x)$ and $G(x)$ both are absolutely continuous.

$\Rightarrow$ $f(x)\cdot G(x)$ is absolutely continuous.   ($\because$ Product of two absolutely continuous functions is absolutely continuous)

$\Rightarrow$ $f(x)\cdot G(x)$ is L-integrable.

($\because$ Every absolutely continuous function is L-integrable)

$\Rightarrow$ $\int_a^b f(x)G(x)dx$ exists.

Now, $f(t)$ is indefinite integral therefore, $f(t)$ is absolutely continuous.

$\Rightarrow$ $f(t)$ is indefinite integral of $f'(t)$

$\Rightarrow$ $f'(t)$ is integrable.

$\Rightarrow$ $f'(t)G(t)$ is integrable.

$\Rightarrow$ $\int_a^b f'(t)G(t)dt$ exists.

Now from (1), we have $G'(x) = g(x)$ a.e. on $[a, b]$.

$$\int_a^b \frac{d}{dx}[f(x)G(x)dx = [f(x) \cdot G(x)]_a^b \qquad \ldots(2)$$

But $\frac{d}{dx}[f(x)G(x)] = f'(x)G(x) + f(x)G'(x) = f'(x)G(x) + f(x)g(x)$

Using this value in (2) we get

$$\int_a^b [f'(x)g(x) + f(x)g(x)]dx = [f(x)G(x)]_a^b$$

$$\Rightarrow \int_a^b f'(x)G(x)dx + \int_a^b f(x)g(x)dx = [f(x) \cdot G(x)]_a^b$$

Hence, $\int_a^b f(x)g(x)dx = [f(x) \cdot G(x)]_a^b - \int_a^b f'(x)G(x)dx$

THEOREM 2. (Generalised First Mean Value Theorem)

Let $f(x)$ be bounded and $g(x) \geq 0$ in a measurable set E and are integrable over E then there exists a number k between the bounds of $f(x)$ in E such that

$$\int_E f(x)g(x)dx = k\int_E g(x)dx$$

PROOF. It is given that $f(x)$ is bounded in E.

$\Rightarrow$ infimum (greatest lower bound) α and supremum (least upper bound) β exists such that $\alpha \leq f(x) \leq \beta$.

So, $\alpha \cdot g(x) \leq f(x)g(x) \leq \beta \cdot g(x)$ $\qquad [\because g(x) \geq 0 \text{ (given)}]$

$\Rightarrow \quad \alpha \int_E g(x)dx \leq \int_E f(x)g(x)dx \leq \beta \int_E g(x)dx$

$\Rightarrow \quad \int_E fgdx = k\int_E gdx$ for $\alpha \leq k \leq \beta$

DEDUCTION. $\int_E fgdx = f(t)\int_E gdx$

PROOF. Since f is integrable, therefore f is continuous $\Rightarrow \exists x, y \in E$ such that

$$f(x) = \alpha, f(y) = \beta$$

Also, $f(x)$ takes every value between α and β

$\Rightarrow \quad \exists t \in E$ such that $f(t) = k, \alpha \leq k \leq \beta$

Therefore, from (1) $\int_E fgdx = f(t)\int_E gdx$

THEOREM 3. (Second Mean Value Theorem)

If $f(x)$ is integrable over $[a, b]$ and $g(x)$ is positive bounded and non-increasing then

$$\int_a^b f(x)g(x)dx = g(a+0)\int_a^t f(x)dx \qquad t \in]a, b[$$

PROOF. Fix arbitrary small positive number $\varepsilon > 0$ such that

$$\varepsilon < g(a+0) - g(b-0)$$

$\Rightarrow \quad \exists$ a point x_1 such that $g(a+0) - g(x) < \varepsilon$, for $a < x < x_1$

$$\geq \varepsilon_1 \text{ for } x > x_1$$

Similarly, $\exists x_2, x_3, \ldots, x_r$ such that

$g(x_{r-1} + 0) - g(x) < \varepsilon$, for $x_{r-1} < x < x_r$

$$\geq \varepsilon, \text{ for } x > x_r$$

Also, $g(x_{r-1} + 0) - g(b - 0) > \varepsilon$, otherwise take $x_n = b$

$\Rightarrow \quad$ We get the point b after a finite number of steps, because the variation of $g(x)$ in each interval $]x_{r-1}, x_r[$ is atleast ε.

Let us write $\phi(x) = g(x_{r+0})$ in each interval $x_r \leq x < x_{r+1}$.

$\Rightarrow \quad 0 \leq \phi(x) - g(x) < \varepsilon$, except possibly at the points $a = x_0, x_1, x_2, \ldots x_r$

and $\qquad \int_a^b \phi(x)f(x)dx = \sum_{r=0}^{n-1} g(x_r + 0)\int_{x_r}^{x_{r+1}} f(x)dx$

Further, suppose that $F(x) = \int_a^x f(\xi)d\xi$ $\qquad\qquad$ ...(1)

Let m and M be the lower and upper bound of F(x) respectively, then by Abel's lemma

$$mg(a+0) \le \int_a^b \phi(x)f(x)dx \le Mg(a+0) \qquad\qquad ...(2)$$

But, we have

$$\left| \int_a^b \phi(x)f(x)dx - \int_a^b g(x)f(x)dx \right| \le \epsilon \int_a^b | f(x)|\,dx$$

$$\rightarrow 0 \text{ as } \epsilon \rightarrow 0$$

Therefore, $\quad \lim_{\epsilon \to 0} \left| \int_a^b \phi f dx - \int_a^b f g dx \right| = 0$

$\Rightarrow \qquad\qquad \lim_{\epsilon \to 0} \int_a^b \phi f dx = \lim_{\epsilon \to 0} \int_a^b f g dx \qquad\qquad ...(3)$

Letting $\epsilon \rightarrow 0$ in (2) and then from (3) we get

$$mg(a+0) \le \int_a^b g(x)f(x)dx \le Mg(a+0)$$

$\Rightarrow \qquad\qquad m \le \dfrac{1}{g(a+0)} \int_a^b g(x)f(x)dx \le M$

We know that indefinite integral is a continuous function and therefore, F(x) is a continuous function. Hence, F(x) takes every value between m and M so that at x = t, we have

$$F(t) = \frac{1}{g(a+0)} \int_a^x g(x)f(x)dx \qquad\qquad ...(4)$$

But $\qquad\qquad F(x) = \int_a^x f(\xi)d\xi$

$\Rightarrow \qquad\qquad \int_a^t f(t)dt = \dfrac{1}{g(a+0)} \int_a^b g(x)f(x)dx \qquad\qquad \text{(By (4) and (5))}$

$\Rightarrow \qquad\qquad \int_a^b f(x)g(x)dx = g(a+0)\int_a^t f(x)dx \text{ where } a < t < b$

☛ **REMARK**

• When g(x) is a positive non-decreasing function then formula reduces to

$$\int_a^b f(x)g(x)dx = g(b-0)\int_t^b f(x)dx, a < t < b$$

13.3 BERNSTEIN POLYNOMIAL

Let f be a function defined on the closed interval [0, 1].

Then the polynomial

$$B_n(x) = \sum_{k=0}^{n} {}^nC_k \, x^k (1-x)^{n-k} f\left(\frac{k}{n}\right)$$

is called Bernstein's polynomial of degree n for the function f.

THEOREM I. (Bernstein Theorem)

Let f(x) be a function which is continuous on the segment [0, 1] then $B_n(x) \rightarrow f(x)$ uniformly w.r.t. x as $n \rightarrow \infty$.

PROOF.   Before proving the main theorem, first we shall prove that

$$\sum_{k=0}^{n} n_{C_k} (k-nx)^2 \cdot x^k (1-x)^{n-k} \leq \frac{n}{4}, \; x \in [0, 1]$$

By Binomial theorem, we have

$$(a+b)^n = \sum_{k=0}^{n} {}^nC_k a^k b^{n-k} \qquad \qquad \ldots(1)$$

Differentiate partially w.r.t. a, we get

$$\sum_{k=0}^{n} {}^nC_k k a^{k-1} \cdot b^{n-k} = n(a+b)^{n-1}$$

$$\Rightarrow \qquad \sum_{k=0}^{n} {}^nC_k k a^k b^{n-k} = na(a+b)^{n-1} \qquad \qquad \ldots(2)$$

Again differentiating w.r.t. a, we get

$$\sum_{k=0}^{n} {}^nC_k k^2 \cdot a^{k-1} b^{n-k} = n(a+b)^{n-1} + n(n-1)a(a+b)^{n-2}$$

$$\Rightarrow \sum_{k=0}^{n} {}^nC_k k^2 a^k b^{n-k} = na(a+b)^{n-1} + n(n-1)a^2(a+b)^{n-2} \qquad \ldots(3)$$

Setting $a = x$, $b = 1 - x$ so that $a + b = 1$

Then equation (2), (3) and (4) becomes respectively

$$\sum_{k=0}^{n} {}^nC_k (1-x)^{n-k} = 1 \qquad \qquad \ldots(5)$$

$$\sum_{k=0}^{n} {}^nC_k k x^k (1-x)^{n-k} = nx$$

$$\sum_{k=0}^{n} {}^nC_k \cdot k^2 \cdot x^k (1-x)^{n-k} = nx + n(n-1)x^2 = nx[1 + nx - x]$$

$$\Rightarrow \sum_{k=0}^{n} {}^nC_k k^2 \cdot x^k (1-x)^{n-k} = nx(1 + nx - x) \qquad \qquad \ldots(7)$$

Now, multiplying (5), (6) and (7) by n^2x^2, $- 2nx$, 1 respectively and then adding we get

$$\sum_{k=0}^{n} {}^nC_k (k-nx)^2 \cdot x^k (1-x)^{n-k} = nx(1-x) \qquad \qquad \ldots(8)$$

Further, we know that

$$(2x - 1)^2 \geq 0$$

$$\Rightarrow \qquad \qquad 4x - 4x^2 \leq 1$$

$$\Rightarrow \qquad \qquad x(1-x) \leq 1/4$$

$$\Rightarrow \qquad \qquad nx(1-x) \leq \frac{n}{4}$$

Then from (8) we get

$$\sum_{k=0}^{n} (k-nx)^2 \, {}^nC_k x^k (1-x)^{n-k} \leq \frac{n}{4} \qquad \qquad \ldots(9)$$

Now, we prove the main theorem

Since, f is continuous, so by definition given $\varepsilon > 0 \; \exists \; \delta > 0$ such that

$|f(x) - f(y)| < \varepsilon$ whenever $|x - y| < \delta,\; x, y \in [0, 1]$

Set $M = \max \{|f(x)| : x \in [0, 1]\}$

Multiplying (5) by $f(x)$ and then subtracting (1) from this we get

$$f(x) - B_n(x) = \sum_{k=0}^{n} \left[f(x) - f\left(\frac{k}{n}\right) \right] {}^nC_k x^k (1-x)^{n-k}$$

$$= \Sigma_1 + \Sigma_2 \qquad \qquad \ldots(10)$$

There Σ_1 is the sum over those values of k such that $\left|\frac{k}{n} - x\right| < \delta$ and Σ_2 is the sum

over those values of k such that $\left|\frac{k}{n} - x\right| \geq \delta$.

Now divide all the numbers $k = 0, 1, 2, \ldots, n$ into two parts A and B such that

$$k \in A \text{ if } \left|\frac{k}{n} - x\right| < \delta \Rightarrow A \text{ corresponds to } \Sigma_1$$

and $k \in B$ if $\left|\frac{k}{n} - x\right| \geq \delta \Rightarrow B$ corresponds to Σ_2

If $k \in A$ then clearly $\left| f\left(\frac{k}{n}\right) - f(x) \right| < \varepsilon$

$$|\Sigma_1| = \left| \Sigma_1 \left[f(x) - f\left(\frac{k}{n}\right) \right] {}^nC_k \cdot x^k (1-x)^{n-k} \right|$$

$$\leq \Sigma_1 \left[\left| f(x) - f\left(\frac{k}{n}\right) \right| \right] {}^nC_k x^k (1-x)^{n-k}$$

$$< \varepsilon \cdot \Sigma_1 \; {}^nC_k x^k (1-x)^{n-k} = \varepsilon \qquad \qquad \text{(By (8))}$$

$$\Rightarrow \qquad |\Sigma_1| < \varepsilon \qquad \qquad \ldots(11)$$

Now if $k \in B$, then $\left|\frac{k}{n} - x\right| \geq \delta \Rightarrow \left|\frac{k - nx}{n\delta}\right| \geq 1$

$$\Rightarrow \qquad \frac{(k - nx)^2}{n^2\delta^2} \geq 1$$

Further if $k \in B$, then

$$|\Sigma_2| = \Sigma_2 \left| f(x) - f\left(\frac{k}{n}\right) \right| {}^nC_k x^k (1-x)^{n-k}$$

$$\leq \Sigma_2 \left[|f(x)| + \left| f\left(\frac{k}{n}\right) \right| \right] {}^nC_k x^k (1-x)^{n-k}$$

$$\leq 2M\Sigma_2 \frac{(k - nx)^2}{n^2\delta^2} {}^nC_k x^k (1-x)^{n-k}$$

$$\leq \frac{2M}{n^2\delta^2}\cdot\frac{n}{4} = \frac{M}{2n\delta^2} \qquad \text{(By (9))}$$

$$\Rightarrow \qquad |\Sigma_2| \leq \frac{M}{2n\delta^2} \qquad \ldots(12)$$

Using (11) and (12) in (10) we get

$$\left|f(x) - B_n(x)\right| < \varepsilon + \frac{M}{2n\delta^2} \qquad \ldots(13)$$

If we choose $n_0 \in N$ such that $n_0 > \dfrac{M}{2\varepsilon\delta^2}$

Then $n \geq n_0 \Rightarrow \quad n \geq n_0 > \dfrac{M}{2\varepsilon\delta^2}$

$$\Rightarrow \quad n > \frac{M}{2\varepsilon\delta^2}$$

$$\Rightarrow \quad \frac{M}{2n\delta^2} < \varepsilon$$

$$\Rightarrow \quad \frac{M}{2n\delta^2} + \varepsilon < 2\varepsilon$$

Hence, from (13)

$$\left|f(x) - B_n(x)\right| < 2\varepsilon \ \forall n \geq n_0$$

$\Rightarrow f(x)$ converges uniformly to $f(x)$ w.r.t. $x \in [0, 1]$ as $n \to \infty$.

13.4 WEIRSTRASS APPROXIMATION AND SEMI CONTINUOUS FUNCTIONS

THEOREM I. (Weirstrass Approximation Theorem)

Let $f(x)$ be a continuous function defined on the closed interval $[a, b]$ then for every $\varepsilon > 0$ there exists a polynomial $P(x)$ such that

$$|f(x) - P(x)| < \varepsilon \ \forall \ x \in [a, b]$$

ALTERNATIVE STATEMENT.

For each continuous function $f(x)$, there exists a sequence $<P_n(x)>$ of polynomials such that $<P_n>$ converges unifomly to $f(x)$ w.r.t. $x \in [a, b]$ as $n \to \infty$.   [MEERUT–2012, AVADH–2008, KANPUR–2005, 06]

PROOF.   By Bernstein's theorem, we can write for continuous function $f(x)$ defined on the closed interval $[0, 1]$ there exists a sequence of polynomials $<P_n(x)>$, $n \in N$ such that $<P_n(x)>$ converges uniformly to the function $f(x)$ w.r.t. $x \in [0, 1]$ as $n \to \infty$.

Let $f(x)$ is continuous on $[a, b]$. If $[a, b] = [0, 1]$ then by above results theorem is obvious.

Further, suppose that $[a, b] \neq [0, 1]$.

Let us define a function

$$g(y) = f[a + (b - a)y] \qquad \text{(Remember)}$$

Then clearly, $g(0) = f(a)$ and $g(1) = f(b)$

Also, f is continuous on $[a, b]$ then $g(y)$ is continuous on $[0, 1]$. Then again by Bernstein's theorem (stated above) there exists a polynomial $Q(y)$ such that

$$|g(y) - Q(y)| < \varepsilon, \; 0 \le y \le 1 \qquad \ldots(1)$$

Now, if $x \in [a, b]$ and $y \in [0, 1]$ then set

$$y = \frac{x-a}{b-a}$$

So, that $\qquad g(y) = g\left(\frac{x-a}{b-a}\right) = f\left[a + (b-a)\left(\frac{x-a}{b-a}\right)\right] = f(x)$

Then, $\qquad \left| f(x) - Q\left(\frac{x-a}{b-a}\right) \right| < \varepsilon, \qquad a \le x \le b \qquad \qquad$ (By (11))

Clearly, the polynomial $Q\left(\dfrac{x-a}{b-a}\right)$ satisfies our requirements.

13.4.1 SEMI CONTINUOUS FUNCTION

Let $f(x)$ be a function defined on a closed interval $[0, 1]$. Then it is said to be lower semi continuous or upper semi-continuous at the point x_0 if

$$\underline{\lim}_{x \to x_0} f(x) = f(x_0) \; \text{ or } \; \overline{\lim}_{x \to x_0} f(x) = f(x_0) \text{ respectively.}$$

Definition. *A function f is said to be lower semi-continuous on the segment $[a, b]$ if it is lower semi continuous at each point of this segment. Similarly, we can define upper semi continuity of a function on a segment $[a, b]$.*

13.4.2 AN IMPORTANT DISCUSSION

If f is continuous at a point x_0, then it will be both upper and lower continuous. On the other hand, for f is continuous at x_0 we have,

$$f(x_0) = \overline{\lim}_{x \to x_0} f(x) = \underline{\lim}_{x \to x_0} f(x)$$

Conversely, if f is lower and upper both continuous at the point x_0 then f is continuous at x_0 provided f is a finite function.

☛ REMARK
- Lower semicontinuity of a function at a point x_0 is equivalent to upper semi-continuity of the function $-(f)$ at the same point x_0.

THEOREM 2.

Let $f(x)$ be a function defined on a closed interval $[a, b]$ and $x_0 \in [a, b]$. If $<x_n>$ be an arbitrary sequence of points in $[a, b]$ such that $<x_n>$ converges to x_0. Then a necessary and sufficient condition that f be lower semicontinuous at x_0 is that

$$f(x_0) \le \underline{\lim}_{x \to x_0} f(x_n)$$

PROOF. We know that $\lim_{n \to \infty} x_n = x_0$ implies that there exists a subsequence $<x_{n_k} : k \in N>$

such that

$$\lim_{n \to \infty} f(x_{n_k}) = \underline{\lim}_{n \to \infty} f(x_n) \qquad \ldots(1)$$

Further, we know that the limit superior of the function f at the point x_0 is the greatest of the numbers which are limits of the sequence of the form.

$$f(x_1), f(x_2), f(x_3),\ldots, x_n \in [a,b] \text{ and } x_n \to x_0$$

We see that $\varlimsup_{x \to x_0} f(x) \le \lim_{n \to \infty} f < x_{n_K} >$

Using (1) we get

$$\varlimsup_{x \to x_0} f(x) \le \lim_{n \to \infty} f(x_{n_K}) \qquad \ldots(2)$$

Necessary Condition: Let us suppose that $f(x)$ be lower semi continuous at x_0 so that

$$f(x_0) = \varliminf_{x \to x_0} f(x) \qquad \ldots(3)$$

We have to prove that

$$f(x_0) \le \varliminf_{n \to \infty} f(x)$$

Using (3) in (2) we get

$$f(x_0) \le \varliminf_{n \to \infty} f(x_n)$$

Sufficient Condition: Let us suppose that

$$f(x_0) \le \varliminf_{x \to \infty} f(x_n) \qquad \ldots(4)$$

We have to prove that f is lower semicontinuous at x_0.
Now, from (2) we have

$$\varliminf_{x \to x_0} f(x) \le \varliminf_{n \to \infty} f(x_n)$$

But we have $x_n \to x_0 \Rightarrow f(x_n) \to f(x_0)$
Therefore, $\varliminf_{x \to x_0} f(x) \le f(x_0) \qquad \ldots(5)$

Finally, from (4) and (5) we get

$$\varliminf_{x \to x_0} f(x) = f(x_0)$$

Hence $f(x)$ is lower continuous at $x = x_0$.

THEOREM 3.

Let $f(x)$ be a function defined on $[a, b]$ and $x_0 \in [a, b]$ and $f(x_0) > -\infty$. Then a necessary and sufficient condition that f be lower continuous at x_0 is that to every $f(x_0) > A$, there correspond a $\delta > 0$ such that $f(x) > A$, provided $|x - x_0| < \delta, x \in [a, b]$.

PROOF. Let $f(x)$ be a function defined on $[a, b]$ and $x_0 \in [a, b]$ and $f(x_0) > -\infty$.

Necessary Condition: Let f be lower semi continuous, so by definition

$$f(x_0) = \varliminf_{x \to x_0} f(x) \qquad \ldots(1)$$

where $\varliminf_{x \to x_0} f(x) = m(x_0) = \lim_{x \to x_0} m_\delta(x_0)$ for $\delta > 0 \qquad \ldots(2)$

with $m_\delta(x_0) = \inf\{f(x) : x \in]x_0 - \delta, x_0 + \delta[\cap [a, b]\}$
Let $f(x_0) > A$.
We have to prove that there exists $x \in [a, b]$ such that $f(x) > A$, when $|x - x_0| < \delta$.
Clearly, from (1) and (2) there exists $x \in]x_0 - \delta, x_0 + \delta[\cap [a, b]$ such that

$$m_\delta(x_0) > A \qquad \ldots(3)$$

Since, $f(x) \geq m_\delta(x_0)$ for $|x - x_0| < \delta$

Then from (3)

$f(x) > A$ for $|x - x_0| < \delta$

Sufficient Condition: Let us suppose that $f(x_0) > A$. We have to prove that $f(x)$ is lower semi continuous at x_0.

Since, $f(x_0) > A$, so we can find a $\delta > 0$ corresponding to A such that

$$m_\delta(x_0) \geq A$$

$\Rightarrow$ $m(x_0) \geq A$

Now letting $A \to f(x_0)$, we get $m(x_0) \geq f(x_0)$ ...(4)

But $f(x_0) \geq m(x_0)$ ...(5)

Thus, from (4) and (5), we conclude that

$$f(x_0) = m(x_0) = \lim_{x \to x_0} f(x_0)$$

Hence, $f(x)$ is lower semi-continuious at x_0.

CORROLLARY-I RELATION BETWEEN CONTINUITY AND SEMICONTINUITY

If $f(x_0)$ is a finite number, then above theorem can be restated as follows:

A necessary and sufficient condition such that $f(x)$ be lower semi-continuous at the point x_0 is that to every $\varepsilon > 0$ $\exists$ a number $\delta > 0$ such that $(f(x_0) - \varepsilon) < f(x)$, provided $|x - x_0| < \delta$, $x \in [a, b]$.

THEOREM 4.

A necessary and sufficient condition that a function f defined on the segment E = [a, b] be lower semi continuous on E is that the set E[f ≤ c] be closed for arbitrary real number c.

PROOF. Let $f(x)$ be a function defined the segment $E = [a, b]$ and $c \in R$

Let us first suppose, $f(x)$ be lower semi continuous on E.

Define $A = E[f \leq c]$

We have to prove that A is closed. For this we shall prove that $D(A) \subseteq A$. If the points of the sequence $<x_n>$ belongs to A and if $x_n \to x_0$ then lower semi continuity of f implies that

$$f(x_0) \leq \lim_{n \to \infty} f(x_n)$$

Also, $x_n \in A$ $\Rightarrow$ $f(x_n) \leq c \ \forall \ n$

$\Rightarrow$ $\lim_{n \to \infty} f(x_n) \leq c$

Therefore, $f(x_0) \leq \lim_{n \to \infty} f(x_n) \leq c$

$\Rightarrow$ $f(x_0) \leq c$

$\Rightarrow$ $x_0 \in A$

So, $x_n \to x_0 \in A$

Therefore, limit point of the set $\{x_n : 1, 2, 3, ...\} \subset A$ belons to A.

$\Rightarrow$ $D(A) \subseteq A \Rightarrow A$ contains all its limit points.

Hence, A is closed.

Conversely, let us suppose that A is closed. We have to prove that f is lower semi continuous on E.

Let us write $B = \varliminf_{x \to x_0} f(x)$

Let if possible $f(x_0) > B$ ...(1)

By our assumption, there exists a sequence $\langle x_n \rangle$ in E such that $x_n \to x_0$.

If we suppose that c is any number between B and $f(x_0)$, i.e.,

$$B < c < f(x_0) \qquad \qquad ...(2)$$

Then $f(x_n) < c$ for sufficiently large n, i.e., $x_n \in A$

Now, $x_0 \in A$ and A is closed therefore, $f(x_0) \le c$, which contradict (2)

So, our assumption is wrong. Therefore,

$$f(x_0) \le B = \varliminf_{x \to x_0} f(x)$$

$$\Rightarrow \qquad f(x_0) \le \varliminf_{x \to x_0} f(x)$$

Hence, f is lower semi continuous at x_0.

13.5 PICARD'S EXISTENCE THEOREM FOR DIFFERENTIAL EQUATIONS

STATEMENT

If $f(x)$ is continuous on some rectangle $D \subset \mathbf{R}^2$ whose interior contain (x_0, y_0) and if there exist $m > 0$ such that it satisfy Lipditz condition, i.e.,

$$\left| f(x, y_1) - f(x, y_2) \right| \le m(y_1 - y_2), \text{ for } [(x, y_1), (x, y_2) \in D] \qquad ...(1)$$

Then there exists $\delta > 0$ and a unique function ψ such that

$$\psi(x) = y_0 + \int_{x_0}^{x} f[t, \psi(t)]dt, \text{ for } |x - x_0| \le \delta \qquad ...(2)$$

where $\dfrac{dy}{dx} = f(x, y)$ is the differential equation with initial condition

$$y(x_0) = y_0 \qquad \qquad ...(3)$$

PROOF. Let $f(x)$ is continuous on a compact set D, then there exists $k > 0$ such that

$$|f(x, y)| \le k \; \forall \; (x, y) \in D$$

Choose $\delta > 0$ such that $(x, y) \in D$ if $|x - x_0| < \delta$, $|y - y_0| \le k\delta$ and $m\delta < 1$, $m > 1$

...(4)

If C^* denote the subset of $C[x_0 - \delta, x_0 + \delta]$ consisting of all function ψ which are continuous on $[x_0 - \delta, x_0 + \delta]$ and such that

$$|x - x_0| \le \delta \quad \Rightarrow \quad |\psi(x) - y_0| \le k\delta$$

Clearly, C^* is a complete metric space. Also, $(t, \psi(t)) \in D$ if $|t - x_0| \le \delta$ and $\psi \in C^*$

Further define a function T on C^* such that for $\psi \in C^*$, we define

$$T_\psi = \phi \text{ as } \phi(x) = y_0 + \int_{x_0}^{x} f[t, \psi(t)]dt, \; |x - x_0| < \delta \qquad ...(5)$$

$\Rightarrow \quad \psi$ satisfies (2) if and only if $T_\psi = \psi$.

We claim that T is a contradiction on the complete metric space C^*. For this we shall prove that T maps C^* into C^*.

If $\psi \in C^*$ and $\phi = T_\psi$ then we can easily shows that ϕ is continuous on the closed interval $[x_0 - \delta, x_0 + \delta]$. Also, if $|x - x_0| < \delta$, then

$$\left| \phi(x) - y_0 \right| \le \left| \int_{x_0}^{x} f[t, \psi(t)]dt \right| \le k|x - x_0| \le k\delta$$

$$\Rightarrow \quad |\phi(x) - y_0| \le k\delta \text{ if } |x - x_0| \le \delta$$

$\Rightarrow \quad \phi \in C^*$

$\Rightarrow \quad T$ maps C^* into C^*.

Let $\psi_1, \psi_2 \in C^*$ and $T_{\psi_1} = \phi_1, T_{\psi_2} = \phi_2$

Then from (5) if $|x - x_0| \leq \phi$ then

$$\phi_1(x) - \phi_2(x) \leq \int_{x_0}^{x} \{f[t, \psi_1(t) - f[t, \psi_2(t)]\}dt$$

and therefore

$$\left|\phi_1(x) - \phi_2(x)\right| \leq \left|\int_{x_0}^{x} \left|f[t, \psi_1(t)] - f[t, \psi_2(t)\right| dt\right|$$

Using (1) we get

$$\left|\phi_1(x) - \phi_2(x)\right| \leq \left|m\int_{x_0}^{x} \left|T_{\psi_1}(t) - T_{\psi_2}(t)\right| dt\right|$$

$$\leq \left|m\int_{x_0}^{x} |T_{\psi_1 - \psi_2}| dt\right|$$

$$\leq m\delta \|\psi_1 - \psi_2\|$$

So, $\quad \|\phi_1 - \phi_2\| \leq m\delta \|\psi_1 - \psi_2\|$

or $\quad \left\|T_{\psi_1} - T_{\psi_2}\right\| \leq m\delta \|\psi_1 - \psi_2\|$

If d is a metric on C^*, then above inequality can be written as

$$d[T_{\psi_1}, T_{\psi_2}] \leq m\delta d(\psi_1, \psi_2)$$

$\Rightarrow \quad T$ is a contraction on C^*.

$\Rightarrow \quad$ There is one and only one point $\psi \in C^*$ such that $T_\psi = \psi$.

$\Rightarrow \quad \psi$ satisfies (2).

13.6 EQUICONTINUOUS FAMILIES AND ARZELA'S THEOREM

Let $[a, b]$ be a closed and bounded interval. Then, a subset C^* of $C[a, b]$ is said to be equicontinuous if for given $\varepsilon > 0 \ \exists \ \delta > 0$ such that

$$|f(x) - f(y)| < \varepsilon \text{ whenever } |x - y| < \delta, f \in C^*$$

☞ REMARK

• In the above definition, δ is independent of the choice of the function f.

THEOREM I. (Arzela's Theorem)

Let C^* be a bounded equicontinuous subset of the metric space $C[a, b]$, then C^* is totally bounded.

PROOF. Let C^* be a bounded equicontinuous subset of the metric space $C[a, b]$.

Since, C^* is bounded $\Rightarrow \exists \ m > 0$ such that

$$f \in C^*, d[f, 0] = \|f\| \leq m$$

Also, since C^* is equicontinuous, then there exist a $\delta > 0$ such that

$$f \in C^*, |x - x'| < \delta \Rightarrow |f(x) - f(x')| < \frac{\varepsilon}{15} \qquad \qquad ...(1)$$

Divide $[a, b]$ by means of points $a = x_0 < x_1 < ... < x_n = b$ where $x_{j+1} - x_j < \delta$
$(j = 0, 1, 2, ..., n - 1)$. In a similar way subdivide $[-m, m]$ by means of points
$-m = y_0 < y_1 < y_2 < ... < y_m = m$ such that

$$y_{k+1} - y_k < \frac{\varepsilon}{15}, k = 0, 2, ..., m - 1$$

Therefore, the rectangle $a \leq x \leq b, -m \leq y \leq m$ is subdivided into subrectangles of base less than δ and height less than $\left(\dfrac{\varepsilon}{15}\right)$.

Now, let $f \in C^*$ be arbitrary.

Define $g \in C[a, b]$ as given below

For each $x_j, j = 0, 1, 2, \dots, n$, $g(x_j) = y_{k(j)}$ where $k(j)$ is choosen such that

$$\left| g(x_j) - f(x_j) \right| = \left| y_{k(j)} + f(x_j) \right| < \frac{\varepsilon}{15} \qquad \qquad \dots(2)$$

Also, the graph of g consists of straight line segments joining successively the points $(x_0, g(x_0)), (x_1, g(x_1)), \dots, (x_n, g(x_n))$

Then $\left| g(x_{j+1}) - g(x_j) \right| \leq \left| g(x_{j+1}) - f(x_{j+1}) \right| + \left| f(x_{j+1}) - f(x_j) \right| + \left| f(x_j) - g(x_j) \right|$ $\quad \dots(3)$

Using (1) and (2) in (3) we get

$$\left| g(x_{j+1}) - g(x_j) \right| < \frac{\varepsilon}{15} + \frac{\varepsilon}{15} + \frac{\varepsilon}{15} = \frac{\varepsilon}{5}$$

$$\Rightarrow \left| g(x_{j+1}) - g(x_j) \right| < \frac{\varepsilon}{5}, \text{ for } x_j \leq x \leq x_{j+1} \qquad \qquad \dots(4)$$

Now, for any $x \in [a, b]$ choose j such that $x_j \leq x < x_{j+1}$, therefore,

$$\left| g(x) - f(x) \right| \leq \left| g(x) - g(x_j) \right| + \left| g(x_j) - f(x_j) \right| + \left| f(x_j) - f(x) \right|$$

So, by (1), (2) and (4) we get

$$\left| g(x) - f(x) \right| < \frac{\varepsilon}{5} + \frac{\varepsilon}{15} + \frac{\varepsilon}{15} = \frac{\varepsilon}{3}$$

$$\Rightarrow \quad \left| g(x) - f(x) \right| < \frac{\varepsilon}{3}$$

$$\Rightarrow \quad \quad \| g - f \| < \frac{\varepsilon}{3}$$

$\Rightarrow$ Open sphere of radius $\dfrac{\varepsilon}{3}$ centred at g includes $f \in C^*$ and therefore their union will contain C.

Now it remains to prove that there can be only a finite number of distinct g's. For each j, $g(x_j)$ must be one of the $(n + 1)$ numbers $y_0, y_1, \dots, y_n$.

So, there are atmost $(m + 1)n + 1$ function g. Therefore, there are a finite number of the open spheres each with diameter $0 \leq \dfrac{2\pi}{3} < \varepsilon$ such that their union contains C^*. Hence, C^* is totally bounded.

Exercise 13.1

1. Show that the family $\langle \sin nx \rangle, n = 1$ to ∞ is not an equicontinuous subset of $C[a, b]$.

2. If $\langle \psi_n \rangle$ be any sequence of functions on $[0, 1]$ such that $\left| \psi_n'(x) \right| \leq M; 0 \leq x \leq 1, x \in Z$.

3. If the function f, g defined on $[a, b]$ are both lower semicontinuous at $x = x_0$ then show that $f + g$ is also lower semicontinuous at x_0 provided $f + g$ is defined on $[a, b]$.

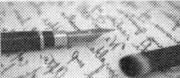 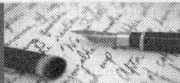
CHAPTER Summary

✎ KEY TERMS

- **POLYNOMIAL FUNCTION:** A function which is expressible as

$$P(x) = a_0 + a_1x + a_2x^2 + \dots + a_nx^n$$

  where n is some non-negative integer and a_0, $a_1, a_2, \dots, a_n$ are constant is called a polynomial function.

- **BERNSTEIN'S POLYNOMIAL:** The polynomial

$$B_n(x) = \sum_{k=0}^{n} {}^nC_k \, x^k (1-x)^{n-k} f\left(\frac{k}{n}\right)$$

  is called Bernstein's polynomial of degree n.

- **SEMICONTINUOUS FUNCTION:** A function f defined on the closed interval $[a, b]$ is said to be lower semi continuous or upper semi continuous at x_0 according as

$$\varliminf_{x \to x_0} f(x) = f(x_0) \text{ or } \varlimsup_{x \to x_0} f(x) = f(x_0)$$

- **LOWER SEMICONTINUOUS FUNCTION IN A SEGMENT:** A function f is said to be lower semi continuous on the segment $[a, b]$ if it is defined and lower semicontinuous at each point of this segment.

✎ RESULTS

- Let $f(x)$ be an indefinite integral and if $G(x)$ is an indefinite integral of $g(x)$ then

$$\int_a^b f(x)g(x)dx = \left[f(x)\cdot G(x)\right]_a^b - \int_a^b f'(x)G(x)dx$$

- Let $f(x)$ be bounded and $g(x) \geq 0$ in a measurable set E and are integrable over E then there exists a number k between the bounds of $f(x)$ in E such that

$$\int_E f(x)g(x)dx = k\int_E g(x)dx$$

- If $f(x)$ is integrable over $[a, b]$ and $g(x)$ is positive bounded and non-increasing then

$$\int_a^b f(x)g(x)dx = g(a+0)\int_a^t f(x)dx \,,\, t \in \,]a, b[$$

- Let $f(x)$ be a function which is continuous on the segment $[0, 1]$ then $B_n(x) \to f(x)$ uniformly w.r.t. x as $n \to \infty$.

- Let $f(x)$ be a continuous function defined on the closed interval $[a, b]$ then for every $\varepsilon > 0$ there exists a polynomial $P(x)$ such that

$$|f(x) - P(x)| < \varepsilon \, \forall \, x \in [a, b]$$

- Let $f(x)$ be a function defined on a closed interval $[a, b]$ and $x_0 \in [a, b]$. If $<x_n>$ be an arbitrary sequence of points in $[a, b]$ such that $<x_n>$ converges to x_0. Then a necessary and sufficient condition that f be lower semi-continuous at x_0 is that $f(x_0) \leq \varliminf_{x \to x_0} f(x_n)$.

- Let $f(x)$ be a function defined on $[a, b]$ and $x_0 \in [a, b]$ and $f(x_0) > -\infty$. Then a necessary and sufficient condition that f be lower continuous at x_0 is that to every $f(x_0) > A$, there correspond a $\delta > 0$ such that $f(x) > A$, provided $|x - x_0| < \delta, x \in [a, b]$.

- A necessary and sufficient condition that a function f defined on the segment $E = [a, b]$ be lower semi continuous on E is that the set $E[f \leq c]$ be closed for arbitrary real number c.

- If $f(x)$ is continuous on some rectangle $D \subset R^2$ whose interior contain (x_0, y_0) and if there exist $m > 0$ such that it satisfy Lipchitz condition, i.e.,

$$\left|f(x, y_1) - f(x, y_2)\right| \leq m(y_1 - y_2),$$

  for $[(x, y_1), (x, y_2) \in D]$ ...(1)

  Then there exists $\delta > 0$ and a unique function ψ such that

$$\psi(x) = y_0 + \int_{x_0}^x f[t, \psi(t)]dt \,, \text{ for } |x - x_0| \leq \delta$$

  ...(2)

  where $\dfrac{dy}{dx} = f(x, y)$ is the differential equation

  with initial condition

$$y(x_0) = y_0 \qquad \qquad ...(3)$$

- Let C^* be a bounded equicontinuous subset of the metric space $C[a, b]$, then C^* is totally bounded.

WORTHY READINGS

☞ The set of all polynomials is dense in the metric space $C[a, b]$, the metric space of all continuous, real valued functions on the closed bounded interval $[a, b]$ with metric d.

☞ For each $f \in C[a, b]$, there exists a sequence of polynomials $<P_n>$ such that $<P_n>$ converges uniformly to f on $[a, b]$.

☞ Every continuous real valued function on a closed bounded interval $[a, b]$ can be uniformly approximated by polynomials.

☞ Let f be any continuous function in $[a, b]$ then given $\varepsilon > 0$ there exists a polynomial P such that

$$|P(x) - f(x)| < \varepsilon, a \leq x \leq b$$

FURTHER READINGS

☞ The space C^* is totally bounded, if for given $\varepsilon > 0 \, \exists$ a finite number of subsets A_i of $C[a, b]$ such that dia. $(A_i) < \varepsilon$ and $C^* \subset \cup A_i$.

☞ Lower semi-continuity of a function at a point x_0 is equivalent to upper semi-continuity of the function $(-f)$ at x_0.

Chapter

14 Fourier Series

14.1 INTRODUCTION

In this section, we shall study a special type of functional series extensively studied by Joseph Fourier. Joseph Fourier represented expansions in trigonometrical series in connection with boundary value problem in conduction of heat. Although such expansions had been studied earlier, these series bear the name 'Fourier series' because of the major contributions of Fourier in this field.

14.2 PERIODIC FUNCTIONS

A function $f(x)$ which satisfies the relation $f(x + T) = f(x)$ for all real x and some fixed T is called a periodic function. The smallest positive number T, for which this relation holds, is called the period of $f(x)$.

If T is the period of $f(x)$. Then

$$f(x) = f(x + T) = f(x + 2T) = ... = f(x + nT) = ...$$

Also, $\qquad f(x) = f(x - T) = f(x - 2T) = ... = f(x - nT) = ...$

$\therefore \qquad f(x) = f(x \pm nT)$, where n is a positive integer.

For example: Consider the function $f(x) = \sin x$. We have

$$\sin x = \sin (x + 2\pi) = \sin (x + 4\pi) = ...$$

Here, $f(x) = \sin x$ is a periodic function with period 2π. This function is also called sinusoidal periodic function.

We have studied about the Macluarian's theorem which is used to expand a function provided the function's derivative are continuous. Now, the need arise to expand functions which have discontinuities in their derivatives. By Fourier series, we can expand both types of functions under certain conditions as an infinite series of sine and cosine of x and it's integral multiple of a function $f(x)$ is defined in the interval $c < x < c + 2\pi$.

Then, Fourier series of $f(x)$ is given by

$$f(x) = \frac{a_0}{2} + \sum_{n=1}^{\infty} a_n \cos nx + \sum_{n=1}^{\infty} b_n \sin nx \qquad ...(1)$$

where a_0, a_n and b_n are called Fourier coefficient of $f(x)$ and their values are given as :

$$a_0 = \frac{1}{\pi} \int_{c}^{c+2\pi} f(x)dx \qquad ...(2)$$

$$a_n = \frac{1}{\pi} \int_c^{c+2\pi} f(x)\cos nx \, dx \qquad \qquad \text{...(3)}$$

$$b_n = \frac{1}{\pi} \int_c^{c+2\pi} f(x)\sin nx \, dx \qquad \qquad \text{...(4)}$$

The series (1) with coefficients a_0, a_n and b_n given by (2), (3) and (4) respectively is called the Fourier series of $f(x)$ and the coefficients a_0, a_n and b_n are called the Fourier coefficients corresponding to $f(x)$.

(i) When $c = 0$, the interval becomes $0 < x < 2\pi$ and formula for a_0, a_n, b_n is obtained by putting $c = 0$.

(ii) When $c = -\pi$, then interval becomes $-\pi < x < \pi$. In this interval, the formula for a_0, a_n and b_n becomes as under :

(a) When $f(x)$ is an odd function, then

$$a_0 = \frac{1}{\pi} \int_{-\pi}^{\pi} f(x)dx = 0$$

$$a_n = \frac{1}{\pi} \int_{-\pi}^{\pi} f(x)\cos nx \, dx = 0 \qquad \text{[By property of definite integral]}$$

$$b_n = \frac{1}{\pi} \int_{-\pi}^{\pi} f(x)\sin nx \, dx = \frac{2}{\pi} \int_0^{\pi} f(x)\sin x \, dx$$

Hence, if function $f(x)$ is odd, its Fourier expansion contains only sine series,

i.e., $\qquad f(x) = \sum_{n=1}^{\infty} b_n \sin nx,$ where $b_n = \frac{2}{\pi} \int_0^{\pi} f(x)\sin nx \, dx.$

(b) When $f(x)$ is even function, then formula for a_0, a_n and b_n are given by

$$a_0 = \frac{1}{\pi} \int_{-\pi}^{\pi} f(x)dx = \frac{2}{\pi} \int_0^{\pi} f(x)dx$$

$$a_n = \frac{1}{\pi} \int_{-\pi}^{\pi} f(x)\cos nx \, dx = \frac{2}{\pi} \int_0^{\pi} f(x)\cos nx \, dx$$

and $\qquad b_n = \frac{1}{\pi} \int_{-\pi}^{\pi} f(x)\sin nx \, dx = 0 \qquad \qquad [\because f(x) \sin nx \text{ is odd.}]$

Hence, if a periodic function $f(x)$ is even, its Fourier expansion contains only cosine terms, i.e., $f(x) = \frac{a_0}{2} + \sum_{n=1}^{\infty} \int_0^{\pi} f(x)dx,$ where

$$a_0 = \frac{2}{\pi} \int_0^{\pi} f(x)dx \text{ and } a_n = \frac{2}{\pi} \int_0^{\pi} f(x).\cos nx \, dx$$

14.3 SOME IMPORTANT RESULTS

The following results are useful in the Fourier series :

(i) $\sin n\pi = 0, \cos n\pi = (-1)^n, \cos\left(n + \frac{1}{2}\right)\pi = 0,$ where $n \in Z.$

(ii) $\int uv = uv_1 - u'v_2 + u''v_3 - u'''v_4 + ...,$ where $u' = \dfrac{du}{dx}, u'' = \dfrac{d^2u}{dx^2}, ...$

$v_1 = \int v\,dx, v_2 = \int v_1\,dx, ...$

(iii) $\int\limits_0^{2\pi} \sin nx\,dx = 0$ (iv) $\int\limits_0^{2\pi} \cos nx\,dx = 0$

(v) $\int\limits_0^{2\pi} \sin^2 nx\,dx = \pi$ (vi) $\int\limits_0^{2\pi} \cos^2 nx\,dx = \pi$

(vii) $\int\limits_0^{2\pi} \sin nx.\sin mx\,dx = 0$ (viii) $\int\limits_0^{2\pi} \cos nx.\cos mx\,dx = 0$

(ix) $\int\limits_0^{2\pi} \sin nx.\cos mx\,dx = 0$ (x) $\int\limits_0^{2\pi} \sin mx.\cos nx\,dx = 0$

(xi) $\int e^{ax} \sin bx\,dx = \dfrac{e^{ax}}{a^2 + b^2}(a\sin bx - b\cos bx) + c$

(xii) $\int e^{ax} \cos bx\,dx = \dfrac{e^{ax}}{a^2 + b^2}(a\cos bx + b\sin bx) + c$

14.4 DETERMINATION OF FOURIER COEFFICIENTS: EULER'S FORMULAE

The fourier series is given by

$$f(x) = \frac{a_0}{2} + a_1 \cos x + a_2 \cos 2x + ... + a_n \cos nx$$

$$+ b_1 \sin x + ... + b_2 \sin 2x + ... + b_n \sin nx + ...$$

or $f(x) = \dfrac{a_0}{2} + \sum\limits_{n=1}^{\infty} a_n \cos nx + \sum\limits_{n=1}^{\infty} b_n \sin nx.$ ...(i)

To find a_0 : Integrating both sides of equation (1) from $x = c+0$, $x = c+2\pi$

$$\int\limits_c^{c+2\pi} f(x)dx = \frac{a_0}{2} \int\limits_c^{c+2\pi} dx + \int\limits_c^{c+2\pi} \left(\sum\limits_{n=1}^{\infty} a_n \cos nx \right) dx + \int\limits_c^{c+2\pi} \left(\sum\limits_{n=1}^{\infty} b_n \sin nx \right) dx$$

$$= \frac{a_0}{2}(c + 2\pi - c) + 0 + 0 = a_0\pi$$

$\Rightarrow$ $a_0 = \dfrac{1}{\pi} \int\limits_c^{c+2\pi} f(x)\,dx$.

To find a_n : Multipling each side of equation (1) by $\cos nx$ and integrate w.r.t. x., between the limit c to $c+2\pi$.

$$\int\limits_c^{c+2\pi} f(x)\cos nx\,dx = \frac{a_0}{2} \int\limits_c^{c+2\pi} \cos nx\,dx + \int\limits_c^{c+2\pi} \left(\sum\limits_{n=1}^{\infty} a_n \cos nx \right) \cos nx\,dx$$

$$+ \int\limits_c^{c+2\pi} \left(\sum\limits_{n=1}^{\infty} b_n \sin nx \right) \cos nx\,dx$$

$$= 0 + a_n\pi + 0 = a_n\pi$$

$$\Rightarrow \qquad a_n = \frac{1}{\pi} \int_c^{c+2\pi} f(x)\cos nx\,dx \;.$$

To find b_n : Multiplying each side of equation (1) by $\sin nx$ and integrate w.r.t. x between the limit c to $c + 2\pi$.

$$\int_c^{c+2\pi} f(x)\sin nx\,dx = \frac{a_0}{2}\int_c^{c+2\pi}\sin nx\,dx + \int_c^{c+2\pi}\left(\sum_{n=1}^{\infty} a_n \cos nx\right)\sin nx\,dx +$$

$$+ \int_c^{c+2\pi}\left(\sum_{n=1}^{\infty} b_n \sin nx\right)\sin nx\,dx$$

$$= 0 + 0 + b_n\pi = b_n\pi$$

$$\Rightarrow \qquad b_n = \frac{1}{\pi}\int_c^{c+2\pi} f(x)\sin nx\,dx$$

These values of a_0, a_n and b_n are called Euler's formulae.

14.5 DIRICHLET'S CONDITIONS

Any function $f(x)$ can be expressed as a Fourier series

$$\frac{a_0}{2} + \sum_{n=1}^{\infty} a_n \cos nx + \sum_{n=1}^{\infty} b_n \sin nx, \text{ where } a_0, a_n \text{ and } b_n \text{ are constants.}$$

(i) $f(x)$ is finite and single valued in the interval $c < x < c + 2\pi$.
(ii) $f(x)$ is periodic with period 2π
(iii) $f(x)$ and $f'(x)$ are piecewise continuous in the interval $c < x < c + 2\pi$.
The Fourier series with its coefficients converge to
(a) $f(x)$ if x is a point of continuity.
(b) $\dfrac{f(x+0)+f(x-0)}{2}$, if x is a point of discontinuity.

The conditions (i), (ii) and (iii) imposed on $f(x)$ are sufficient but not necessary. *i.e.,* if the conditions are satisfied, the convergence is guaranteed. However, if they are not satisfied the series may or may not converge.

Solved Examples

EXAMPLE 1. *Expand the function $f(x) = x \sin x$ as a Fourier series in interval $-\pi \le x \le \pi$. Deduce*

that $\dfrac{1}{1.3} - \dfrac{1}{3.5} + \dfrac{1}{5.7} - \dfrac{1}{7.9} + ... = \dfrac{\pi-2}{4}$.

SOLUTION. Since $x \sin x$ is an even function of x, so $b_n = 0$, then Fourier series is given by

$$f(x) = x \sin x = \frac{a_0}{2} + \sum_{n=1}^{\infty} a_n \cos nx,$$

where $$a_0 = \frac{2}{\pi}\int_0^\pi x \sin x\,dx = \frac{2}{\pi}\left[-x\cos x + \sin x\right]_0^\pi = \frac{2}{\pi}(-\pi\cos\pi) = 2$$

$$a_n = \frac{2}{\pi}\int_0^\pi x\sin x\cos nx\,dx = \frac{1}{\pi}\int_0^\pi x.2\cos nx\sin x\,dx$$

$$= \frac{1}{\pi} \int_0^\pi x\{\sin(n+1)x - \sin(n-1)x\}\,dx$$

$$= \frac{1}{\pi}\left[x\left\{\frac{-\cos(n+1)x}{n+1} + \frac{\cos(n+1)x}{n-1}\right\}\right.$$

$$\left. -1\left\{\frac{-\sin(n+1)x}{(n+1)^2} + \frac{\sin(n-1)x}{(n+1)^2}\right\}\right]_0^\pi$$

$$= \frac{1}{\pi}\left[\pi\left\{\frac{-\cos(n+1)\pi}{n+1} + \frac{\cos(n-1)\pi}{n-1}\right\}\right]$$

$$= \frac{\cos(n-1)\pi}{n-1} - \frac{\cos(n+1)\pi}{n+1}; n \neq 1$$

$$= \begin{cases} \dfrac{1}{n-1} - \dfrac{1}{n+1} = \dfrac{2}{n^2-1} & \text{if } n \text{ is odd } n \neq 1 \\[2ex] \dfrac{-1}{n-1} + \dfrac{1}{n+1} = \dfrac{-2}{n^2-1} & \text{if } n \text{ is even} \end{cases}$$

When $n=1$, then

$$a_1 = \frac{2}{\pi}\int_0^\pi x\sin x\cos x\,dx = \frac{1}{\pi}\int_0^\pi x\sin 2x\,dx$$

$$= \frac{1}{\pi}\left[x\left(\frac{-\cos 2x}{2}\right) - \left(\frac{-\sin 2x}{4}\right)\right]_0^\pi = \frac{1}{\pi}\left[\frac{-\pi\cos 2\pi}{2}\right] = -\frac{1}{2}$$

$$\therefore \qquad x\sin x = 1 - \frac{1}{2}\cos x - 2\left[\frac{\cos 2x}{2^2-1} - \frac{\cos 3x}{3^2-1} + \frac{\cos 4x}{4^2-1} - \frac{\cos 5x}{5^2-1} + \dots\right]$$

Putting $\qquad x = \dfrac{\pi}{2}$, we get $\dfrac{\pi}{2} = 1 - 2\left(\dfrac{-1}{2^2-1} + \dfrac{1}{4^2-1} - \dfrac{1}{6^2-1} + \dots\right)$

$$\Rightarrow \qquad \frac{\pi}{2} - 1 = 2\left(\frac{1}{3} - \frac{1}{15} + \frac{1}{35} - \dots\right) \Rightarrow \frac{\pi-2}{4} = \left(\frac{1}{1.3} - \frac{1}{3.5} + \frac{1}{5.7} - \dots\right).$$

EXAMPLE 2. Find the Fourier series to represent e^{ax} in interval $-\pi < x < \pi$.

SOLUTION. Let

$$f(x) = e^{ax} = \frac{a_0}{2} + \sum_{n=1}^\infty a_n \cos nx + \sum_{n=1}^\infty b_n \sin nx$$

$$a_0 = \frac{1}{\pi}\int_{-\pi}^\pi f(x)\,dx = \frac{1}{\pi}\int_{-\pi}^\pi e^{ax}\,dx = \frac{1}{\pi}\left[\frac{e^{ax}}{a}\right]_{-\pi}^\pi$$

$$= \frac{1}{a\pi}(e^{a\pi} - e^{-a\pi}) = \frac{2\sinh a\pi}{\pi a}$$

$$a_n = \frac{1}{\pi}\int_{-\pi}^\pi f(x)\cos nx\,dx = \frac{1}{\pi}\int_{-\pi}^\pi e^{ax}\cos nx\,dx$$

$$= \left[\frac{e^{ax}}{\pi(a^2 + n^2)} a\cos nx + a\sin nx \right]_{-\pi}^{\pi}$$

$$= \frac{a\cos n\pi(e^{a\pi} - e^{-a\pi})}{\pi(a^2 + n^2)} = \frac{2a(-1)^n \sinh a\pi}{\pi(a^2 + n^2)}$$

Similarly, we can set

$$b_n = \frac{2n(-1)^n \sinh a\pi}{\pi(a^2 + n^2)}$$

$$\therefore \qquad e^{ax} = \frac{\sinh a\pi}{a\pi} + \sum_{n=1}^{\infty} \frac{2a(-1)^n \sinh a\pi}{\pi(a^2 + n^2)} \cos nx + \sum_{n=1}^{\infty} \frac{2n(-1)^n \sinh a\pi}{\pi(a^2 + n^2)} \sin n\pi$$

$$= \frac{2\sinh a\pi}{\pi} \left[\frac{1}{2a} - a\left(\frac{\cos x}{a^2 + 1^2} - \frac{\cos 2x}{a^2 + 2^2} + \frac{\cos 3x}{a^2 + 3^2} - \cdots \right) \right.$$

$$\left. - \left(\frac{\sin x}{a^2 + 1^2} - \frac{2\sin 2x}{a^2 + 2^2} + \frac{3\sin 3x}{a^2 + 3^2} - \cdots \right) \right]$$

EXAMPLE 3. *Obtain the Fourier series for the function $f(x) = x^2$, $-\pi < x < \pi$. Sketch the graph f function f(x). Hence, show that*

(i) $\dfrac{1}{1^2} + \dfrac{1}{2^2} + \dfrac{1}{3^2} + \dfrac{1}{4^2} + \cdots = \displaystyle\sum_{n=1}^{\infty} \frac{1}{n^2} = \frac{\pi^2}{6}$

(ii) $\dfrac{1}{1^2} - \dfrac{1}{2^2} + \dfrac{1}{3^2} - \dfrac{1}{4^2} + \cdots = \dfrac{\pi^2}{12}$

(iii) $\dfrac{1}{1^2} + \dfrac{1}{3^2} + \dfrac{1}{5^2} + \cdots = \displaystyle\sum_{n=1}^{\infty} \frac{1}{(2n-1)^2} = \frac{\pi^2}{8}$

SOLUTION. $f(x) = x^2$ is an even function, therefore $b_n = 0$

Now $\qquad f(x) = x^2 = \dfrac{a_0}{2} + \displaystyle\sum_{n=1}^{\infty} a_n \cos nx$. Then

$$a_0 = \frac{2}{\pi} \int_0^\pi f(x)\,dx = \frac{2}{\pi} \int_0^\pi x^2\,dx = \frac{2}{\pi}\left[\frac{x^3}{3} \right]_0^\pi = \frac{2}{3}\pi^2$$

$$a_n = \frac{2}{\pi} \int_0^\pi f(x)\cos nx\,dx = \frac{2}{\pi} \int_0^\pi x^2 \cos nx\,dx$$

$$= \frac{2}{\pi}\left[x^2\left(\frac{\sin nx}{n}\right) - 2x\left(\frac{-\cos nx}{n^2}\right) + 2\left(\frac{-\sin nx}{n^2}\right) \right]_0^\pi$$

$$= \frac{2}{\pi}\left[2\pi \frac{\cos n\pi}{n^2} \right] = 4\frac{(-1)^n}{n^2}$$

$$\therefore \qquad x^2 = \frac{\pi^2}{3} - 4\left(\frac{\cos x}{1^2} - \frac{\cos 2x}{2^2} + \frac{\cos 3x}{3^2} - \frac{\cos 4x}{4^2} + \cdots \right)$$

$$\Rightarrow \qquad x^2 = \frac{\pi^2}{3} + 4\sum_{n=1}^{\infty} \frac{(-1)^n}{n^2}\cos nx \qquad \qquad \dots(1)$$

Put $x = \pi$ in (1), we get

$$\pi^2 = \frac{\pi^2}{3} - 4\left(-\frac{1}{1^2} - \frac{1}{2^2} - \frac{1}{3^2} - \frac{1}{4^2} - \cdots\right)$$

$$\Rightarrow \qquad \frac{2\pi^2}{3} = -4\left(-\frac{1}{1^2} - \frac{1}{2^2} - \frac{1}{3^2} - \frac{1}{4^2} - \cdots\right)$$

$$\therefore \quad \frac{1}{1^2} + \frac{1}{2^2} + \frac{1}{3^2} + \frac{1}{4^2} \cdots = \frac{\pi^2}{6} \qquad \qquad \dots(2)$$

Put $x = 0$ in (1), we get

$$0 = \frac{\pi^2}{3} - 4\left(-\frac{1}{1^2} - \frac{1}{2^2} - \frac{1}{3^2} - \frac{1}{4^2} - \cdots\right)$$

$$\therefore \quad \frac{1}{1^2} - \frac{1}{2^2} - \frac{1}{3^2} - \frac{1}{4^2} - \cdots = \frac{\pi^2}{12} \qquad \dots(3)$$

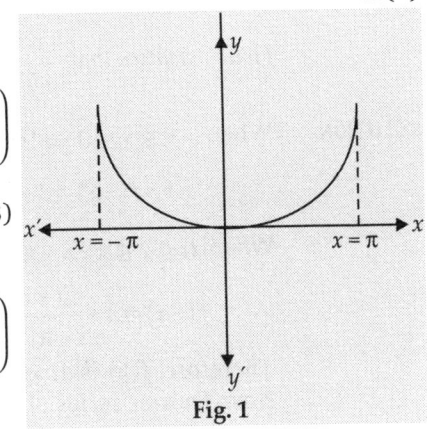

Adding (2) and (3), we get

$$\frac{\pi^2}{4} = 2\left(\frac{1}{1^2} + \frac{1}{3^2} + \frac{1}{5^2} + \cdots\right)$$

$$\therefore \quad \frac{1}{1^2} + \frac{1}{3^2} + \frac{1}{5^2} + \cdots = \frac{\pi^2}{8} \,.$$

Fig. 1

EXAMPLE 4. *Obtain the Fouries series for $f(x) = e^{-x}$ in the interval $0 < x < 2\pi$.*

SOLUTION. Let $f(x) = e^{-x}$. The Fourier series of $f(x)$ can be written as

$$f(x) = e^{-x} = \frac{a_0}{2} + \sum_{n=1}^{\infty} a_n \cos nx + \sum_{n=1}^{\infty} b_n \sin nx$$

Then,

$$a_0 = \frac{1}{2} \int_0^{2\pi} f(x) dx = \frac{1}{\pi} \int_0^{2\pi} e^{-x} dx = \frac{1}{\pi}\cdot\left[-e^{-x}\right]_0^{2\pi} = \frac{1 - e^{-2\pi}}{\pi}$$

$$a_n = \frac{1}{\pi} \int_0^{2\pi} f(x) \cos nx \, dx = \frac{1}{\pi} \int_0^{2\pi} e^{-x} \cos nx \, dx$$

$$= \frac{1}{\pi(1+n^2)}[e^{-x}(-\cos nx + n \sin nx)]_0^{2\pi} = \frac{1 - e^{-2\pi}}{\pi(1+n^2)}$$

$$b_n = \frac{1}{\pi} \int_0^{2\pi} f(x) \sin nx \, dx = \frac{1}{\pi} \int_0^{2\pi} e^{-x} \sin nx \, dx$$

$$= \frac{e^{-x}}{\pi(1+n^2)}\left[-\sin nx - n \cos nx\right]_0^{2\pi} = \frac{1 - e^{-2\pi}}{\pi} \cdot \frac{n}{1+n^2}$$

$$\therefore \quad e^{-x} = \frac{1 - e^{-2\pi}}{\pi}\left[\frac{1}{2} + \left(\frac{1}{2}\cos x + \frac{1}{5}\cos 2x + \frac{1}{10}\cos 3x + \cdots\right)\right]$$

$$+ \left(\frac{1}{2}\sin x + \frac{2}{5}\sin 2x + \frac{3}{10}\sin 3x + \cdots\right)$$

$$= \frac{1-e^{-2\pi}}{2\pi} + \frac{1-e^{-2\pi}}{\pi} \sum_{n=1}^{\infty} \frac{\cos nx}{1+n^2} + \frac{1-e^{-2\pi}}{\pi} \sum_{n=1}^{\infty} \frac{n\sin nx}{1+n^2}$$

EXAMPLE 5. *Obtain Fourier series for the function f(x), given by*

$$f(x) = \begin{cases} 1 + \dfrac{2x}{\pi}; & -\pi \le x \le 0 \\ 1 - \dfrac{2x}{\pi}; & 0 \le x \le \pi \end{cases}$$

Hence, deduce that $\dfrac{1}{1^2} + \dfrac{1}{3^2} + \dfrac{1}{5^2} + \ldots = \dfrac{\pi^2}{8}$

SOLUTION. When $-\pi \le x \le 0 \Rightarrow 0 \le -x \le \pi$

$$\therefore \qquad f(-x) = 1 - \frac{2(-x)}{\pi} = 1 + \frac{2x}{\pi} = f(x)$$

When $0 \le x \le \pi \Rightarrow -\pi \le -x \le 0$

$$\therefore \qquad f(-x) = 1 + \frac{2(-x)}{\pi} = 1 - \frac{2x}{\pi} = 1 - \frac{2x}{\pi} = f(x)$$

Therefore, $f(x)$ is an even function of x in the interval $[-\pi, \pi]$. Hence $b_n = 0$. Now, Fourier series of $f(x)$ is given by

$$f(x) = \frac{a_0}{2} + \sum_{n=1}^{\infty} a_n \cos nx$$

Then, $\qquad a_0 = \dfrac{2}{\pi} \int_0^{\pi} f(x)\,dx = \dfrac{2}{\pi} \int_0^{\pi} \left(1 - \dfrac{2x}{\pi}\right) dx = \dfrac{2}{\pi}\left[x - \dfrac{x^2}{\pi}\right]_0^{\pi} = 0$

$$a_n = \frac{2}{\pi} \int_0^{\pi} f(x) \cos nx\,dx = \frac{2}{\pi} \int_0^{\pi} \left(1 - \frac{2x}{\pi}\right) \cos nx\,dx$$

$$= \frac{2}{\pi}\left[\left(1 - \frac{2x}{\pi}\right)\sin\frac{nx}{n} - \left(-\frac{2}{\pi}\right)\left(-\frac{\cos nx}{n^2}\right)\right]_0^{\pi}$$

$$= \frac{2}{\pi}\left[-\frac{2\cos n\pi}{\pi n^2} + \frac{2}{\pi n^2}\right] = \frac{4}{\pi^2 n^2}[1 - (-1)^n]$$

$$\Rightarrow \qquad f(x) = \frac{4}{\pi^2} \sum_{n=1}^{\infty} [1 - (-1)^n] \frac{\cos nx}{n^2}$$

$$= \frac{4}{\pi^2}\left(\frac{2\cos x}{1^2} + \frac{2\cos 3x}{3^2} + \frac{2\cos 5x}{5^2} + \ldots\right)$$

$$= \frac{8}{\pi^2}\left(\frac{\cos x}{1^2} + \frac{\cos 3x}{3^2} + \frac{\cos 5x}{5^2} + \ldots\right)$$

Putting $x = 0$, we get $\dfrac{1}{1^2} + \dfrac{1}{3^2} + \dfrac{1}{5^2} + \ldots = \dfrac{\pi^2}{8}$ \qquad [Since $f(0) = 1$]

EXAMPLE 6. *Find a Fourier series to represent* $x - x^2$ *from* $x = -\pi$ *to* $x = \pi$.

Deduce that $\dfrac{1}{1^2} - \dfrac{1}{2^2} + \dfrac{1}{3^2} - \dfrac{1}{4^2} + \ldots = \dfrac{\pi^2}{12}$.

SOLUTION. The Fourier series for $f(x)$ in $(-\pi, \pi)$ is

$$f(x) = a_0 + \sum_{n=1}^{\infty} a_n \cos nx + \sum_{n=1}^{\infty} b_n \sin nx$$

Here, $\quad a_0 = \dfrac{1}{2\pi} \int_{-\pi}^{\pi} (x - x^2)\,dx = \dfrac{1}{2\pi}\left[\dfrac{x^2}{2} - \dfrac{x^3}{3}\right]_{-\pi}^{\pi} = -\dfrac{\pi^2}{3}$

$$a_n = \dfrac{1}{\pi} \int_{-\pi}^{\pi} (x - x^2) \cos nx\, dx$$

$$= \dfrac{1}{\pi}\left[(x - x^2)\dfrac{\sin nx}{n} - (1 - 2x)\left(-\dfrac{\cos nx}{n^2}\right) + (-2)\left(-\dfrac{\sin nx}{n^3}\right)\right]_{-\pi}^{\pi}$$

$$= \dfrac{-4(-1)^n}{n^2}$$

and $\quad b_n = \dfrac{1}{\pi}\int_{-\pi}^{\pi}(x - x^2)\sin nx\, dx$

$$= \dfrac{1}{\pi}\left[(x - x^2)\left(-\dfrac{\cos nx}{n}\right) - (1 - 2x)\cdot\left(-\dfrac{\sin nx}{n^2}\right) + (-2)\left(\dfrac{\cos nx}{n^3}\right)\right]_{-\pi}^{\pi}$$

$$= \dfrac{(-2)(-1)^n}{n}$$

∴ The required Fourier series is

$$x - x^2 = -\dfrac{\pi^2}{3} + 4\left[\dfrac{\cos x}{1^2} - \dfrac{\cos 2x}{2^2} + \dfrac{\cos 3x}{3^2} - \dfrac{\cos 4x}{4^2} + \ldots\right]$$

$$+ 2\left[\dfrac{\sin x}{1} - \dfrac{\sin 2x}{2} + \dfrac{\sin 3x}{3} - \dfrac{\sin 4x}{4} + \ldots\right] \qquad \ldots(1)$$

Deduction. Putting $x = 0$ in (1), we get $0 = -\dfrac{\pi^2}{3} + 4\left(\dfrac{1}{1^2} - \dfrac{1}{2^2} + \dfrac{1}{3^2} - \dfrac{1}{4^2} + \ldots\right)$

or $\quad \dfrac{1}{1^2} - \dfrac{1}{2^2} + \dfrac{1}{3^2} - \dfrac{1}{4^2} + \ldots = \dfrac{\pi^2}{12}$.

EXAMPLE 7. *Find the Fourier series of the function defined as*

$$f(x) = \begin{cases} x + \pi & ; \quad 0 \le x \le \pi \\ -x - \pi & ; \quad -\pi \le x \le 0 \end{cases} \quad \text{and } f(x + 2\pi) = f(x)$$

SOLUTION. Let $\quad f(x) = \dfrac{a_0}{2} + \sum_{n=1}^{\infty} a_n \cos nx + \sum_{n=1}^{\infty} b_n \sin nx$

Then, $\quad a_0 = \dfrac{1}{\pi}\int_{-\pi}^{\pi} f(x)\,dx = \dfrac{1}{\pi}\int_{-\pi}^{0} f(x)\,dx + \dfrac{1}{\pi}\int_{0}^{\pi} f(x)\,dx$

$$= \frac{1}{\pi} \int_{-\pi}^{0} (-x-\pi)\,dx + \frac{1}{\pi}\int_{0}^{\pi} (x+\pi)\,dx$$

$$= \frac{1}{\pi}\left[\left(-\frac{x^2}{2} - \pi x \right)_{-\pi}^{0} + \left(\frac{x^2}{2} + \pi x \right)_{0}^{\pi} \right]$$

$$= \frac{1}{\pi}\left\{ \left(\frac{\pi^2}{2} - \pi^2 \right) + \left(\frac{\pi^2}{2} + \pi^2 \right) \right\} = \pi$$

$$a_n = \frac{1}{\pi}\int_{-\pi}^{\pi} f(x)\cos nx\,dx = \frac{1}{\pi}\int_{-\pi}^{0} f(x).\cos nx\,dx + \frac{1}{\pi}\int_{0}^{\pi} f(x).\cos nx\,dx$$

$$= \frac{1}{\pi}\int_{-\pi}^{0} (-x-\pi)\cos nx\,dx + \frac{1}{\pi}\int_{0}^{\pi} (x+\pi)\cos nx\,dx$$

$$= \frac{1}{\pi}\left[(-x-\pi)\frac{\sin nx}{n} - (-1)\left\{ -\frac{\cos nx}{n^2} \right\} \right]_{-\pi}^{0}$$

$$+ \frac{1}{\pi}\left[(x+\pi)\frac{\sin nx}{n} - (-1)\left\{ -\frac{\cos nx}{n^2} \right\} \right]_{0}^{\pi}$$

$$= \frac{1}{\pi}\left[-\frac{1}{n^2} + \frac{(-1)^n}{n^2} \right] + \frac{1}{\pi}\left[\frac{(-1)^n}{n^2} - \frac{1}{n^2} \right]$$

$$= \frac{2}{n^2 \pi}[(-1)^n - 1] = \begin{cases} -\dfrac{4}{n^2 \pi} & ; \quad \text{if } n \text{ is odd} \\ 0 & ; \quad \text{if } n \text{ is even} \end{cases}$$

Also, $b_n = \dfrac{1}{\pi}\int_{-\pi}^{\pi} f(x)\sin nx\,dx$

$$= \frac{1}{\pi}\left\{ \int_{-\pi}^{0} f(x).\sin nx\,dx + \int_{0}^{\pi} f(x).\sin nx\,dx \right\}$$

$$= \frac{1}{\pi}\left\{ \int_{-\pi}^{0} (-x-\pi)\sin nx\,dx + \int_{0}^{\pi} (x+\pi)\sin nx\,dx \right\}$$

$$= \frac{1}{\pi}\left[(-x-\pi)\left(-\frac{\cos nx}{n} \right) - (-1)\left\{ -\frac{\sin nx}{n^2} \right\} \right]_{-\pi}^{0}$$

$$+ \frac{1}{\pi}\left[(x+\pi)\left(-\frac{\cos nx}{n} \right) - (-1)\left\{ -\frac{\sin nx}{n^2} \right\} \right]_{0}^{\pi}$$

$$= \frac{1}{\pi}\left[\frac{\pi}{n} \right] + \frac{1}{\pi}\left[\frac{-2\pi}{n}(-1)^n + \frac{\pi}{n} \right] = \frac{1}{n}[1-2(-1)^n+1] = \frac{2}{n}[1-(-1)^n]$$

$$= \begin{cases} \dfrac{4}{n} & , \quad \text{if } n \text{ is odd} \\ 0 & , \quad \text{if } n \text{ is even} \end{cases}$$

The required Fourier series is given by

$$f(x) = \frac{a_0}{2} + a_1 \cos x + a_2 \cos 2x + \dots + b_1 \sin x + b_2 \sin 2x + \dots$$

$$= \frac{\pi}{2} - \frac{4}{\pi}\left(\frac{\cos x}{1^2} + \frac{\cos 3x}{3^2} + \dots\right) + 4\left(\frac{\sin x}{1} + \frac{\sin 3x}{3} + \dots\right)$$

EXAMPLE 8.   *Find the Fourier series for the function* $f(x) = x + x^2$, $-\pi < x < \pi$. *Hence, show that*

(i) $\dfrac{\pi^2}{6} = 1 + \dfrac{1}{2^2} + \dfrac{1}{3^2} + \dfrac{1}{4^2} + \dots$ (ii) $\dfrac{\pi^2}{12} = \dfrac{1}{1^2} - \dfrac{1}{2^2} + \dfrac{1}{3^2} - \dfrac{1}{4^2} + \dots$

SOLUTION.   Let the Fourier series be

$$x + x^2 = \frac{a_0}{2} + \sum_{n=1}^{\infty} a_n \cos nx + \sum_{n=1}^{\infty} b_n \sin nx \qquad \dots(1)$$

Here,

$$a_0 = \frac{1}{\pi}\int_{-\pi}^{\pi}(x + x^2)dx$$

$$= \frac{1}{\pi}\left[\int_{-\pi}^{\pi}x\,dx + \int_{-\pi}^{\pi}x^2\,dx\right] = \frac{2}{\pi}\int_0^\pi x^2 dx = \frac{2}{3}\pi^2$$

$$a_n = \frac{1}{\pi}\int_{-\pi}^{\pi}(x + x^2)\cos nx\,dx$$

$$= \frac{1}{\pi}\left[\int_{-\pi}^{\pi}x\cos nx\,dx + \int_{-\pi}^{\pi}x^2\cos nx\,dx\right] = \frac{2}{\pi}\int_0^\pi x^2 \cos nx\,dx$$

$$= \frac{2}{\pi}\left[\left(x^2\frac{\sin nx}{n}\right)_0^\pi - \int_0^\pi 2x.\frac{\sin nx}{n}dx\right] = -\frac{4}{n\pi}\int_0^\pi x\sin nx\,dx$$

$$= -\frac{4}{n\pi}\left[\left\{x\left(-\frac{\cos nx}{n}\right)\right\}_0^\pi - \int_0^\pi 1.\left(-\frac{\cos nx}{n}\right)dx\right]$$

$$= -\frac{4}{n\pi}\left(-\frac{\pi}{n}\cos nx\right) = \frac{4}{n^2}\cos n\pi = \frac{4}{n^2}(-1)^n$$

and

$$b_n = \frac{1}{\pi}\int_{-\pi}^{\pi}(x + x^2)\sin nx\,dx$$

$$= \frac{2}{\pi}\int_0^\pi x\sin nx\,dx + \frac{2}{\pi}\int_0^\pi x^2 \sin nx\,dx \qquad \left[\because \int_0^\pi x^2 \sin nx\,dx = 0\right]$$

$$= \frac{2}{\pi}\left(-\frac{\pi}{n}\cos n\pi\right) = -\frac{2}{n}(-1)^n.$$

From (1),

$$x + x^2 = \frac{\pi^2}{3} + 4\sum_{n=1}^{\infty}\frac{(-1)^n}{n^2}\cos nx - 2\sum_{n=1}^{\infty}\frac{(-1)^n}{n}\sin nx$$

$$f(x) = \frac{\pi^2}{3} + 4\left[-\frac{1}{1^2}\cos x + \frac{1}{2^2}\cos 2x - \frac{1}{3^2}\cos 3x + \dots\right]$$

$$-2\left[-\frac{1}{1}\sin x + \frac{1}{2}\sin 2x - \frac{1}{3}\sin 3x + \dots\right]. \qquad \dots(2)$$

We observe that the series on the R.H.S. given by equation (2), always represents $x + x^2$ for all values of x except the end points $-\pi$ or π.

At the point of discontinuity

$$f(-\pi) = \frac{1}{2}(\text{L.H.L.} + \text{R.H.L.})$$

$$= \frac{1}{2}[f(-\pi - 0) + f(-\pi + 0)] = \frac{1}{2}[f(\pi - 0) + f(-\pi + 0)]$$

$$= \frac{1}{2}[\pi + \pi^2 + (-\pi) + (-\pi)^2] = \pi^2.$$

Putting $x = -\pi$ in equation (2), we get

$$\pi^2 = \frac{\pi^2}{3} + 4\left[\frac{1}{1^2} + \frac{1}{2^2} + \frac{1}{3^2} + \frac{1}{4^2} + ...\right]$$

Therefore, $\dfrac{\pi^2}{6} = 1 + \dfrac{1}{2^2} + \dfrac{1}{3^2} + \dfrac{1}{4^2} + ...$ ...(3)

Again, putting $x = 0$ in equaton (2), we get

$$0 = \frac{\pi^2}{3} + 4\left[-\frac{1}{1^2} + \frac{1}{2^2} - \frac{1}{3^2} + \frac{1}{4^2} - ...\right]$$

$\Rightarrow \qquad \dfrac{\pi^2}{12} = \dfrac{1}{1^2} - \dfrac{1}{2^2} + \dfrac{1}{3^2} - \dfrac{1}{4^2}...$

EXAMPLE 9.   *Express $f(x) = |x|$, $-\pi < x < \pi$, as Fourier series. Hence, show that*

$$\frac{1}{1^2} + \frac{1}{3^2} + \frac{1}{5^2} + ... = \frac{\pi^2}{8}.$$

SOLUTION.   Here, $f(-x) = |-x| = |x| = f(x)$

$\therefore$ $f(x)$ is an even function and hence $b_n = 0$.

Let $f(x) = |x| = \dfrac{a_0}{2} + \sum\limits_{n=1}^{\infty} a_n \cos nx$

Then, $a_0 = \dfrac{2}{\pi}\int_0^\pi f(x)dx = \dfrac{2}{\pi}\int_0^\pi |x|\, dx$

$$= \frac{2}{\pi}\int_0^\pi x\, dx = \frac{2}{\pi}\left[\frac{x^2}{2}\right]_0^\pi = \pi$$

and $a_n = \dfrac{2}{\pi}\int_0^\pi f(x)\cos nx\, dx$

$$= \frac{2}{\pi}\int_0^\pi |x|.\cos nx\, dx = \frac{2}{\pi}\int_0^\pi x\cos nx\, dx$$

$$= \frac{2}{\pi}\left[x\left(\frac{\sin nx}{n}\right) - 1\left(-\frac{\cos nx}{n^2}\right)\right]_0^\pi = \frac{2}{\pi}\left[\frac{\cos nx}{n^2} - \frac{1}{n^2}\right]$$

$$= \frac{2}{\pi n^2}[(-1)^n - 1] = \begin{cases} 0 & , \text{ if } n \text{ is even} \\ -\dfrac{4}{\pi n^2} & , \text{ if } n \text{ is odd} \end{cases}$$

Hence, $|x| = \dfrac{\pi}{2} - \dfrac{4}{\pi}\left(\cos x + \dfrac{\cos 3x}{3^2} + \dfrac{\cos 5x}{5^2} + ... \right)$ ...(1)

Deduction. Putting $x = 0$, in equation (1), we get

$$\dfrac{1}{1^2} + \dfrac{1}{3^2} + \dfrac{1}{5^2} + ... = \dfrac{\pi^2}{8}$$

EXAMPLE 10. *Find the Fourier series expansion of f(x), if* $f(x) = \begin{cases} -\pi & , & -\pi < x < 0 \\ x & , & 0 < x < \pi \end{cases}$

Deduce that $\dfrac{1}{1^2} + \dfrac{1}{3^2} + \dfrac{1}{5^2} + ... = \dfrac{\pi^2}{8}$.

SOLUTION. Let the Fourier series be

$$f(x) = \dfrac{a_0}{2} + \sum_{n=1}^{\infty} a_n \cos nx + \sum_{n=1}^{\infty} b_n \sin nx$$

Then, $a_0 = \dfrac{1}{2\pi} \int_{-\pi}^{\pi} f(x)dx = \dfrac{1}{2\pi}\left[\int_{-\pi}^{0}(-\pi)dx + \int_{0}^{\pi} x\,dx \right]$

$= \dfrac{1}{\pi}\left[-\pi(x)_{-\pi}^{0} + \left(\dfrac{x^2}{2} \right)_{0}^{\pi} \right] = \dfrac{1}{\pi}\left[-\left(\pi^2 + \dfrac{\pi^2}{2} \right) \right] = -\dfrac{\pi}{2}$

$a_n = \dfrac{1}{\pi} \int_{-\pi}^{\pi} f(x) \cos nx\, dx = \dfrac{1}{\pi}\left[\int_{-\pi}^{0}(-\pi) \cos nx\,dx + \int_{0}^{\pi} x \cos nx\, dx \right]$

$= \dfrac{1}{\pi}\left[-\pi\left(\dfrac{\sin nx}{n} \right)_{-\pi}^{0} + \left(\dfrac{x \sin nx}{n} + \dfrac{\cos nx}{n^2} \right)_{0}^{x} \right]$

$= \dfrac{1}{\pi}\left[0 + \dfrac{1}{n^2} \cos n\pi - \dfrac{1}{n^2} \right] = \dfrac{1}{\pi n^2}(\cos n\pi - 1)$

and $b_n = \dfrac{1}{\pi} \int_{-\pi}^{\pi} f(x) \sin nx\, dx = \dfrac{1}{\pi}\left[\int_{-\pi}^{0}(-\pi) \sin nx\,dx + \int_{0}^{\pi} x \sin nx\, dx \right]$

$= \dfrac{1}{\pi}\left[\left(\dfrac{\pi \cos nx}{n} \right)_{-\pi}^{0} + \left(-\dfrac{\cos nx}{n} + \dfrac{\sin nx}{n^2} \right)_{0}^{\pi} \right]$

$= \dfrac{1}{\pi}\left[\dfrac{\pi}{n}(0 - \cos n\pi) - \dfrac{\pi}{n} \cos n\pi \right] = \dfrac{1}{n}(1 - 2\cos n\pi)$

The required Fourier series is

$$f(x) = -\dfrac{\pi}{4} - \dfrac{2}{\pi}\left(\cos x + \dfrac{\cos 3x}{3^2} + \dfrac{\cos 5x}{5^2} + ... \right)$$

$$+ \left(3\sin x - \dfrac{\sin 2x}{2} + \dfrac{3\sin 3x}{3} - \dfrac{\sin 4x}{4} + ... \right) \qquad ...(1)$$

Deduction. Putting $x = 0$ in (1), we get

$$f(0) = \dfrac{\pi}{4} - \dfrac{2}{\pi}\left(1 + \dfrac{1}{3^2} + \dfrac{1}{5^2} + ... \right) \qquad ...(2)$$

But $f(x)$ is continuous at $x = 0$, and we have $f(0 - 0) = -\pi$ and $f(0 + 0) = 0$

$$\therefore \qquad f(0) = \frac{1}{2}[f(0-0) + f(0+0)] = -(\pi/2) \qquad \qquad ...(3)$$

Hence, from (2) and (3), we have

$$-\frac{\pi}{2} = -\frac{\pi}{4} - \frac{2}{\pi}\left[\frac{1}{1^2} + \frac{1}{3^2} + \frac{1}{5^2} + ...\right] \text{or} \frac{1}{1^2} + \frac{1}{3^2} + \frac{1}{5^2} + ... = \frac{\pi^2}{8}.$$

Exercise 14.1

1. Express $f(x) = \frac{1}{2}(\pi - x)$ in a Fourier series in the interval $0 < x < 2\pi$.

2. Find the Fourier series to represent the function $f(x) = |\sin x|, -\pi < x < \pi$.

3. Obtain the Fourier series to represent $f(x) = \frac{1}{4}(\pi - x)^2, 0 < x < 2\pi$. Hence, obtain the following results :

   (i) $\dfrac{1}{1^2} + \dfrac{1}{2^2} + \dfrac{1}{3^2} + \dfrac{1}{4^2} + ... = \dfrac{\pi^2}{6}$

   (ii) $\dfrac{1}{1^2} - \dfrac{1}{2^2} + \dfrac{1}{3^2} - \dfrac{1}{4^2} + ... = \dfrac{\pi^2}{12}$

   (iii) $\dfrac{1}{1^2} + \dfrac{1}{3^2} + \dfrac{1}{5^2} + ... = \dfrac{\pi^2}{8}$

4. Expand in a Fourier series the function $f(x) = x$ in the interval $0 < x < 2\pi$, sketch its graph from $x = -4\pi$ to $x = 4\pi$.

5. Show that for $-\pi < x < \pi$

   $\sin ax =$

   $\dfrac{2\sin a\pi}{\pi}\left(\dfrac{\sin x}{1^2 - a^2} - \dfrac{2\sin 2x}{2^2 - a^2} + \dfrac{3\sin 3x}{3^2 - a^2} - ...\right)$

6. Obtain a Fourier expansion for $\sqrt{1 - \cos x}$ in the interval $-\pi < x < \pi$.

7. Obtain a Fourier series to represent e^{-ax} from $x = -\pi$ to $x = \pi$. Hence derive the series for $\dfrac{\pi}{\sinh \pi}$.

8. Find the Fourier series to represent the periodic function:

   $$f(x) = \begin{cases} x & , \quad -\pi/2 < x < \pi/2 \\ \pi - x & , \quad \pi/2 < x < 3\pi/2 \end{cases}$$

9. Find a series of sines and cosines to multiples of x which will represent $\dfrac{\pi}{\sinh \pi}e^x$ in the interval $-\pi < x < \pi$.

10. Prove that

    $$x^2 = \frac{\pi^2}{3} + 4\sum_{n=1}^{\infty}(-1)^n\frac{\cos nx}{n^2}, -\pi < x < \pi.$$

11. Prove that in the interval

    $$x\cos x = -\frac{1}{2}\sin x + 2\sum_{n=2}^{\infty}\frac{n(-1)^n}{n^2-1}\sin nx$$

12. If $f(x) = \cos \omega x, -\pi < x < \pi$, where ω is a fraction as a Fourier series, prove that

    $$\cot\theta = \frac{1}{\theta} + \frac{2\theta}{\theta^2 - \pi^2} + \frac{2\theta}{\theta^2 - 4\pi^2} + ...$$

ANSWERS

1. $f(x) = \displaystyle\sum_{n=1}^{\infty}\frac{\sin nx}{n}$

2. $|\sin x| = \dfrac{2}{\pi} - \dfrac{4}{\pi}\left(\dfrac{\cos 2x}{3} + \dfrac{\cos 4x}{15} + ... + \dfrac{\cos 2nx}{4n^2 - 1} + ...\right)$

3. $f(x) = \dfrac{\pi^2}{12} + \displaystyle\sum_{n=1}^{\infty}\frac{\cos nx}{n^2} = \dfrac{\pi^2}{12} + \dfrac{\cos x}{1^2} + \dfrac{\cos 2x}{2^2} + \dfrac{\cos 3x}{3^2} + ...$

4. $f(x) = \pi - 2 \cdot \displaystyle\sum_{n=1}^{\infty}\frac{\sin nx}{n}$

5. $\sin ax = \dfrac{2\sin a\pi}{\pi}\displaystyle\sum_{n=1}^{\infty}\frac{(-1)^{n+1}}{n^2 - a^2}\sin nx$

6. $\sqrt{1 - \cos x} = \dfrac{2\sqrt{2}}{\pi} - \dfrac{4\sqrt{2}}{\pi}\displaystyle\sum_{n=1}^{\infty}\frac{\cos nx}{4n^2 - 1}$

7. $e^{-ax} = 2\dfrac{\sinh a\pi}{\pi}\left[\left(\dfrac{1}{2a} - \dfrac{a\cos x}{1^2 + a^2} + \dfrac{a\cos 2x}{2^2 + a^2} - ...\right) - \left(\dfrac{\sin x}{1^2 + a^2} - \dfrac{2\sin 2x}{2^2 + a^2} + \dfrac{3\sin 3x}{3^2 + a^2} ...\right)\right]$

$\dfrac{\pi}{\sinh \pi} = 2\left[\dfrac{1}{2^2 + 1} - \dfrac{1}{3^2 + 1} + \dfrac{1}{4^2 + 1} - ...\right]$

8. $f(x) = \dfrac{4}{\pi}\left[\dfrac{\sin x}{1^2} - \dfrac{\sin 3x}{3^2} + \dfrac{\sin 5x}{5^2} - \ldots\right]$

9. $\dfrac{\pi}{2\sin n\pi}e^x = \dfrac{1}{2} + \displaystyle\sum_{n=1}^{\infty}\dfrac{\cos n\pi}{1+n^2}\cos nx - \sum_{n=1}^{\infty}\left\{\dfrac{n}{1+n^2}\cos nx\sin n\pi\right\}$

$\qquad = \dfrac{1}{2} - \left(\dfrac{1}{2}\cos x - \dfrac{1}{2}\cos 2x + \dfrac{1}{10}\cos 3x - \dfrac{1}{17}\cos 4x + \ldots\right)$

14.6 THE L^2-THEORY OF FOURIER SERIES

We know that a function f is said to be square integrable over $[0, 2\pi]$ if f is measurable and $\int_0^{2\pi} f^2 dx$ is finite. Here, we write $f^2 \in [0, 2\pi]$ or $f \in L^2[0, 2\pi]$.

THEOREM I. (Parsevel's Identity Theorem)

Consider the Fourier series $\dfrac{a_0}{2} + \displaystyle\sum_{n=1}^{\infty}(a_n\cos nx + b_n\sin nx)$ *. If $f(x)$ converges uniformly to $f(x)$ at every point of the interval $(0, 2\pi)$, then*

$$\dfrac{1}{\pi}\int_0^{2\pi}\{f(x)\}^2 dx = \dfrac{a_0^2}{2} + \sum_{n=1}^{\infty}(a_n^2 + b_n^2)$$

PROOF. Let the series $\dfrac{a_0}{2} + \displaystyle\sum_{n=1}^{\infty}(a_n\cos nx + b_n\sin nx)$ represent the Fourier series of $f(x)$.

Also, let this series converges uniformly to $f(x)$ at every point of the interval $(0, 2\pi)$ so that

$$f(x) = \dfrac{a_0}{2} + \sum_{n=1}^{\infty}(a_n\cos nx + b_n\sin nx) \qquad\qquad \ldots(1)$$

and that term by term integration is possible.

To prove that $\dfrac{1}{\pi}\int_0^{2\pi}\{f(x)\}^2 dx = \dfrac{a_0^2}{2} + \Sigma(a_n^2 + b_n^2)$

We have $\quad a_n = \dfrac{1}{\pi}\int_0^{2\pi} f(x).\cos nx\, dx \quad (n = 0, 1, 2, 3, \ldots)$

$$b_n = \dfrac{1}{\pi}\int_0^{2\pi} f(x).\sin nx\, dx \quad (n = 0, 1, 2, 3 \ldots)$$

Multiplying (1) by $f(x)$ and then integrating from $x = 0$ to $x = 2\pi$, we get

$$\int_0^{2\pi}\{f(x)\}^2 dx = \dfrac{a_0}{2} + \int_0^{2\pi} f(x)\, dx + \sum_{n=1}^{\infty}\left(a_n\int_0^{2\pi} f(x).\cos nx\, dx + b_n\int_0^{2\pi} f(x)\sin nx\, dx\right)$$

$$= \dfrac{a_0}{2}.\pi a_0 + \sum_{n=1}^{\infty}(\pi a_n^2 + \pi b_n^2)$$

Dividing by π, we get $\dfrac{1}{\pi}\int_0^{2\pi}\{f(x)\}^2 dx = \dfrac{a_0^2}{2} + \displaystyle\sum_{n=1}^{\infty}(a_n^2 + b_n^2)$.

Solved Examples

EXAMPLE 1. *Obtain the Fourier series expansion of* $f(x) = x^2$ *in* $-\pi < x < \pi$ *and prove that*

$$\sum_{n=1}^{\infty} \frac{1}{n^4} = \frac{\pi^4}{90} \text{ by using Parsevel's theorem.}$$

SOLUTION. Since $f(x) = x^2$ is even function so $b_n = 0$

Let the Fourier series expansion of $f(x)$ is given by

$$f(x) = x^2 = \frac{a_0}{2} + \sum_{n=1}^{\infty} a_n \cos nx \qquad \ldots (1)$$

where, $\qquad a_0 = \frac{2}{\pi}\int_0^{\pi} f(x)dx = \frac{2}{\pi}\int_0^{\pi} x^2 dx = \frac{2\pi^2}{3}$

$$a_n = \frac{2}{\pi}\int_0^{\pi} f(x)\cos nx\,dx = \frac{2}{\pi}\int_0^{\pi} x^2 \cos nx\,dx$$

$\Rightarrow \qquad a_n = \frac{2}{\pi}\left[x^2 \frac{\sin nx}{n} + 2x.\frac{\cos nx}{n^2} - 2\frac{\sin nx}{n^2} \right]_0^{\pi} = \frac{\pi(-1)^2}{n^2}$

$\therefore$ (1) becomes, $x^2 = \frac{\pi^2}{3} + 4\sum_{n=1}^{\infty} \frac{(-1)^n \cos nx}{n^2}$ $\qquad \ldots(2)$

which is the required Fourier expansion.

Now, by Parsevel's theorem, we have

$$\int_{-\pi}^{\pi}\{f(x)\}^2 dx = \pi\left[\frac{a_0^2}{2} + \sum_{n=1}^{\infty} (a_n^2 + b_n^2) \right]$$

Hence, $\qquad \int_{-\pi}^{\pi} x^4 dx = \pi\left[\frac{4\pi^4}{2.9} + \sum_{n=1}^{\infty}\frac{16}{n^4} \right]$

$\Rightarrow \qquad \left(\frac{x^5}{5}\right)_{-\pi}^{\pi} = \frac{2\pi^5}{9} + \pi\sum_{n=1}^{\infty}\frac{16}{n^4}$ or $\frac{2\pi^5}{5} - \frac{2\pi^5}{9} = \pi\sum_{n=1}^{\infty}\frac{16}{n^4}$

$\Rightarrow \qquad \frac{\pi^4}{90} = \sum_{n=1}^{\infty}\frac{1}{n^4}.$

EXAMPLE 2. *By using the sine series for* $f(x) = 1$ *in* $0 < x < \pi$, *show that*

$$\frac{\pi^2}{8} = 1 + \frac{1}{3^2} + \frac{1}{5^2} + \frac{1}{7^2} + \ldots.$$

SOLUTION. The Fourier sine series for $f(x) = 1$ in $(0, \pi)$ is $f(x) = \sum b_n \sin nx$,

where, $\qquad b_n = \frac{2}{\pi}\int_0^{\pi} f(x)\sin nx\,dx = \frac{2}{\pi}\int_0^{\pi}(1).\sin nx\,dx = \frac{2}{\pi}\left(-\frac{\cos nx}{n}\right)_0^{\pi}$

$$= -\frac{2}{n\pi}[\cos n\pi - 1] = -\frac{2}{n\pi}[(-1)^n - 1] = \begin{cases} \dfrac{4}{n\pi} & \text{, if } n \text{ is odd} \\ 0 & \text{, if } n \text{ is even} \end{cases}$$

The Fourier sine series is

$$1 = \frac{4}{\pi}\sin x + \frac{4}{3\pi}\sin 3x + \frac{4}{5\pi}\sin 5x + \frac{4}{7\pi}\sin 7x + \dots$$

By Parsevel's formula, we get

$$\int_0^\pi [f(x)]^2 dx = \frac{c}{2}[b_1^2 + b_2^2 + b_3^2 + b_4^2 + b_5^2 + \dots]$$

$$\Rightarrow \qquad \int_0^\pi (1)^2 dx = \frac{\pi}{2}\left[\left(\frac{4}{\pi}\right)^2 + \left(\frac{4}{3\pi}\right)^2 + \left(\frac{4}{5\pi}\right)^2 + \left(\frac{4}{7\pi}\right)^2 + \dots\right]$$

$$\Rightarrow \qquad [x]_0^\pi = \left(\frac{\pi}{2}\right)\left(\frac{16}{\pi^2}\right)\left[1 + \frac{1}{3^2} + \frac{1}{5^2} + \frac{1}{7^2} + \dots\right]$$

$$\Rightarrow \qquad \pi = \frac{\pi}{2}\left(\frac{16}{\pi^2}\right)\left[1 + \frac{1}{3^2} + \frac{1}{5^2} + \frac{1}{7^2} + \dots\right]$$

Hence, $\qquad \dfrac{\pi^2}{8} = 1 + \dfrac{1}{3^2} + \dfrac{1}{5^2} + \dfrac{1}{7^2} + \dots$

EXAMPLE 3. If $f(x) = \begin{cases} \pi x &, \quad 0 < x < 1 \\ \pi(2-x) &, \quad 1 < x < 2 \end{cases}$

Using half range cosine series, show that $\dfrac{1}{1^4} + \dfrac{1}{3^4} + \dfrac{1}{5^4} + \dots = \dfrac{\pi^4}{96}$

SOLUTION The half range cosine series for $f(x)$ in $(0, c)$ is

$$f(x) = \frac{a_0}{2} + \sum_{n=1}^{\infty} a_n \cos\frac{n\pi x}{c}$$

Here, $\qquad a_0 = \dfrac{2}{c}\int_0^c f(x)dx = \dfrac{2}{2}\left[\int_0^1 \pi x\, dx + \int_1^2 \pi(2-x)dx\right]$

$$= \pi\left[\frac{x^2}{2}\right]_0^1 + \pi\left[2x - \frac{x^2}{2}\right]_0^1 = \frac{\pi}{2} + \pi\left[(4-2) - \left(2 - \frac{1}{2}\right)\right] = \pi$$

$$a_n = \frac{2}{c}\int_0^c f(x)\cdot\cos\frac{n\pi x}{c}dx$$

$$= \frac{2}{2}\left[\int_0^1 \pi x \cos\frac{n\pi x}{2}dx + \int_1^2 \pi(2-x)\cos\frac{n\pi x}{2}dx\right]$$

$$= \pi\left[\frac{x\sin\frac{n\pi x}{2}}{\frac{n\pi}{2}} - \left(\frac{\cos\frac{n\pi x}{2}}{\frac{n^2\pi^2}{4}}\right)\right]_0^1 + \pi\left[(2-x)\frac{\sin\frac{n\pi x}{2}}{\frac{n\pi}{2}} - (-1)\left(\frac{\cos\frac{n\pi x}{2}}{\frac{n^2\pi^2}{4}}\right)\right]_1^2$$

$$= \pi \left[\frac{2}{n\pi} \sin \frac{n\pi}{2} + \frac{4}{n^2\pi^2} \cos \frac{n\pi}{2} - \frac{4}{n^2\pi^2} \right]$$

$$+ \pi \left[0 - \frac{4}{n^2\pi^2} \cos n\pi - \frac{2}{n\pi} \sin \frac{n\pi}{2} + \frac{4}{n^2\pi^2} \cos \frac{n\pi}{2} \right]$$

$$= \pi \left[\frac{8}{n^2\pi^2} \cos \frac{n\pi}{2} - \frac{4}{n^2\pi^2} - \frac{4}{n^2\pi^2} \cos n\pi x \right] = \frac{4}{n^2\pi} \left[2\cos \frac{n\pi}{2} - 1 - \cos n\pi \right]$$

Putting $n = 1, 2, 3, \ldots$, we get

$$a_1 = 0, a_2 = \frac{-4}{\pi}, a_3 = 0, a_4 = 0, a_5 = 0, a_6 = -\frac{4}{9\pi}$$

By Parsevel's formula, we get

$$\int_0^c \{f(x)\}^2 dx = \frac{c}{2} \left[\frac{a_0^2}{2} + a_1^2 + a_2^2 + a_3^2 + \ldots \right]$$

$$\int_0^1 (\pi x)^2 dx + \int_1^2 \pi^2 (2-x)^2 dx = \frac{2}{2} \left[\frac{\pi^2}{2} + \frac{16}{\pi^2} + \frac{16}{81\pi^2} + \ldots \right]$$

$$\pi^2 \left[\frac{x^3}{3} \right]_0^1 - \pi^2 \left[\frac{(2-x)^3}{3} \right]_1^2 = \frac{\pi^2}{2} + \frac{16}{\pi^2} + \frac{16}{81\pi^2} + \ldots$$

$$\Rightarrow \quad \frac{\pi^2}{3} - \pi^2 \left(0 - \frac{1}{3} \right) = \frac{\pi^2}{3^2} + \frac{16}{\pi^2} \left[1 + \frac{1}{81} + \ldots \right]$$

$$\Rightarrow \quad \frac{2\pi^2}{3} - \frac{\pi^2}{2} = \frac{16}{\pi^2} \left[1 + \frac{1}{3^4} + \frac{1}{5^4} + \ldots \right]$$

$$\Rightarrow \quad \frac{\pi^2}{6} = \frac{16}{\pi^2} \left[1 + \frac{1}{3^4} + \frac{1}{5^4} + \ldots \right] \Rightarrow \frac{\pi^4}{96} = 1 + \frac{1}{3^4} + \frac{1}{5^4} + \ldots$$

THEOREM 2. (Riemann-Lebesgue Theorem)

If $f \in L[-\pi, \pi]$ and if $<a_n>$ and $<b_n>$ are Fourier coefficients of a function f then

$$\lim_{n \to \infty} a_n = 0, \lim_{n \to \infty} b_n = 0$$

PROOF. Define an unbounded measurable function g on $(-\pi, \pi)$ such that

$$\int_{-\pi}^{\pi} |f(x) - g(x)| \, dx < \frac{\pi\varepsilon}{2} \text{ for arbitrary small } \varepsilon > 0. \qquad \ldots(1)$$

Then $g \in L^2[-\pi, \pi]$ so that

$$\sum_{n=1}^{\infty} (A_n^2 + B_n^2) < \infty \qquad \ldots(2)$$

where, $$A_n = \frac{1}{\pi} \int_{-\pi}^{\pi} g(x) \cos nx \, dx$$

and $\qquad B_n = \frac{1}{\pi}\int_{-\pi}^{\pi}g(x)\sin nxdx$

Now, (2) implies

$$\Sigma A_n^2 < \infty$$

$\Rightarrow \qquad \lim_{n\to\infty} A_n = 0$

$\Rightarrow \quad \exists \; n_0 \in N$ such that $|A_n| < \frac{\varepsilon}{2} \; \forall n \geq n_0$ $\qquad$ ...(3)

Thus, for any n,

$$|a_n - A_n| = \left|\frac{1}{\pi}\int_{-\pi}^{\pi}[f(x)-g(x)]\cos nxdx\right|$$

$$\leq \frac{1}{\pi}\int_{-\pi}^{\pi}|f-g|\,dx < \frac{1}{\pi}\cdot\frac{\pi\varepsilon}{2}=\frac{\varepsilon}{2} \qquad ...(4)$$

$\Rightarrow \qquad (a_n) = (a_n - A_n) + A_n$

$\Rightarrow \qquad |a_n| \leq |a_n - A_n| + |A_n|$

$$< \frac{\varepsilon}{2}+\frac{\varepsilon}{2}=\varepsilon, \text{ for } n \geq n_0 \qquad \text{(Using (3) and (4))}$$

So, $\qquad |a_n| < \varepsilon \; \forall \; n \geq n_0$

Therefore, $\qquad \lim_{n\to\infty} a_n = 0$

Similarly, we can prove that $\lim_{n\to\infty} b_n = 0$.

Exercise 14.2

1. If a function
$$f(x) = \frac{a_0}{2} + \sum_{n=1}^{\infty}(a_n\cos nx + b_n\sin nx)$$
is Lebesgue integrable and uniformly convergent in $[c, c+2\pi]$ then show that
$$a_n = \frac{1}{\pi}\int_c^{c+2\pi}f(x)\cos nxdx, n = 0,1,2,...$$
and $\quad b_n = \frac{1}{\pi}\int_c^{c+2\pi}f(x)\sin nxdx, n = 1,2,3,...$

2. Prove that $\dfrac{a_0^2}{2} + \sum_{n=1}^{\infty}(a_n^2 + b_n^2) \leq \dfrac{1}{l}\int_{-l}^{l}[f(x)]^2 dx$.

3. Establish the Fejer's integral
$$\sigma_n = \frac{1}{2\pi n}\int_0^{\pi}\frac{\sin^2\left(\dfrac{nu}{2}\right)}{\sin^2\left(\dfrac{u}{2}\right)}[f(x+u)+f(x-u)]du$$

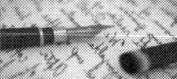 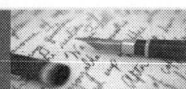

CHAPTER Summary

☙ KEY TERMS

- **PERIODIC FUNCTIONS:** A function $f(x)$ which satisfies the relation $f(x + T) = f(x)$ for all real x and some fixed T is called a periodic function. The smallest positive number T, for which this relation holds, is called the period of $f(x)$.

- **DIRICHLET'S CONDITIONS:** Any function $f(x)$ can be expressed as a Fourier series

$$\frac{a_0}{2} + \sum_{n=1}^{\infty} a_n \cos nx + \sum_{n=1}^{\infty} b_n \sin nx,$$

where a_0, a_n and b_n are constants.

(i) $f(x)$ is finite and single valued in the interval $c < x < c + 2\pi$.

(ii) $f(x)$ is periodic with period 2π

(iii) $f(x)$ and $f'(x)$ are piecewise continuous in the interval $c < x < c + 2\pi$.

☙ RESULTS

- Consider the Fourier series $\frac{a_0}{2} + \sum_{n=1}^{\infty} (a_n \cos nx + b_n \sin nx)$. If $f(x)$ converges uniformly to $f(x)$ at every point of the interval

$(0, 2\pi)$, then $\frac{1}{\pi}\int_0^{2\pi}\{f(x)\}^2 dx = \frac{a_0^2}{2} + \sum_{n=1}^{\infty}(a_n^2 + b_n^2)$

- If $f \in L[-\pi, \pi]$ and if $<a_n>$ and $<b_n>$ are Fourier coefficients of a function f then

$$\lim_{n \to \infty} a_n = 0, \lim_{n \to \infty} b_n = 0$$

☙ WORTHY READINGS

- ☞ A function f is said to be square integrable over the interval $[-\pi, \pi]$ if f is measurable and $f^2 \in L[-\pi, \pi]$.

- ☞ The space of square integrable function is denoted by $L^2[-\pi, \pi]$.

- ☞ If the trigonometric series

$$\frac{a_0}{2} + \sum_{k=1}^{\infty} (a_x \cos kx + b_x \sin kx)$$

converges uniformly on $[-\pi, \pi]$ to the integrable function f, then it is Fourier series of f.

☙ FURTHER READINGS

- ☞ At the point of discontinuity, the value of the function for Fourier series is obtained by the average of left hand limit and right hand limit of functions at that point of discontinuity.

- ☞ If $f, g \in L^2[-\pi, \pi]$ such that they have the same

Fourier coefficients then $f = g$, i.e., $f(x) = g(x)$ for almost all x.

- ☞ If f is an even function and g is an odd function then fg is an odd function.

- ☞ Function fg is even if either f and g are both even or if both are odd.

BIBLIOGRAPHY

1.	Barra, G.D.	2011	*Measure theory and Integration* New Age International
2.	Goldberg, R.R.	1961	*Fourier Transforms,* Cambridge University Press
3.	Jain, P.K. and Gupta, V.P.	1989	*Lebesgue Measure and Integration* Willy Eastern Limited, New Delhi.
4.	Royden, H.L.	1968	*Real Analysis,* Macmillan, New York.
5.	Rudin, W	1964	*Principles of Mathematical Analysis,* McGraw-Hill, New York.
6.	Rudin, W	1964	*Real and Complex Analysis,* McGraw-Hill, New York.
7.	Taylor, A.E. and Lay, D.C.	1963	*Introduction to Functional Analysis,* McGraw-Hill, New York.
8.	Wheeden, R.L. and Zygmund, A.	1977	*Measure and Integral,* Mercel Dekker, Inc. New York.

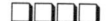

Index